Methods in Molecular Biology™

Series Editor
John M. Walker
School of Life Sciences
University of Hertfordshire
Hatfield, Hertfordshire, AL10 9AB, UK

For further volumes:
http://www.springer.com/series/7651

Single Domain Antibodies

Methods and Protocols

Edited by

Dirk Saerens and Serge Muyldermans

Department of Molecular and Cellular Interactions, VIB, Brussels, Belgium

Laboratory of Cellular and Molecular Immunology, Vrije Universiteit Brussel, Brussels, Belgium

Humana Press

Editors
Dirk Saerens
Department of Molecular
and Cellular Interactions
VIB, Brussels, Belgium

Laboratory of Cellular
and Molecular Immunology
Vrije Universiteit Brussel
Brussels, Belgium

Serge Muyldermans
Department of Molecular
and Cellular Interactions
VIB, Brussels, Belgium

Laboratory of Cellular
and Molecular Immunology
Vrije Universiteit Brussel
Brussels, Belgium

ISSN 1064-3745 ISSN 1940-6029 (electronic)
ISBN 978-1-4939-5915-0 ISBN 978-1-61779-968-6 (eBook)
DOI 10.1007/978-1-61779-968-6
Springer New York Heidelberg Dordrecht London

Softcover re-print of the Hardcover 1st edition 2012

Printed on acid-free paper

Humana Press is a brand of Springer
Springer is part of Springer Science+Business Media (www.springer.com)

Preface

The development of the hybridoma technology created the possibility to obtain unlimited amounts of monoclonal antibodies (mAb) with high specificity and affinity for any target and to introduce mAbs in a wide range of applications. Examples of antibody-based drugs in therapeutic settings and antibody-based probes in diagnostics are infinite. However, the bulky size of mAbs, costly production, and cumbersome engineering retarded or hampered regularly their streamlined development in some applications. Consequently, mAbs became the focus of many attempts to minimize the size and complexity of their antigen-binding fragments. Eventually, these efforts led to the recombinant production of smaller antigen-binding fragments such as Fab or scFv (where a synthetic linker connects the variable domains of heavy and light chain, i.e., VH and VL), and even sdAbs (single domain antibodies derived mostly of the VH). Although the first set of sdAbs offered significant advantages, they also suffered from multiple shortcomings, all of which have been remediated by elegant engineering. Interestingly, while scientists were designing, engineering, and shaping the ideal sdAb, a serendipitous discovery showed that a similar engineering occurred already in nature in the camelids, and later on, it was found that cartilaginous fish antibodies performed the exercise even earlier on in evolution. These animals have in their blood functional antibody isotype composed of heavy chains—only that lack light chains, in addition to the classical antibodies containing two heavy and two light chains. These heavy-chain antibodies (HCAbs) recognize the antigen via a single variable domain, referred to as VHH or V-NAR. The VHH or V-NAR is the smallest intact antigen-binding fragment that can be produced recombinantly at low cost.

The valuable properties of man-made sdAbs, VHHs, and V-NARs including solubility and stability, high affinity and specificity for their cognate antigen, small size and strict monomeric behavior offer many opportunities. As a result, several spin-off companies have been founded in Australia, Belgium, England, Germany, Netherlands, and Scotland that introduced these proteins successfully in a wide range of applications to cover a special need in research or even to produce next-generation therapeutics in the clinic.

Brussels, Belgium

Dirk Saerens
Serge Muyldermans

Contents

Contributors

VISHAL AGRAWAL • *Biotechnology Research Institute, National Research Council of Canada, Montreal, QC, Canada*
MEHDI ARBABI-GHAHROUDI • *Institute for Biological Sciences, National Research Council Canada, Ottawa, ON, Canada; School of Environmental Sciences, University of Guelph, Guelph, ON, Canada; Department of Biology, Carleton University, Ottawa, ON, Canada*
PATRICK DE BAETSELIER • *Laboratory of Cellular and Molecular Immunology (CMIM), Vrije Universiteit Brussel (VUB), Brussels, Belgium; Department of Molecular and Cellular Interactions, Vlaams Instituut voor Biotechnologie (VIB), Brussels, Belgium*
TOYA NATH BARAL • *Institute for Biological Sciences, National Research Council of Canada, Ottawa, ON, Canada*
LOUIS BISSON • *Biotechnology Research Institute, National Research Council of Canada, Montreal, QC, Canada*
SYLVIE DE BUCK • *Department of Plant Systems Biology, VIB, Ghent, Belgium; Department of Plant Biotechnology and Bioinformatics, Ghent University, Ghent, Belgium*
NICO CALLEWAERT • *Unit for Medical Biotechnology, Department for Molecular Biomedical Research, VIB, Ghent, Belgium; Laboratory for Protein Biochemistry and Biomolecular Engineering (L-ProBe), Department of Biochemistry and Microbiology, Ghent University, Ghent, Belgium*
VICKY CAVELIERS • *In Vivo Cellular and Molecular Imaging (ICMI) Laboratory, Vrije Universiteit Brussel (VUB), Brussels, Belgium; Department of nuclear Medicine, UZ Brussel, Brussels, Belgium*
DANIEL CHARLIER • *Erfelijkheidsleer en Microbiologie, Vrije Universiteit Brussel, Brussels, Belgium*
DANIEL CHRIST • *Garvan Institute of Medical Research, Darlinghurst/Sydney, NSW, Australia*
ANN DEPICKER • *Department of Plant Systems Biology, VIB, Ghent, Belgium; Department of Plant Biotechnology and Bioinformatics, Ghent University, Ghent, Belgium*
NICK DEVOOGDT • *In Vivo Cellular and Molecular Imaging (ICMI) Laboratory, Vrije Universiteit Brussel (VUB), Brussels, Belgium*
MATTHIAS D'HUYVETTER • *In Vivo Cellular and Molecular Imaging (ICMI) Laboratory, Vrije Universiteit Brussel (VUB), Brussels, Belgium*
WEN DING • *Institute for Biological Sciences, National Research Council Canada, Ottawa, ON, Canada*
CHRISTOPHER M. DOBSON • *Department of Chemistry, University of Cambridge, Cambridge, UK*
EDWARD DOLK • *QVQ, Utrecht, The Netherlands*

TRONG NGUYEN DUC • *Department of Molecular and Cellular Interactions, VIB, Brussels, Belgium; Laboratory of Cellular and Molecular Immunology, Brussels, Belgium*
KIP DUDGEON • *Garvan Institute of Medical Research, Darlinghurst/Sydney, NSW, Australia*
YVES DUROCHER • *Biotechnology Research Institute, National Research Council of Canada, Montreal, QC, Canada*
KRISTOFFER FAMM • *Centre for Protein Engineering, MRC Centre, Cambridge, UK; GlaxoSmithKline, Middlesex, UK*
ERWIN DE GENST • *Department of Chemistry, University of Cambridge, Cambridge, UK*
ANDREA GORLANI • *Department of Biomolecular Imaging, Utrecht University, Utrecht, The Netherlands; Biomolecular Imaging, Faculty of Science, Department of Biology, Universiteit Utrecht, Utrecht, The Netherlands*
JACQUELINE GREGOR • *ChromoTek GmbH, Martinsried, Germany*
ANDREW GRIFFITHS • *Laboratoire de Biologie Chimique, Institut de Science et d'Ingenierie Supramoleculaires, Université Louis Pasteur, Strasbourg, France*
HANS DE HAARD • *Cell Biology, Utrecht University, Utrecht, The Netherlands*
YOSHIHISA HAGIHARA • *National Institute of Advanced Industrial Science and Technology (AIST), Ikeda, Osaka, Japan*
GHOLAMREZA HASSANZADEH-GHASSABEH • *Department of Molecular and Cellular Interactions, VIB, Brussels, Belgium; Laboratory of Cellular and Molecular Immunology, Brussels, Belgium*
SOPHIE HERNOT • *In Vivo Cellular and Molecular Imaging (ICMI) Laboratory, Vrije Universiteit Brussel (VUB), Brussels, Belgium*
LUCY J. HOLT • *Biopharm R&D, GlaxoSmithKline, Cambridge, UK*
GREG HUSSACK • *Institute for Biological Sciences, National Research Council Canada, Ottawa, ON, Canada; Department of Biochemistry, Microbiology and Immunology, University of Ottawa, Ottawa, ON, Canada*
OLGA IGNATOVICH • *Biopharm R&D, GlaxoSmithKline, Cambridge, UK*
LAURENT JESPERS • *Biopharm R&D, GlaxoSmithKline, Cambridge, UK*
DAE YOUNG KIM • *Institute for Biological Sciences, National Research Council Canada, Ottawa, ON, Canada*
RINSE KLOOSTER • *Department of Human and Clinical Genetics, Medical Genetics Center, Leiden University Medical Center, Leiden, The Netherlands*
AKIKO KOIDE • *Department of Biochemistry and Molecular Biology, The University of Chicago, Chicago, IL, USA*
SHOHEI KOIDE • *Department of Biochemistry and Molecular Biology, The University of Chicago, Chicago, IL, USA*
JYOTHI KUMARAN • *Institute for Biological Sciences, National Research Council of Canada, Ottawa, ON, Canada; School of Environmental Sciences, University of Guelph, Guelph, ON, Canada*
TOON LAEREMANS • *Structural Biology Brussels, VIB/VUB, Brussels, Belgium*
TONY LAHOUTTE • *In Vivo Cellular and Molecular Imaging (ICMI) Laboratory, Vrije Universiteit Brussel (VUB), Brussels, Belgium; Nuclear Medicine Department, UZ Brussel, Brussels, Belgium*

Els Van Lerberge • *Department of Plant Systems Biology, VIB, Ghent, Belgium; Department of Plant Biotechnology and Bioinformatics, Ghent University, Ghent, Belgium*

Heinrich Leonhardt • *CIPS, Center for Integrated Protein Science at the Department of Biology II, Ludwig Maximilians University Munich, Planegg-Martinsried, Germany*

Silvère M. van der Maarel • *Department of Human and Clinical Genetics, Medical Genetics Center, Leiden University Medical Center, Leiden, The Netherlands*

C. Roger MacKenzie • *Institute for Biological Sciences, National Research Council Canada, Ottawa, ON, Canada; School of Environmental Sciences, University of Guelph, Guelph, ON, Canada*

Kien T. Maik • *Division of Anatomical Pathology, Department of Pathology and Laboratory Medicine, The Ottawa Hospital, Ottawa, ON, Canada; University of Ottawa, Ottawa, ON, Canada*

Ario de Marco • *University of Nova Gorica (UNG), Rožna Dolina, Nova Gorica, Slovenia*

Sam Massa • *In Vivo Cellular and Molecular Imaging (ICMI) Laboratory, Vrije Universiteit Brussel (VUB), Brussels, Belgium; Laboratory of Cellular and Molecular Immunology (CMIM), Vrije Universiteit Brussel (VUB), Brussels, Belgium; Department of Molecular and Cellular Interactions, Vlaams Instituut voor Biotechnologie (VIB), Brussels, Belgium*

Thomas De Meyer • *Department of Plant Systems Biology, VIB, Ghent, Belgium; Department of Plant Biotechnology and Bioinformatics, Ghent University, Ghent, Belgium*

Yanal Murad • *Institute for Biological Sciences, National Research Council of Canada, Ottawa, ON, Canada*

Serge Muyldermans • *Department of Molecular and Cellular Interactions, VIB, Brussels, Belgium; Laboratory of Cellular and Molecular Immunology, Vrije Universiteit Brussel, Brussels, Belgium*

Jonah Nolf • *Department of Plant Systems Biology, VIB, Ghent, Belgium; Department of Plant Biotechnology and Bioinformatics, Ghent University, Ghent, Belgium*

Stewart D. Nuttall • *CSIRO Materials Science and Engineering, Parkville, VIC, Australia*

Aurelien Olichon • *INSERM U563—Institut Claudius Regaud, Toulouse, France*

Annelies De Paepe • *Department of Plant Systems Biology, VIB, Ghent, Belgium; Department of Plant Biotechnology and Bioinformatics, Ghent University, Ghent, Belgium*

Eveline Peeters • *Erfelijkheidsleer en Microbiologie, Vrije Universiteit Brussel, Brussels, Belgium*

Mireille Pellis • *Department of Molecular and Cellular Interactions, VIB, Brussels, Belgium; Laboratory of Cellular and Molecular Immunology, Vrije Universiteit Brussel, Brussels, Belgium*

Sylvie Perret • *Biotechnology Research Institute, National Research Council of Canada, Montreal, QC, Canada*

GARWIN PICHLER • *CIPS, Center for Integrated Protein Science at the Department of Biology II, Ludwig Maximilians University Munich, Planegg-Martinsried, Germany*
ROBIN PIRON • *Department of Plant Systems Biology, VIB, Ghent, Belgium; Department of Plant Biotechnology and Bioinformatics, Ghent University, Ghent, Belgium*
TERENCE H. RABBITTS • *Weatherall Institute of Molecular Medicine, MRC Molecular Haematology Unit, University of Oxford, John Radcliffe Hospital, Headington, Oxford, UK*
ULRICH ROTHBAUER • *Natural and Medical Science Institute at the University of Tuebingen, University of Tuebingen, Reutlingen, Germany; ChromoTek GmbH, Planegg-Martinsried, Germany*
ROMAIN ROUET • *Garvan Institute of Medical Research, Darlinghurst/Sydney, NSW, Australia*
KIM S. RUTGERS • *Department of Human and Clinical Genetics, Medical Genetics Center, Leiden University Medical Center, Leiden, The Netherlands*
LUCY RUTTEN • *Biomolecular Imaging, Department of Biology, Utrecht University, Utrecht, The Netherlands*
DANIEL RYCROFT • *Biopharm R&D, GlaxoSmithKline, Cambridge, UK*
DIRK SAERENS • *Department of Molecular and Cellular Interactions, VIB, Brussels, Belgium; Laboratory of Cellular and Molecular Immunology, Vrije Universiteit Brussel, Brussels, Belgium*
KRISTOF DE SCHUTTER • *Unit for Medical Biotechnology, Department for Molecular Biomedical Research, VIB, Ghent, Belgium; Ghent University, Ghent (Zwijnaarde), Belgium*
ARMIN SEPP • *Innovation Biopharm Discovery Unit, Biopharm R&D, GlaxoSmithKline Plc, Cambridge, UK*
SACHDEV S. SIDHU • *Terrence Donnelly Center for Cellular and Biomolecular Research and Banting and Best Department of Medical Research, University of Toronto, Toronto, ON, Canada; Department of Molecular Genetics, University of Toronto, Toronto, ON, Canada*
IGOR SLIVAC • *Biotechnology Research Institute, National Research Council of Canada, Montreal, QC, Canada*
GILLES ST-LAURENT • *Biotechnology Research Institute, National Research Council of Canada, Montreal, QC, Canada*
TOMOYUKI TANAKA • *Leeds Institute of Molecular Medicine, St. James's University Hospital, University of Leeds, Leeds, UK*
JAMSHID TANHA • *Institute for Biological Sciences, National Research Council Canada, Ottawa, ON, Canada; Department of Biochemistry, Microbiology, and Immunology, University of Ottawa, Ottawa, ON, Canada; School of Environmental Sciences, University of Guelph, Guelph, ON, Canada*
JEAN-LUC TEILLAUD • *Cordeliers Research Center/INSERM U.872, Paris Descartes University and Pierre et Marie Curie University (UPMC), Paris, France*
IAN M. TOMLINSON • *Biopharm R&D, GlaxoSmithKline, Cambridge, UK*

RAFFI TONIKIAN • *Terrence Donnelly Center for Cellular and Biomolecular Research and Banting and Best Department of Medical Research, University of Toronto, Toronto, ON, Canada; Department of Protein Engineering, Biogen Idec, Cambridge, MA, USA*

ILSE VANEYCKEN • *In Vivo Cellular and Molecular Imaging (ICMI) Laboratory, Vrije Universiteit Brussel (VUB), Brussels, Belgium*

PETER VERHEESEN • *Structural Biology Brussels, VIB/VUB, Brussels, Belgium*

THEO VERRIPS • *QVQ, Utrecht, The Netherlands*

CÉCILE VINCKE • *Department of Molecular and Cellular Interactions, VIB, Brussels, Belgium; Laboratory of Cellular and Molecular Immunology, Vrije Universiteit Brussel, Brussels, Belgium*

VIKRAM VIRDI • *Department of Plant Systems Biology, VIB, Ghent, Belgium; Department of Plant Biotechnology and Bioinformatics, Ghent University, Ghent, Belgium*

JENS DE VOS • *In Vivo Cellular and Molecular Imaging (ICMI) Laboratory, Vrije Universiteit Brussel (VUB), Brussels, Belgium; Laboratory of Cellular and Molecular Immunology (CMIM), Vrije Universiteit Brussel (VUB), Brussels, Belgium; Department of Molecular and Cellular Interactions, Vlaams Instituut voor Biotechnologie (VIB), Brussels, Belgium*

KIRSTEN DE WILDE • *Department of Plant Systems Biology, VIB, Ghent, Belgium; Department of Plant Biotechnology and Bioinformatics, Ghent University, Ghent, Belgium*

RUUD M.T. DE WILDT • *Biopharm R&D, GlaxoSmithKline, Cambridge, UK*

CATARINA XAVIER • *In Vivo Cellular and Molecular Imaging (ICMI) Laboratory, Vrije Universiteit Brussel (VUB), Brussels, Belgium*

JIANBING ZHANG • *Institute for Biological Sciences, National Research Council of Canada, Ottawa, ON, Canada; University of Ottawa, Ottawa, ON, Canada*

KOUROSH ZOLGHADR • *Natural and Medical Science Institute at the University of Tuebingen, University of Tuebingen, Reutlingen, Germany; ChromoTek GmbH, Martinsried, Germany*

Part I

Overview of Single Domain Antibodies

Chapter 1

From Whole Monoclonal Antibodies to Single Domain Antibodies: Think Small

Jean-Luc Teillaud

Abstract

The development of therapeutic monoclonal antibodies over the last 35 years has led to the emergence of a new class of useful therapeutic molecules. These "first generation" antibodies have been obtained thanks to the conjugated and huge efforts of both academic and biotech researchers. About 30 monoclonal antibodies are currently approved for therapeutic use in Europe, USA, and China. Strikingly, only a restricted number of these antibodies are immunoglobulin fragments, single variable domains, or multiunit formats based on the engineering of immunoglobulin variable domains. In the present chapter, we will review the major steps of the therapeutic antibodies history and we will highlight the enormous potential of antibody fragments, either used as multiunits such as bispecific antibodies, single units, or as cell modifiers such as intrabodies or cell surface-expressed molecules.

Key words: Bispecific antibody, Chimeric antibody, Humanized antibody, Intrabody, Monoclonal antibody, Nanobody, Phage display, Single chain Fv, Single domain antibody

1. Introduction

Since their discovery by Köhler and Milstein 37 years ago (1), a lot of efforts have been devoted to optimize the functional properties of monoclonal antibodies (mAbs), to reduce their immunogenicity and to increase their clinical efficacy. In the early 1980s, the vast majority of mAbs was of rodent origin. This became quickly a major concern as high titers of human anti-mouse antibodies (HAMAs) were detected when mAbs of murine origin were infused to patients. Such HAMAs lower or block the therapeutic efficacy of mAbs and provoke side effects related to the formation of immune complexes. Although it was already well established at that time that the Fc region of murine IgG was mostly responsible for the immunogenicity, the strategies that were then explored barely focused on the use of antibody fragments but mostly on the generation of fully

Dirk Saerens and Serge Muyldermans (eds.), *Single Domain Antibodies: Methods and Protocols*,
Methods in Molecular Biology, vol. 911, DOI 10.1007/978-1-61779-968-6_1, © Springer Science+Business Media, LLC 2012

human antibodies using cellular engineering or, in parallel, on the use of molecular engineering techniques to reduce the immunogenicity of the murine mAbs by introducing sequences of human origin as much as possible. The choice of developing whole IgG rather than antibody fragments for therapeutics was based on the fact that the Fc region is critical for IgG effector functions, e.g., complement activation and binding to Fcgamma receptors (FcγRs), as well as for the control of IgG serum half-life, due to the Fc-dependent binding of IgG to the human neonatal FcRn. This receptor rescues IgG from degradation and, hence, increases their serum half-life. Thus, the goal of getting a clinically efficient mAb was closely associated with its ability to recruit effector functions and to exhibit a sufficient half-life. Even though a number of approaches focused already on the capacity of mAbs to neutralize the biological activity of cytokines, toxins, or viruses or on the use of antibodies as a cargo to deliver payloads to the targeted cells (toxins, drugs, radionucleids), hence not requiring the presence of an Fc region, the use of IgG fragments was very limited. The production of IgG-derived fragments at an industrial scale was a considerable challenge at that time, as no easy-to-perform recombinant technology was available and one has to rely on time-consuming and costly biochemical processes to produce such fragments. Thus, mostly whole IgG molecules have been developed for therapeutic use in humans so far. Although one of the first therapeutic mAbs to receive approval by the regulatory agencies was a Fab fragment [abciximab, an anti-GPIIb/IIIa mAb (1994)], only recently, three other antibody fragments have been approved for clinical use [the anti-CD147 ^{131}I-F(ab′)$_2$ mAb metuximab (2005, China), the anti-Vascular Endothelium Growth Factor A (VEGF-A) Fab mAb ranibizumab (2006), the anti-TNFα Fab′ mAb certolizumab pegol (PEG) (2008)]. In the present chapter, we will review the major steps that have marked the history of therapeutic antibodies and of their formats, from the whole mouse IgG molecule to the single domain human antibody format.

2. Monoclonal Antibodies: The Mouse That Wanted to Become Human

No technology was available in the late 1970s to generate fully human antibodies, except the infection of human B cells by Epstein–Barr virus (EBV), which allows the generation of immortalized cells producing mAbs (2). However, the use of this method has been limited by important problems. These include the difficulty to get stable cell clones, the low amount of antibodies produced, and the limited capacity to select antibodies with the desired antigen specificity. A few human mAbs have been nevertheless obtained using EBV transformation combined with molecular engineering [anti-Rhesus D, anti-Tetanus Toxoïd, anti-Human Immunodeficiency Virus (HIV)], some of these mAbs being currently developed for therapeutic use (3). Other approaches based on cellular engineering (such as the use of optimized fusion partners, of in vitro cellular immunization, or of long-term growth of human B lymphocytes (4–6)) were shown to be poorly efficient. Molecular engineering of mAbs therefore rapidly developed in the early 1980s and has been the leading force for antibody engineering since then. However, cellular engineering has made recently a remarkable comeback, based on advance in the definition of memory B cells and of new signaling pathways leading to sustained proliferation of hypermutated switched B cells. Notably, the transformation of memory B cells by EBV from virus-infected patients and their stimulation with CpG (which triggers TLR9-mediated B-cell proliferation) allowed the generation of a large number of EBV-transformed cell lines which produce high-affinity specific IgG mAbs (7). Moreover, the ability to repopulate immuno-deficient mice ($Rag2^{-/-}$ $\gamma c^{-/-}$) with functional immune cells following injection of $CD34^{+}$ human cord blood cells has allowed to generate fully human mAbs following immunization with the desired antigen (8). Thus, the combination of more sophisticated cellular engineering with powerful molecular engineering techniques makes it possible to generate now fully human antibodies more easily, at least when antibodies directed against viruses or other pathogens are searched and when hyperimmunized volunteers are available.

The development of molecular engineering techniques has been made possible by a better knowledge of Ig gene organization and of immunoglobulin 3-D structure. It allowed the engineering of chimeric antibodies and humanized antibodies. Chimeric antibodies comprise the variable domains derived from rodent mAbs fused to the constant domains of human heavy and light chains (9). In most cases, the human CH1-CH2-CH3 $\gamma 1$ and human Cκ domains have been used. Six chimeric mAbs are on the market, including the anti-GPIIb/IIIa abciximab Fab and the ^{131}I-Vivatuxin/^{131}I-chTNT (China). Humanized antibodies are obtained by grafting complementarity determining regions (CDRs) derived from murine antibodies with desired specificity onto carefully chosen human VH and VL frameworks (FRs). The human FRs are selected based on structural models of the variable domains of the mouse parental antibodies (10). However, the humanization technology is far more complex than the chimerization. A strong decrease in antibody affinity or even a loss of antigen binding of the resulting humanized variable domains is often observed. To overcome this major drawback, one has to develop lengthy and costly molecular analyses of antigen–antibody interactions such as alanine scanning and cocrystallization studies, when possible (11). Nevertheless, this approach has proved to be powerful. Thirteen humanized mAbs are currently on the market, including the Fab ranibizumab and the Fab′ pegylated certolizumab fragments. Of note, all these mAbs are humanized IgG1 antibodies, but one (eculizumab, an anti-C5 mAb). The gemtuzumab (an anti-CD33 humanized IgG4 coupled to the ozogamycin antibiotic) has been recently withdrawn, due to an unfavorable benefit/risk ratio. Many different protocols to generate humanized antibodies have been described over the years. An alternative method to CDRs grafting has been developed to humanize variable domains. It is based on the detailed analysis of the amino-acids of the murine and human variable domains exposed to solvents. The use of a peculiar amino-acid at a given exposed position allows the determination of well-defined «surface residues patterns», specific to each antibody. It is then possible to switch from a murine to a human profile by site-directed mutagenesis targeting a limited number of amino-acids, without modifying the antigen-binding capacity. This technique, termed «variable domain resurfacing» has been used to generate a number of humanized mAbs (12).

An elegant technique for generating fully human antibodies has been the skillful adaptation of the filamentous phage display technique (13) to the expression of antibody fragments (14). It allowed the establishment of large combinatorial libraries of human VH and VL and made it possible to select for specific Fab′ or single chain Fv (scFv) fragments (see below) which are then used to format a whole recombinant human mAb. This technique has become popular and has been largely used because the display of antibody fragments fused to the phage pIII coat protein on the surface of filamentous phages allows the rapid selection of specific antibodies among billions of VH/VL pairs. In addition, it has been extensively used to select high-affinity variants using site-directed or random mutagenesis (11, 15). An alternative technique that uses the λ lytic phage instead of a filamentous phage had been described earlier, but has not been proved useful. It allows the screening of only a few hundred thousand clones and requires the use of duplicate lifts with nitrocellulose for detecting the binding of specific antibody fragments to radiolabeled antigens (16). An alternative to phage display is the yeast display where antibody scFv fragments fused to the yeast protein Aga2p are exposed on the surface of yeasts (*Saccharomyces cerevisiae*). It allows the screening of scFv libraries by cell sorting using fluorochrome-labeled target molecules and the isolation of the relevant VH/VL encoding cDNA (17).

Another molecular approach developed to select human antibodies has been the «ribosome display», which is based on the production of mRNA derived from scFv libraries. mRNA are then translated in vitro and selected as a ribosome-polypeptide (the nascent scFv chain) complex, allowing the selection of the encoding sequences of the VH/VL domains of interest, which then can be reformatted as a whole IgG. This technique has been successfully used to select high-affinity antibodies from naïve libraries (18).

Finally, techniques that allow mouse D and/or J mini-gene inactivation and insertion of large human DNA fragments from yeast artificial chromosome in mouse germline have made it possible to generate transgenic mice capable of producing fully human antibodies following immunization (19, 20). Later on, an alternative to these approaches has been the generation of double trans-chromosomic (Tc) mice that harbor two individual "mini-chromonosomes," containing the complete germline loci of immunoglobulin heavy and κ-light chains (21). Humanized mice can mount an antigen-specific human antibody response following immunization, and human antigen-specific mAbs can be generated. Further refinement to these approaches has included the use of hyperimmunized humanized mice to build immune phage libraries.

Two antibodies obtained from phage display libraries (including the ranibizumab Fab fragment which was affinity-matured using filamentous phage display) and seven from humanized mice are now on the market. Many others are currently being tested in clinical trials. Although only less than a quarter of the mAbs approved and marketed are fully human antibodies, about 20–25% of the mAbs currently in clinical development are human antibodies derived either from phage display libraries or from transgenic mice.

3. The Monoclonal Antibody Fragments: Many Formats for Many Uses

Although the development of useful therapeutic antibody fragments has been very slow since the discovery of mAbs in 1975, it is striking to note that the use of antibody fragments by immunologists started as early as in the late 1950s after the publication of the pioneering work of Porter (22). It made it possible to understand the topology of an IgG molecule and to introduce the concept of Fab (for fragment antigen binding) and Fc (for fragment crystallizable) fragments (22, 23). Treatment of immunoglobulins (Ig) with proteolytic enzymes was first used to remove the species-specific antigenic determinants of horse anti-tetanus antibodies used in passive immunization of humans. It was then used to elucidate Ig structure. The studies of Porter showed that rabbit IgG can be cleaved by papain into three well-defined fragments (two Fabs and one Fc) (23). Proteolytic cleavage became then a basic research tool in the elucidation of Ig structure. It was used to solve the three-dimensional structure of the Fab′ fragment by crystallography (24) and made it possible to define functions associated with the different fragments. Due to their monovalency or bivalency, Fab and $F(ab)'_2$ fragments have been widely used for research, in particular for receptors studies, their lack of Fc region allowing to avoid the nonspecific binding to cells through FcγRs.

Although both Fab and Fc fragments exert important biological functions, mostly antigen-binding fragments have been developed for therapeutic purpose. Fc fragments have been successfully used instead of intravenous immunoglobulins (IVIg) for the treatment of acute immune thrombocytopenic purpura (ITP) in a clinical trial (25), but their clinical development was discontinued. Only recently, Fc fragments have been proposed as therapeutic molecules for intravenous IVIg replacement, with improved activity and availability (26). By contrast, Fab fragments have been used to generate radio-conjugated molecules for imaging and for radio-immuno-therapy (RIT). In the early 1980s, they started being used as building block of bispecific antibodies (BsAb), a format that overcome the absence of the Fc portion by recruiting activating molecules expressed on effector cells of the immune system (27). The careful selection of mAbs directed against stimulatory molecules such as CD3 (expressed on T cells), FcγRI (expressed on neutrophils and activated macrophages), and FcγRIII (expressed on NK cells, activated macrophages, and subsets of monocytes and T cells) made it possible to generate BsAbs that exhibited powerful anti-tumor activities (28, 29). However, it rapidly appeared that the mass production of therapeutic BsAbs by a biochemical process (that includes the GMP preparation of large amounts of Fab′ from the two parental purified mAbs, the coupling of the two Fab′ by a chemical linker, and the purification of the resulting BsAb) was difficult to perform, time-consuming, and costly. Thus, alternative molecular approaches were explored in the early 90s based on the pioneering observation of Inbar and coworkers (30) showing that an intact antigen-binding site of about 25 kDa, representing VH-VL heterodimer, termed Fv fragment, could be obtained by proteolytic digestion (see Fig. 1a). The demonstration that Fv format can be produced, eventually as a single polypeptide chain (single chain Fv, sFv, or scFv), in bacteria (31–33) led to the generation of new bispecific formats such as diabodies (34) (see Fig. 1a). ScFv are made of one heavy chain variable domain (VH) linked through a flexible spacer (usually a repeated motif of 3 × GGGGS, although some others have been also described) (35), to one light chain variable domain (VL). The VH-linker-VL sequence can be inverted without any loss of the binding. Shortened linkers have been used to produce scFvs under divalent or bispecific forms (35, 36). However, this first generation of "molecular" BsAbs has proved to be unstable, prone to aggregation, and difficult to produce at a large scale. Only recently, BsAb molecular constructs have appeared to be promising therapeutic molecules, with the advent of a new format (the "BiTE" antibody) that could induce a significant clinical response in cancer patients, while being used at very low doses as compared to whole IgG mAbs (37). Further clinical studies are however needed to confirm this exciting observation.

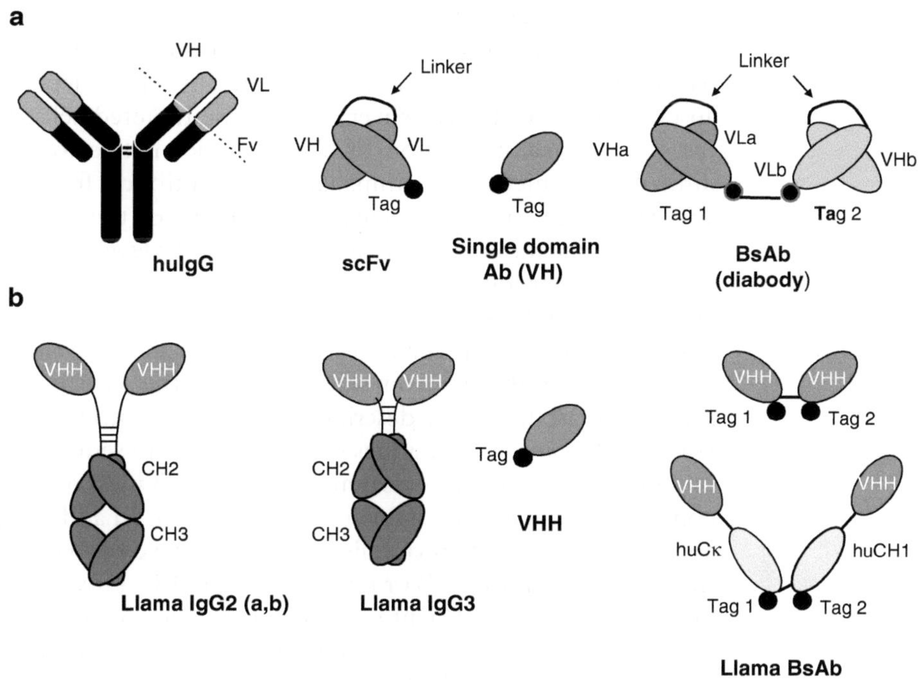

Fig. 1. Molecular engineering of single domain molecules and of multiunit formats. (**a**) Single domain antibody (sdAb), made of a single stable VH domain, and single chain Fv (scFv), made of one VH and one VL domains fused to each other through a flexible hydrophilic linker, can be used as single monovalent molecules or further engineered to generate multiunit formats such as bispecific antibodies (BsAbs). (**b**) Single VHH domains can be derived from llama IgG2 and IgG3 antibodies that do not exhibit light chains. They can be then used as a single domain (Nanobody) or as a modular unit to build more complex molecules such as BsAbs. Tag sequences are usually inserted at the C-terminus or at the N-terminus for research use (in vitro detection and purification of the recombinant molecule, intracellular tracking).

The production of scFv fragments by molecular engineering has also led to the concept of intrabodies, i.e., the intracellular expression of antibody fragments within a mammalian cell, a kind of "intracellular immunization" (38). Intrabodies have been mostly derived from neutralizing monoclonal antibodies (mAbs) and have provided the basis for phenotypic knock-outs (that we termed "Antibody-Mediated Knock-Out," AMKO) via the binding and sometimes the relocalization of the targeted antigen. They can be easily directed to various subcellular compartments by adding appropriate localization sequences to target viral proteins, oncogene or tumor suppressor gene products, or cell surface receptors (39–42). Intrabodies have been used mostly as neutralizing antibody fragments [HIV gp120, $p21^{Ras}$, IL-2Rα, human papilloma virus type 16 (HPV Type 16) E7 protein…], although the restoration of function (i.e., transcriptional activity) has been also achieved with an anti-p53 scFv (42). More recently, a study by Nizak et al. (43) has shown that intrabodies represent also remarkable conformation sensors and can be used to track specific conformers within a cell, suggesting that they represent also a powerful tool for basic science. However, the use of antibody fragments as intrabodies has encountered important problems. First, this approach is a combination of antibody therapy and gene therapy and is dependent on an efficient scFv cDNA delivery within the targeted cells. Second, the intracellular expression of a scFv under native form can be difficult to achieve in mammalian cells. Antibody fragments can aggregate due to the reducing environment of the cytosol (44). Moreover, the monomeric or divalent forms, the levels of expression, and the cellular localization have also an impact on the functional efficacy of intrabodies. A selection assay for functional intracellular antibodies using an in-cell two-hybrid system allowing the de novo selection of intrabodies from scFv libraries in the reducing environment of yeast has been described (45). A common signature of conserved amino-acid residues was deduced from sequence analysis of scFv isolated using this assay allowing the definition of a candidate consensus sequence for stable intrabodies (46). In addition, stable and functional scFv without disulfide bonds have been obtained by molecular evolution (47) or rational design (48). However, how to deliver intrabodies efficiently within a target cell in vivo remains to be solved. If so, this class of molecules will make undoubtedly its comeback in the field of targeted therapy, due to the exquisite specificity and high affinity of antibodies.

Another interesting use of scFv has been developed based on the observation that recombinant antibody fragments can be also expressed on the surface of effector or target cells. In both settings, the aim is to recruit and activate immune cells thanks to the antibody fragment being expressed on the cell surface. On the one hand, the expression on T cells of scFv fused to a transmembrane domain and to a T-cell receptor-signaling chain (49) has been explored. T cells retrovirally transduced with such a construct, termed T-bodies, can recognize antibody-defined antigens, which leads to T-cell activation, specific lysis, and cytokine release (49). This approach has led to adoptive immunotherapy trials (50), some of them being still ongoing. However, it has encountered important technical challenges that remain to be solved (cell transduction/infection efficacy, cell homing, cell survival…). On the other hand, tumor cells have been also engineered to express scFv directed against activating receptors expressed on different cell types of the immune system (36, 51). Antibodies expressed on tumor cells and directed against activating molecules present on immune cells could act as a trigger to induce a reverse cytotoxicity and other biological effects. Ideally, the targeted antigen should be expressed on a variety of immune cells harboring different effector functions, by contrast to the T-bodies that are restricted to a small subset of cytotoxic T cells. An interesting target candidate that has been explored is FcγRIII (51). Cells from both innate and adaptative immunity can be activated following the binding of anti-FcγRIIII scFv expressing tumor cells. FcγRIII$^+$ NK cells can be recruited to kill tumor cells through the activation of these receptors. Furthermore, the enhancement of phagocytosis of tumor cells or cell extracts by FcγRIII$^+$ antigen-presenting cells (APCs) could induce a protective long-term immunity to tumors by allowing recruitment of T cells (52). This approach, based on the expression on the tumor cell membrane of a scFv specifically directed against FcγRIII, prevented tumor growth in mice (51). It has been called the "Hooking tumor strategy" (51) and could represent a potent antibody-based gene therapy strategy for cancer therapy, as it does not require a high efficiency of tumor cell transduction.

Finally, the use of antibody fragments as therapeutics has been also stimulated by two major observations. First, in 1990, it was demonstrated that isolated VH domains (about 13 kDa) with good antigen-binding affinities (in the 20 nM range) can be isolated from libraries of VH domains expressed and secreted from *Escherichia coli* (53) (see Fig. 1a). This led to the concept that single domain antibodies (dAbs or sdAbs) may represent useful diagnosis and/or therapeutic tools, easy to use as building blocks for various formats of antibody-based therapeutic molecules. Second, the discovery that antibodies composed of heavy-chain dimers and devoid of light chains, but exhibiting nevertheless an extensive antigen-binding repertoire, are present in the serum of camelids (54) (see Fig. 1b) paved the way to new molecular engineering approaches based on the cloning and engineering of the variable domains of these antibodies termed VHH (also called Nanobodies due to their small size of 4 nm by 2.5 nm in diameter). The easy generation and selection of these single domain antibodies following immunization of a dromedary or of a llama and phage display (55), as well as their remarkable biophysical properties (very stable and highly soluble, strict monomeric behavior), make them, as the dAbs described by Ward and coworkers (53), particularly attractive for a clinical use in humans under various formats (56) (see Fig. 1). Notably, the small size of dAbs and of Nanobodies should allow them to penetrate tissues more readily or to block cell/protein functions by binding to epitopes otherwise difficult to reach for a whole antibody molecule. The generation and the expression of single domain antibodies, as well as some of their research, diagnosis, and clinical use, are detailed in the following chapters.

Acknowledgments

The author wishes to thank the INSERM, the Paris Descartes University, the Pierre and Marie Curie University (UPMC), and the Cordeliers Research Center for their financial support.

References

1. Köhler G, Milstein C (1975) Continuous cultures of fused cells secreting antibody of predefined specificity. Nature 256:495–497
2. Steinitz M et al (1977) Virus induced B lymphocyte cell lines producing specific antibodies. Nature 269:420–422
3. Béliard R et al (2008) An anti-D monoclonal antibody selected for enhanced FcγRIII engagement clears RhD-positive autologous red cells in human volunteers as efficiently as polyclonal anti-D antibodies. Br J Haematol 141:109–119
4. Olsson L, Kaplan HS (1980) Human-human hybridomas producing monoclonal antibodies of predefined antigenic specificity. Proc Natl Acad Sci U S A 77:5429–5431
5. Borrebaeck CA, Möller SA (1986) In vitro immunization. Effect of growth and differentiation factors on antigen-specific cell activation and production of monoclonal antibodies to autologous antigens and immunogens. J Immunol 13:3710–3715
6. Banchereau J et al (1989) Long-term human B cell lines dependent on interleukin-4 and antibody to CD40. Science 251:70–72
7. Traggiai E et al (2004) An efficient method to make human monoclonal antibodies from memory B cells: potent neutralization of SARS coronavirus. Nat Med 8:871–875
8. Traggiai E et al (2004) Development of a human adaptive immune system in cord blood cell-transplanted mice. Science 304:104–107
9. Morrison SL et al (1984) Chimeric human antibody molecules: mouse antigen-binding domains with human constant region domains. Proc Natl Acad Sci U S A 81:6851–6855
10. Queen C et al (1989) A humanized antibody that binds to the interleukin 2 receptor. Proc Natl Acad Sci U S A 86:10029–10035
11. Chen Y et al (1999) Selection and analysis of an optimized anti-VEGF antibody: crystal structure of an affinity-matured Fab in complex with antigen. J Mol Biol 293:865–881
12. Roguska MA et al (1994) Humanization of murine monoclonal antibodies through variable domain resurfacing. Proc Natl Acad Sci U S A 91:969–973
13. Smith GP (1985) Filamentous fusion phage: novel expression vectors that display cloned antigens on the virion surface. Science 228:1315–1317
14. McCafferty J et al (1990) Phage antibodies: filamentous phage displaying antibody variable domains. Nature 348:552–554
15. Hawkins RE, Russell SJ, Winter G (1992) Selection of phage antibodies by binding affinity: mimicking affinity maturation. J Mol Biol 226:889–896
16. Huse WD et al (1989) Generation of a large combinatorial library of the immunoglobulin repertoire in phage lambda. Science 246: 1275–1281
17. Feldhaus MJ et al (2003) Flow-cytometric isolation of human antibodies from a nonimmune *Saccharomyces cerevisiae* surface display library. Nat Biotechnol 21:163–170
18. Hanes J et al (2000) Picomolar affinity antibodies from a fully synthetic naive library selected and evolved by ribosome display. Nat Biotechnol 18:1287–1292
19. Lonberg N et al (1994) Antigen-specific human antibodies from mice comprising four distinct genetic modifications. Nature 368:856–859
20. Green LL et al (1994) Antigen-specific human monoclonal antibodies from mice engineered with human Ig heavy and light chain YACs. Nat Genet 7:13–21
21. Tomizuka K et al (2000) Double trans-chromosomic mice: maintenance of two individual human chromosome fragments containing Ig heavy and kappa loci and expression of fully human antibodies. Proc Natl Acad Sci U S A 97:722–727
22. Porter RR (1958) Separation and isolation of fractions of rabbit gamma-globulin containing the antibody and antigenic combining sites. Nature 182:670–671
23. Porter RR (1959) The hydrolysis of rabbit gamma-globulin and antibodies with crystalline papain. Biochem J 73:119–26
24. Poljak RJ et al (1973) Three-dimensional structure of the Fab' fragment of a human immunoglobulin at 2.8 A resolution. Proc Natl Acad Sci U S A 70:3305–3310
25. Debré M et al (1993) Infusion of Fc gamma fragments for treatment of children with acute immune thrombocytopenic purpura. Lancet 342:945–949
26. Anthony RM et al (2008) Recapitulation of IVIG anti-inflammatory activity with a recombinant IgG Fc. Science 320:373–376
27. Brennan M (1985) Preparation of bispecific antibodies by chemical recombination of monoclonal immunoglobulin G1 fragments. Science 229:81–83
28. Weiner LM et al (1993) A human tumor xenograft of therapy with a bispecific monoclonal antibody targeting c-erbB-2 and CD16. Cancer Res 53:94–100
29. Michon J et al (1995) In vitro killing of neuroblastoma cells by neutrophils derived from granulocyte colony-stimulating factor-treated cancer patients using an anti-disialoganglioside/anti-Fc gamma RI bispecific antibody. Blood 86:1124–1130

30. Inbar D et al (1972) Localization of antibody-combining sites within the variable portions of heavy and light chains. Proc Natl Acad Sci U S A 69:2659–2662
31. Skerra A, Plückthun A (1988) Assembly of a functional immunoglobulin Fv fragment in *Escherichia coli*. Science 240:1038–1041
32. Huston JS et al (1988) Protein engineering of antibody binding sites: recovery of specific activity in an anti-digoxin single-chain Fv analogue produced in *Escherichia coli*. Proc Natl Acad Sci U S A 85:5879–5883
33. Bird RE et al (1988) Single-chain antigen-binding proteins. Science 242:423–426
34. Holliger P et al (1993) "Diabodies": small bivalent and bispecific antibody fragments. Proc Natl Acad Sci U S A 90:6444–6448
35. Huston JS et al (1991) Protein engineering of single-chain Fv analogs and fusion proteins. Methods Enzymol 203:46–88
36. Kontermann RE, Muller R (1999) Intracellular and cell surface displayed single-chain diabodies. J Immunol Methods 226:179–188
37. Bargou R et al (2008) Tumor regression in cancer patients by very low doses of a T cell-engaging antibody. Science 321:974–977
38. Marasco WA (1997) Intrabodies: turning the humoral immune system outside in for intracellular immunization. Gene Ther 4:11–15
39. Marasco WA, Haseltine WA, Chen S (1993) Design, intracellular expression, and activity of a human anti-human immunodeficiency virus type 1 gp120 single-chain antibody. Proc Natl Acad Sci U S A 90:7889–7893
40. Cochet O et al (1998) Intracellular expression of an antibody fragment neutralizing $p21^{ras}$ promotes tumor regression. Cancer Res 58: 1170–1176
41. Richardson JH et al (1995) Phenotypic knockout of the high-affinity human interleukin 2 receptor by intracellular single-chain antibodies against the alpha sub-unit of the receptor. Proc Natl Acad Sci U S A 92:3137–3141
42. Caron de Fromentel C et al (1999) Restoration of transcriptional activity of p53 mutants in human tumor cells by intracellular expression of anti-p53 single chain Fv fragments. Oncogene 18:551–557
43. Nizak C et al (2003) Recombinant antibodies to the small GTPase Rab6 as conformation sensors. Science 300:984–987
44. Cardinale A, Filesi I, Biocca S (2001) Aggresome formation by anti-Ras intracellular scFv fragments. The fate of the antigen-antibody complex. Eur J Biochem 268:268–277
45. Visintin M et al (1999) Selection of antibodies for intracellular function using a two-hybrid in vivo system. Proc Nat Acad Sci U S A 9:11723–11728
46. Visintin M et al (2002) The intracellular antibody capture technology (IACT): towards a consensus sequence for intracellular antibodies. J Mol Biol 317:73–83
47. Proba K et al (1998) Antibody scFv fragments without disulfide bonds made by molecular evolution. J Mol Biol 275:245–253
48. Wirtz P, Steipe B (1999) Intrabody construction and expression III: engineering hyperstable V(H) domains. Protein Sci 8:2245–2250
49. Ross G, Waks T, Eshhar Z (1989) Expression of immunoglobulin-T-cell receptor chimeric molecules as functional receptors with antibody-type specificity. Proc Natl Acad Sci U S A 86:10024–10028
50. Pinthus JH et al (2004) Adoptive immunotherapy of prostate cancer bone lesions using redirected effector lymphocytes. J Clin Invest 114:1774–1781
51. Gruel N, Fridman WH, Teillaud JL (2001) By-passing tumor-specific and bispecific antibodies: triggering of antitumor immunity by expression of anti-FcγR scFv on cancer cell surface. Gene Ther 8:1721–1728
52. Kalergis AM, Ravetch JV (2002) Inducing tumor immunity through the selective engagement of activating Fcγ receptors on dendritic cells. J Exp Med 195:1653–1659
53. Ward ES et al (1989) Binding activities of a repertoire of single immunoglobulin variable domains secreted from *Escherichia coli*. Nature 341:544–546
54. Hamers-Casterman C et al (1993) Naturally occurring antibodies devoid of light chains. Nature 363:446–448
55. Behar G et al (2008) Isolation and characterization of anti-FcgammaRIII (CD16) llama single-domain antibodies that activate natural killer cells. Protein Eng Des Sel 21:1–10
56. Els Conrath K et al (2001) Camel single-domain antibodies as modular building units in bispecific and bivalent antibody constructs. J Biol Chem 276:7346–7350

Chapter 2

Introduction to Heavy Chain Antibodies and Derived Nanobodies

Cécile Vincke and Serge Muyldermans

Abstract

The immune response of infected or immunized dromedaries contains a diverse repertoire of conventional and heavy chain-only antibodies, both functional in antigen binding. By definition, a heavy chain antibody is devoid of a light chain and in the case of the heavy chain antibodies in camelids the CH1 domain is also missing. Consequently a camelid heavy chain antibody associates with its cognate antigen via a single domain, the variable heavy chain domain of a heavy chain antibody or VHH. An antigen-specific VHH, also known as Nanobody, with excellent biochemical properties can be obtained in various ways. Their recombinant expression provides access to user-friendly tools for a wide variety of applications.

Key words: Camels, Llamas, Heavy chain antibodies, Single domain antibodies, Nanobodies

1. Introduction

Immunoglobulin (Ig) molecules evolve naturally towards molecular recognition units that associate specifically and with high affinity with their cognate target. The basic structure of an Ig, a polypeptide tetramer of approximately150 kDa, comprises two identical pairs of heavy (50 kDa) and light polypeptide chains (25 kDa), linked by interchain disulfide bonds (1). The light chain consists of one variable domain (VL) at the N-terminal end and a single constant domain (CL) at the C-terminal end, whereas the heavy chain contains four or five domains: one variable domain (VH) at the N-terminal end followed by three or four constant domains (CH1, CH2, CH3, and possibly CH4) (see Fig. 1a) (1).

Immunoglobulins are bifunctional molecules that (1) bind antigens and, in addition, (2) initiate secondary biologic processes that are independent of the antigen specificity. These two independent aspects of immunoglobulin function reside in separate regions

Dirk Saerens and Serge Muyldermans (eds.), *Single Domain Antibodies: Methods and Protocols*,
Methods in Molecular Biology, vol. 911, DOI 10.1007/978-1-61779-968-6_2, © Springer Science+Business Media, LLC 2012

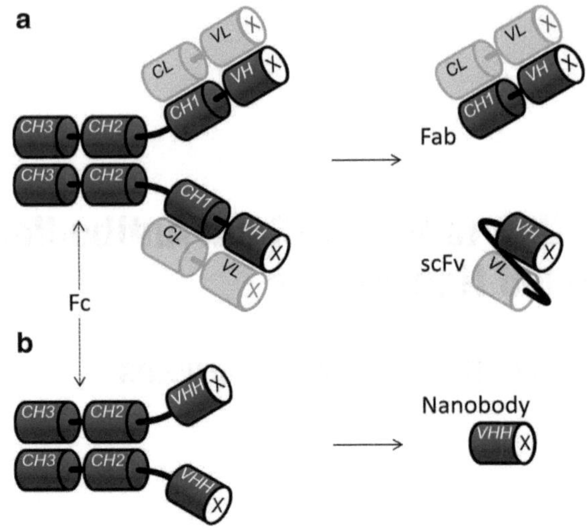

Fig. 1. Schematic representation of (**a**) a conventional and (**b**) a camelid heavy chain IgG antibody and their respective antigen-binding fragments (Fab or scFv for classical antibodies and VHH for HCAbs, respectively). The antigen-binding site of the VH–VL pair or of the VHH (or Nanobody) is denoted by crossed white surfaces.

of each protein. Indeed, these Y- or T-shaped molecules contain two antigen-binding fragments (Fabs), linked via a flexible hinge region located between the CH1 and CH2 domains, to a constant Fc region, responsible for effector functions. The flexibility of the hinge, conferred by a typically loose secondary structure, enables the two Fab arms to move relatively freely with respect to each other. This composition in independent modules and the overall structure of Igs is remarkably well conserved among mammals.

Throughout animal evolution, several classes of Igs have emerged; however, it is the IgG class that is the most abundant immunoglobulin in serum of mammals. It is the product of an affinity-matured immune response and thus, in general, highly specific antibodies with high affinity for their cognate antigen are generated. These antibodies are also very stable and easily purified by a variety of techniques of which affinity-chromatography on Protein A or Protein G is most convenient and well established. For all these reasons IgG is the most important class of antibodies from a biotechnological and medical perspective.

1.1. The Fc Fragment

The Fc portion of antibodies, which comprises the CH2 and CH3 domains of both heavy chains, recruits cytotoxic effector functions through antibody-dependent cellular cytotoxicity (ADCC) and/or complement-dependent cytotoxicity (CDC) (2). In ADCC, antibodies bind to Fc receptors (FcγRs) located in the membrane of various effector cells, such as natural killer cells, dendritic cells, and macrophages, and trigger phagocytosis or lysis of the targeted cells. In CDC, antibodies kill the targeted cells by triggering the complement cascade at the cell surface. Each Ig class and subclass has a different Fc fragment with its own specific set of properties. The Fc region also mediates the serum half-life/clearance through binding of antibodies to the neonatal Fc receptor (FcRn) by facilitating their recycling and preventing their catabolism (3). Therefore, the half-life of human IgG1 in blood is generally approximately 3 weeks.

1.2. The Antigen-Binding Site

Located at the N-terminal end of each polypeptide chain, the paired VH and VL domains form the antigen-combining site (Fv) of an antibody. Each domain is made of about 110 amino acids and features the characteristic immunoglobulin fold consisting of a sandwich of two antiparallel β-sheets connected by a conserved intramolecular disulfide bond (1). Within each variable domain, three regions are highly variable in length and/or sequence and are referred to as complementarity determining regions (CDRs) or antigen-binding loops. These regions are separated by relatively invariant stretches, known as framework regions that act as scaffold to support the CDRs. Noncovalent association of the VH and VL domains clusters the hypervariable loops at the N-terminal side of the folded Fv fragment to form an extended interface that interacts with the antigen, the so-called paratope (1). At a structural level, the hypervariable regions fold into a limited number of canonical loop structures, determined by the loop length and the presence of conserved residues at key positions within the hypervariable and framework regions (4). For the CDR3 of VH, the most variable CDR in length and amino acid composition, it is more difficult to predict its structure. Antigen binding is mediated by noncovalent interactions that primarily involve amino acids in the CDRs (especially CDR3) of each chain, but nearby residues in the framework regions may also participate in antigen recognition.

1.3. The Generation of Antigen-Binding Site Diversity

The efficiency of the humoral immune response relies on its ability to generate an almost infinite variety of antibody molecules, each having a unique antigen-binding site. Thus, the immune system must have the genetic capacity to produce a very large number of different variable domain sequences. Immunoglobulin *V* genes in the germline, do not exist as intact, functional genes but as linear arrays of widely separated gene segment clusters: variable (*V*), diversity (*D*), and joining (*J*) gene segments (5). The great diversity of the VL and VH sequences results from a (more or less) random rearrangement of these germline gene segments (combinatorial diversity) whereby one single *VH*, one *D* and one *JH* mini-gene are selected from a set of multiple mini-genes to join and to produce a functional VH polypeptide. Similarly, a *VL-JL* joining leads to the VL domain production. Following successful assembly, producing a single functional heavy or light chain gene, the *V(D)J* rearrangement machinery on the second allele is turned off. This allelic exclusion ensures that a single B cell produces only one type of antibody.

An even greater variety in the region arises because the DNA recombination mechanisms are imprecise and occur in conjunction with deletion of nucleotides at the splice junctions of the recombining *VH-D-JH* or *VL-JL* gene segments. In addition, during assembly of the VH region, nontemplated nucleotides (called N-region) are often added by terminal deoxynucleotidyl transferase (TdT), a template-independent DNA polymerase, at the junction of the *V*, *D*, and *J* segments (6). Moreover, coding joints also contain short deletions and palindromic nucleotide segments. This junctional diversity is achieved at the CDR3 which is a major determinant of the specific interaction between antigen-receptor and antigen (1). Additional diversification of the antigen-binding site (VH–VL) may be introduced by somatic hypermutation (SHM). These mutations are not entirely random as they target preferred sequence motifs known as mutational hotspots (7). These hotspots occur preferentially near or within the antigen-binding site and consequently influence the affinity of the resulting immunoglobulin for its target antigen (8). Individual cells that express higher-affinity mutants have a selective advantage and will proliferate resulting in a continual positive selection for cells bearing higher affinity antibodies, a process called affinity maturation.

2. Heavy Chain Antibodies

The composition and overall structure of antibodies is remarkably well conserved among mammals. Three deviations from the classic heterotetrameric structure have been described over the years, and all of them consist of a homodimer of an immunoglobulin heavy chain. The first described heavy chain antibody is linked to a pathological disorder, known as heavy chain disease (9), and occurs in sera of patients. These truncated antibodies result from a somatic event that removes various parts of the *VH* and *CH1* region from the expressed Ig gene. These human heavy chain antibodies (or those that have been identified in mouse hybridomas) are not functional in antigen binding since the VL and part of the VH domain are missing.

The second type of heavy chain antibodies naturally devoid of light chains were found by serendipity in sera of species from the family of Camelidae (10). The Camelidae (Old World camelids including *Camelus dromedarius* and *Camelus bactrianus*, and New World camelids including *Lama glama*, *Lama pacos*, *Lama guanicoe*, and *Lama vicugna*) belong to the suborder of the Tylopoda that constitutes together with Ruminantia and Suiformes the order of the Artiodactyla. Ruminantia and Suiformes do not possess heavy chain antibodies in their blood, whereas the sera of all camelids contain in addition to the classic isotypes a unique class of heavy chain antibodies (HCAbs). In sharp contrast with the human HCAbs from patients with heavy chain disease, the camelid HCAbs are bona fide antibodies, which evidently contribute to the immune response of these animals (10). The genetic evidence indicates that the origin of HCAbs is not to be found in remnants of a putative primordial HCAb form but that they are apparently the outcome of more recent adaptive changes occurring in the compartment of the conventional antibodies within the Camelidae lineage (11).

The third type of heavy chain-only antibodies is occurring naturally in shark (12) (see Chapter 3).

2.1. HCAbs in Camelids

Three fractions containing IgG of distinct molecular weight can be isolated from the dromedary serum by differential adsorption on Protein A and Protein G columns. The so-called "IgG1" fraction contains the conventional antibodies comprising two heavy and two light chains. The "IgG2" and "IgG3" fraction contains HCAbs composed of heavy chains that are approximately 10 and 12 kDa smaller than the heavy chain of conventional antibodies (10). This reduced MW of the heavy chain in HCAbs is due to the absence of the entire CH1 domain (see Fig. 1b). The CH1, which functions as an anchor for the light chain in conventional antibodies is encoded in the gene of the heavy chain isotype for the HCAb but is removed during mRNA splicing, due to a point mutation in the splice signal at the 3′ end of the *CH1* exon (13, 14). Hence, the variable domain is joined directly to the hinge region in HCAbs. The removal of the CH1 domain is critical for the secretion of the HCAbs, since intact heavy chains are retained in the endoplasmic reticulum by specific chaperones interacting with the CH1 domain, and it is the displacement of these chaperones by the light chain that allows secretion of classic antibodies (15).

Based on cDNA analysis two isotypes are distinguished within the IgG1 fraction, one encoding a hinge of 19 amino acids (IgG1a) and one encoding a hinge of 12 amino acids (IgG1b) downstream the *CH1* exon. Likewise, the IgG2 fraction from dromedary sera contains two isotypes, one with a hinge of 35 amino acids (IgG2a) and one with a hinge of 15 amino acids (IgG2c). A third type of hinge with 29 amino acids was identified in llama and attributed to the IgG2b subclass (16). Heavy chain antibodies of the IgG3 fraction contain a hinge of 12 amino acids. The relative proportion of heavy chain antibodies to conventional antibodies seems to vary, but an average of 50% of each type is common for Old World camelids, this percentage is somewhat lower (approximately 30%) for New World camelids.

2.2. The Antigen-Binding Site of HCAbs

Since the homodimeric HCAbs lack a light chain and thus a VL domain, the antigen is recognized by one single domain, i.e., the variable domain of the heavy chain of a heavy chain antibody abbreviated as VHH. The recombinant expression of the VHH yields a soluble single domain antibody (sdAb) fragment with dimensions in the single digit nanometer range, and has been referred to as Nanobody (Nb). These Nanobodies with a MW of only 15 kDa, which is at least half the size of the intact antigen-binding site of a conventional antibody (i.e., the VH–VL pair), are the smallest, intact antigen-binding fragments derived from a functional immunoglobulin (see Fig. 1). Obviously, the VHHs are expected to have acquired important adaptations to remain soluble and functional in the absence of an associated light chain variable domain.

2.3. Sequence Adaptations of VHHs

Nanobodies are distinct from conventional VHs by the substitution of five amino acids that are very well conserved in all VH domains of classic antibodies of vertebrates (17). These VH-VHH hallmark substitutions are as follows: Leu12Ser, Val42Phe/Tyr, Gly49Glu, Leu50Arg/Cys, and Trp52Gly (the last substitution is less well conserved) (numbers refer to the amino acid positions numbered according to IMGT (The International ImMunoGeneTics information system; http://www.imgt.org/)). The substitution of Leu12Ser in dromedary VHH (a considerable fraction of the llama VHH still has a Leu at position 12) is seen as an adaptation to deal with the absence of the CH1 domain (16). The substitution of the hydrophobic side chain of Leu with the smaller, hydrophilic Ser undoubtedly also increases the solubility of the Nanobodies in an aqueous environment. The residues at positions 42, 49, 50, and 52 of the VH domain are part of the large interface with the VL domain. Removal of the VL domain from an Fv would expose a large hydrophobic surface of the VH domain to the solvent, leading to stickiness and aggregation. The hydrophobic to hydrophilic amino acid substitutions observed in Nanobodies explain both their failure to associate with a VL domain and their increased solubility (18).

Three distinctive features of Nanobodies are to be found in the hypervariable regions. First, the CDR1 of Nanobodies is extended towards the N-terminal end (16). The greater variability in this region compared to the corresponding region in VH domains results from the presence of mutational hotspots for SHM imprinted in the germline *VHH* sequences at the codons for residues 28 and 30 (19). This hypervariability suggests that these residues of a VHH participate in antigen binding and that the somatic mutations in this area will be selected during the affinity maturation process. Second, Nanobodies have on average a longer CDR3. The average CDR3 length in dromedary VHHs is 18 amino acids compared to 14 and 11 residues in human and mouse VHs, respectively (17). Third, in addition to the conserved intradomain disulphide bond, the CDR3 of Nanobodies also often harbors a cysteine that forms an additional disulfide bond with a cysteine in the CDR1 or the framework-2 (16, 17). This second cystine constrains the antigen-binding loops and restrains the flexibility of the long CDR3 loop, which might otherwise impede the antigen-binding capacity of the paratope (18).

All these adaptations enlarge the antigen-interaction surface of Nanobodies and offer an additional diversity to their antigen-binding repertoire which probably compensates in part for the absence of the VL domain with its three antigen-binding loops.

2.4. Structural Adaptations of VHHs

Crystal structures confirm that Nanobodies adopt a normal immunoglobulin fold consisting of nine β-strands spread over two β-sheets packed against each other and linked with a conserved disulphide bond. The organization of the Cα-atoms within the β-strands scaffold of the Nanobody superimposes nicely with that in a human or mouse VH (17).

The region interacting with the VL in the conventional VH domains is resurfaced by the VHH specific amino acid substitutions clustered in this region and exhibits therefore a quite different architecture. The nonpolar to polar amino acid substitutions (Gly49Glu and Leu50Arg) increase the hydrophilicity of the surface of the VHH. This effect is even enhanced by the rotation of the hydrophobic side chains of adjacent residues to expose their most hydrophilic parts to the solvent, without deforming the Cα backbone (e.g., Trp118 in cAb-Lys3) (18). Furthermore, the substitutions at positions 42 and 52 cause a net shift of the bulky hydrophobic groups towards the centre of the five-stranded β-sheet. In addition, the CDR3 loop usually folds over these residues and makes them solvent inaccessible.

However, the largest structural differences between the VH and a VHH occur at the level of the antigen-binding loops. Indeed, the CDR1 and CDR2 of Nanobodies adopt a larger number of possible loop structures that deviate fundamentally from the canonical loop structures defined for conventional antibodies (4, 20). This additional structural diversity is attributed to the presence of novel residues at key sites for the loop conformation, the variable length of the CDRs and the formation of an interloop cystine between an additional Cys present in the CDR1 or framework-2 and a Cys located in the CDR3. All these features increase the structural repertoire of Nanobodies by allowing a wide variety of geometrical presentations of the paratope.

Apparently, Nanobodies employ different strategies to interact with their cognate antigen depending on the size and type of the target. As expected, planar paratopes are observed to interact with a proteinaceous antigen (21). Nanobodies are also able to form a cavity with their three CDRs to accommodate binding with a hapten (22). Besides the standard architectures of the paratope such as cavities, grooves or flat surfaces, Nanobodies are also able to form large protruding loops (18). For example, part of the long CDR3 of a lysozyme binder folds over the former VL side while the other part protrudes from the remaining paratope and penetrates into the active site of lysozyme. This large convex paratope provides over 70% of the contacts with lysozyme and the interaction area with lysozyme is as large as the interface between an antigen and a

VH–VL pair. This feature allows Nanobodies to recognize epitopes that are usually not antigenic for classical antibodies, such as the catalytic site of enzymes and canyons in viral and infectious disease biomarkers (18, 23). Hence, it seems that the paratope of HCAbs and conventional antibodies recognize different antigenic sites on their target. It is therefore possible that HCAbs have been selected and maintained in the camelid species for a complementary function in their humoral immune response (11).

Despite the single domain nature of Nanobodies with three antigen binding loops in the paratope of which the CDR3 is the most important, their antigen-binding surface is as large as that of a scFv where the paratope is equally spread over the CDRs of the VH and VL domains (24). As a result the antigen specificity and the affinity or kinetic binding properties of a VHH or a scFv with its cognate antigen are within the same range.

2.5. Diversity of VHH in HCAbs

Identification of germline *VH* (approximately 50) and *VHH* (approximately 40) segments in dromedary demonstrates that VHHs, with their characteristic key residues substitutions, are encoded by a dedicated set of *V* genes, and do not result from an ontogenic process of SHM starting from a *VH* gene (19). Additional support for a dedicated set of *VHH* germline genes is provided by the presence of a codon for a noncanonical cysteine at different possible positions in the *VHH* germline segments, but not in the dromedary *VH* germline segments. Both *VH* and *VHH* gene segments are accommodated in the *V* gene cluster of the heavy chain locus and rearrange with the same *D* and *JH* gene segments to form either a conventional antibody or a HCAb (25). These dromedary *VHHs* can be categorized into seven *VHH* subfamilies, based on the position of the extra cysteine within the CDR1 or the framework-2 region and the length of the CDR2 (either 16 or 17 amino acids) (19). Since extra cysteines are rare in llama VHH sequences, they cannot be used as a subfamily-hallmark and alternative subfamily divisions had to be proposed for llama VHHs (25, 26).

The VH and VHH amino acid sequence share a high degree of identity and are most similar (approximately 80% sequence identity) to the human VH of family 3 (16). Dromedary also possesses a *VH* germline gene sharing a high degree of sequence homology with human *VH* of family 4. Surprisingly, although these genes do not comprise the VHH hallmarks (framework-2 and Cys to form an extra intradomain disulphide bond) their V-D-J recombination products can be part of the heavy chain isotypes of both, classic antibodies and HCAbs. However, current data suggests that this *VH-4* gene is only sporadically expressed in dromedary B cells (27). Thus, the preferential employment of one major subgroup (*VHH-3*) might pose restrictions on the complexity of antigen-binding site of HCAbs. However, the family 3 is the most widespread human VH family in terms of both expression and genome complexity. Random association of heavy and light variable domains contributes considerably to the expansion of the conventional antibody repertoire. It appears that the HCAbs lacking this VH–VL combinatorial diversity developed multiple diversity mechanisms to acquire a complex repertoire of antigen-binding sites. Indeed, analysis of the *VHH* gene segments evidenced that *VHH* genes exhibits a larger diversity than the *VH* segments. This is attributed to a higher frequency of mutation hotspots and DNA recombination signal sequences in *VHH* germline sequences than in *VH* germline genes (19). The variation in sequence is mainly clustered near or within the paratope at codons whose encoded residues are determinants for the antigen-binding loop structures.

In conclusion, the sequence of Nanobodies is readily diversified by the introduction of an additional disulphide bridge, the high incidence of nucleotide insertions/deletions, gene replacement and extensive somatic point mutations (21, 28).

3. Importance of VHH

Antibodies, either polyclonal or monoclonal, from animal or human origin are essential for a very broad range of applications, as a research tool for target detection or purification, or as a medical tool for diagnosis and therapy. Consequently, the demand for a cheap and renewable source of antibodies is continuously increasing (29). The highly organized and modular structure of antibodies provides a great flexibility for their modification and tailoring to meet special requirements imposed by the envisaged application. Advances in antibody engineering allow fine-tuning of the various features of antibodies, such as valency or avidity, stability, intrinsic affinity, and size.

Whole antibodies, with a molecular weight of about 150 kDa, sometimes lead to practical drawbacks, such as a slow production at high cost, or a weak tissue penetration of the antibody. In addition, for a range of applications, such as radioimmunotherapy or in vivo imaging, the Fc-mediated cellular effects or prolonged half-life in blood are usually serious bottlenecks. Consequently, smaller recombinant antibody fragments become top listed as an emerging new class of drugs. The smallest fragment of a classical antibody that retains the antigen binding specificity of a whole antibody is the scFv in which the VH and VL domains are tethered by a synthetic linker. However, the expression of a single variable domain of an Fv (VH or VL) further reduces the size and might in some instances still produce a fragment retaining residual antigen binding (30). Unfortunately, an isolated VH (or VL) domain exposes a large hydrophobic side to the aqueous environment that renders this type of sdAb rather difficult to handle. Nowadays this shortcoming has been remediated either by a prior selection of a "soluble and well behaving" (human) VH scaffold (31), or after engineering the VL-binding side of the VH domain according to a man-made design (32) or using the VHH hallmarks in the framework-2 as template. Evidently, an alternative, fast, and convenient source of antigen-specific sdAbs consists in the direct cloning and selection of VHHs from affinity matured HCAbs (from an immunized camelid).

Apart from the size advantages, the recombinant expression of sdAbs turned out to be favorable as well, as validated in various expression systems. Nanobodies are preferentially expressed in *Escherichia coli* where they can be produced economically as soluble and nonaggregating recombinant proteins (33). Higher production levels of Nanobodies are obtained in yeast systems such as *Saccharomyces cerevisiae* and *Pichia pastoris* (34). Finally, functional Nanobodies expressed in tobacco plants have been shown to constitute up to about 1.6% of the total leave soluble fraction, demonstrating the feasibility to use transgenic plants as an economic source of Nanobodies (35).

Nanobodies, because of their single domain nature, offer several advantages for biotechnological applications. Libraries of Nanobodies from immunized camels and llamas can be generated through a straightforward cloning procedure (36). The VHHs within these libraries retain full functional diversity resulting in the isolation of high-affinity antigen-binding Nanobodies after phage display. However, a naïve VHH library or a synthetic library on any autonomous (human) VH might also be used to retrieve specific antigen-binders. Also, the higher stability compared to scFvs, with the feature of reversible denaturation offers an additional asset to these Nanobodies (37, 38). This regained functionality after chemical or thermal denaturation is mainly attributed to an efficient refolding. The adaptations at the former VL interface and the packing of extended CDR3 loops against this interface contributes to the domain stability. These adaptations also confer a high level of solubility to these sdAbs. Furthermore, the single domain nature and the small gene fragment size (350–380 bp) of an sdAb facilitate subsequent molecular manipulation to engineer multivalent formats.

The short serum half-life due to a rapid renal clearance might limit the efficacy of Nanobodies in therapeutic applications. Therefore, Nanobodies have been targeted to normally long-lived serum proteins such as albumin or immunoglobulin using bispecific Nanobodies recognizing these serum proteins in addition to the therapeutic target, resulting in increased half-lives (39). The well-known approach of PEGylation was also successfully used to increase the half-life of a foot-and-mouth disease virus-neutralizing Nanobody (40). Constructing multivalent molecules or engineering the Nanobodies back into full HCAbs by addition of an Fc region is a third possibility to extend serum residence times because of the increased size of the molecule or its interaction with Fc receptors (41).

References

1. Padlan EA (1994) Anatomy of the antibody molecule. Mol Immunol 31:169–217
2. Greenwood J, Clark M, Waldmann H (1993) Structural motifs involved in human IgG antibody effector functions. Eur J Immunol 23: 1098–1104
3. Ghetie V, Hubbard JG, Kim JK, Tsen MF, Lee Y, Ward ES (1996) Abnormally short serum half-lives of IgG in beta 2-microglobulin-deficient mice. Eur J Immunol 26:690–696
4. Chothia C, Lesk AM (1987) Canonical structures for the hypervariable regions of immunoglobulins. J Mol Biol 196:901–917
5. Matsuda F, Ishii K, Bourvagnet P, Kuma K, Hayashida H, Miyata T, Honjo T (1998) The complete nucleotide sequence of the human immunoglobulin heavy chain variable region locus. J Exp Med 188:2151–2162
6. Desiderio SV, Yancopoulos GD, Paskind M, Thomas E, Boss MA, Landau N, Alt FW, Baltimore D (1984) Insertion of N regions into heavy-chain genes is correlated with expression of terminal deoxytransferase in B cells. Nature 311:752–755
7. Betz AG, Neuberger MS, Milstein C (1993) Discriminating intrinsic and antigen-selected mutational hotspots in immunoglobulin V genes. Immunol Today 14:405–411
8. Tomlinson IM, Walter G, Jones PT, Dear PH, Sonnhammer EL, Winter G (1996) The imprint of somatic hypermutation on the repertoire of human germline V genes. J Mol Biol 256: 813–817
9. Alexander A, Steinmetz M, Barritault D, Frangione B, Franklin EC, Hood L, Buxbaum JN (1982) gamma Heavy chain disease in man: cDNA sequence supports partial gene deletion model. Proc Natl Acad Sci U S A 79:3260–3264
10. Hamers-Casterman C, Atarhouch T, Muyldermans S, Robinson G, Hamers C, Songa EB, Bendahman N, Hamers R (1993) Naturally occurring antibodies devoid of light chains. Nature 363:446–448
11. Flajnik MF, Deschacht N, Muyldermans S (2011) A case of convergence: why did a simple alternative to canonical antibodies arise in sharks and camels? PLoS Biol 9:e1001120
12. Greenberg AS, Avila D, Hughes M, Hughes A, McKinney EC, Flajnik MF (1995) A new antigen receptor gene family that undergoes rearrangement and extensive somatic diversification in sharks. Nature 374:168–173
13. Nguyen VK, Hamers R, Wyns L, Muyldermans S (1999) Loss of splice consensus signal is responsible for the removal of the entire C(H)1 domain of the functional camel IGG2A heavy-chain antibodies. Mol Immunol 36:515–524
14. Woolven BP, Frenken LG, van der Logt P, Nicholls PJ (1999) The structure of the llama heavy chain constant genes reveals a mechanism for heavy-chain antibody formation. Immunogenetics 50:98–101
15. Lee YK, Brewer JW, Hellman R, Hendershot LM (1999) BiP and immunoglobulin light chain cooperate to control the folding of heavy chain and ensure the fidelity of immunoglobulin assembly. Mol Biol Cell 10:2209–2219
16. Vu KB, Ghahroudi MA, Wyns L, Muyldermans S (1997) Comparison of llama VH sequences from conventional and heavy chain antibodies. Mol Immunol 34:1121–1131
17. Muyldermans S, Atarhouch T, Saldanha J, Barbosa JA, Hamers R (1994) Sequence and structure of VH domain from naturally occurring camel heavy chain immunoglobulins lacking light chains. Protein Eng 7:1129–1135
18. Desmyter A, Transue TR, Ghahroudi MA, Thi MH, Poortmans F, Hamers R, Muyldermans S, Wyns L (1996) Crystal structure of a camel single-domain VH antibody fragment in complex with lysozyme. Nat Struct Biol 3:803–811
19. Nguyen VK, Hamers R, Wyns L, Muyldermans S (2000) Camel heavy-chain antibodies: diverse germline V(H)H and specific mechanisms enlarge the antigen-binding repertoire. EMBO J 19:921–930
20. Decanniere K, Muyldermans S, Wyns L (2000) Canonical antigen-binding loop structures in immunoglobulins: more structures, more canonical classes? J Mol Biol 300:83–91
21. Conrath KE, Wernery U, Muyldermans S, Nguyen VK (2003) Emergence and evolution of functional heavy-chain antibodies in Camelidae. Dev Comp Immunol 27:87–103
22. Spinelli S, Frenken LG, Hermans P, Verrips T, Brown K, Tegoni M, Cambillau C (2000) Camelid heavy-chain variable domains provide efficient combining sites to haptens. Biochemistry 39:1217–1222
23. Lauwereys M, Arbabi GM, Desmyter A, Kinne J, Holzer W, De Genst E, Wyns L, Muyldermans S (1998) Potent enzyme inhibitors derived from dromedary heavy-chain antibodies. EMBO J 17:3512–3520
24. De Genst E, Silence K, Decanniere K, Conrath K, Loris R, Kinne J, Muyldermans S, Wyns L (2006) Molecular basis for the preferential cleft recognition by dromedary heavy-chain antibodies. Proc Natl Acad Sci U S A 103:4586–4591

25. Achour I, Cavelier P, Tichit M, Bouchier C, Lafaye P, Rougeon F (2008) Tetrameric and homodimeric camelid IgGs originate from the same IgH locus. J Immunol 181:2001–2009
26. Harmsen MM, Ruuls RC, Nijman IJ, Niewold TA, Frenken LG, de Geus B (2000) Llama heavy-chain V regions consist of at least four distinct subfamilies revealing novel sequence features. Mol Immunol 37:579–590
27. Deschacht N, De Groeve K, Vincke C, Raes G, De Baetselier P, Muyldermans S (2010) A novel promiscuous class of camelid single domain antibody contributes to the antigen-binding repertoire. J Immunol 184:5696–5704
28. De Genst E, Silence K, Ghahroudi MA, Decanniere K, Loris R, Kinne J, Wyns L, Muyldermans S (2005) Strong in vivo maturation compensates for structurally restricted H3 loops in antibody repertoires. J Biol Chem 280: 14114–14121
29. Taussig MJ, Stoevesandt O, Borrebaeck CA, Bradbury A, Cahill D, Cambillau C, de Daruvar A, Dubel S, Eichler J, Frank R, Gibson TJGD, Gold L, Herberg FW, Hermjakob H, Hoheisel JD, Joos TO, Kallioniemi O, Koegl M, Konthur Z, Kremmer E, Krobitsch S, Landegren U, van der Maarel S, McCafferty J, Muyldermans S, Nygren PA, Palcy S, Pluckthun A, Polic B, Przybylski M, Saviranta P, Sawyer A, Sherman DJ, Skerra A, Templin M, Ueffing M, Uhlen M (2007) ProteomeBinders: planning a European resource of affinity reagents for analysis of the human proteome. Nat Methods 4:13–17
30. Ward ES, Gussow D, Griffiths AD, Jones PT, Winter G (1989) Binding activities of a repertoire of single immunoglobulin variable domains secreted from *Escherichia coli*. Nature 341: 544–546
31. Jespers L, Schon O, Famm K, Winter G (2004) Aggregation-resistant domain antibodies selected on phage by heat denaturation. Nat Biotechnol 22:1161–1165
32. Barthelemy PA, Raab H, Appleton BA, Bond CJ, Wu P, Wiesmann C, Sidhu SS (2008) Comprehensive analysis of the factors contributing to the stability and solubility of autonomous human VH domains. J Biol Chem 283:3639–3654
33. Arbabi-Ghahroudi M, Tanha J, MacKenzie R (2005) Prokaryotic expression of antibodies. Cancer Metastasis Rev 24:501–519
34. Frenken LG, van der Linden RH, Hermans PW, Bos JW, Ruuls RC, de Geus B, Verrips CT (2000) Isolation of antigen specific llama VHH antibody fragments and their high level secretion by *Saccharomyces cerevisiae*. J Biotechnol 78:11–21
35. Rajabi-Memari H, Jalali-Javaran M, Rasaee MJ, Rahbarizadeh F, Forouzandeh-Moghadam M, Esmaili A (2006) Expression and characterization of a recombinant single-domain monoclonal antibody against MUC1 mucin in tobacco plants. Hybridoma 25:209–215
36. Arbabi Ghahroudi M, Desmyter A, Wyns L, Hamers R, Muyldermans S (1997) Selection and identification of single domain antibody fragments from camel heavy-chain antibodies. FEBS Lett 414:521–526
37. Dumoulin M, Conrath K, Van Meirhaeghe A, Meersman F, Heremans K, Frenken LG, Muyldermans S, Wyns L, Matagne A (2002) Single-domain antibody fragments with high conformational stability. Protein Sci 11:500–515
38. van der Linden RH, Frenken LG, de Geus B, Harmsen MM, Ruuls RC, Stok W, de Ron L, Wilson S, Davis P, Verrips CT (1999) Comparison of physical chemical properties of llama VHH antibody fragments and mouse monoclonal antibodies. Biochim Biophys Acta 1431:37–46
39. Coppieters K, Dreier T, Silence K, de Haard H, Lauwereys M, Casteels P, Beirnaert E, Jonckheere H, Van de WC, Staelens L, Hostens J, Revets H, Remaut E, Elewaut D, Rottiers P (2006) Formatted anti-tumor necrosis factor alpha VHH proteins derived from camelids show superior potency and targeting to inflamed joints in a murine model of collagen-induced arthritis. Arthritis Rheum 54:1856–1866
40. Harmsen MM, van Solt CB, Fijten HP, van Keulen L, Rosalia RA, Weerdmeester K, Cornelissen AH, De Bruin MG, Eble PL, Dekker A (2007) Passive immunization of guinea pigs with llama single-domain antibody fragments against foot-and-mouth disease. Vet Microbiol 120:193–206
41. Hmila I, Abdallah RB, Saerens D, Benlasfar Z, Conrath K, Ayeb ME, Muyldermans S, Bouhaouala-Zahar B (2008) VHH, bivalent domains and chimeric Heavy chain-only antibodies with high neutralizing efficacy for scorpion toxin AahI'. Mol Immunol 45:3847–3856

Chapter 3

Overview and Discovery of IgNARs and Generation of VNARs

Stewart D. Nuttall

Abstract

Immunoglobulin new antigen receptors (IgNARs) from sharks are a distinct class of immune receptors, consisting of homodimers with no associated light chains. Antigen binding is encapsulated within single VNAR immunoglobulin domains of 13–14 kDa in size. This small size and single domain format means that they exhibit considerable stability and are readily produced in heterologous protein expression systems. In this chapter, I describe the history and discovery of IgNARs, the development of VNAR biotechnology, and highlight important factors in VNAR protein production.

Key words: Shark antibody, VNAR protein expression, Biosensor, Crystallographic structure

1. The Search for Single-Domain Antibodies

During the 1990s the search was on for single domain antibody-like binding reagents. Conventional antibodies could be readily engineered into single-chain Fv and Fab fragments, and the logical next step was smaller entities. Multiple approaches included but were by no means limited to VH engineering, V-like domains, fibronectins, and T-cell receptors (1). The discovery of the camelid VHH isotype illustrated that nature had already reached at least one solution to the problem of how to produce stable and functional single domain antibodies (2). Subsequent VHH structural studies only emphasized the elegance and utility of employing an extended CDR3 loop region, stabilized by interloop disulphide bridges, to enhance stability, solubility, and the binding interface (3). Against this background, the shark immunoglobulin new antigen receptor (IgNAR) antibody isotype went relatively unnoticed and underexploited in a rapidly developing field.

Dirk Saerens and Serge Muyldermans (eds.), *Single Domain Antibodies: Methods and Protocols*,
Methods in Molecular Biology, vol. 911, DOI 10.1007/978-1-61779-968-6_3, © Springer Science+Business Media, LLC 2012

2. The Discovery of the IgNARs

In 1995, Martin Flajnik and colleagues published the first description of the IgNAR isotype in *Nature* (4). Complementary DNA libraries from Florida nurse sharks (*Ginglymostoma cirratum*), originally screened for immunoglobulin/T-cell receptor type molecules, revealed the presence of the novel IgNAR isotype. It was immediately apparent that these molecules were different from previously identified immunoglobulins. While initially clustering with TCRs, they exhibited significant variability within the CDR1 (complementarity determining region-1) and CDR3 loops, analogous to antibody variable domains. At the domain level, IgNARs consist of homodimers containing one variable and five constant domains with no associated light chains (see Fig. 1a).

The primary sequences of the IgNAR variable domains (VNARs; approximately 13 kDa) suggested that residues thought important in domain–domain contact (for example antibody VH-VL dimerization) were mutated or missing (4). In a second manuscript Flajnik and coworkers demonstrated by immune electron microscopy that the individual VNAR domains were indeed independent in solution and that the intact IgNAR molecule was likely to have enhanced avidity (functional affinity) through dimeric antigen binding (5). The reader is strongly encouraged to study these two early papers in order to gain an understanding of how basic research into the nature of the antibody/TCR progenitor leads to our current shark antibody technologies.

But were VNARs true antibodies? The variability within the CDR1 and CDR3 regions certainly suggested so, as did the general organization into a variable-constant domain format, and the occurrence of transmembrane and secretory forms of the protein (6). However, formal validation did not occur until the successful immunization of sharks and demonstration of a specific VNAR response (7). The in vitro generation of antigen-specific clones further strengthened this argument (8). Later, histology clearly identified shark immune organs and tissues responsible for VNAR production and maturation, which paralleled those involved in, for example, shark IgM and IgW isotype generation (9).

3. The Three Types of VNAR

Primary sequence analysis of nurse shark VNARs identified two different types of VNARs based upon the number and pattern of cysteine residues (4). Type I VNARs have additional framework cysteines in the immunoglobulin C and J strands, as well as

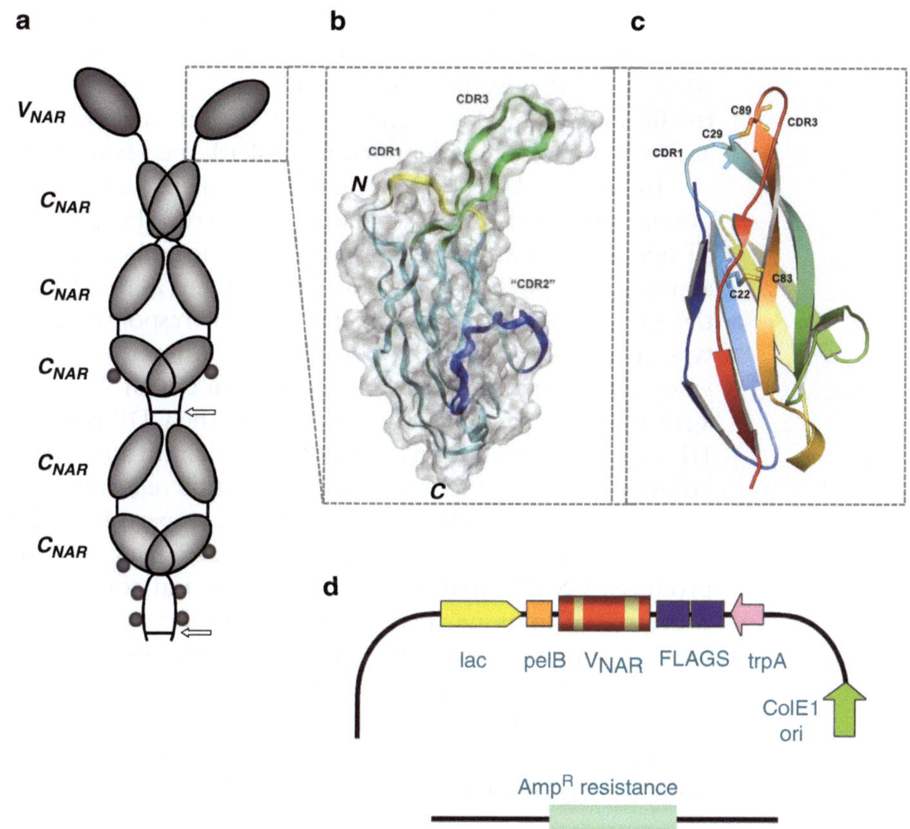

Fig. 1. (**a**) The intact IgNAR antibody consists of one variable (VNAR) and five constant (CNAR) domains. Two protein chains are disulphide bonded (*arrows*) to form a homodimer. *Circles* represent potential N-linked glycosylation sites. (**b**) Crystallographic structure of the 12Y-2 VNAR (PDB: 1VES), illustrating the positions of the CDR1, CDR3, and "CDR2" loop regions. Note the positions of the N-terminus of the protein chain adjacent to the antibody paratope, compared to the C-terminus at the bottom of the molecule. (**c**) For the 12A-9 VNAR (PDB: 2COQ) the CDR1 and CDR3 regions are linked by a disulphide bridge (29–89). The canonical (22–83) disulphide bridge is also illustrated. (**d**) The pGC *E. coli* expression vector allows for protein export to the periplasmic space through the subsequently cleaved *PelB* leader, and purification through dual C-terminal FLAG affinity tags.

apparently paired cysteines within the extended CDR3 loops. Despite much protein modeling, elucidation of the disulphide bridge arrangements of these multiple half-cystines was not possible until three dimensional structural determinations (see later). In contrast, Type II VNARs appeared to have a more straightforward pairing of cysteine residues, with approximately two thirds of cases having a half-cystine in the CDR1 loop matched by a similar residue within the CDR3. By analogy with the structure of camelid nanobodies, it took little imagination to hypothesize that these formed inter-CDR disulphide bridges. The function of these various additional disulphide linkages is almost certainly stabilization of the extended CDR3 loops, providing a degree of rigidity to what would otherwise be fairly flexible structures. Interestingly, in a study of Wobbegong sharks (*Orectolobus maculatus*) in my own laboratory (10), we failed to identify any Type I variants. To date, to the best of my knowledge, Type II, but not Type I, IgNAR antibodies have been identified in all shark species studied.

In 2002, a Type III VNAR was identified during an investigation into the early IgNAR immune repertoire, which is expressed in all neonatal tissues (11). This version is of limited variability and appears to be phased out in most shark organs as the shark ages and the Type I and II VNAR adaptive immune response matures. This type may represent an early broad-spectrum antibody which provides the immunologically immature shark with early protection against pathogens. While the variability in the CDR regions of Type III VNARs is low in terms of CDR3 loop length and sequence heterogeneity, protein modeling suggests that there is sufficient conformational freedom to allow at least a minimal repertoire of differential antigen binding (12). The study of how the shark immune system produces VNAR variability is a fascinating and complex field. The processes of immune maturation in response to antigen and the immunogenetics of diversity and joining have been extensively dissected and described in several papers (11, 13–15). Interestingly, the shark immune response appears to generate a diverse primary immune response and rely less on affinity maturation, whereas for camelid VHHs, the converse appears to be the case (14, 16).

3.1. The VNAR Structure

VNAR sequence alignments demonstrated both extended CDR3 loop regions compared to conventional VH and VL antibodies, and also "missing" sequence in the vicinity of the CDR2 loop (Ig strands C′–C″). Notwithstanding, our models and those produced by other laboratories still fitted the CDR2 loop adjacent to and supporting the CDR1 and CDR3 regions (5, 10). In these models the absent residues were compensated by a compacted loop at the bottom of the molecule. However, at least in our hands, there was lingering doubt that something was "not quite right" with these interpretations.

In 2004, two sets of crystallographic structures were published that both disproved these models, and provided significant insight into VNAR structure–function. My colleague Victor Streltsov and I were able to crystallize and solve the structures of two related Type II VNARs (see Fig. 1b) (17). These VNARs, designated 12Y-1 and 12Y-2, target the Apical Membrane Antigen 1 found on the merozoite stage of malarial (*Plasmodium falciparum*) parasites (18). In this instance both VNARs were crystallized in the absence of antigen. The data sets initially resisted solution by conventional molecular replacement techniques, emphasizing the evolutionary distance from other immunoglobulins, and resolution required the use of multiwavelength anomalous dispersion (MAD) data sets to obtain the initial structures. Our efforts were closely followed by publication of a Type I VNAR structure, this time in complex with lysozyme (19).

Here, co-crystallization with a well-characterized model antigen allowed fairly straightforward structural solution. The underlying immunoglobulin frameworks for both Type I and Type II variants were essentially identical, and both structures revealed significant and unusual VNAR-specific traits. These included:

3.1.1. The Missing CDR2 and the Origin of the VNARs

The VNAR framework exhibits a folding topology that resembles both V- and I-set immunoglobulin families (17). V-set features include a cis-proline mediated kink in the A chain and bulges in the C-terminal portion of the G strand. I-set features include a short C′ strand and very short C″ strand which result in the "CDR2" loop snaking across the bottom of the molecule, and not adjacent to the other CDR loops, in a manner very reminiscent of I-set cell adhesion molecules. With various such analyses alternatively grouping VNARs with TCRs, VL domains, and I-sets, we have now regrettably probably gleaned as much evidence as we can as to the evolutionary origin of the VNARs from structural analysis, without an unequivocally accepted theory as to their origin (14, 20).

3.1.2. Features Contributing to Stability and Solubility

In VH-VL antibodies the interdomain interface is predominantly of a hydrophobic character, suited to a buried surface. This interface has retroevolved in the camelid VHH to a more hydrophilic surface, with solubility improvements also contributed by the CDR3 loop (21, 22). Reflecting evolution to a single domain format over a far longer evolutionary period, this region in the VNARs consists of a conserved and satisfyingly elegant pattern of criss-crossing charged residues (residues Glu46; Lys82; Gln84; Arg101; Lys104) providing both a hydrophilic face to the surrounding medium, and shielding conserved immunoglobulin hydrophobic framework residues (17).

3.1.3. CDR Loop Stability

In approximately two thirds of cases, the Type II VNAR CDR3 loop is stabilized by a disulphide linkage to the adjacent CDR1 (see Fig. 1c). In other cases, loop stability appears to be maintained either by internal packing (23) or in the case of the 12Y-2 VNAR, by formation of a two-stranded extended β-hairpin structure (17). The Type I VNAR is stabilized by interesting C strand-CDR3 and J strand-CDR3 disulphide bridges (19).

3.1.4. Targeting of Cryptic Epitopes and "Induced Fit" Binding

Conventional antibodies efficiently target a range of epitopes, with the possible exception of cleft structures (24). In contrast the extended loop structures of VNARs appear ideal conformations to penetrate such otherwise cryptic epitopes. For the as yet limited VNAR-antigen co-crystallographic complexes, a feature is the targeting of such epitopes, for example naturally occurring Type 1 and Type 2 VNARs raised against lysozyme penetrate the enzyme active site (19, 25, 26). For the 12Y-2 family of VNARs, the non-disulphide stabilized CDR3 also accesses an evolutionarily conserved and biologically vital canyon which bisects the AMA1 molecule, and bypasses surface-exposed polymorphic regions which attract the majority of human antibody immune surveillance (27). Notably, where unliganded VNAR structures are also available, they suggest that the CDR3 loop undergoes significant conformational rearrangement upon antigen binding, and in particular the flipping of tyrosine residues from internal to external loop positions (a result not readily predictable by protein modeling) (26, 27). Thus, despite the various strategies for loop stabilization, there appears to be significant freedom for CDR3 rearrangement upon binding.

4. Production of VNARs in Heterologous Expression Systems

When I began working on the VNARs in 1999/2000, my group focused on their potential biotechnological applications, driven by the potential suggested in their small size and long evolution towards protein stability. We immediately cloned the Type II repertoire from Wobbegong sharks, one of our indigenous species, and tested individual clones for expression, purification, and stability qualities in comparison to in-house single domain immunoglobulins and antibody scFv and Fab fragments. While the expected clone-to-clone variability was observed, the VNARs performed extremely well in these comparisons.

Thenceforth, our protein production strategies were driven by use of established cassette-based systems compatible with bacteriophage antibody display and selection vectors. First, VNAR libraries were cloned into the fd phage display vector pFAB5c.HIS at the 5′ *Sfi*I and 3′ *Not*I sites (28). The *Sfi*I site is a component of the *Pel*B N-terminal leader sequence, which directs export to the oxidizing environment of the *E. coli* periplasmic space (allowing formation of the important canonical framework and inter- and intra-CDR disulphide bridges). An added advantage of cloning the VNAR downstream of the *Pel*B leader is that precise cleavage by the secretory protease allows exact reconstitution of the VNAR N-terminus, an important consideration for paratope formation. For example, wobble at positions 1–3 in the naturally occurring VNAR repertoire suggests that residues at the extreme N-terminus play a general role in antigen binding, consistent with evolutionary pressure to maximize antigen binding in the absence of contributions from a CDR2 loop (10, 29). We have also demonstrated that residues Ala1 and Trp2 of the 12Y-2 family of VNARs contact the antigen at distances of less than 4 Å, confirming this hypothesis (27).

The 3′ *Not*I site adds three alanine residues to the C-terminus of the VNAR G-strand, and forms a peptide linker to the N-terminus of the bacteriophage gene3 protein (for phage vectors). Upon completion of phage-based selection, the *Sfi*I-*Not*I fragment is readily liberated from purified pFAB5c.HIS DNA and subcloned into similarly cut protein expression vectors. Our vector of choice, pGC, is a pUC derivative with the identical N-terminal *Pel*B signal sequence, and dual C-terminal FLAG epitope tags for affinity purification (see Fig. 1d) (30). Alternative vector configurations incorporate in line FLAG-HIS affinity tags. Realistically any good C-terminal affinity tag sequence can be utilized, depending upon laboratory preferencces, systems, and availability of affinity purification procedures. Our rationales for using FLAG epitopes included availability of such reagents, as well as the fact that many of the recombinant antigens used for library screening at the time were (and still are) purified through hexahistidine tags and metal affinity chromatography. This is an important consideration for downstream analysis of recombinant antibody clones by conventional ELISA-based assays.

In our hands, this simple protein expression system worked well for VNAR production at "cottage industry" levels. Other laboratories have utilized similar systems, for example pHEN2 for library construction and pIMS100 Human C-kappa (HuCκ) and pIMSΔHuCκ for expression (7), followed by metal-affinity chromatography and further purification by HEL-Sepharose column (possible because of the lysozyme-binding of this particular VNAR) (25, 26). Similarly, other groups have utilized well-established or in-house bacteriophage display and protein expression vectors utilizing N-terminal leader sequences and C-terminal tags for affinity purification (31–33). Following the example of VHH scale-up production, there is every reason to suggest that VNARs will be amendable to large-scale purification in a variety of heterologous expression systems, for example those based around yeast (*Saccharomyces* and *Pichia*), mammalian expression, and plant systems, when accompanied by appropriate codon modification and expression condition optimization.

5. Downstream Modifications and Affinity Maturation

VNARs are susceptible to affinity maturation, both by the natural shark immune system, and in vitro (18, 25). We have demonstrated the utility of error prone mutagenesis followed by selection in bacteriophage and ribosome display systems (34, 35). Interestingly, both ribosome display and the natural shark process appear to target a hot-spot in so-called loop region 2, and specifically residue 61 where the side chain is oriented upward and outward toward the antigen. As described above, the N-terminus also appears to play an antigen-binding role, suggesting that downstream modifications such as N-terminal coupling of functional moieties will be deleterious to function. In contrast the C-terminus, at the bottom of the molecule and normally connected to the constant domains for effector functions (see Fig. 1a–c) is the logical location for more sophisticated modifications beyond coupling to affinity tags, bacteriophages, and sensor/microarray surfaces. Preliminary reconstitution of the VNAR domain, e.g., into dimeric formats, is deleterious to expression levels but results in functional molecules (36).

6. VNAR Humanization

The question from the human therapeutics community is: will there be an adverse human antishark response upon administration of therapeutic VNARs, and will this limit their utility? Whatever the answer to this question, it is important that the field addresses approaches to limit potential immunogenicity of the VNAR domain. One approach is algorithm-based identification of immunogenic residues involved in the T-cell response, together with recognition of hallmark VNAR residues (33). To what extent the VNAR scaffold can be modified without reducing its favorable antigen-binding and structural stability characteristics remains to be seen. An alternative approach, identified by Victor Streltsov and myself, is based on the structural homology between VNAR domains and the "intermediate" or I-set family of immunoglobulins (20). Upon overview of the general structures it is apparent that VNARs and I-sets share a truncated C′–C″ loop in place of the more conventional antibody CDR2 loop. The ability to align VNAR framework-CDR take-off angles for I-set immunoglobulins such as domain I of the human neural cell adhesion molecule (NCAM) means that we can directly translate the protein engineering principles from an IgNAR to an I-set, including a now extended and extensively randomized CDR3 loop (which may have cysteine residues positioned to interact with similar half-cystines in the newly randomized CDR1) to produce a fully human single domain antibody repertoire.

7. The Future for VNARs

VNAR technology has moved rapidly, over the last one and a half decades, from discovery research through to adoption by the biotechnology industry. Companies such as Pfizer (United Kingdom) and AdAlta (Australia) are actively pursuing shark antibody research and applications. There is still more to be learnt: are there further types of VNARs present in different species of sharks, and are there more surprises like the recent identification of an apparent TCR-VNAR hybrid molecule of unknown function (37)? Whether the

VNARs can successfully compete in the human therapy space with conventional antibodies and the increasing number of alternative scaffolds remains to be seen (38). However, with their small size, high stability, and possible advantages in cryptic epitope recognition, VNARs are natural candidates for future niche biotechnological and diagnostic applications.

Acknowledgements

I thank all my colleagues and collaborators who have worked with me to develop the VNAR technology. The author acts as a consultant to AdAlta Pty Ltd.

References

1. Nuttall SD, Irving RA, Hudson PJ (2000) Immunoglobulin VH domains and beyond: design and selection of single-domain binding and targeting reagents. Curr Pharm Biotechnol 1:253–263
2. Hamers-Casterman C et al (1993) Naturally occurring antibodies devoid of light chains. Nature 363:446–448
3. Desmyter A et al (1996) Crystal structure of a camel single-domain VH antibody fragment in complex with lysozyme. Nat Struct Biol 3:803–811
4. Greenberg AS et al (1995) A new antigen receptor gene family that undergoes rearrangement and extensive somatic diversification in sharks. Nature 374:168–173
5. Roux KH et al (1998) Structural analysis of the nurse shark (new) antigen receptor (NAR): molecular convergence of NAR and unusual mammalian immunoglobulins. Proc Natl Acad Sci U S A 95:11804–11809
6. Rumfelt LL et al (2004) Unprecedented multiplicity of Ig transmembrane and secretory mRNA forms in the cartilaginous fish. J Immunol 173:1129–1139
7. Dooley H, Flajnik MF, Porter AJ (2003) Selection and characterization of naturally occurring single-domain (IgNAR) antibody fragments from immunized sharks by phage display. Mol Immunol 40:25–33
8. Nuttall SD et al (2001) Isolation of the new antigen receptor from wobbegong sharks, and use as a scaffold for the display of protein loop libraries. Mol Immunol 38:313–326
9. Rumfelt LL et al (2002) The development of primary and secondary lymphoid tissues in the nurse shark *Ginglymostoma cirratum*: B-cell zones precede dendritic cell immigration and T-cell zone formation during ontogeny of the spleen. Scand J Immunol 56:130–148
10. Nuttall SD et al (2003) Isolation and characterization of an IgNAR variable domain specific for the human mitochondrial translocase receptor Tom70. Eur J Biochem 270: 3543–3554
11. Diaz M et al (2002) Structural analysis, selection, and ontogeny of the shark new antigen receptor (IgNAR): identification of a new locus preferentially expressed in early development. Immunogenetics 54:501–512
12. Streltsov VA, Carmichael JA, Nuttall SD (2005) Structure of a shark IgNAR antibody variable domain and modeling of an early-developmental isotype. Protein Sci 14:2901–2909
13. Diaz M et al (1999) Mutational pattern of the nurse shark antigen receptor gene (NAR) is similar to that of mammalian Ig genes and to spontaneous mutations in evolution: the translesion synthesis model of somatic hypermutation. Int Immunol 11:825–833
14. Dooley H, Flajnik MF (2006) Antibody repertoire development in cartilaginous fish. Dev Comp Immunol 30:43–56
15. Diaz M, Greenberg AS, Flajnik MF (1998) Somatic hypermutation of the new antigen receptor gene (NAR) in the nurse shark does not generate the repertoire: possible role in antigen-driven reactions in the absence of germinal centers. Proc Natl Acad Sci U S A 95:14343–14348
16. De Genst E et al (2005) Strong in vivo maturation compensates for structurally restricted H3 loops in antibody repertoires. J Biol Chem 280:14114–14121

17. Streltsov VA et al (2004) Structural evidence for evolution of shark Ig new antigen receptor variable domain antibodies from a cell-surface receptor. Proc Natl Acad Sci U S A 101: 12444–12449
18. Nuttall SD et al (2004) Selection and affinity maturation of IgNAR variable domains targeting *Plasmodium falciparum* AMA1. Proteins 55: 187–197
19. Stanfield RL et al (2004) Crystal structure of a shark single-domain antibody V region in complex with lysozyme. Science 305:1770–1773
20. Streltsov V, Nuttall S (2005) Do sharks have a new antibody lineage? Immunol Lett 97: 159–160
21. Saerens D et al (2005) Identification of a universal VHH framework to graft non-canonical antigen-binding loops of camel single-domain antibodies. J Mol Biol 352:597–607
22. Riechmann L, Muyldermans S (1999) Single domain antibodies: comparison of camel VH and camelised human VH domains. J Immunol Methods 231:25–38
23. Simmons DP et al (2008) Shark IgNAR antibody mimotopes target a murine immunoglobulin through extended CDR3 loop structures. Proteins 71:119–130
24. MacCallum RM, Martin AC, Thornton JM (1996) Antibody-antigen interactions: contact analysis and binding site topography. J Mol Biol 262:732–745
25. Dooley H et al (2006) First molecular and biochemical analysis of in vivo affinity maturation in an ectothermic vertebrate. Proc Natl Acad Sci U S A 103:1846–1851
26. Stanfield RL et al (2007) Maturation of shark single-domain (IgNAR) antibodies: evidence for induced-fit binding. J Mol Biol 367: 358–372
27. Henderson KA et al (2007) Structure of an IgNAR-AMA1 complex: targeting a conserved hydrophobic cleft broadens malarial strain recognition. Structure 15:1452–1466
28. Engberg J et al (1995) Phage-display libraries of murine and human antibody Fab fragments. Methods Mol Biol 51:355–376
29. Nuttall SD et al (2002) A naturally occurring NAR variable domain binds the Kgp protease from *Porphyromonas gingivalis*. FEBS Lett 516: 80–86
30. Coia G, Hudson PJ, Lilley GG (1996) Construction of recombinant extended single-chain antibody peptide conjugates for use in the diagnosis of HIV-1 and HIV-2. J Immunol Methods 192:13–23
31. Liu JL et al (2007) Selection of cholera toxin specific IgNAR single-domain antibodies from a naive shark library. Mol Immunol 44:1775–1783
32. Liu JL, Anderson GP, Goldman ER (2007) Isolation of anti-toxin single domain antibodies from a semi-synthetic spiny dogfish shark display library. BMC Biotechnol 7:78
33. Fennell BJ et al (2010) Dissection of the IgNAR V domain: molecular scanning and orthologue database mining define novel IgNAR hallmarks and affinity maturation mechanisms. J Mol Biol 400:155–170
34. Kopsidas G et al (2006) In vitro improvement of a shark IgNAR antibody by Qbeta replicase mutation and ribosome display mimics in vivo affinity maturation. Immunol Lett 107:163–168
35. Hosse RJ et al (2009) Kinetic screening of antibody-Im7 conjugates by capture on a colicin E7 DNase domain using optical biosensors. Anal Biochem 385:346–357
36. Simmons DP et al (2006) Dimerisation strategies for shark IgNAR single domain antibody fragments. J Immunol Methods 315:171–184
37. Criscitiello MF, Saltis M, Flajnik MF (2006) An evolutionarily mobile antigen receptor variable region gene: doubly rearranging NAR-TcR genes in sharks. Proc Natl Acad Sci U S A 103:5036–5041
38. Nuttall SD, Walsh RB (2008) Display scaffolds: protein engineering for novel therapeutics. Curr Opin Pharmacol 8:609–615

Part II

Single Domain Antibody Library Construction

Chapter 4

Creation of the Large and Highly Functional Synthetic Repertoire of Human VH and Vκ Domain Antibodies

Olga Ignatovich, Laurent Jespers, Ian M. Tomlinson, and Ruud M.T. de Wildt

Abstract

This protocol describes a method for creation of a highly diverse and functional synthetic phage-displayed repertoire of fully human domain antibodies (dAbs). The repertoire is based on two human frameworks (one VH and one Vκ) that express well in bacteria and are frequently used in human antibodies. To achieve this, we first build dAb libraries, containing full synthetic diversity at key positions in the complementarity-determining regions (CDRs). We then use an antigen-independent preselection of this primary dAb repertoire on generic ligands of the VH and the Vκ scaffolds (namely, the bacterial superantigens, protein A and L) to enrich for folded dAbs. Finally, the CDRs of these preselected dAbs are randomly recombined to further expand genetic diversity. The resulting phage repertoire is in excess of 10^{10} clones and is largely populated by correctly folded (over 50%) functional dAbs.

Key words: Antibody, Phage display, Single domain antibody, Combinatorial repertoire, Single scaffold

1. Introduction

Monoclonal antibodies (mAbs) are well established as therapeutic drugs being highly potent, highly specific, long-lived in serum, and well tolerated. More than 20 mAbs have now been approved and many more are currently in clinical trials. However, these large proteins (approximately 150 kDa) are confined to the extracellular environment and do not rapidly penetrate into solid tumors, they may recruit unwanted effector functions through their Fc part, and are complex to manufacture through expression in mammalian cell lines. Recombinant antibodies have therefore been progressively reduced in size (50 kDa for a Fab, 25 kDa for a scFv, 12–15 kDa for single VH and VL domains, dAbs). These molecules offer promising new formats because they are very specific and potent, can be produced in high yields in bacterial or yeast expression systems,

Dirk Saerens and Serge Muyldermans (eds.), *Single Domain Antibodies: Methods and Protocols*, Methods in Molecular Biology, vol. 911, DOI 10.1007/978-1-61779-968-6_4, © Springer Science+Business Media, LLC 2012

and because they can be reformatted into conjugates or multimers to adjust their pharmacodynamic profiles. A growing number of these new antibody fragments are currently in clinical trials (1).

Here we describe creation of a large and highly functional synthetic phage-displayed repertoire of fully human dAbs based on two human frameworks (one VH and one Vκ) that express well in bacteria and that are frequently used in human antibodies.

The VH repertoire is built on a single scaffold encoded by human germline genes V3-23/DP-47 and JH4b. DP47, a VH3 family member, is the most frequently used germline gene in natural antibodies and is also frequently selected from human antibody phage display libraries (2–4). The Vκ repertoire is encoded by germline genes O12/O2/DPK9 and Jκ1. DPK9 is a Vκ1 member, which is the most frequently used family in natural antibodies. Among joining (J) genes, JH4b and Jκ1 are the most frequently used. The canonical structures of the CDRs (VH: 1–3 and Vκ: 2-1-1) encoded by DP47 or DPK9 are used by approximately 50% of human antibodies (5). These frameworks have been shown to express well in *E. coli* either as scFv (6) or on their own as a single domain (7). It has been shown that VH3 family members bind protein A (8, 9), and Vκ1 members bind protein L (10). The crystal structures of protein A or L in complex with their respective V domains (8, 11) show that the contact residues do not involve loops comprising CDRs, but are mainly located in conserved FR1 and FR3 residues of VH3 members (binding to protein A) and in conserved FR1 residues in Vκ1 members (binding to protein L). These ligands bind only folded V domains, independently of antigen binding. Here we exploit these generic ligands to construct highly functional dAb libraries.

The libraries are created in three steps (see Fig. 1). In the first step we perform primary PCR reactions using oligonucleotides with NNK diversified codons that encode all 20 amino acids. Diversity is incorporated in the CDRs at positions that make contacts to antigen in known structures and are highly diverse in the mature repertoire (12). Primary PCR products are then assembled into a full dAb sequence by three-way SOE PCR (splicing by overlap extension PCR) whereby the CDR regions are randomly combined. These products are then cloned into a phage vector to create primary libraries (approximately 10^9 transformants). These primary libraries are tested for their ability to bind anti *c-myc* antibody (to detect clones that are in frame) and they are tested for binding to protein A or protein L (to detect clones that are correctly folded). Seventy to ninety percent of these primary libraries contain clones that are in frame, however on average only 5% of these libraries are functional, which confirms that full amino acid diversity often encodes residues that are incompatible with the overall dAb structure. Therefore, we perform a second step whereby we preselect our primary synthetic VH and Vκ dAb repertoires on

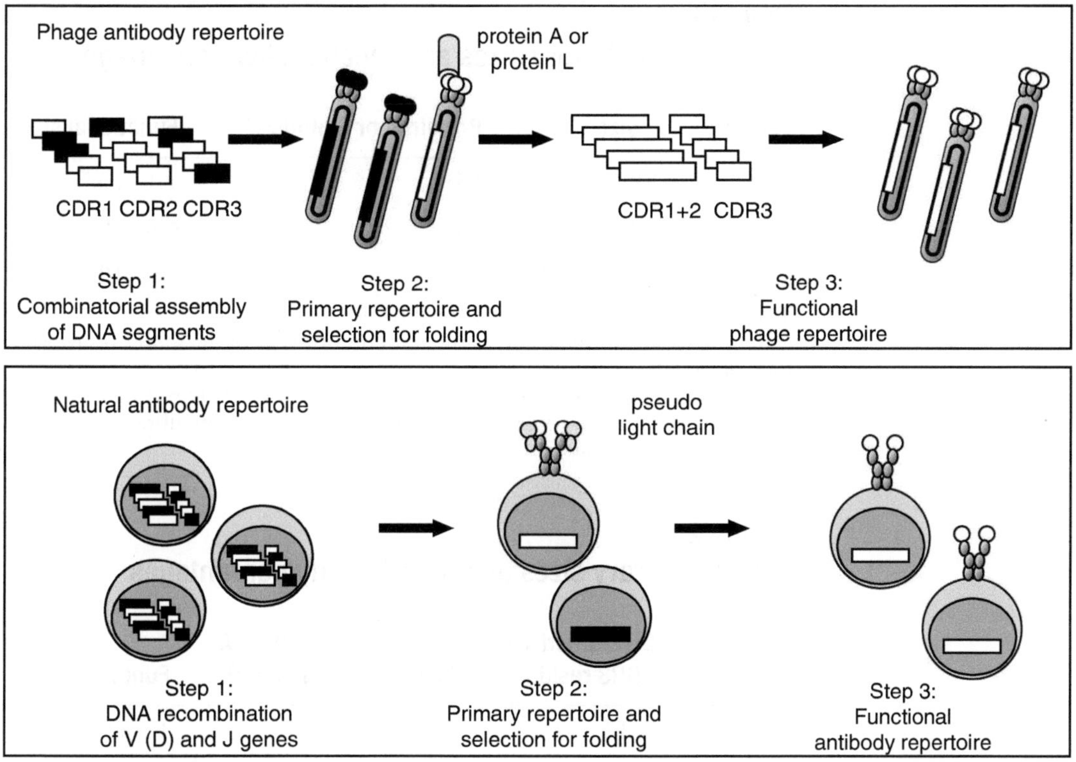

Fig. 1. Schematic overview of library construction. *Step 1*: Combinatorial synthetic diversity was introduced to create a primary repertoire using a three-way assembly PCR. *Step 2*: "Clean Up" of the primary phage repertoire, by selection on protein A (for the VH library) or protein L (for the Vκ library). *Step 3*: Further combinatorial diversity is introduced by recombining DNA segments encoding CDR1 + 2 and CDR3 amplified from a cleaned up library. This strategy mimics parts of the immune system, in that only diversified CDRs compatible with functional and stable antibodies are retained in the final repertoire. Code: *white boxes*: DNA fragments or proteins that are functional; *black boxes*: DNA fragments or proteins which are nonfunctional.

protein A and protein L, respectively, that only recognize well folded VH and Vκ scaffolds. The vast majority of phage (>95%) bind protein A or L after this selection procedure. However, the output of such selection is only approximately 1% of input phage thereby reducing the primary repertoire to approximately 10^7, which is too small for a final repertoire. We therefore perform a third step whereby we increase again the combinatorial diversity of each of these repertoires by DNA recombination: the fragments comprising the repertoires of CDR1 + 2 and CDR3 are amplified separately and randomly reassembled by SOE-PCR to form the full dAb sequence (see Fig. 1). This strategy mimics parts of *in vivo* antibody diversification whereby diversity is created in a combinatorial manner and an antigen-independent checkpoint for functional rearrangements ensures that only diversified CDRs compatible with functional and stable antibodies are retained in the final antibody repertoire (see Fig. 1).

Table 1
Summary of library sizes and functionality percentages

Library	Size[a]	Protein A or L binders[b]	Functional size[c]
Vκ	1.7×10^{10}	65	1.1×10^{10}
VH	1.6×10^{10}	45	6.5×10^{9}
Total	3.3×10^{10}	55	1.7×10^{10}

The library is enriched for functional dAbs
[a]The library size is calculated as the total number of colonies after transformation of the libraries
[b]The percentage of phages in the library that bind to protein A or L
[c]The functional library size is estimated by multiplying the library size by the fraction of functional clones

Table 2
VH sub-library sizes and functionality percentages

Library	Diversified VH CDR3 residues	Size[a]	Protein A binders[b]	Functional size
H10	4–12	2.6×10^{9}	58	1.5×10^{9}
H1	4	1.9×10^{9}	46	8.7×10^{8}
H2	5	1.0×10^{9}	54	5.4×10^{8}
H3	6	1.6×10^{9}	45	7.2×10^{8}
H4	7	1.2×10^{9}	40	4.8×10^{8}
H5	8	1.7×10^{9}	30	5.1×10^{8}
H6	9	1.6×10^{9}	43	6.9×10^{8}
H7	10	1.0×10^{9}	48	4.8×10^{8}
H8	11	1.0×10^{9}	39	3.9×10^{8}
H9	12	1.0×10^{9}	34	3.4×10^{8}
VH		1.6×10^{10}	45	6.5×10^{9}

The library is enriched for functional dAbs
[a]The library size is calculated as the total number of colonies after transformation of the libraries
[b]The percentage of phages in the library that bind to protein A or L

The resulting phage repertoire is in excess of 10^{10} clones and is largely populated by correctly folded (over 50%) functional dAbs (see Tables 1 and 2). Our repertoire is routinely used for rapid generation of human dAbs against a variety of targets with potencies ranging from low micromolar to low nanomolar. These dAbs are expressed at high levels and have good biophysical properties making them ideal leads for human therapy.

2. Materials

Prepare all solutions using Millipore-filtered water and analytical grade reagents. Prepare and store all reagents at room temperature (unless indicated otherwise). Use Millipore-filtered water in all experiments.

2.1. Template DNA and Diversifying Oligonucleotides

1. Oligonucleotide primers.
2. DNA Miniprep kit (Qiagen, Crawley, UK).

2.2. Primary Diversifying PCRs

1. Thermal cycler (0.5 mL tube or 96 well plate model).
2. 10× PCR buffer: 500 mM KCl, 100 mM Tris–HCl, pH 8.8, 15 mM $MgCl_2$, 1% Triton X-100.
3. dNTP mix (Qiagen, Crawley, UK).
4. Taq polymerase (Qiagen, Crawley, UK).
5. 1.2% Agarose gel.
6. 1 kb plus DNA ladder (Invitrogen, Paisley, UK).

2.3. DpnI Digestion and Gel Purification of Primary PCR Products

1. *Dpn*I restriction enzyme (New England Biolabs, Hitchin, UK).
2. 1.2% Agarose gel.
3. DNA Gel Extraction kit (Qiagen, Crawley, UK).
4. 1 kb plus DNA ladder.

2.4. PCR Assembly of Primary PCR Products

1. Thermal cycler (0.5 mL tube or 96 well plate model).
2. 10× PCR buffer: 500 mM KCl, 100 mM Tris–HCl, pH 8.8, 15 mM $MgCl_2$, 1% Triton X-100.
3. dNTP mix.
4. Taq polymerase.
5. Mineral oil.
6. 1.2% Agarose gel.
7. 1 kb plus DNA ladder.

2.5. Preparation of the Library dAb Insert

1. PCR purification kit (Qiagen, Crawley, UK).
2. *Sal*I and *Not*I restriction enzymes (New England Biolabs, Hitchin, UK).
3. Streptavidin M-280 magnetic beads (Dynal, Paisley, UK).
4. 2× W+B buffer: 2 M NaCl, 10 mM Tris–HCl pH7.5, 1 mM EDTA.
5. 1.2% Agarose gel.
6. 1 kb plus DNA ladder.

2.6. Test Library Ligation and Transformation

1. *Sal*I, *Not*I, *Pst*I restriction enzymes (New England Biolabs, Hitchin, UK).
2. T4 DNA ligase (New England Biolabs, Hitchin, UK).
3. TB1 *E. coli* (New England Biolabs, Hitchin, UK).
4. TB1 *E. coli* electrocompetent cells (Agilent, Wokingham, UK).
5. 2xTY medium: 16 g Tryptone, 10 g yeast extract, and 5 g NaCl in 1 L of H_2O.
6. Gene Pulser (Bio-Rad, Hemel Hempstead, UK).
7. 2xTYE Tet plates: 15 g Bacto-agar, 10 g Tryptone, 8 g NaCl, 5 g yeast extract in 1 L of H_2O, pH 7.0, 15 μg/mL Tetracycline.
8. pUC18 vector (Sigma, Dorset, UK).

2.7. Functionality Protein A/L Phage ELISA

1. 96 Well Cell Culture Cluster with round bottom and lid.
2. 2xTY Tet medium: 16 g Tryptone, 10 g yeast extract, and 5 g NaCl in 1 L of H_2O, 15 μg/mL Tetracycline.
3. Maxisorp 96 well immunoplate (Nunc, Langenselbold, Germany).
4. PBS: 10 mM Phosphate buffer, 2.7 mM KCl, 137 mM NaCl, pH 7.4.
5. Recombinant Protein A (Sigma, Dorset, UK).
6. Recombinant Protein L (Actigen, Oslo, Norway).
7. 2% MPBS: PBS with 2% Marvel (dried skimmed milk powder). Prepare fresh and do not store.
8. 4% MPBS: PBS with 4% Marvel (dried skimmed milk powder). Prepare fresh and do not store.
9. 0.05% TPBS: PBS with 0.05% Tween-20.
10. Sheep anti M13 antibody (GSK, in-house reagent).
11. Chicken anti sheep HRP conjugated antibody (Immunsystem AB, Uppsala, Sweden).
12. SureBlue TMB 1-component microwell peroxidase substrate (KPL, Gaithersburg, Maryland, USA).
13. 1 M Sulphuric acid.

2.8. Anti c-myc Antibody Binding Phage ELISA

1. 96 Well cell culture cluster with round bottom and lid.
2. 2xTY Tet: 16 g Tryptone, 10 g yeast extract and 5 g NaCl in 1 L of H_2O, 15 μg/mL Tetracycline.
3. Maxisorp 96 well immunoplate (Nunc, Langenselbold, Germany).
4. PBS: 10 mM Phosphate buffer, 2.7 mM KCl, 137 mM NaCl, pH 7.4.
5. 2% MPBS: PBS with 2% Marvel (dried skimmed milk powder). Prepare fresh and do not store.

6. 4% MPBS: PBS with 4% Marvel (dried skimmed milk powder). Prepare fresh and do not store.
7. 0.05% TPBS: PBS with 0.05% Tween-20.
8. Anti c-myc 9E10 mAb (Sigma, Dorset, UK).
9. Anti M13-HRP conjugated mAb (Pharmacia, Milton Keynes, UK).
10. SureBlue TMB 1-component microwell peroxidase substrate (KPL, Gaithersburg, Maryland, USA).
11. 1 M Sulphuric acid.

2.9. Full-Scale Primary Library Ligation and Transformation

1. T4 DNA ligase.
2. TB1 *E. coli* (New England Biolabs, Hitchin, UK).
3. TB1 *E. coli* electrocompetent cells (Agilent, Wokingham, UK).
4. 2xTY medium: 16 g Tryptone, 10 g yeast extract and 5 g NaCl in 1 L of H_2O.
5. Gene Pulser (Bio-Rad, Hemel Hempstead, UK).
6. 2xTYE Tet plates: 15 g Bacto-agar, 10 g Tryptone, 8 g NaCl, 5 g yeast extract in 1 L of H_2O, pH 7.0, 15 μg/mL Tetracycline.
7. "Microcon YM-50" concentrating columns (Millipore, Watford, UK).
8. 2xTY with 15% glycerol.

2.10. Production of Recombinant Phage Particles from Primary VH and Vκ Libraries

1. 2xTY Tet medium: 16 g Tryptone, 10 g yeast extract, and 5 g NaCl in 1 L of H_2O, 15 μg/mL Tetracycline.
2. PEG–NaCl: 20% Polyethylene glycol 8000, 2.5 M NaCl pre-chilled to 4°C.
3. PBS: 10 mM Phosphate buffer, 2.7 mM KCl, 137 mM NaCl, pH 7.4.
4. 0.45 μm filters.
5. PBS with 15% glycerol.
6. *E. coli* TG1 cells.

2.11. Preselection of the Primary VH and Vκ Libraries on Protein A and L

1. MaxiSorp immuno test tubes (Nunc, Langenselbold, Germany).
2. Recombinant Protein A (Sigma, Dorset, UK).
3. Recombinant Protein L (Actigen, Oslo, Norway).
4. PBS: 10 mM Phosphate buffer, 2.7 mM KCl, 137 mM NaCl, pH 7.4.
5. 2% MPBS: PBS with 2% Marvel (dried skimmed milk powder). Prepare fresh and do not store.

6. 1,000 ppm free chlorine bleach solution (Precept, J & J Medical, New Brunswick, New Jersey, USA).
7. 0.1% TPBS: PBS with 0.1% Tween-20.
8. Trypsin stock solution: 5 mg/mL Trypsin in 50 mM Tris–HCl pH 7.4, 1 mM $CaCl_2$. Aliquote and store at −20°C to avoid autoproteolysis.
9. *E. coli* TG1 cells.
10. 2xTY Tet medium: 16 g Tryptone, 10 g yeast extract, and 5 g NaCl in 1 L of H_2O, 15 μg/mL Tetracycline.
11. 2xTY with 15% glycerol.
12. DNA Midi prep kit (Qiagen, Crawley, UK).

2.12. CDR Reamplification and Reassembly of the Final Library

All materials are as described previously (see Subheadings 2.1, 2.2, 2.3, 2.4, 2.5, 2.6, 2.7, 2.8, 2.9, and 2.10).

2.13. Analysis of dAb/gIII Display Levels

1. NuPAGE LDS Sample Buffer (Invitrogen, Paisley, UK).
2. NuPAGE Sample Reduction Agent (Invitrogen, Paisley, UK).
3. NuPAGE 4–12% Bis-Tris gel (Invitrogen, Paisley, UK).
4. XCell *SureLock* Mini-Cell (Invitrogen, Paisley, UK).
5. NuPAGE MES SDS Running Buffer (Invitrogen, Paisley, UK).
6. NuPAGE Antioxidant (Invitrogen, Paisley, UK).
7. PVDF, 0.2 μm pore size (Invitrogen, Paisley, UK).
8. XCell II Blot Module (Invitrogen, Paisley, UK).
9. NuPAGE transfer buffer (Invitrogen, Paisley, UK).
10. Methanol/NuPAGE transfer buffer: 10 or 20% methanol in NuPAGE transfer buffer.
11. PBS: 10 mM Phosphate buffer, 2.7 mM KCl, 137 mM NaCl, pH 7.4.
12. 5% MPBS: PBS with 5% Marvel (dried skimmed milk powder). Prepare fresh and do not store.
13. Anti-pIII (g3p) antibody (MoBiTec GmbH, Göttingen, Germany).
14. 0.2% TPBS: PBS with 0.2% Tween-20.
15. HRP conjugated goat-anti-mouse IgG (Fc specific) (Sigma, Dorset, UK).
16. ECL Plus Western Blotting Detection Reagents (Amersham Biosciences, Little Chalfont, UK).
17. Hyperfilm ECL (Amersham Biosciences, Little Chalfont, UK).

3. Methods

3.1. Template DNA and Diversifying Oligonucleotides

1. Human VH and Vκ germline genes (see Fig. 2) cloned into pDOM5 vector (see Fig. 3) were used as template DNA for library construction. Prepare template DNA according to the DNA miniprep kit manufacturer.

a

```
                                                H10
       E   V   Q   L   L   E   S   G   G   G   L   V   Q   P   G   G
1     GAG GTG CAG CTG TTG GAG TCT GGG GGA GGC TTG GTA CAG CCT GGG GGG
      CTC CAC GTC GAC AAC CTC AGA CCC CCT CCG AAC CAT GTC GGA CCC CCC

                  H20                                       H30
       S   L   R   L   S   C   A   A   S   G   F   T   F   S   S   Y
49    TCC CTG CGT CTC TCC TGT GCA GCC TCC GGA TTC ACC TTT AGC AGC TAT
      AGG GAC GCA GAG AGG ACA CGT CGG AGG CCT AAG TGG AAA TCG TCG ATA
                                                               HCDR1

                                    H40
       A   M   S    W   V   R   Q   A   P   G   K   G   L   E   W   V
97    GCC ATG AGC  TGG GTC CGC CAG GCT CCA GGG AAG GGT CTA GAG TGG GTC
      CGG TAC TCG  ACC CAG GCG GTC CGA GGT CCC TTC CCA GAT CTC ACC CAG
        HCDR1

         H50     H52  a  H53                          H60
       S   A   I   S   G   S   G   G   S   T   Y   Y   A   D   S   V
145   TCA GCT ATT AGT GGT AGT GGT GGT AGC ACA TAC TAC GCA GAC TCC GTG
      AGT CGA TAA TCA CCA TCA CCA CCA TCG TGT ATG ATG CGT CTG AGG CAC
                                      HCDR2

                                 H70
       K   G    R   F   T   I   S   R   D   N   S   K   N   T   L   Y
193   AAG GGC  CGG TTC ACC ATC TCC CGT GAC AAT TCC AAG AAC ACG CTG TAT
      TTC CCG  GCC AAG TGG TAG AGG GCA CTG TTA AGG TTC TTG TGC GAC ATA
       HCDR2

      H80     H82  a   b   c  H83                         H90
       L   Q   M   N   S   L   R   A   E   D   T   A   V   Y   Y   C
241   CTG CAA ATG AAC AGC CTG CGT GCC GAG GAC ACC GCG GTA TAT TAC TGT
      GAC GTT TAC TTG TCG GAC GCA CGG CTC CTG TGG CGC CAT ATA ATG ACA

                          H98     H101
       A   K   X   X   X   X   F   D   Y   W   G   Q   G   T   L   V
289   GCG AAA NNK NNK NNK NNK TTT GAC TAC TGG GGC CAG GGA ACC CTG GTC
      CGC TTT NNM NNM NNM NNM AAA CTG ATG ACC CCG GTC CCT TGG GAC CAG
                            HCDR3

      H110        H113
       T   V   S   S
337   ACC GTC TCG AGC
      TGG CAG AGC TCG
```

Fig. 2. (**a**) Sequence of VH framework based on germline sequence DP47—JH4b. Randomized positions are indicated in *bold* text. (**b**) Sequence of Vκ framework based on germline sequence DPκ9—Jκ1. Randomized positions are indicated in *bold* text.

b

```
                                      L10
       D   I   Q   M   T   Q   S   P   S   S   L   S   A   S   V   G
1      GAC ATC CAG ATG ACC CAG TCT CCA TCC TCC CTG TCT GCA TCT GTA GGA
       CTG TAG GTC TAC TGG GTC AGA GGT AGG AGG GAC AGA CGT AGA CAT CCT

                   L20                                     L30
       D   R   V   T   I   T   C   R   A   S   Q   S   I   S   S   Y
49     GAC CGT GTC ACC ATC ACT TGC CGG GCA AGT CAG AGC ATT AGC AGC TAT
       CTG GCA CAG TGG TAG TGA ACG GCC CGT TCA GTC TCG TAA TCG TCG ATA
                                                     LCDR1
                                      L40
       L   N   W   Y   Q   Q   K   P   G   K   A   P   K   L   L   I
97     TTA AAT TGG TAC CAG CAG AAA CCA GGG AAA GCC CCT AAG CTC CTG ATC
       AAT TTA ACC ATG GTC GTC TTT GGT CCC TTT CGG GGA TTC GAG GAC TAG

           L50                                 L60
       Y   A   A   S   S   L   Q   S   G   V   P   S   R   F   S   G
145    TAT GCT GCA TCC AGT TTG CAA AGT GGG GTC CCA TCA CGT TTC AGT GGC
       ATA CGA CGT AGG TCA AAC GTT TCA CCC CAG GGT AGT GCA AAG TCA CCG
                   LCDR2
                           L70                                     L80
       S   G   S   G   T   D   F   T   L   T   I   S   S   L   Q   P
193    AGT GGA TCT GGG ACA GAT TTC ACT CTC ACC ATC AGC AGT CTG CAA CCT
       TCA CCT AGA CCC TGT CTA AAG TGA GAG TGG TAG TCG TCA GAC GTT GGA

                                              L90
       E   D   F   A   T   Y   Y   C   Q   Q   S   Y   S   T   P   N
241    GAA GAT TTT GCT ACG TAC TAC TGT CAA CAG AGT TAC AGT ACC CCT AAT
       CTT CTA AAA CGA TGC ATG ATG ACA GTT GTC TCA ATG TCA TGG GGA TTA
                                                         LCDR3
                   L100                        L107
       T   F   G   Q   G   T   K   V   E   I   K   R
289    ACG TTC GGC CAA GGG ACC AAG GTG GAA ATC AAA CGG
       TGC AAG CCG GTT CCC TGG TTC CAC CTT TAG TTT GCC
```

Fig. 2. (continued)

2. The libraries have been diversified using NNK side chains in positions chosen to mirror those which are diverse in the human antibody repertoire (where N represents nucleotides A, C, G, or T and K represents G or T). The diversified positions are indicated below, numbered according to Kabat (13, 14) and are shown in the context of the complete dAb sequences in Fig. 2.

   Vκ:

   Vκ CDR1: L28, L30, L31, L32, L34.

   Vκ CDR2: L50, L51, L53.

   Vκ CDR3: L91, L92, L93, L94, and L96.

   13 residues randomized in total

   VH:

   VH CDR1: H30, H31, H33, H35.

   VH CDR2: H50, H52, H52a, H53, H55, and H56.

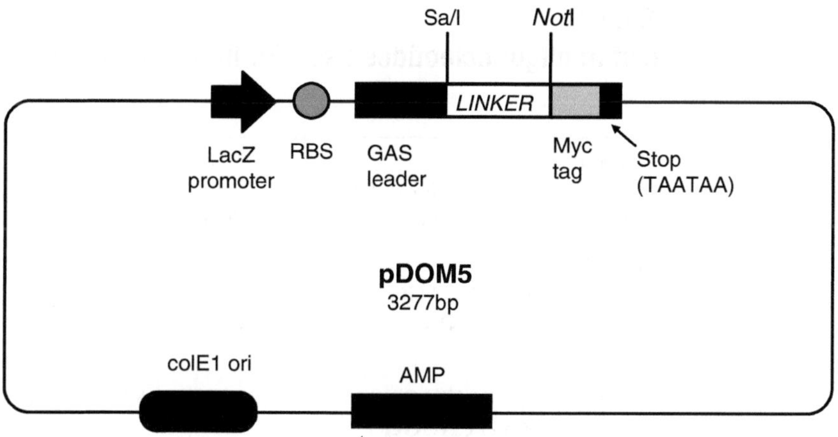


```
1      AGCGGATAAC AATTTCACAC AGGAAACAGC TATGACCATG ATTACGCCAA

                                                  M   L   F   K
51     GCTTGCATGC AAATTCTATT TCAAGGAGAC AGTCATAATG TTATTTAAAT
       HindIII

                             GAS leader      DOM172 PCR primer
        S  L  S  K   L  A  T   A  A  A   F  F  A  G   V  A  T
101    CATTATCAAA ATTAGCAACC GCAGCAGCAT TTTTTGCAGG CGTGGCAACA

                                                 c-myc tag
        A  S  T                A  A  A   E  Q  K  L   I  S  E
151    GCGTCGACAC ACTGCAGGAG GCGGCCGCAG AACAAAAACT CATCTCAGAA
          SalI       PstI       NotI

        E  D  L   N  *  *                 DOM173 PCR primer
201    GAGGATCTGA ATTAATAAGA ATTCACTGGC CGTCGTTTTA CAACGTCGTG
                           EcoRI

251    ACTGGGAAAA CCCTGGCG
```

Fig. 3. Vector map and multiple cloning site sequence of vector pDOM5, a pUC119-based expression vector under control of the LacZ promoter. dAbs are fused to the universal yeast glycolipid anchored surface protein (GAS) leader signal peptide at the N-terminal end. In addition, a myc-tag is appended at the C-terminal end of the dAbs.

VH CDR3: 4–12 diversified residues: e.g., H95, H96, H97, and H98 in VH H11 and H95, H96, H97, H98, H99, H100, H100a, H100b, H100c, H100d, H100e, and H100f in VH H19. The last three CDR3 residues are FDY so CDR3 lengths vary from 7 to 15 residues.

14–22 residues randomized in total

3. Oligonucleotides used for library generation are summarized in Table 3.

Table 3
List of oligonucleotides used for library generation

DOM163 AGACCCTTCCCTGGAGCCTGGCGGACCCAMNNCATMNNATAMNNMNNAAAGGTGAATCCGGAGGCTGC
DOM164 CCGCCAGGCTCCAGGGAAGGGTCTAGAGTGGGTCTCANNKATTNNKNNKNNKGGTNNKNNKACATACTACGCAGACTCCG
DOM165A ACCGCGGTATATTACTGTGCGAAANNKNNKNNKNNKTTTGACTACTGGGGTCAGGG
DOM165B ACCGCGGTATATTACTGTGCGAAANNKNNKNNKNNKNNKTTTGACTACTGGGGTCAGGG
DOM165C ACCGCGGTATATTACTGTGCGAAANNKNNKNNKNNKNNKNNKTTTGACTACTGGGGTCAGGG
DOM165D ACCGCGGTATATTACTGTGCGAAANNKNNKNNKNNKNNKNNKNNKTTTGACTACTGGGGTCAGGG
DOM165E ACCGCGGTATATTACTGTGCGAAANNKNNKNNKNNKNNKNNKNNKNNKTTTGACTACTGGGGTCAGGG
DOM165F ACCGCGGTATATTACTGTGCGAAANNKNNKNNKNNKNNKNNKNNKNNKNNKTTTGACTACTGGGGTCAGGG
DOM165G ACCGCGGTATATTACTGTGCGAAANNKNNKNNKNNKNNKNNKNNKNNKNNKNNKTTTGACTACTGGGGTCAGGG
DOM165H ACCGCGGTATATTACTGTGCGAAANNKNNKNNKNNKNNKNNKNNKNNKNNKNNKNNKTTTGACTACTGGGGTCAGGG
DOM165I ACCGCGGTATATTACTGTGCGAAANNKNNKNNKNNKNNKNNKNNKNNKNNKNNKNNKNNKTTTGACTACTGGGGTCAGGG
DOM167 TAGGGGCTTTCCCTGGTTTCTGCTGGTACCAMNNTAAMNNMNNMNNAATMNNCTGACTTGCCCGGCAAGTG
DOM168 CAGCAGAAACCAGGGAAAGCCCCTAAGCTCCTGATCTATNNKNNKTCCNNKTTGCAAAGTGGGGTCCCATCACG
DOM169 GCTACGTACTACTGTCAACAGNNKNNKNNKNNKCCTNNKACGTTCGGCCAAGGGACCAAGG

(continued)

Table 3 (continued)

DOM172/Biotin TTGCAGGCGTGGCAACAGCG
DOM173/Biotin CACGACGTTGTAAAACGACGGCC
DOM174 ACCGCGGTATATTACTGTGCG
DOM175 GCTACGTACTACTGTCAACAG
DOM166 CGCACAGTAATATACCGCGGTGTCC
DOM170 GTTGACAGTAGTACGTAGCAAAATC

3.2. Primary Diversifying PCRs

1. Set up three primary PCRs to amplify CDR1, 2, and 3 of the Vκ dAb and set up 11 primary PCRs to amplify CDR1, 2, and 3 of the VH dAb. The combinations of oligonucleotides used for these amplifications are summarized below.

	Oligo pair	
Diversification required	**Forward**	**Reverse**
Vκ CDR1	DOM172	DOM167
Vκ CDR2	DOM168	DOM170
Vκ CDR3	DOM169	DOM173
VH CDR1	DOM172	DOM163
VH CDR2	DOM164	DOM166
VH CDR3	DOM165A,B,C,D,E,F,G, H, or I	DOM173

2. Make up 50 μL PCR mixes containing the following (see Note 1):

Master mix	**1×**
10× PCR buffer	5 μL
dNTP stock (10 mM each)	1 μL
Forward primer (10 μM stock)	2 μL
Reverse primer (10 μM stock)	2 μL
Taq polymerase	0.25 μL
Template DNA (in pDOM5)	1 μL (see Note 2)
dH_2O	38.75 μL (to final volume 50 μL)

3. Perform PCR cycling as outlined below (see Note 3):

Initial denaturation	5 min	94°C
Denaturation	1 min	94°C
Annealing (25 cycles)	1 min	55°C
Extension	1 min	72°C
Final extension	10 min	72°C

4. Confirm successful PCR amplified DNA by running 3–5 μL of the PCR product on a 1.2% agarose gel. The presence of a single band and the correct product sizes should be confirmed (this will vary according to PCR). Typical yields are 5–10 μg/100 μL reaction.

3.3. DpnI Digestion and Gel Purification of Primary PCR Products

1. Set up a *Dpn*I digest (see Note 4) in a 200 μL reaction volume and incubate at 37°C for at least 2 h. This can be added directly to the primary PCR reactions without purification.

	Total volume = 250 μL
PCR product (10–20 μg)	200 μL
NEB buffer 4	25 μL
*Dpn*I (20 U/μL)	5 μL
dH_2O	20 μL

2. Run after *DpnI* digest all PCR products on a preparative 1.2% agarose gel.
3. After electrophoresis, visualize the gel under UV and excise the PCR products carefully from the gel. Bands should be excised in the minimum volume of gel and placed into 2 mL eppendorf tubes taking care to avoid cross-contamination.
4. Perform gel purification using DNA Gel Extraction kit. A single cleanup column should be sufficient per 50 μL PCR reaction. Elute DNA in 50 μL of elution buffer. Analyze 3–5 μL of the purified product on a 1.2% agarose gel. Typical yields are 5 μg/100 μL reaction.

3.4. PCR Assembly vof Primary PCR Products

1. Set up assembly PCRs (see Note 5) as follows:

Extension reaction	1×
10× PCR buffer	8 μL
dNTP stock (10 mM each)	2 μL
Taq polymerase	1 μL
CDR1 cleaned PCR product	200 ng

(continued)

Extension reaction	**1×**
CDR2 cleaned PCR product	200 ng
CDR3 cleaned PCR product	200 ng
dH_2O	to final volume of 80 μL
Primer mix (added later)	1×
Biotinylated DOM172 (10 μM stock)	2 μL
Biotinylated DOM173 (10 μM stock)	2 μL
10× PCR Buffer	2 μL
dH_2O (to final volume of 20 μL)	14 μL

2. The assembled products will be used in the final library construction. For this reason, two 100 μL PCR reactions are required per library which will generate sufficient product (typically 5–10 μg/100 μL).
3. PCRs can be overlaid with mineral oil to prevent evaporation during pausing and addition of the primer mix. The PCR reactions are performed using the program described below. After the initial assembly the PCR machine should be set to pause at 94°C. Twenty microliters of primer mix should be added to each reaction and mixed.

   Step 1 Assembly

Initial denaturation	5 min	94°C
Denaturation	1 min	94°C
Annealing (10 cycles)	1 min	55°C
Extension	1 min	72°C

   At this stage a sample of 10 μL can be taken from the control PCR reaction. This 10 μL should be analyzed on an agarose gel (together with the final amplified product) to monitor correct assembly without amplification.

   Step 2 Amplification (*Pause at 94°C, Primers are now added*)

Denaturation	1 min	94°C
Annealing (25 cycles)	1 min	55°C
Extension	1 min	72°C

4. Check PCR products by running 3–5 μL of each reaction on a 1.2% agarose gel. The assembled PCR product of about 600–700 bp should be observed with only minimal additional nonspecific bands.

3.5. Preparation of the Library dAb Insert

1. Purify PCR assembly products using PCR purification kit.
2. Digest the cleaned PCR products first with *Sal*I enzyme and then with *Not*I enzyme (approximately 10 U of enzyme should be used per digest per μg of DNA). Perform each digest for a minimum of 4 h (or overnight) at 37°C and clean DNA using PCR purification kit following each digest.
3. Remove undigested products and digested ends from the cut product via the biotinylated PCR primer ends using streptavidin beads (see Note 6). Sixty-five microliters of M-280 streptavidin-coated beads is sufficient for each 10–20 μg of assembly PCR product.
4. Place the beads in a 1.5 mL eppendorf tube and capture the beads using the magnetic rack. Remove the supernatant and wash the beads twice in 2× W+B Buffer.
5. Resuspend the beads in 100 μL of 2× W+B Buffer and add the digested inserts (100 μL to give a final 1× concentration of W+B buffer)
6. Rotate the bead–DNA mix at room temperature for 5 min after which the beads are captured on the magnetic rack.
7. Remove the supernatant (containing purified insert) from the beads for subsequent clean up using PCR purification kit.
8. Monitor the efficiency of the digests and purification by running 3–5 μL of the following products side by side on a 1.2% agarose gel: the assembled PCR product before digest, after digest, and after beads purification.

3.6. Test Library Ligation and Transformation

1. It is essential that test ligations are performed prior to library ligations. These are done using approximately 100 ng of *Sal*I/*Pst*I/*Not*I digested pDOM4 vector (see Fig. 4) and varying amounts of insert (1:3, 1:1, and 3:1 molar ratios of insert/vector are typically used).
2. Perform test ligations in 20 μL volume, using 200 U of T4 DNA ligase and are incubate at room temperature for >30 min or for >3 h at 16°C.
3. Transform the test ligations into TB1 electrocompetent cells (see Note 7). Transform 2 μL of each ligation. Recover the cells by adding 1 mL of prewarmed 2xTY and incubate for 1 h at 37°C shaking at 250 rpm followed by plating of the full transformation onto 2xTYE Tet plates. Controls should include the following: cut vector control (to determine background of uncut vector in vector prep), pUC18 control (at known concentration to monitor competency of cells), and ligated cut vector control (to determine background religation without insert).
4. Test library ligations should give approximately 100-fold more colonies than the vector only ligation (see Note 8). Check the

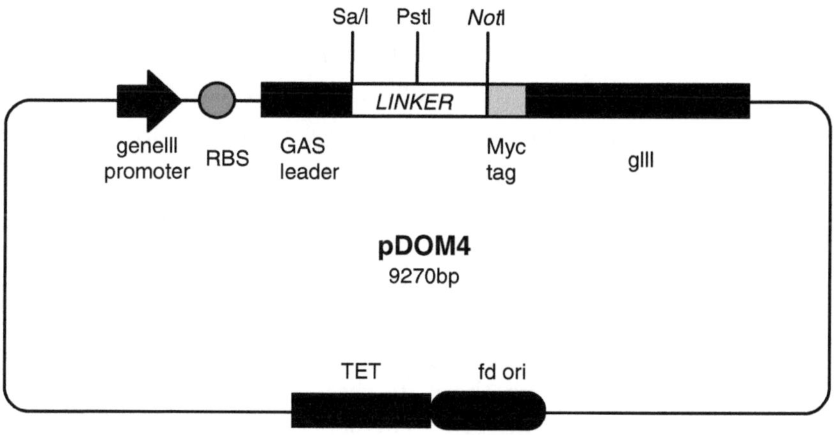


```
                      GAS leader
  M  L  F   K  S  L   S  K  L   A  T  A  A   A  F  F
TAATGTTATT TAAATCATTA TCAAAATTAG CAACCGCAGC AGCATTTTTT

 A  G  V   A  T  A  S   T               A  A   A  E  Q
GCAGGCGTGG CAACAGCGTC GACACACTGC AGGAGGCGGC CGCAGAACAA
                  SalI       PstI       NotI

         MYC tag
 K  L  I   S  E  E  D   L  N
AAACTCATCT CAGAAGAGGA TCTGAATTCG
                         EcoRI
```

Fig. 4. Vector map and multiple cloning site sequence of vector pDOM4, a derivative of the Fd phage vector in which the gene III signal peptide sequence is replaced with the GAS leader signal peptide.

transformants for the presence of insert by PCR screening with primers DOM172 and DOM173 (see Subheading 3.2 for PCR protocol) and sequence at least ten clones from each library to check the dAb sequence is in-frame with no deletions or insertions. At this stage analyze the functionality of the library by protein A/L binding phage ELISA (to detect clones that are correctly folded) and anti *c-myc* antibody binding phage ELISA (to detect clones that are in frame).

3.7. Functionality Protein A/L Phage ELISA

1. Following transformation of test ligations, pick individual bacterial clones into 96 well cell culture plates containing 200 μL per well of 2xTY with 15 μg/mL tetracycline and are incubated overnight in a humidified atmosphere at 37°C with shaking at 250 rpm.
2. Following overnight incubation of the plates, pellet the bacterial cells by centrifugation at 1,800 × *g* for 10 min at 4°C. The supernatant can be stored at 4°C for up to 2 days.

3. Coat a 96 well Maxisorp assay plate overnight at 4°C with 100 μL per well of Protein L/Protein A (at 1 μg/mL in PBS).
4. Wash the plate wells three times with PBS.
5. Add 200 μL per well of 2% MPBS to block and incubate plate for 1–2 h at room temperature.
6. Wash the wells three times with PBS and then add 50 μL of 4% MPBS followed by 50 μL of the appropriate bacterial supernatant, containing the phage-dAbs. Incubate for 1 h at room temperature.
7. Discard phage-dAb solution by inverting plate and shaking, then wash the plate three times with 0.05% TPBS and three times with PBS. The supernatants and wash solution are discarded into 1,000 ppm free chlorine bleach solution. Add 100 μL of sheep anti M13 antibody, prediluted 1/1,000 in 2% MPBS, to each well and incubate for 1 h at room temperature.
8. Discard the antibody conjugate solution and wash three times with 0.05% TPBS and three times with PBS. Add 100 μL of chicken anti sheep HRP conjugated antibody, prediluted 1/1,000 in 2% MPBS, to each well and incubate for 1 h at room temperature.
9. Discard the antibody conjugate solution and wash three times with 0.05% TPBS followed by three washes with PBS.
10. Add 50 μL of SureBlue 1-Component TMB MicroWell Peroxidase solution, prewarmed to room temperature, to each well, mix by gently tapping the plate and leave at room temperature for 2–60 min (see Note 9). The reaction is stopped by the addition of 50 μL of 1 M sulphuric or hydrochloric acid. (The blue color will turn yellow.)
11. Read the $OD_{450\ nm}$ of the plate in a 96 well plate reader within 30 min of acid addition. The $OD_{450\ nm}$ is proportional to the amount of bound HRP conjugate.

3.8. Anti c-myc Antibody Binding Phage ELISA

The protocol is the same as previously described (see Subheading 3.7) except that a 96 well Maxisorp assay plate is coated overnight at 4°C with 100 μL per well of anti c-myc 9E10 mAb (1 μg/mL in PBS) and the detection of the bound dAb-phage is performed using anti M13-HRP conjugated antibody (1:4,000 dilution).

3.9. Full-Scale Primary Library Ligation and Transformation

1. Scale up the amount of vector and insert (at the correct ratio) as well as the total volume for the library ligation. Amounts typically used for library ligations are 5–10 μg of digested vector and 1–2 μg of purified insert and typically result in $>5\times10^8$ transformants. Ligations are performed in a volume of 500 μL to 1 mL using 15 μL of T4 DNA Ligase (400 U/μL) overnight at 16°C.
2. Inactivate the ligase by incubation of the ligation at 70°C on a hotblock for 30 min.

3. Extract DNA once with phenol–chloroform and once with chloroform.
4. Transfer the supernatant then to an Amicon 50 K concentrating column (see Note 10).
5. Spin the column at 3,000 × *g* for 9–15 min until 30–50 μL is left on top of the column and discard the spin-through. The columns must not be allowed to run dry.
6. Discard the solution in the collection tube and add a further 400 μL of HPLC grade dH_2O to the concentrator and mix with the remaining sample before the procedure is repeated.
7. Repeat steps 5–6 a total of four times.
8. Pipet off the remaining sample at the top of the column (containing concentrated ligated library DNA) carefully (typically approximately 30 μL). Reverse the filter and spin any remaining sample into a fresh collection tube and combine with the initial 30 μL. This is typically split between 5 and 10 library transformations.
9. Perform electroporations using TB1 electrocompetent cells. Ligations and cells are premixed prior to aliquoting to prechilled cuvettes (0.1 mL per cuvette).
10. Add 0.9 mL of prewarmed 2xTY immediately after electroporation and resuspend cells gently.
11. Combine the electroporated cell samples in a sterile disposable flask and top up to 50 mL using prewarmed 2xTY.
12. Incubate the culture for 1 h by shaking at 250 rpm at 37°C.
13. Plate out dilutions of the electroporated cells at -10^{-5}, 10^{-7} and 10^{-9} to determine the size of the library. Centrifuge the remaining cultures at 3,300 × *g* for 10 min. Discard the supernatant and resuspend the cell pellet in 2 mL of 2xTY. Each 1 mL is plated onto one large square (22 cm) Bio-Assay plate containing 2xTYE Tet agar.
14. Incubate plates at 37°C overnight, then scrape off cells into 2–5 mL of 15% glycerol/2xTY and freeze in cryogenic vials to create glycerol stocks of the libraries. Store glycerol stocks at –70°C. The primary VH and Vκ libraries should contain approximately 10^9 transformants.

3.10. Production of Recombinant Phage Particles from Primary VH and Vκ Libraries

1. Take sufficient *E. coli* glycerol stock to ensure complete representation of the library diversity. Typically a 10–100 fold excess of cells to the library diversity is used (i.e., a minimum of 1×10^{10} cells from the glycerol stock for a library with a diversity of 1×10^9 unique dAbs). Inoculate 2 L volumes of 2xTY containing 15 μg/mL tetracycline for each primary library (see Note 11). The culture is incubated at 37°C with shaking at 250 rpm for between 18 and 24 h.

2. Centrifuge the overnight culture at 3,300 × *g* for 15 min. Recover the supernatant and add 100 mL of prechilled PEG–NaCl per 400 mL of supernatant. Incubate the mixture on ice for at least 1 h to precipitate the phages.
3. Centrifuge the mixture at 3,300 × *g* for 30 min and discard the supernatant.
4. Resuspend each resulting pellets in 8 mL of PBS and add 2 mL of prechilled PEG–NaCl. Mix the solution well by inversion and leave on ice for 1 h.
5. Centrifuge the mixture at 3,300 × *g* for 30 min and discard the supernatant. Recentrifuge the pellets briefly and remove any remaining PEG–NaCl by pipette.
6. Resuspend each pellet in 5 mL of PBS, aliquot into 2 mL microfuge tubes and centrifuge at 11,600 × *g* for 10 min in a microcentrifuge to remove any remaining bacterial debris.
7. Pool the supernatant for each primary library and pass through a 0.45 μm filter using a syringe.
8. Store the phages in PBS with 15% glycerol at –70°C.
9. Determine the phage titer by infecting log phase *E. coli* TG1 cells with serial dilutions of the phage stock (see Note 12).

3.11. Preselection of the Primary VH and Vκ Libraries on Protein A and L

1. Coat immunotubes overnight at 4°C with 4 mL of protein A (for preselection of the primary VH libraries) or protein L (for preselection of the primary Vκ library) at 50 μg/mL in PBS.
2. Next day wash the tubes three times with PBS.
3. Block the tubes to prevent nonspecific binding of phages. Fill the tubes to the brim with 2% MPBS and incubate for at least 1 h, typically at room temperature.
4. Wash the tubes three times with PBS.
5. Add the primary phage libraries (10^{11} TU) in 4 mL of 2% MPBS to the coated tubes and incubate for 60 min at room temperature rotating using an under-and-over turntable. The tubes are left to stand for a further 60 min at room temperature. Discard the supernatant into 1,000 ppm free chlorine bleach solution.
6. Wash the tubes ten times with 0.1% TPBS. Excess wash solution is shaken out of the tube.
7. Elute phages by adding 500 μL of trypsin-PBS (100 μL of trypsin stock solution added to 400 μL of PBS) and rotating for 10 min at room temperature using an under-and-over turntable.
8. Use eluted phage to infect log phase *E. coli* TG1 cells that are then plated onto plates containing 2xTYE, 15 μg/mL tetracycline.

9. Determine phage titer by infecting log phase *E. coli* TG1 cells with serial dilutions of the eluted phage (see Note 12).
10. Grow plates at 37°C overnight.
11. After overnight growth, add 2 mL of 2xTY with 15% glycerol to the plates and loosen cells with a glass spreader and then mix thoroughly. Fifty microliters of the scraped bacteria are inoculated into 50 mL of 2xTY containing 15 μg/mL tetracycline and 1 mL stored at −70°C in 15% glycerol.
12. Grow the 50 mL culture overnight at 37°C, with shaking.
13. Centrifuge the overnight culture at 3,300×*g* for 15 min to pellet the bacteria.
14. The bacterial pellet is used to isolate DNA using plasmid Midi Prep kit.

3.12. CDR Reamplification and Reassembly of the Final Library

1. Set up PCRs to reamplify CDR1+2 and CDR3 regions of the VH and Vκ libraries selected on Protein A/L. The combinations of oligonucleotides used for these amplifications are summarized below.

	Oligo pair	
Amplification required	**Forward**	**Reverse**
Vκ CDR1+2	DOM172	DOM170
Vκ CDR3	DOM175	DOM173
VH CDR1+2	DOM172	DOM166
VH CDR3	DOM174	DOM173

2. PCR mixes are made up and PCRs carried out using template DNA as described previously (see Subheadings 3.2 and 3.11).
3. Purify PCR products as described previously (see Subheading 3.3).
4. Perform PCR assembly as described previously (see Subheading 3.4) with exception that a two way SOE PCR is required at this stage using CDR1+2 and CDR3 fragments.
5. Repeat steps described in Subheadings 3.5, 3.6, 3.7, 3.8, and 3.9 to create final VH and Vκ libraries in excess of 10^{10} clones (see Tables 1 and 2).

3.13. Analysis of dAb/gIII Display Levels

To determine the efficiency of display levels polyclonal phage is prepared from the final VH and Vκ libraries (as described in Subheading 3.10) and subjected to SDS-PAGE followed by Western blotting and detection using anti-pIII antibody (see Fig. 5).

1. Denature purified phage samples by mixing with NuPAGE LDS sample buffer, NuPAGE sample reduction agent and

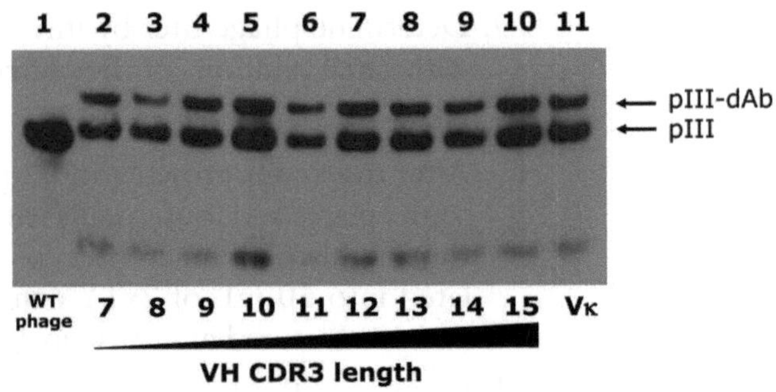

Fig. 5. Western blot analysis of dAb phage libraries. Approximately 10^{10} phage particles were loaded per lane and detected with anti-coat protein III antibody. Lane 1, wild-type Fd phage; lane 2–10: VH H1-VH H9 phage; lane 11, Vκ phage. The amount of dAb-pIII fusion protein is approximately 25% compared to pIII protein indicating that the majority of phage carries a dAb (each phage has 3–5 copies of pIII). For comparison, only 1–5% of phage particles produced from phagemid vectors carry an antibody fusion (15).

heating at 70°C for 10 min. Ideally, 1×10^{10} phage should be loaded onto each lane of the gel.

2. Load denatured samples onto NuPAGE 4–12% Bis-Tris gel. The gel is run in a *X*Cell SureLock Electrophoresis Cell. Two hundred milliliters of MES running buffer containing 500 μL of the NuPAGE antioxidant is added to the inner buffer chamber and 600 mL of running buffer is added to the outer buffer chamber. The gel is run at 200 V for 35 min.
3. Blot the electrophoresed gel onto PVDF membrane using *X*Cell II Blot Module in methanol/NuPAGE transfer Buffer at 30 V for 1 h. Ten percent methanol in NuPAGE transfer buffer is used for single gel-transfer and 20% methanol in NuPAGE transfer buffer is required for double gel-transfer to ensure even and efficient transfer.
4. Block the membrane with an excess volume of 5% MPBS overnight at 4°C with gentle rocking.
5. Incubate the membrane with 20 mL of a 1:20,000 dilution of anti-pIII (g3p) antibody in 5% MPBS for 1 h at room temperature with shaking.
6. Wash the membrane three times with 20 mL of 0.2% TPBS for 10 min per wash.
7. Incubate the blot with 20 mL of a 1:10,000 dilution of HRP conjugated goat-anti-mouse IgG (Fc-specific) in 5% MPBS for 1 h at room temperature with shaking.
8. Wash the blot four times with 20 mL of 0.2% TPBS for 10 min per wash.
9. Dry the blot gently by touching the corner onto clean tissue and develop using the ECL Plus Western Blotting Detection Reagents following manufacturers' instructions on Hyperfilm ECL.

4. Notes

1. As large quantities of primary PCR products will be required for the subsequent PCR assemblies, it is recommended to set up at least 4 × 50 μL PCRs per CDR.
2. Template DNA should be kept to a minimum to avoid its presence in the final library. About 10 pg to 1 ng of template should be used per reaction. A good starting point is to set up reactions with 1 μL of a 1:1,000 dilution of the parental miniprep DNA.
3. *Taq* polymerase is added after the initial denaturation step (HotStart PCR). This results in more specific amplification.
4. *Dpn* I cleaves only when its restriction site is methylated. It will therefore only cleave DNA purified from dam + strain (TG1, HB2151, etc.) and therefore reduce the contamination of parental template DNA in the library. *Dpn* I will digests efficiently in the presence of most buffers used for PCR.
5. Assembly PCR (also known as "pull-through") or SOE (splicing by overlap extension) allows the three primary PCR products (CDR1, CDR2, and CDR3) to be brought together without digest or ligation, making use of their complementary ends. During this process the three primary products are brought together and denatured and their complementary ends are allowed to anneal together in the presence of Taq polymerase and dNTPs. Several cycles of reannealing and extension result in fill-in of the complementary strands and the production of a full-length library template. Primers that flank the now full-length dAb cassette are then added and a conventional PCR program initiated to amplify the assembled product. It is important that equimolar amounts of the primary PCR products are used for the assembly reaction. These primary PCR products have to be quantified using $OD_{260\ nm}$.
6. DOM172 and DOM173 are biotinylated primers that should be used during assembly PCR to allow easy postdigest cleanup.
7. Electroporation conditions are 2.5 kV, 25 μF and 200 Ω.
8. Test ligations may be run on a 1.2% agarose gel to check ligation efficiency. Controls on the gel should include cut and uncut vector and insert.
9. High background signals can be observed when detecting protein A binding phage. This can be about 10–20% of the foreground signal and is due to a small proportion of protein A binding Igs in the sheep antiserum. Low background signal will be observed when detecting protein L binding phage.
10. One Amicom 50 K column should be used per 500 μL of ligation—the volume should be made up to 500 μL if some loss occurs during phenol–chloroform steps.

11. The $OD_{600\ nm}$ immediately following inoculation should never exceed 0.1 to allow growth of the library. To achieve this, typically 5×10^{10} cells are grown in 2 L of 2xTY medium.

12. The eluted phage titer is determined by preparing a tenfold dilution series of the phage stock from 10^{-1} to 10^{-8} in sterile PBS. This is achieved by adding 10 μL of eluted phage to 90 μL of PBS in a microtiter plate and mixing by pipetting (this is the 10^{-1} dilution). Ten microliters of the phage dilution is then added to the next 90 μL of PBS using fresh tips, mixed by pipetting (creating the 10^{-2} dilution), and repeated down to a dilution of 10^{-8}. Ten microliters from each dilution is then mixed with 90 μL of log phase *E. coli* TG1 that has been pre-dispensed in a microtiter plate and incubated, covered with a lid, for 30–45 min at 37°C in an air incubator. Ten microliters from each infection is spotted onto dried TYE plates containing 15 μg/mL tetracyclin (several spots can be added to an individual TYE plate). As a control, 10 μL of uninfected *E. coli* TG1 must be spotted. Incubate the plates overnight at 37°C.

    The number of phage (from 1 mL) is determined by:
    Number of colonies in a spot × dilution factor ($10–10^8$) × 10 (10 μL from dilution used to infect 90 μL of *E. coli*) × 100 (10 μL eluted phage used).

Acknowledgements

The authors were all employees of Domantis Ltd at the time this work was carried out. dAb™ and Domain Antibody™ are all registered trademarks in the name of Domantis Limited.

References

1. Enever C et al (2009) Next generation immunotherapeutics-honing the magic bullet. Curr Opin Biotechnol 20:405–411
2. Sheets MD et al (1998) Efficient construction of a large nonimmune phage antibody library: the production of high-affinity human single-chain antibodies to protein antigens. Proc Natl Acad Sci U S A 95:6157–6162
3. Vaughan TJ et al (1996) Human antibodies with sub-nanomolar affinities isolated from a large non-immunized phage display library. Nat Biotechnol 14:309–314
4. Griffiths AD et al (1994) Isolation of high affinity human antibodies directly from large synthetic repertoires. EMBO J 13:3245–3260
5. de Wildt RMT et al (1999) Analysis of heavy and light chain pairings indicates that receptor editing shapes the human antibody repertoire. J Mol Biol 285:895–901
6. de Wildt RMT et al (2000) Antibody arrays for high-throughput screening of antibody-antigen interactions. Nat Biotechnol 18:989–994
7. Ewert S et al (2003) Biophysical properties of human antibody variable domains. J Mol Biol 325:531–553
8. Graille M et al (2000) Crystal structure of a *Staphylococcus aureus* protein A domain complexed with the Fab fragment of a human IgM antibody: structural basis for recognition of B-cell receptors and superantigen activity. Proc Natl Acad Sci USA 97: 5399–5404
9. Potter KN, Li Y, Pascual V, Capra JD (1997) Staphylococcal protein A binding to VH3

encoded immunoglobulins. Int Rev Immunol 14:291–308
10. Bjorck L (1988) Protein L. A novel bacterial cell wall protein with affinity for Ig L chains. J Immunol 140:1194–1197
11. Graille M et al (2001) Complex between *Peptostreptococcus magnus* protein L and a human antibody reveals structural convergence in the interaction modes of Fab binding proteins. Structure (Camb) 9:679–687
12. Tomlinson IM et al (1996) The imprint of somatic hypermutation on the repertoire of human germline V genes. J Mol Biol 256:813–817
13. Kabat EA, Wu TT (1971) Attempts to locate complementarity-determining residues in the variable positions of light and heavy chains. Ann N Y Acad Sci 190:382–393
14. Wu TT, Kabat EA (1970) An analysis of the sequences of the variable regions of Bence Jones proteins and myeloma light chains and their implications for antibody complementarity. J Exp Med 132:211–250
15. O'Connell D et al (2002) Phage versus phagemid libraries for generation of human monoclonal antibodies. J Mol Biol 321: 49–56

Chapter 5

Preparation of a Naïve Library of Camelid Single Domain Antibodies

Aurelien Olichon and Ario de Marco

Abstract

The preparation of antibody libraries starting from lymphocytes recovered from immunized members of the *Camelidae* enables to collect binders that underwent somatic maturation. However, the time and costs necessary to prepare a library for each new antigen may urge to look for alternatives such as those offered by large one-pot libraries. Here we describe how to obtain a suitable naïve library using material from nonimmunized llamas. Despite the lack of somatic maturation, the selection based on phage display allowed to isolate from such naïve libraries VHHs with affinity in the subnanomolar range and suitable for the standard immunoapplications.

Key words: Competitive elution, Nanobody, One-pot library, Panning, Recombinant antibodies, Somatic maturation, VHH

1. Introduction

The preparation of naïve libraries does not significantly differ from the protocol otherwise used for recovering immune libraries (1). Their specificity is that they are one-pot collections (2) from which it is possible directly fishing out the desired reagents and this opportunity allows saving the time and costs related to preparing a new library for any new project. On the other side, the lack of somatic maturation stimulated in vivo by repeated immunization makes the antibody collection, by definition, unspecific. This means that there should be no preferred antigen for any antibody subpopulations and that the selection of suitable binders will happen randomly. Consequently it is necessary to create large libraries in terms of diversity to increase the chance of identifying at least one antibody with the requested features of specificity for any given antigen.

In practical terms, the theoretical diversity and, therefore, potential utility of a naive library increases with the number of

Dirk Saerens and Serge Muyldermans (eds.), *Single Domain Antibodies: Methods and Protocols*, Methods in Molecular Biology, vol. 911, DOI 10.1007/978-1-61779-968-6_5, © Springer Science+Business Media, LLC 2012

animals and lymphocytes initially collected. Furthermore, all the steps necessary to clone the library should be performed with the highest care to avoid material loss, a drawback that leads to diversity reduction. Since a reliable naïve library has the potentialities for being a long-lasting tool, it is worthy to make an extra effort during its preparation for preserving the largest genetic diversity. However, for practical reasons related to material handling, it is not feasible to start with blood samples larger than 1 L without risking of compromising the accuracy of each library preparation step. As an alternative, it could be more beneficial increasing the final library size by mixing independently prepared collections.

In the following protocol, the critical steps are commented with appropriate notes and the characteristics of the naïve libraries prepared in our groups using llama lymphocytes are critically discussed. Finally, the specific panning conditions and binder applications are illustrated taking examples from the lab praxis.

2. Materials

Prepare all solutions using Millipore-filtered water and analytical grade reagents. Prepare and store all reagents at room temperature (unless indicated otherwise). Use Millipore-filtered water in all experiments.

2.1. Lymphocyte Isolation

1. 1 L of blood, possibly collected from several naïve animals (for instance, 50 mL of blood from 20 different young animals).
2. 2% Sodium citrate plus 1.8% dextrose or 2% EDTA solubilized in Tris acetate, pH 8.0, as anticoagulant.
3. Lymphoprep (Axis-Shield, Dundee, UK) or Ficoll-Paque PLUS (GE Healthcare, Pollards Wood, UK) kits.
4. Centrifuge and 50 × 25 mL tubes.

2.2. RNA Extraction and cDNA Preparation

1. MilliQ H_2O.
2. Nucleospin RNA II (Machery-Nagel, Düren, Germany).
3. Oligo(dT) 12–18 primers (Invitrogen, Carlsbad, CA, USA).
4. Random primers (Invitrogen, Carlsbad, CA, USA).
5. RNAse OUT ribonuclease inhibitor (Invitrogen, Carlsbad, CA, USA).
6. 10 mM dNTPs in MilliQ H_2O.
7. Diethylpyrocarbonate (DEPC) water. It was prepared dissolving 1 mL of DEPC into 1 L of MilliQ H_2O. The solution was mixed overnight at room temperature and autoclaved before use.

8. Agarose.
9. Superscript III reverse transcriptase (Invitrogen, Carlsbad, CA, USA).
10. Bench centrifuge with adaptors for 96-well plates.
11. Vortex.
12. Spectrophotometer with cuvettes for measuring volumes of 1 μL.
13. Multichannel micropipettes.
14. Electrophoresis cuvette for agarose gels, ideally adapted to multichannel pipette loading.

2.3. VHH Amplification: PCR1

1. 100 μM Universal primers for VHH region amplification, in MilliQ H_2O
   CaLl 01 (GTC.CTG.GCT.GCT.CTT.CTA.CAA.GG) and CaLl 02 (GGT.ACG.TGC.TGT.TGA.ACT.GTT.CC).
2. Homemade Taq polymerase.
3. Polymerase buffer 10× (Fermentas, St. Leon-Roth, Germany).
4. 10 mM dNTPs in MilliQ H_2O.
5. DMSO.
6. 3.6 M Betaine in MilliQ H_2O.
7. MilliQ H_2O.
8. Qiaquick gel extraction kit (Qiagen, Hilden, Germany).
9. PCR thermal cycler.

2.4. VHH Amplification: PCR2 and PCR3

1. 100 μM VHH P1 primer, HPLC purification grade: CCAGCCGGCCATGGCTGA**K**GT**B**CAGCTGGTGGAGTCTGG (see Note 1).
2. 100 μM VHH P2 primer, HPLC purification grade: GGACTAGTGCGGCCGCGTGAGGAGACGGTGACC**W**GGGT.
3. 50 μM VHH for2 primer, HPLC purification grade: AACATGCCATGACTCGCGGCTCAACCGG<u>CCATGG</u>CTGA**K**GT**B**CAG<u>CTGCAG</u>GC GTCTGG**R**GGAGG (*Nco*I and *Pst*I recognition sites are underlined) (see Note 2).
4. 50 μM VHH rev2 primer, HPLC purification grade: GTTATTATTATTCAGATTATTAGT<u>GCGGCCGC</u>TGGAGACGGTGACC**W**GGGTCC (*Not*I recognition site is underlined).
5. Homemade Taq polymerase.
6. Polymerase buffer 10× (Fermentas, St. Leon-Roth, Germany).
7. 10 mM dNTPs in MilliQ H_2O.

8. DMSO.
9. 3.6 M Betaine in MilliQ H_2O.
10. MilliQH_2O.
11. Qiaquick gel extraction kit (Qiagen, Hilden, Germany).
12. 96-Well PCR plates with lid.
13. PCR thermal cycler.
14. Bench centrifuge with adaptors for 96-well plates.
15. Multichannel micropipettes.

2.5. Preparation of DNA Inserts and Vector and Subsequent Ligation

1. Phenol.
2. 24:1 v/v chloroform–isoamylalcohol solution.
3. Ethanol.
4. TE buffer: 10 mM Tris–HCl, 1 mM EDTA, pH 8.0.
5. Acetate buffer: 3 M Na acetate, pH 5.2.
6. Round-bottom glass (Schott, Mainz, Germany) or clear polypropylene tubes (35 mL, Nalgene, Roskilde, Denmark).
7. *Pst*I, *Nco*I, *Not*I restriction enzymes plus corresponding buffers.
8. QIAquick (Qiagen, Hilden, Germany) or Nucleospin Extract II (Macherey Nagel, Düren, Germany) purification kit.
9. MilliQ water.
10. pHEN4 vector with a staffer sequence larger than 1.2 kbp between *Pst*I and *Not*I restriction sites.
11. Quick ligase kit (Fermentas, St. Leon-Rot, Germany).

2.6. Transformation and Library Recovery

1. Electrocompetent TG1 cells.
2. TYE medium: 16 g Bacto Tryptone (Difco, Sparks, MD, USA), 10 g Bacto Yeast Extract (Difco, Sparks, MD, USA), 5 g NaCl, MilliQ H_2O to 1 L. Autoclave to sterilize.
3. Solid TYE medium: TYE medium plus 15 g Bacto agar (Difco, Sparks, MD, USA). Autoclave to sterilize, cool down to 55°C, add 100 mg/L ampicillin and 1% w/v sterile glucose.
4. SOC medium: 20 g Bacto tryptone, 5 g Bacto yeast extract, 0.5 g NaCl, 2.5 mL KCl 1 M, MilliQH_2O to 1 L. Adjust the pH to 7.0 with NaOH, autoclave to sterilize and add 20 mL of 1 M sterile glucose.
5. Electroporator system.
6. Large square dishes (500 cm^2).
7. Scrapers.
8. LB medium: 10 g Bacto tryptone, 5 g Bacto yeast extract, 10 g NaCl, add MilliQH_2O to 1 L and adjust the pH to 7.0. Autoclave and add 50% glycerol.

2.7. Library Evaluation

1. 100 μM M13rev primer, desalted: 5′-CAGGAAACAGCTATG ACC-3′.
2. 100 μM pHen4rev primer, desalted: 5′-CAACTTTCAACAG TCTATGC-3′.
3. Restriction enzyme *Hinf*I.

3. Methods

3.1. Lymphocyte Isolation

1. Immediately add an anticoagulant (see Subheading 2.1, item 2) to the blood recovered from the animals.
2. Recover the lymphocytes by gradient separation according to the manufacturers' instructions (see Note 3). Consider that 1 L blood can yield up to 2×10^9 lymphocytes and that 50 tubes could be necessary for this step.

3.2. RNA Extraction and cDNA Preparation

1. Load Lymphocytes on Nucleospin RNA II columns to recover total RNA. Load an amount of 5×10^7 cells onto each column (40 columns total for an initial yield of 2×10^9 lymphocytes) and perform the extraction according to the manufacturer's instructions. Keep eluted total RNA from each column separated to minimize the loss of diversity in the next amplification steps due to mix of large amount of material with very variable efficiency for PCR reaction.
2. Determine RNA concentration by measuring the absorbance at 260 nm. An $OD_{260\ nm}$ value of 1 corresponds to 40 μg/mL of total RNA. The expected yields are 500–600 μg/column in a volume of 500 μL (approximately 1 μg/μL).
3. Check RNA integrity by running a sample of 2 μg on an agarose gel. All the material must be RNase free to avoid degradation during the run.
4. Verify the success of the reverse transcriptase reaction first by using 0.5 μg of total RNA (0.5 μL of an elution fraction) (see Note 4). Use the resulting cDNA as a template for amplifying the VHH domains (see Subheading 3.3) and control the final PCR product after its run on an agarose gel (see Fig. 1).
5. Scale-up the reverse transcriptase reaction, after having successfully accomplished previous step (see Subheading 3.2, item 4) is. Use each RNA sample separately at three RNA concentrations (0.5, 1, and 2 μg) and in duplicate with both sets of primers (Oligo(dT) 12–18 and random primers) (see Note 5). The reaction mixtures are, respectively: (a) 1 μL Oligo(dT) 12–18 primers (0.5 μg/μL), 1 μL dNTPs (10 mM), 8 μL ddH_2O, 0.5, and 1, or 2 μL template RNA; (b) 0.2 μL random primers (3 μg/μL), 1 μL dNTPs (10 mM), 8.5 μL ddH_2O, and 0.5, 1,

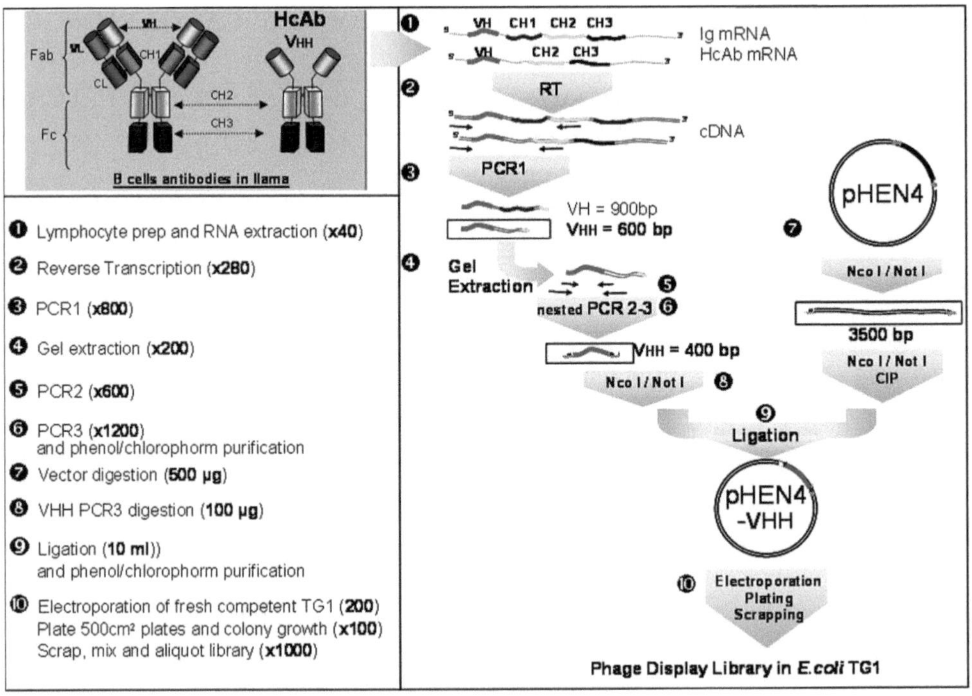

Fig. 1. Schematic representation of the protocol steps. *Top left*: Schematic structure of conventional and heavy chain antibodies produced in llama lymphocytes (B cells). *Bottom left*: summary of the major protocol steps. *Right panel*: (1) Lymphocytes from Ficoll-Paque™ gradient are isolated and RNA is extracted; (2) cDNA is produced by reverse transcription (RT) using random primers; (3) PCR1 amplification is performed starting from the CH2 domain of IgG cDNA and leads to 900 and 600 bp products corresponding to VHs and VHHs, respectively; (4) The VHH-specific PCR1 product is extracted from the gel; (5) The VHH domain sequences are amplified with PCR2; (6) The restriction sites *Nco*I, *Pst*I and *Not*I are introduced with the nested PCR3; (7) pHEN4 phagemid vector is first digested *Nco*I (or *Pst*I)-*Not*I and then dephosphorylated; (8) The PCR3 products are purified and digested *NcoI* (or *Pst*I)-*Not*I; (9) PCR3 VHHs are ligated into the digested pHEN4; (10) The resulting ligation product is transformed into freshly prepared electrocompetent TG1 bacteria and plated on 2XTY agar plates containing ampicillin and 1% glucose. After overnight growth at 30°C, colonies are scrapped, pooled, 50% glycerol is added and the library aliquots are stored at –80°C.

or 2 µL template RNA. Denature RNA by heating 5 min at 65°C, then transfer the tubes to 0°C and incubated 5 min before adding of the cDNA synthesis mix: RT buffer 10× (2 µL), 25 mM $MgCl_2$ (4 µL), RNAse OUT (1 µL), DTT 0.1 M (2 µL), and Superscript III reverse transcriptase (1 µL). Only the tubes containing the random hexamers plates needs an extra incubation (10 min at 25°C) before starting the cDNA synthesis reaction (50 min at 50°C) followed by enzymatic denaturation (5 min at 85°C) and RNA removal (20 min at 37°C) in the presence of 1 µL RNase. Store the cDNA at –20°C.

3.3. VHH Amplification: PCR1

Three different amounts (2, 5, and 10 µL) of each one of the cDNA samples will be used as templates for the PCR reaction aimed at amplifying the common VH-VHH sequence spanning between the conserved CH2 domain and the leader region (see Note 5).

1. Perform the PCR reactions in a total volume of 40 μL: 4 μL polymerase buffer 10×, 0.3 μL primer CaLl1, 0.3 μL primer CaLl2, 1 μL dNTPs, 0.4 μL DMSO, 13.5 μL betaine, 1 μL Taq polymerase, cDNA (2, 5, or 10 μL), and ddH_2O to reach the final volume.
2. Set the reaction conditions at: 5 min at 94°C, 22 cycles of (1 min at 94°C, 90 s at 52°C, 85 s at 72°C), 10 min at 72°C, cooling at 4°C.
3. Check the PCR1 products by means of a 2% agarose gel. Two distinct bands corresponding to VHs and VHHs should be clearly visible at 850–900 and 550–600 bp, respectively. Cut out the band corresponding to VHHs (lower band at 550–600 bp) and purify with a gel extraction kit eluting the DNA in water. It is possible to pool four PCR1 products obtained using comparable conditions and to purify them together. This procedure will allow reducing the total sample number to process in the next steps.

3.4. VHH Amplification: PCR2 and PCR3

In this double PCR step the VHH sequences are specifically amplified by using primers that anneal to the conserved regions of the frameworks 1 and 4 of the variable domain and, at the same time, the sequences recognized by the restriction enzymes *Nco*I, *Pst*I, and *Not*I are introduced for enabling the successive cloning in the pHEN4 phagemid vector.

1. Set the conditions for the nested PCR reactions using a linear gradient of template (0.5, 1, 2, 4, 8 μL of PCR1 product) for PCR2 and vary the cycle number of both PCR2 and PCR3 (8–12 cycles). The outcome of the PCR2 reaction could be too diluted to be visible in a 2% agarose gel and, therefore, it is directly used for the PCR3 and only this second product is analyzed (see Note 6). Determine the optimal cycle number.
2. Use 2, 4 and 6 μL of PCR1 product as a template and run the PCR2 amplification in a total volume of 40 μL: 4 μL polymerase buffer 10×, 0.075 μL primer VHH P1, 0.075 μL primer VHH P2, 1 μL dNTPs, 0.4 μL DMSO, 13.5 μL betaine, 1 μL Taq polymerase, PCR1 template (2, 5, or 10 μL), and ddH_2O to reach the final volume.
3. Set the PCR2 reaction conditions at 5 min at 95°C, 8–10 cycles of (30 s at 94°C, 30 s at 52°C, 60 s at 72°C), 10 min at 72°C, cooling at 4°C.
4. Use the PCR2 products as templates (0.5 and 2 μL) for the PCR3 amplification and the VHHfor2 and VHHrev2 primers in a total volume of 40 μL: 4 μL polymerase buffer 10×, 0.25 μL primer VHHfor2, 0.25 μL primer VHHrev2, 1.2 μL dNTPs, 0.5 μL DMSO, 13.5 μL betaine, 1 μL Taq polymerase, PCR1 template (2, 5, or 10 μL), and ddH_2O to reach the final volume.

5. Set the PCR3 conditions at 5 min at 95°C, 12 cycles of (50 s at 94°C, ramp to 55°C at 0.3°C/s, 30 s at 55°C, ramp to 72°C at 0.5°C/s, 60 s at 72°C), 10 min at 72°C, cooling at 4°C (see Note 6).
6. Analyze one PCR3 product for each experimental condition after separation on a 2% agarose gel. DNA corresponding to VHH sequences has roughly 400 bp.
7. Purify the band using a gel extraction kit according to the manufacturer's instructions.

3.5. Preparation of DNA Insert and Vector and Subsequent Ligation

The PCR products must be digested and inserted in the phagemid vector pHEN4. Two digestion combinations are possible, namely two libraries can be created cloned *Nco*I-*Not*I and *Pst*I-*Not*I, respectively (see Note 7).

1. Purify the remaining PCR3 products by phenol–chloroform extraction and ethanol precipitation to obtain highly pure material and maximize the ligation yields.
2. Pool the PCR3 products (35–50 mL) and quantify the DNA by running a sample on a 2% agarose gel. Purify the band of the sample.
3. Under a fume hood, add phenol to the DNA fraction (1:1 v/v) in a round bottom glass or polypropylene tube, vortex and centrifuge the tubes 10 min at 20,500 × *g*.
4. Transfer the upper phases to fresh tubes.
5. Add TE buffer (1:1 volumes) to the lower phase, vortex, centrifuge the tubes 10 min at 20,500 × *g*, and transfer the upper phases to fresh tubes. This step should allow recovering any DNA still present in the phenol fraction.
6. Prepare a chloroform–isoamylalcohol solution (24:1 v/v) and add it to the recovered aqueous phases (1:1 v/v). Vortex and centrifuge the tubes 10 min at 20,500 × *g*.
7. Transfer the upper phases to fresh 13 mL polypropylene tubes.
8. Precipitate the DNA by adding 3 M Na acetate, pH 5.2 (1:10 v/v, in average 0.2 mL), and 100% ethanol (2.5:1 v/v, in average 5 mL). After having vigorously mixed, store the tubes overnight at −80°C.
9. Centrifuge 30 min at 20,500 × *g*, mark the tube area in which the pellet should accumulate, discard the supernatant, and dry the tube (see Note 8).
10. Recover the DNA from the pellet identified by the marked area by gently rinsing with 1 mL of 80% ethanol (see Note 9).

11. Transfer the DNA into an eppendorf tube and centrifuge 10 min at 20,500 × *g*.
12. Wash the pellet with 70% ethanol and let dry.
13. Resuspend the DNA in 1 mL of MilliQ water and quantify the yield.
14. Digest two aliquots of 100 μg of DNA (more than 10^{13} molecules) in a total volume of 1 mL, one using *Pst*I-*Not*I restriction enzymes, the second in the presence of *Nco*I-*Not*I (see Note 7).
15. Run a 2% agarose gel and purify the digested inserts using a standard kit.
16. Produce 1 mg of pHEN4 vector and digest two aliquots of 500 μg, one using *Pst*I-*Not*I restriction enzymes, the second in the presence of *Nco*I-*Not*I (see Note 10).
17. Ligation conditions should be tested in small scale using a Quick ligase kit, three insert/vector molar ratios and the vector alone as a control for self-ligation. Electroporate the ligation products in TG1 cells, culture the bacteria in SOC medium and plate at different dilutions on TYE dishes (see Subheading 3.6). This step is aimed at: (a) identifying the optimal fragment/vector molar ration to use for the large scale ligation and transformation; (b) controlling the homogeneity of the cloned inserts; (c) estimating the library dimension and diversity (see Note 11).
18. Once defined the optimal ligation conditions, incubate the corresponding DNA amounts of double digested vector and inserts (indicatively, 60 μg of the vector and 50 μg of the insert) in the presence of ligase buffer and 500 units of T4 DNA ligase in a total volume of 10 mL. Incubate 1 h at 24°C and overnight at 16°C before inactivating the enzyme by heating 10 min at 70°C. Cool down to room temperature, purify the DNA using the phenol–chloroform protocol (see Subheading 3.5, items 3–12), and resuspend it in 800 μL of MilliQ water.

3.6. Transformation and Library Recovery

1. Prepare 200 aliquots of 4 μL each of the purified ligation product and chill the tubes on ice.
2. Add 65 μL of freshly prepared electrocompetent TG1 cells and transfer to electroporation cuvettes.
3. Set the electroporator at 200 Ω, 2.5 kV, and 25 μF.
4. Transform and immediately add 950 μL of SOC medium prewarmed at 40°C to the cuvette, then transfer to culture tubes.
5. Incubate the cultures 1 h at 37°C under constant shaking.

6. Pool all samples (200–220 mL). In duplicate, take an aliquot of 20 μL, perform serial dilutions and plate on dishes prepared with TYE medium plus ampicillin and 1% glucose (TYEAG). The colonies grown using bacteria from the successive dilutions will be counted for estimating the library size. It should be around 10^9–10^{10}.
7. Prepare 100 Nunclon large square dishes (500 cm^2) with TYEAG and prewarm them at 37°C before plating 2.2 mL on each dish.
8. Incubate the plates overnight at 30°C (see Note 12).
9. Add 10 mL of TYE medium to each plate and thoroughly scrap the bacterial colonies. Repeat the step using further 10 mL of TYE medium.
10. Pool all the bacterial suspensions (volume >2 L), mix accurately for 10 min, and centrifuge 20 min at 660×*g*.
11. Discard the supernatant and wash the bacteria by resuspending the pellets in 200 mL of TYE.
12. Centrifuge 20 min at 660×*g*, discard the supernatant, and resuspend the pellets into 650 mL of LB medium+50% glycerol.
13. Measure the $OD_{600\ nm}$ of the suspension and calculate the bacterial concentration. Accordingly, prepare aliquots that have a number of cells 5–15 times higher than the library size and flash-freeze in liquid nitrogen (see Note 13).
14. Store the library aliquots at −80°C (see Note 14).

3.7. Library Evaluation

1. Evaluate the functional dimension of the library. For analyzing religation and insertion of contaminant DNA, pick-up 190 random colonies from the dishes used for estimating the library size (see Subheading 3.6, item 6) and use them for colony PCR (see Note 11) to detect the presence of inserts corresponding to the single domain variable region (400–450 bp). Add positive and negative TG1 controls to fill two PCR plates.
2. For estimating the total diversity, digest 192 colony PCR products with *HinfI*, compare the digestion patterns separating the samples in a 2% agarose gel, and sequence the clones sharing the same pattern (see Note 15).
3. For evaluating the effective expression capability of the selected clones, grow 50 colonies with inserts of the correct size in LB medium at 28°C until the $OD_{600\ nm}$ reaches 0.6, induce the recombinant expression with 1 mM IPTG and collect the bacteria after 16 h. Recover the periplasmic fractions by osmotic shock and detect the presence of HA-tagged VHH fragments by dot blot or Western blot (see Note 16 and Note 17).

4. Notes

1. Degenerated nucleotides have been used to cope with natural sequence variability. R is for A+G, K for G+T, W for A+T, and B for G+T+C.
2. Long 5′ extensions have been used since they improve significantly the digestion yields.
3. The two most used kits for lymphocyte recovery have been recently compared and they assure similar results in terms of composition and quantity of yielded cells (3). Lymhocytes should be aliquoted, pelleted, and flash-frozen in liquid nitrogen before being stored at minus 80°C.
4. The standard protocols for recombinant antibody library preparation usually consider a step for mRNA purification before starting the reverse transcriptase step. We preferred to skip on this procedure for the reason that any protocol passage can potentially be detrimental for maintaining the initial diversity.
5. It means a total of 480 reaction tubes whether 40 RNA samples were initially collected from 2×10^9 lymphocytes. In the lab praxis, however, the lymphocyte yield per liter of blood is lower than the optimal and, consequently, all the numbers are lower than the theoretical values. Anyhow, in our experience 240–360 samples are collected at the cDNA preparation step and it means 720–1,080 PCR-1 products, with random primers that give better results. This might be explained because VHH domains are encoded by 5′ coding sequences that are distant from the polyA tail.
6. It must be underlined that this step is crucial since it must yield enough material for the final ligation, but the PCR cycles should be limited to avoid overamplification of a limited number of sequences structurally more suitable for replication. In other words, the total diversity will strongly depend on the accuracy of this double amplification step.

   For estimating the optimal PCR cycle number, two parameters must be considered. First, the amount of final PCR3 products obtained using increasing amounts of template in PCR2 should increase linearly. Among conditions that accomplish to this requisite, select the one that assure higher DNA yields. Remember that PCR1 products have been produced by cDNA at different concentrations and, therefore, their own concentrations can significantly vary. Therefore, the necessary cycle number in PCR2 usually changes according to the amount of DNA (PCR1 products) used as a template. In our experience, PCR2 needs ten amplification cycles when the PCR1 templates were generated starting from 2 μL of cDNA, whereas eight amplification cycles are sufficient for PCR1 templates yielded starting from 5 and 10 μL of cDNA.

7. The PCR3 products have long extensions optimized for elevated digestion efficiency using either *Nco*I or *Pst*I. Cloning two independent libraries avoids the loss of VHH clones with internal *Nco*I or *Pst*I sites. VHHs cloned using the *Pst*I share with *Nco*I-cloned VHHs the sequence upstream of the cloning site but can be subcloned using either *Pst*I or *Nco*I. Furthermore, the *Pst*I–*Not*I combination can be exploited to obtain bivalent constructs (4, 5) whilst the *Nco*I–*Not*I restriction sites can be used to direct subcloning into recently developed expression vectors ((6, 7); see Chapter 32). This ease in transferring VHH coding regions results is a clear advantage when selected binders must be produced as recombinant proteins for specific applications.
8. Some DNA may be still present in the supernatant after centrifugation. Therefore, a high-speed centrifugation step can be undertaken for precipitating the remaining DNA from the supernatant fraction recovered after the first centrifugation.
9. DNA is transparent. Consequently, visible pellets are due to salt precipitation and are indicative of poor quality. Marking the area in which the pellet should accumulate (the part of the tube bottom that lays down when the tube is inserted in the rotor) facilitates the blind DNA resuspension using limited solution volumes.
10. The preparation of the host vector is a standard technique. However, the amount of material needed for the ligation of two libraries largely exceeds the norm. We advise to start very soon during library preparation to produce and digest the vector. The linearized plasmid should not self-ligate. Self-ligation resulting in a number of colonies higher than 10% of the positive control needs a further step of digestion and purification. Once having carefully set this parameter, the ready-to-use plasmid can be stored at –20°C.
11. Religation can be estimated indirectly, by comparing the number of the colonies between control and transformed plates, or directly, analyzing by colony PCR the percentage of clones containing the insert amplified by the primers M13rev and pHen4rev. This control will also enable to detect the presence of recombined sequences of wrong size that would indicate suboptimal PCR conditions.

    The library overall size can be evaluated by the number of colonies present on dishes plated with repeated dilutions of the transformation output. Library diversity can be estimated by *HinfI* digestion of the PCR products and successive sequencing of the clones sharing the same pattern.

12. Large plates can easily overdry specially when incubated in ventilated shakers. Keep the necessary moisture by adding a large bucket filled with water or wrap the plates with parafilm.
13. It is important to have any sequence represented at least once in each aliquot. Since the PCR efficiency with templates having different sequences may significantly vary and casual losses may happen during other steps such as electroporation and library recovery, it is important to increase the chances of preserving the complete library representation by assuring a total cell size in excess with respect to that theoretically calculated.
14. Due to the larger amounts of materials needed, naïve libraries are more labor-intensive and expensive to prepare than conventional libraries. However, the effort is limited (approximately 30–50% of overcosts), considering that the library can be used for tens of projects.
15. The protocol used for library preparation should assure the presence of only sequences corresponding to VHH. However, we identified (8) several clones with the VH hallmarks (9) and further experiments have been undertaken to understand this apparently incongruence.
16. We used the protocol proposed by Skerra and Plückthun (10). Although the statistical significance of these analyses is insufficient due to the low number of samples considered with respect to the library global dimension, the result of these tests remains a necessary tool for validating the total functional diversity of the library. A value >95% should result from this calculation.
17. There are some details to consider when panning with naïve libraries. The first is that the initial number of potential binders for an antigen will be lower than in an immune library since the antibodies present in naïve libraries do not undergo, for definition, somatic maturation and, therefore, cannot evolve into a population with improved binding features for a specific antigen. However, the effectiveness of antibodies selected from naive libraries has been recently confirmed by experiments performed using a yeast-display VHH nonimmune collection (11) and it is possible selecting binders with affinity in the subnanomolar range (8). Furthermore, avidity could be significantly improved by cloning solutions that favor molecule dimerization (7).

The recent discovery of a new class of single-domain antibodies (12) could further contribute to increase the diversity of naive libraries since the simple addition of a PCR amplification step using specific primers for the promiscuous VH(4) domains present in *Camelidae* would allow the integration of also these antibodies in the overall repertoire.

In any case, probably, it will be still necessary to screen more clones by ELISA after the second/third panning cycle than when working with immune libraries to recover suitable specific antibodies. Three 96-well plates are sufficient under normal conditions.

Given the low initial number of specific anti-antigen VHHs in the total population, the chances to select and replicate unspecific binders can increase. Therefore, alternate milk and BSA as a blocking medium during the panning cycles, or use one of them for panning and the other for the ELISA screenings.

When possible, competitive elution of the phages by means of a known binder instead of using triethylamine is a reliable method for reducing contaminations with nonspecific binders.

References

1. Arbabi Ghahroudi M et al (1997) Selection and identification of single domain antibody fragments from camel heavy-chain antibodies. FEBS Lett 414:521–526
2. Muyldermans S (2001) Single domain camel antibodies: current status. J Biotechnol 74:277–302
3. Yeo C, Saunders N, Locca D (2009) Ficoll-Paque™ versus Lymphoprep™: A comparative study of two density gradient media for therapeutic bone marrow mononuclear cell preparations. Regen Med 4:689–696
4. Olichon A, Surrey T (2007) Selection of genetically encoded fluorescent single domain antibodies engineered for efficient expression in *Escherichia coli*. J Biol Chem 282: 36314–36320
5. Garaicoechea L et al (2008) Llama-derived single-chain antibody fragments directed to rotavirus VP6 protein possess broad neutralizing activity in vitro and confer protection against diarrhea in mice. J Virol 82:753–764
6. Bossi S et al (2010) Antibody-mediated purification of co-expressed antigen-antibody complexes. Protein Expr Purif 72:55–58
7. Aliprandi M et al (2010) The availability of a recombinant anti-SNAP antibody in VHH format amplifies the application flexibility of SNAP-tagged proteins. J Biomed Biotechnol. doi:10.1155/2010/658954
8. Monegal A et al (2009) Immunological applications of single-domain llama recombinant antibodies isolated from a naive library. Prot Engineer Des Sel 22:273–280
9. Nguyen VK, Muyldermans S, Hamers R (1998) The specific variable domain of camel heavy-chain antibodies is encoded in the germline. J Mol Biol 275:413–418
10. Skerra A, Plückthun A (1988) Assembly of a functional immunoglobulin Fv fragment in *Escherichia coli*. Science 240:1038–1041
11. Dong J et al (2010) A single-domain llama antibody potently inhibits the enzymatic activity of *Botulinum* neurotoxin by binding to the non-catalytic α–exosite binding region. J Mol Biol 397:1106–1118
12. Deschacht N et al (2010) A novel promiscuous class of camelid single-domain antibody contributes to the antigen-binding repertoire. J Immunol 184:5696–5704

Part III

Selection of Single Domain Antibodies

Chapter 6

Selection by Phage Display of Single Domain Antibodies Specific to Antigens in Their Native Conformation

Peter Verheesen and Toon Laeremans

Abstract

Phage display of antibody fragments and other binding molecules is a well-established technique to identify ligands interacting with any molecule of interest. Selection of in vivo matured single domain antibody fragments from phage display libraries is very powerful as in these libraries each clone represents a noncombinatorial functional domain of a naturally circulating antibody, and thus such libraries contain a high number of antigen-specific clones. Consequently, individual binders to antigens of interest are efficiently obtained typically after one or two selection rounds. Furthermore, the large functional diversity within these antibody libraries allows the application of different and more stringent selection conditions resulting in the selection of complementary antibody panels. In this chapter, we present a guide to perform selections against purified antigens and antigens in their native conformation and context.

Key words: Phage display, Single domain antibody, Native conformation, Virus-like particle, Lipoparticle

1. Introduction

Several excellent books on phage display have been published dealing with all aspects of phage biology, the different types of display, library construction and phage rescue, and many applications of phage display techniques (1–3). In this chapter, we describe protocols more specifically for selecting single domain antibodies using phage display. We have opted for an outline of this chapter based on the antigen format and the presentation of the antigen during the selections. Protocols are given to select for binders to pure antigens such as proteins, haptens, or peptides conjugated to carrier proteins and antigens presented in complex matrices such as membrane extracts, lipoparticles, or whole cells. Equally important to the phage display selection is the immunization strategy that precedes library construction. The immunization strategy determines

Dirk Saerens and Serge Muyldermans (eds.), *Single Domain Antibodies: Methods and Protocols*,
Methods in Molecular Biology, vol. 911, DOI 10.1007/978-1-61779-968-6_6, © Springer Science+Business Media, LLC 2012

what antibody repertoire is raised in the animal and, together with the selection protocol, determines the specificity, affinity, and epitope recognition of the selected antibodies. To present integral membrane proteins in their native conformation, it is often advantageous to immunize with whole cells expressing the antigen over immunizing with purified protein, protein domains, or derived peptides. However, it is even more preferred to bias the immune response towards conformational epitopes of the protein of interest while reducing the response against matrix contaminants. Eliciting an immune response to matrix contaminants may cause problems in phage display selections and lead to high backgrounds. Two examples of powerful strategies that minimize eliciting undesired immune responses are genetic immunization administering target-encoding DNA (4, 5), or vaccinating with the target membrane protein expressed on a cell background derived from the same animal species to be used for immunization. Selections can be performed under different conditions depending on the available functional format of the antigen. The most straightforward selection method is by coating pure antigens directly on a solid surface. Selections with purified antigens are preferably performed in 96-well plates allowing parallel selections varying coating conditions stabilizing the antigen conformation (i.e., detergents, pH, cofactors), antigen formats, and elution methods. An alternative to solid phase-coated antigen is using biotinylated antigen and allowing phage to bind in solution. This is advantageous because the antigen concentration can be controlled and conformational changes consequent to solid phase coating of the antigen are avoided. Complexes of phage bound to biotinylated antigen can then be captured using solid phase-coated streptavidin or streptavidin-coated magnetic beads. Typically, after one or two selection rounds with pure antigens, libraries are sufficiently enriched for antigen-specific antibody fragments to screen individual clones for target binding. Selection conditions can then be altered to select for antibodies with more defined characteristics such as binding to complementary epitopes, antibodies that are cross-reactive between antigen orthologs, antibodies blocking protein–protein interactions (e.g., ligand-receptor binding), antibodies with higher affinity, or antibodies that discriminate between closely related molecules. To select for binders against integral membrane proteins, the selection process is more challenging as purified protein presenting the target of interest in its native conformation is often not available (detergent solubilized cell surface protein or purified recombinant ectodomains may contain subtle conformation changes). Tissues, cells, membrane extracts, and virus-like particles (VLPs) present the target protein in its native conformation but also in a matrix of "contaminants" (lipids, extracellular matrix, nonrelated membrane proteins). Important for the enrichment of binders in selections against membrane proteins are (1) presenting a high concentration of the protein of interest in the complex matrix and (2) changing the matrix background in consecutive selection rounds. Combining these will facilitate enrichment of target-specific antibodies over those interacting with matrix contaminants. Panels of binders against native target can be obtained in 1 or 2 weeks by choosing the correct antigen format and appropriate selection conditions.

Selections with naïve or synthetic single domain antibody libraries are performed similarly compared to selections with immune libraries, but are more complex as the libraries are not enriched for the target and often require (1) 1 or 2 more selection rounds, (2) depletion for matrix contaminants by preincubating the phage library with the complex matrix lacking the target of interest and/or (3) performing epitope-specific elutions.

Selection protocols for pure antigens using solid phase-coated antigen or biotinylated antigen in solution and different protocols using complex matrices such as membrane extracts, VLPs, or whole cells for selections are provided below. Each protocol resulted in successful selection of antigen-specific single domain antibodies.

2. Materials

Prepare all components using deionized (MilliQ) water and analytical grade reagents.

2.1. Selection of Single Domain Antibodies by the Biopanning Method

1. Pure antigen, quality controlled (see Note 1) and of known concentration.
2. 96-well Maxisorp plate as selection recipient (Nunc/Thermo Scientific, Roskilde, Denmark).
3. Sealers for 96-well plates (Nunc/Thermo Scientific, Roskilde, Denmark).
4. Library phage, preferably rescued with helper phage VCSM13 (Stratagene/Agilent Technologies, Santa Clara, CA, USA), 10^{11} colony forming units (CFU) library phage for each selection well.
5. M9 minimal agar: To prepare 200 mL of M9 minimal agar, sterilize a 2% bacteriological agar solution and allow cooling until solution is hand-warm. Now, add (all sterilized) 20 mL of 10× M9 minimal salts (Sigma, St. Louis, MO, USA), 200 μL of 0.1 M $CaCl_2$, 400 μL of 1 M $MgSO_4$, 2 mL of 2% glucose, 2 mL of 100 mg/mL thiamine hydrochloride.
6. Phosphate buffered saline (PBS); 0.01 M phosphate buffer, 0.0027 M potassium chloride, and 0.137 M sodium chloride, pH 7.4, at 25°C. Weigh 8 g NaCl, 0.2 g KCl, 1.15 g Na_2HPO_4, 0.24 g KH_2PO_4, adjust to pH 7.4, and fill to 1 L.
7. Carbonate buffer: 50 mM carbonate pH 9.6; Prepare a 0.1 M Na_2CO_3 stock solution and prepare a 0.1 M $NaHCO_3$ stock

solution. Mix 17.5 mL of 0.1 M Na_2CO_3 stock solution with 32.5 mL of 0.1 M $NaHCO_3$ stock solution, fill to 100 mL.

8. *Escherichia coli* TG1 cells (Stratagene/Agilent Technologies, Santa Clara, CA, USA) cultured on solid M9 minimal medium for maintaining F-pili expression and maximum infectivity of phage.
9. Blocking solution: 2–5% skimmed milk or 1% casein dissolved in PBS, the latter solution heat sterilized. Before applying solution to the selection wells, centrifuge suspension at 3,000 × *g* for 10 min and transfer supernatant to a new tube to remove nondissolved components.
10. Washing buffer PBST: PBS containing 0.05% Tween-20.
11. Washing buffer PBS.
12. Elution buffer (see Note 2): 100 mM Triethylamine in water.
13. Neutralization buffer: 1 M Tris–HCl, pH 7.5.
14. Elution buffer (see Note 3): 1 mg/mL trypsin (Sigma, St. Louis, MO, USA) in PBS. Stock solution can be stored as aliquots at −20°C.
15. Trypsin inhibitor 4-(2-Aminoethyl)benzenesulfonyl fluoride hydrochloride (AEBSF) (Sigma, St. Louis, MO, USA): 4 mg/mL in water. Stock solution can be stored as aliquots at −20°C.
16. Low-binding polypropylene 96-well plate for transfer and storage of eluted phage (Nunc/Thermo Scientific, Roskilde, Denmark).
17. Luria Broth (LB) solid agar (see Note 4): 10 g/L Tryptone (pancreatic digest of casein), 5 g/L yeast extract, 5 g/L NaCl; 15 g/L Agar; Autoclave for 15 min at 121°C.
18. 20% glucose: 200 g/L glucose. Autoclave for 15 min at 121°C.
19. 100 mg/mL Ampicillin. Filter sterilize.
20. 2×TY culture medium: 16 g/L Tryptone, 10 g/L yeast extract, 5 g/L NaCl; Autoclave for 15 min at 121°C.
21. Filter tips P1000, P200, P20, P10 (see Note 5).
22. Multichannel pipets 20–200, 5–50, 1–10 μL.

2.2. Selection of Single Domain Antibodies by In-Solution Selections

1. All materials according to the previous section (see Subheading 2.1).
2. Pure biotinylated antigen, quality controlled (see Note 6) and of known concentration.
3. Blocking solution: Preferably use a biotin-free blocking solution, i.e., 1% casein in PBS.
4. If streptavidin or neutravidin-coated plates are used: Streptavidin (Pierce Biotechnology/Thermo Scientific, Rockford, USA) or

Neutravidin (Pierce Biotechnology/Thermo Scientific, Rockford, USA) (see Note 7), prepare a stock solution of 2 mg/mL and store aliquots at −20°C.

5. If streptavidin-coated beads are used: Streptavidin magnetic beads (Dynabeads/ Invitrogen, Carlsbad, CA, USA), DynaMag-Spin or DynaMag-2 magnet (Invitrogen, Carlsbad, CA, USA).

2.3. Whole Cell Selections

1. Selection cells (highly expressing the membrane protein of interest) and null cells (not expressing the target of interest but presenting all matrix components).
2. Phosphate buffered saline, tissue culture grade (PBS).
3. Heat-inactivated fetal calf serum (FCS).
4. Skimmed milk powder (see Note 8).
5. Cell blocking solution: Appropriate culture medium supplementing necessary additives, 10% FCS, 2% milk powder (see Note 9).
6. Phage blocking solution: PBS, 10% FCS, 2% milk powder.
7. Trypsin solution: 1 mg/mL Trypsin in PBS.
8. AEBSF solution: 4 mg/mL AEBSF in water.

2.4. Virus-Like Particle or Lipoparticle Selections

1. 96-well Maxisorp plate as the selection recipient (Nunc/ Thermo Scientific, Roskilde, Denmark).
2. VLPs (target presenting) and null VLPs (see Note 10).
3. Phosphate buffered saline, tissue culture grade (PBS).
4. Skimmed milk powder (see Note 8).
5. Blocking solution: PBS, 2% milk powder.
6. Trypsin solution: 1 mg/mL Trypsin in PBS.
7. AEBSF solution: 4 mg/mL AEBSF in water.

2.5. Membrane Extract Selections

1. 96-well Maxisorp plate as the selection recipient (Nunc/ Thermo Scientific, Roskilde, Denmark).
2. Membrane extracts (MEs) and null MEs.
3. Phosphate buffered saline, tissue culture grade (PBS).
4. Skimmed milk powder (see Note 8).
5. Blocking solution: PBS, 2–4% milk powder.
6. Trypsin solution: 1 mg/mL Trypsin in PBS.
7. AEBSF solution: 4 mg/mL AEBSF in water.

2.6. Selection for Internalizing Single Domain Antibody Fragments

1. Selection cells (cells with high expression levels of the membrane protein of interest) and null cells (not expressing the target of interest but presenting all matrix components).
2. Phosphate buffered saline, tissue culture grade (PBS).

3. Heat-inactivated FCS.
4. Skimmed milk powder (see Note 8).
5. Cell binding solution: Appropriate culture medium supplementing necessary additives, 10% FCS.
6. Cell blocking solution: Cell binding solution containing 2% milk powder (see Note 9).
7. Phage blocking solution: PBS, 10% FCS, 2% milk powder.
8. Cell stripping buffer: 500 mM NaCl, 100 mM glycine-HCl, pH 2.5.
9. Cell lysis solution: 100 mM triethanylamine (TEA).
10. Neutralization buffer: 500 mM Tris–HCl, pH 7.4.

3. Methods

Carry out all procedures at room temperature unless otherwise specified. Working with phage easily causes contamination and all handlings should be performed in such a way that contamination is avoided (see Note 5).

3.1. Selection of Single Domain Antibodies by the Biopanning Method

1. Coat wells of a 96-well Maxisorp plate with antigen in PBS or 50 mM carbonate buffer (pH 9.6) or any suitable buffer that stabilizes the antigen conformation. Fill the wells with 100 μL/well antigen solution in different concentrations [e.g., concentrations 10 μg/mL and 0.1 μg/mL (see Note 1)]. Seal the plate to avoid evaporation (see Note 11) and perform coating overnight at 4°C without shaking.
2. Prepare an overnight culture of *E. coli* TG1. Pick a single colony from a minimal media agar plate and grow in 50 mL liquid 2×TY in a 250-mL flask at 37°C in a rotary incubator (see Notes 12 and 13).
3. Next day, continue coating of the Maxisorp plate for 30 min to 2 h at room temperature on an ELISA shaking platform at 450–900 rpm. Wash the plate three times with ≥200 μL/well PBST (see Note 14). Add minimally 200 μL/well blocking solution (2–5% skimmed milk in PBS or 1% casein in PBS) to each coated well and blank wells (nonantigen containing). Use independent blank wells for each phage library to be selected. Perform blocking for 1–2 h at room temperature.
4. Dilute overnight grown *E. coli* TG1 100-fold in fresh 2×TY and grow at 37°C to $OD_{600\ nm} = 0.5$ (typically 1.5–2 h) (see Notes 12 and 15). When at $OD_{600\ nm} = 0.5$ keep cells on ice and use for infections with dilution series of input library phage and eluted phage.

5. Prepare a premix of phage in blocking solution containing approximately 10^{12} of CFU (mL) (see Note 16) and preincubate by head-over-head rotation at 20 rpm for minimally 30 min (see Note 17).
6. Remove blocking solution from wells and wash five times applying each time 200 μL/well PBST (see Note 14). Add 100 μL/well preincubated phage premixes to the antigen-coated and blank selection wells. Cover the plate with a sealer and incubate for 90–120 min on an ELISA shaking platform at 450–900 rpm.
7. Wash extensively to remove nonspecifically bound phage. Perform 12 washes with ≥200 μL/well PBST and 3 washes with ≥200 μL/well PBS (see Note 14). After the last wash, empty the wells of the washed plate by inverting the plate above a bleach-containing waste recipient and tapping the plate upside down on a paper towel.
8. Elute bound phage at high pH. Add 100 μL/well elution buffer, cover the plate with a sealer, and incubate for 15 min on an ELISA shaking platform at 450–900 rpm. Fill a low-binding 96-well plate with 50 μL/well neutralization buffer. Transfer eluted phage to the wells prefilled with neutralization buffer to neutralize phage eluates. Alternatively, elute bound phage with trypsin (see Notes 3 and 18). Add 100 μL/well of 1 mg/mL trypsin in PBS, cover the plate with a sealer, and incubate for 30 min on an ELISA shaking platform at 450–900 rpm. Fill a low-binding 96-well plate with 5 μL/well of 4 mg/mL AEBSF trypsin inhibitor. Transfer eluted phage to the wells prefilled with trypsin inhibitor to inhibit trypsin activity.
9. Titrate eluted phage and input library phage. Prepare dilutions in a low-binding 96-well plate. Use 45 μL of 2×TY per well (see Note 19) and add 5 μL of neutralized or premix input phage. Make 10^{-1} to 10^{-6} serial dilutions for eluted phage, i.e., fill wells with 45 μL of 2×TY and transfer 5 μL from each previous dilution. For nonselected input library phage premixes, prepare 10^{-1} to 10^{-10} serial dilutions.
10. For infection, add 50 μL of *E. coli* TG1 at $OD_{600\ nm} = 0.5$ to each well and incubate at 37°C without shaking for 20 min (see Note 20). Spot 5 μL droplets of infected *E. coli* from each infection on LB agar plates with 2% glucose and an appropriate antibiotic (depending on the antibiotic resistance marker encoded by the display vector). To verify whether no contamination of *E. coli* TG1 cells occurred, also spot 5 μL of *E. coli* TG1 without phage infection (this spot should not give any colonies).
11. Also use the eluted phage from antigen-coated wells for infection of *E. coli* TG1 cells to amplify the obtained sublibrary and

subsequently to prepare new phage particles for a new round of selection. For infection, transfer half of the neutralized eluted phage volume (75 μL for triethylamine elutions or 50 μL for trypsin elutions) to 1.5-mL tubes and add 1 mL of logarithmically grown *E. coli* TG1 cells ($OD_{600\ nm}=0.5$) (see Note 21). Infect for 20 min at 37°C without shaking. Spin down cells for 5 min at 6,000 × *g* and remove and discard the supernatant. Resuspend cells and transfer to 50-mL tubes containing 10 mL of LB medium, 2% glucose, and the appropriate selective antibiotic. Grow cultures in a rotary incubator at 37°C overnight. Store the remainder of neutralized phage eluate at −20°C (see Note 22).

12. Next day, analyze colony spots and calculate eluted phage numbers. Compare phage numbers eluted from antigen-coated wells to phage numbers eluted from blank control wells and the amount of input phage that was added to each well (see Note 23).
13. Prepare glycerol cell stocks from the overnight cultures to store selection outputs and rescue and prepare new phage pools according to standard protocols (1).

In case target-specific enrichment is observed, screen individual clones for target specificity with ELISA in a setup similar to the selection conditions.

3.2. Selection of Single Domain Antibodies by In-Solution Selections

Streptavidin-coated magnetic beads are preferred over streptavidin-coated micro plates for capturing complexes of biotinylated antigens with bound phage. The binding capacity and efficiency of streptavidin-coated beads is higher than for streptavidin-coated micro plates.

1. Prepare an overnight culture of *E. coli* TG1 the day before selection as described previously (see Subheading 3.1, step 2).
2. If streptavidin-coated micro plates are used for capturing complexes of biotinylated antigens with bound phage, coat a multi well plate with streptavidin the day before selection. Coat wells of a 96-well Maxisorp plate with streptavidin in PBS or 50 mM carbonate buffer (pH 9.6). Fill the wells of a 96-well Maxisorp plate with 100 μL/well 2–5 μg/mL steptavidin solution. Seal the plate to avoid evaporation and perform coating overnight at 4°C without shaking.
3. On the day of selection, prepare a premix of phage in blocking solution as previously described (see Subheading 3.1, step 5). When using streptavidin-coated beads for capturing complexes of biotinylated antigen with bound phage, prepare 1 mL of phage premix for each selection condition and a blank selection (see Note 17). When using a streptavidin-coated micro plate for capturing complexes of biotinylated antigen with

bound phage, prepare 100 μL/well of phage premix for each selection condition and a blank selections (see Note 17).

4. When using streptavidin-coated beads for capturing complexes of biotinylated antigen with bound phage, use 100 μL of streptavidin-coated Dynabead suspension (10 mg/mL) for each selection condition and blank and transfer to a 1.5-mL tube. Draw beads to one side of the tube using a magnet. Remove supernatant and resuspend beads in an equal volume of 1% casein in PBS. Block beads by head-over-head rotation at 20 rpm for minimally 30 min. Alternatively, when capturing complexes on a streptavidin-coated micro plate, continue coating of the Maxisorp plate for 30 min to 2 h at room temperature on an ELISA shaking platform at 450–900 rpm. Wash the plate three to five times with ≥200 μL/well PBST (see Note 14). Add minimally 200 μL/well blocking solution (1% casein in PBS) to each coated well and streptavidin-coated blank wells. Use independent streptavidin-coated blank wells for each phage library to be selected. Perform blocking for 1–2 h at room temperature.

5. Dispense the preincubated phage solution over the number of selection conditions in 1.5-mL tubes (when beads are used for capturing of complexes of biotinylated antigen with bound phage) or wells of a low-binding polypropylene 96-well plate (when a streptavidin-coated micro plate is used for capturing of complexes of biotinylated antigen with bound phage). Add biotinylated antigen (final concentration 1–500 nM) directly into the premix of blocked phage. Incubate tubes by head-over-head rotation at 20 rpm for 1–2 h or seal plates and incubate on an ELISA shaking platform at 450–900 rpm (see Note 24).

6. To capture complexes of biotinylated antigen with bound phage on streptavidin-coated beads, draw the blocked beads to one side of the tube with the magnet and remove the blocking buffer. Resuspend the beads in equal volume of 1% casein and add 100 μL of beads to phage-antigen mixes and incubate by head-over-head rotation at 20 rpm for 1–5 min (see Note 24). Perform a short spin in a micro centrifuge to remove all liquid and beads from the lids of the tubes and place the tubes in a magnetic rack and wait until all beads are pulled to the magnetic side (20 s–1 min). Aspirate the tubes carefully, leaving the beads on the side of the tube. Wash the beads carefully six times with 1 mL of PBST or 1% casein/PBST. Transfer the solutions to new 1.5-mL tubes and wash the beads another six times with 1 mL of PBST or 1% casein/PBST. Transfer solution to a new 1.5-mL tube and wash the beads twice with 1 mL of PBS. Alternatively, to capture complexes of biotinylated antigen with bound phage on streptavidin-coated plates, remove and discard the blocking solution from the plate and

add 100 μL/well of phage-antigen mixes and incubate on a ELISA shaking platform at 450–900 rpm for 5–15 min (see Note 24). Proceed with washes as described for biopanning selections (see Subheading 3.1, step 7).

7. Elutions with complexes of biotinylated antigen and phage captured on beads are performed similarly to those in biopanning selections (see Subheading 3.1, step 8) with the following modifications. Draw the beads to the sides of the tubes with a magnet and carefully remove and discard the wash solution. Elute bound phage at high pH. Add 1 mL/tube elution buffer and incubate with head-over-head rotation at 20 rpm for 15 min. Perform a short spin in a micro centrifuge to remove all beads and liquid from the lids of the tubes and place the tubes in a magnetic rack and wait until all beads are pulled to the magnetic side (20 s–1 min). Fill new tubes with 500 μL/tube neutralization buffer. Transfer eluted phage to the tubes prefilled with neutralization buffer to neutralize phage eluates (see Note 25). Alternatively, elute bound phage with trypsin (see Notes 3 and 18). Add 1 mL of 1 mg/mL trypsin in PBS to each tube and incubate with head-over-head rotation at 20 rpm for 30 min. Perform a short spin in a micro centrifuge to remove all beads and liquid from the lids of the tubes and place the tubes in a magnetic rack and wait until all beads are pulled to the magnetic side (20 s–1 min). Fill new tubes with 50 μL/tube of 4 mg/mL AEBSF trypsin inhibitor. Transfer eluted phage to the tubes prefilled with trypsin inhibitor to inhibit trypsin activity. Alternatively, for complexes of antigen with bound phage captured on streptavidin-coated plates, elutions are performed identical to those in biopanning selections (see Subheading 3.1, step 8).

8. Titration of eluted phage and input phage are performed as described for biopanning selections (see Subheading 3.1, step 9–11). When infecting half of the eluted phage volume, adjust volumes as follows: Use 750 μL for phage eluted from beads by high pH (from 1.5 mL neutralized eluted phage in total) or 500 μL for phage eluted from beads with trypsin (from 1.05 mL eluted and trypsin inhibited phage in total). Add 4.25 or 4.5 mL of *E. coli* TG1 cells ($OD_{600\ nm} = 0.5$) for infection, respectively. Incubate infections at 37°C for 20 min without shaking. Spin down cells for 5 min at 6,000 × *g* and remove and discard the supernatant. Resuspend cells and transfer to 50-mL tubes containing 10 mL of LB medium, 2% glucose, and the appropriate selective antibiotic as previously described (see Subheading 3.1).

9. Proceed as described for biopanning selections (see Subheading 3.1, steps 12–13).

In case target-specific enrichment is observed, screen individual clones for target specificity with ELISA in a setup similar to the selection conditions. Adapt the above selection protocols for pure antigens to select for more specific characteristics such as single domain antibodies binding to complementary epitopes (see Note 26), single domain antibodies that are cross-reactive between antigen orthologs (see Note 27), single antibodies blocking protein–protein interactions (e.g., ligand-receptor binding) (see Note 28), single domain antibodies with high affinity (see Note 29), or single domain antibodies that discriminate between closely related molecules (see Note 30).

3.3. Whole Cell Selections

Different sources of cells can be used to select for antibodies against extracellular epitopes of a membrane protein: Cell lines endogenously expressing the target of interest or stably or transiently transfected cell lines expressing the target of interest. Key is to use cell lines expressing a high density of the protein of interest on the cell surface. Tumor cell lines often overexpress the target and consequently such cell lines are useful selection tools. Avoid rigorous vortexing, foam, or high-speed centrifugation of cell-containing solutions. Carry out all steps at 4°C unless otherwise specified (see Note 31). Selection recipients can be 50-mL or micro centrifuge or FACS tubes. It is critical to assess functional receptor expression (as an indication of its native conformation) before performing whole cell selections (see Note 32).

1. Prepare logarithmically grown TG1 cells as described for biopanning selections (see Subheading 3.1, steps 2 and 4).
2. Pellet freshly harvested and washed cells (see Notes 33 and 34).
3. Resuspend 10^6 selection cells and in a separate tube an identical aliquot of null cells in cell blocking solution and incubate for 30 min. Keep the cells in suspension by head-over-head rotation at 20 rpm.
4. Meanwhile block input phage (see Note 16) by incubating 100 μL of phage library (dissolved in PBS) in 900 μL of phage blocking solution for 30 min by head-over-head rotation at 20 rpm in a micro centrifuge tube.
5. Pellet selection and null cells and resuspend cells in separate tubes in 1 mL of blocked phage solution.
6. Incubate on ice for 1–2 h, while gently shaking or with head-over-head rotation at 20 rpm allowing cells to remain in suspension.
7. Pellet cells, discard supernatant, and wash five times with 1 mL of ice-cold phage blocking solution in micro centrifuge tubes.
8. Wash cell aliquots twice more with 1 mL of ice-cold PBS removing remaining blocking agents (FCS, skimmed milk) and discard supernatant (see Note 35).

9. Elute total cell-bound phage by resuspending cell pellet in 200 μL of trypsin stock solution (see Note 36) and incubate 15 min with head-over-head rotation at 20 rpm at room temperature. Subsequently, spin for 10 min at maximal speed and transfer phage-containing supernatant to a new micro centrifuge tube. Neutralize remaining trypsin activity in phage eluate by adding 10 μL of 4 mg/mL AEBSF stock solution. For epitope-specific phage elution (see Note 37), omit PBS washes (see Subheading 3.3, step 8) and add minimally 100-fold molar excess of epitope competing reagent over estimated cell surface receptor in PBS, 10% FCS, 2% skimmed milk and incubate for minimally 1 h. Following phage elution, pellet cells and collect phage-containing eluate.
10. Infect phage eluate in exponentially grown *E. coli* TG1, titrate the phage output, amplify the phage output, and prepare glycerol stocks similar to described under biopanning selection procedure (see Subheading 3.1, steps 9–13).

In case target-specific enrichment is observed (see Note 38), screen individual clones for target specificity via cell surface binding via flow cytometry, cell ELISA, or (radio-) ligand competition assays on whole cells or membrane extracts. In case no clear enrichment is observed, a consecutive selection round is to be performed following the above-described protocol, but using the target expressed on a different cell background compared to this applied in the previous selection round(s). Alternating cell backgrounds expressing the target of interest during subsequent selection rounds minimizes the selection for background surface cell markers.

3.4. Virus-Like Particle or Lipoparticle Selections

Lipoparticles or VLPs are noninfective, nonreplicative virus-like structures of homogeneous nanometer size, presenting recombinant membrane proteins of interest in a native lipid bilayer after budding from the host cell, often HEK293 cells (6). VLPs present up to 100-fold enriched concentrations of integral membrane proteins compared to the densities on the native cell surface, retaining its native conformation, both structurally and functionally (see Note 39). The lipoparticles are stable at room temperature and can be stored at 4°C for months. VLPs allow similar biopanning procedures as with purified protein (solid phase immobilization of the particles in micro well plates). VLPs present the recombinant membrane proteins in their native configuration, keeping the direction of exposure of the extracellular and intracellular domains of the target protein as on the cell surface. As for whole cells, VLPs are excellent tools to identify single domain antibodies against epitopes on the extracellular domain of the membrane target. The production of VLPs, however, is labor-intensive and requires particular mammalian VLP production vectors and expert skills. Alternatively, certain companies provide (expensive) custom-based

VLP production services presenting the target of interest (Integral Molecular, Philadelphia US or Icosagen, Estonia).

1. Coat optimal quantities (see Note 40) of lipoparticles on a Maxisorp plate overnight at 4°C (see Note 41) as described for biopanning selections (see Subheading 3.1, step 1).
2. Prepare logarithmically grown TG1 cells as described for biopanning selections (see Subheading 3.1, step 2).
3. Next day, wash wells twice with 250 μL of PBS and discard nonimmobilized VLPs in solution.
4. Block noncoated well surface by applying 200 μL of blocking solution and incubation at room temperature on an ELISA shaking platform at 450–900 rpm for 2 h.
5. Meanwhile, preblock input phage by incubating >200 μL of input phage (see Notes 16 and 17) in PBS, 1% skimmed milk for 30 min at room temperature by gentle shaking, or head-over-head rotation at 20 rpm in a micro centrifuge tube.
6. Empty wells and wash wells twice with 250 μL of PBS to remove traces of blocking agent.
7. Add 100 μL of the preblocked phage solution to each well containing VLPs or null VLPs and incubate at room temperature on an ELISA shaking platform at 450–900 rpm for 2 h allowing phage binding.
8. Wash wells 15 times with 250 μL of PBS. Following the last wash, discard washing solution and remove traces of washing solution by gently tapping 96-well plate on paper towel.
9. Elute bound phage using trypsin as described under the biopanning procedure (see Subheading 3.1, step 8). Alternatively, use an epitope-specific competing reagent as described (see Note 28).
10. Infect phage eluate in exponentially grown *E. coli* TG1, titrate the phage output, amplify the phage output, and prepare glycerol stocks similar to described under biopanning selection procedure (see Subheading 3.1, steps 9–13).

In case target-specific enrichment is observed (see Note 42), screen monoclonal antibodies for target specificity via flow cytometry, ELISA (immobilizing VLPs), or (radio)ligand competition assays on whole cells or membrane extracts. In case no clear enrichment is observed, a consecutive selection round is to be performed following the above-described protocol. Using a library derived from an appropriately immunized animal, typically one or two selection rounds are required to identify single domain antibodies against the target of interest.

3.5. Membrane Extract Selections

Membrane extracts (MEs) are whole cell derivatives that present membrane proteins in their native lipid bilayer at target densities similar to those on the native cell surface. As for whole cell selections, the decision to use a particular batch of MEs as selection matrix should only be taken after evaluating the conformation (functionality) of the protein of interest preferably via (radio-) ligand binding assay or any other binding assay using a detection reagent shown to interact with conformational epitopes (mAbs, agonists, …). While a whole cell or VLP selection allows selecting for extracellular epitopes, MEs allow phage binding to both the extracellular and intracellular epitopes. Several companies (e.g., Perkin Elmer, Boston, US) provide broad panels of MEs harboring a multitude of receptors.

Essentially, selections are performed similarly as described under the section using VLPs as selection tool.

1. Coat optimal quantities of MEs (see Note 43), diluted in PBS on a Maxisorp plate overnight at 4°C (see Note 44) as described for biopanning selections (see Subheading 3.1, step 1).
2. Prepare logarithmically grown TG1 cells as described for biopanning selections (see Subheading 3.1, step 2).
3. Next day, wash wells twice with 250 μL of PBS and discard nonimmobilized MEs in solution (see Note 44).
4. Block noncoated well surface by applying 200 μL of blocking solution and incubate at room temperature on an ELISA shaking platform at 450–900 rpm for 2 h.
5. Meanwhile, preblock input phage by incubating > 200 μL of input phage (see Notes 16 and 17) in PBS, 1% skimmed milk for 30 min at room temperature by gentle shaking, or head-over-head rotation at 20 rpm in a micro centrifuge tube.
6. Empty wells and wash wells twice with 250 μL of PBS to remove traces of blocking agent.
7. Add 100 μL of the blocked phage solution to each well containing MEs or null MEs and incubate at room temperature on an ELISA shaking platform at 450–900 rpm for 2 h allowing phage binding.
8. Wash wells 15 times with 250 μL of PBS. Following the last wash, discard washing solution and remove traces of washing solution by gently tapping 96-well plate on paper towel.
9. Elute bound phage using trypsin as described under the biopanning procedure (see Subheading 3.1, step 8). Alternatively, use an epitope-specific competing reagent as described (see Note 28).
10. Infect phage eluate in exponentially grown *E. coli* TG1, titrate the phage output, amplify the phage output, and prepare glycerol stocks similar to described under biopanning selection procedure (see Subheading 3.1, steps 9–13).

In case target-specific enrichment is observed (see Note 45), screen monoclonal antibodies for target specificity. As MEs present both extra- and intracellular epitopes of the target of interest, suitable screening assays should allow detection of binding to intracellular epitopes as well. In case no clear enrichment is observed, a consecutive selection round is to be performed following the above-described protocol, but applying MEs presenting the target on a different cell background compared to the previous selection round(s), reducing the selection for antibodies against background cell surface markers. Using a library derived from an appropriately immunized animal, typically one or two selection rounds are required to identify single domain antibodies against the target of interest.

3.6. Selection for Internalizing Single Domain Antibody Fragments

Complex matrices such as whole cells can be used to select for antibodies that bind a target of interest, but also to select for antibodies with a specific function. An example of such selection for function is based on the ability of receptors to downregulate its signaling function by endocytosis. This method was published by Poul et al. (7) and an adapted protocol, described below, allowed the identification of single domain antibodies that trigger receptor tyrosin kinase endocytosis (9).

Avoid rigorous vortexing, bubbles or foam, or high-speed centrifugation of cell-containing solutions. Precool all buffers to carry out all steps at 4°C unless otherwise specified (see Note 31). Selection recipients can be 50-mL tubes for suspension cells or 10-cm culture Petri dishes for adhering cells.

1. Pellet freshly harvested and washed cells (see Note 33).
2. Mix 2×10^7 freshly harvested null cells (see Note 34) with the input phage library (see Notes 16 and 17) in 5 mL of ice-cold cell binding solution and incubate for 30 min by head-over-head rotation at 20 rpm (see Notes 9 and 46).
3. During preincubation of phage library with null cells, cover (for adhering cells, see Note 47) or resuspend (suspension cells) 5×10^6 selection cells in 5 mL of cell blocking solution. Incubate at 4°C on an orbital ELISA shaking platform at 100–200 rpm or with head-over-head rotation at 20 rpm.
4. Add the phage, recovered via centrifugation from the incubation with the null cell suspension, to the antigen expressing cells and allow phage binding during incubation for minimally for 2 h at 4°C on an ELISA shaking platform at 100–200 rpm to keep cells in suspension.
5. Wash selection cells six times with 10 mL of ice-cold PBS to remove phage not bound to selection cells. After final wash step, discard remaining PBS.
6. Cover or resuspend (see Note 47) cells with prewarmed binding solution and immediately transfer to 37°C for 20 min allowing phage antibodies to internalize.
7. Cool down the cells on ice for 10 min and strip noninternalized, cell surface-bound phage with two subsequent incubations

in 10 mL of ice-cold cell stripping buffer during 10 min. Discard remaining stripping solution.

8. In case selections are performed on a cell suspension, immediately proceed to next step. When working with adhering cells, first trypsinize cells until cells dissociate and a homogeneous cell suspension is obtained and transfer to a new 50-mL Falcon tube. Wash resuspended selection cells twice with ice-cold PBS to remove traces of trypsin (see Note 48).
9. Immediately lyse cells by incubating with 1 mL of cell lysis solution for 4 min and neutralize phage eluate by mixing with half volume of neutralization buffer.
10. Infect phage eluate in exponentially grown *E. coli* TG1, titrate the phage output, amplify the phage output, and prepare glycerol stocks similar to described under biopanning selection procedure (see Subheading 3.1, steps 9–13).

Individual clones can now be screened for target specificity via cell surface binding (e.g., flow cytometry) or immediately for receptor-mediated internalization (via immunofluorescence techniques (7)).

4. Notes

1. Perform a quality control to assess concentration and conformation for each antigen. The molecular weight of the antigen, its concentration, and the presence of protein contaminants in the antigen aliquot can be checked by running a SDS-PAGE and by comparing the intensity of the band of interest with a concentration series of a standard protein (for instance BSA). Also, the optimum coating concentrations and buffer for each antigen are investigated before starting selections. Coat a concentration series of antigen (typically protein dilutions start at 10 μg/mL) in a multi-well plate and analyze optimum concentration and buffer in an ELISA setup. A ligand, a known binding partner, or an anti-tag antibody for recombinantly produced antigens can be used to detect the antigen coated to the plate. Best coating concentrations for selections are a high concentration for which maximum binding of the ligand (or binding partner or antibody) was observed, and a significantly lower coating concentration for which binding was still well above background but below the maximally obtained signal. If a ligand or binding partner is able to bind the antigen coated on the plate, this shows that the epitopes to which the ligand or binding partner binds are also available for phage binding in selections.
2. Phage can be eluted by different methods, e.g., by applying a pH change. Elution by pH change is reversible as eluted phage

can be neutralized. Please note that elution by pH change is sometimes not harsh enough to elute the strongest binders.

3. Phage can be eluted by different methods, e.g., by proteolysis. Elution by proteolysis is irreversible. Trypsin cleaves proteins specifically, mainly after the amino acids lysine or arginine except when either is followed by proline. Please note that phage infectivity is not impaired by short incubation with trypsin (i.e., 0.1–1 mg/mL trypsin at room temperature for 1 h).
4. To prepare LB agar containing 2% glucose supplemented with selective antibiotic. LB agar medium: Prepare LB agar media and autoclave, for example, in 360 mL portions in 500-mL flasks. Cool down media until hand-warm and add 40 mL of 20% glucose and 400 μL of 100 mg/mL ampicillin (final concentration 100 μg/mL) to each flask and poor plates. Plates can be stored at 4°C for approximately 2 weeks.
5. All phage work is preferably carried out in a laminar flow to avoid contaminating the lab with phage. Filter tips are used for all pipetting. Liquid phage waste is immediately discarded in bleach-containing waste recipients. Solid phage waste such as pipette tips or tubes is discarded in a separate plastic bag, kept in the laminar flow during the experiment, and immediately closed and discarded after the experiment. Clean the work area with a solution of bleach in between phage experiments.
6. When biotinylating the antigen for selection, choose an appropriate ratio of biotin incorporation on the antigen. The extent of biotin labeling depends on the distribution of amino groups on the protein, protein concentration, and the amount of reagent used. The biotinylation reaction is a random process. Using too little biotin may result in the presence of nonbiotinylated antigen molecules in the sample. Using too much biotin may result in overbiotinylation of the antigen and may cause conformational changes or modification of epitopes. Adjust the molar ratio of biotin to protein to obtain the level of incorporation desired. Best is to have a random biotinylation and to perform a quality control of the biotinylated antigen before starting selections. Follow the instructions above (see Note 1), but use a Maxisorp plate coated with streptavidin (i.e., 2–5 μg/mL in PBS) to capture the biotinylated antigen. To select antibodies against a wide variety of epitopes, biotinylated antigen can be used in solution, or captured on streptavidin. If the biotinylated antigen is captured on streptavidin before phage are added, follow the biopanning protocol for selections.
7. Neutravidin is a deglycosylated alternative to avidin or streptavidin with neutral isoelectric point (pI) and higher specificity than avidin or streptavidin.

8. Dissolve skimmed milk powder in appropriate blocking solution and remove nonsoluble components by centrifugation at ≥3,000 × *g* at room temperature for 10 min.
9. Additional inclusion of milk powder to reduce specific phage binding to cells does not affect cell viability. Milk powder can be omitted as FCS is also expected to reduce specific phage binding to cells.
10. Null VLPs should be derived from the same cell line of which the target presenting cell line is derived but not presenting the target, or alternatively, presenting a nonrelated target.
11. Avoid drying of wells with coated antigens at all times.
12. It is advised to use dedicated glassware for growing F-pili-expressing *E. coli* TG1 as phage contamination occurs easily.
13. An overnight culture of *E. coli* TG1 started from a M9 minimal medium grown colony can be kept at 4°C for approximately 2 weeks. For growing TG1 cells to early log phase ($OD_{600\,nm} = 0.5$), use the 2×TY overnight grown liquid culture.
14. A 96-well plate is emptied by inverting the plate above a waste recipient and tapping the plate upside down on a paper towel. A single wash cycle consists of filling a plate with wash buffer and emptying the plate above the waste recipient and tapping the plate upside down on a paper towel. A plate to which phage have been added is washed carefully and aerosols are avoided at all times to avoid contamination. The plate is emptied above a bleach-containing waste recipient and tapped upside down on a paper towel, but a new paper towel is used for each wash. Alternatively, wells can be washed by careful pipetting and/or a plate washer.
15. If it takes longer for the culture to reach an $OD_{600\,nm}$ of 0.5, this may indicate that a contamination occurred and a new culture must be started in fresh media and new flask.
16. The number of input phage contains an amount of CFU typically corresponding to 100–1,000-fold the library size and minimally 10^{11} CFU.
17. The blocking of phage reduces backgrounds in phage selections. Prepare phage predilution in excess to make sure that all wells will be incubated with appropriate phage amounts and that sufficient input phage premix is left over for titrations.
18. Phage can be eluted with a pH change using 100 mM TEA or 100 mM glycine-HCl pH 2.5. Phage can also be eluted more stringently by using trypsin or by adding *E. coli* TG1 directly to the selection wells containing bound phage. Trypsin elution or adding *E. coli* TG1 directly to the selection wells are elution methods independent of the strength of phage antibody binding to the antigen. Differences were found in the diversity of

the eluted phage between pH elution and by using trypsin or adding *E. coli* TG1. In some cases, antigen-specific clones that were found with trypsin elution or by adding *E. coli* TG1 were missing from the pools with pH elution. Therefore, it is preferred to elute with trypsin over pH elution. Eluting with trypsin is also preferred over adding *E. coli* TG1 to wells with bound phage. By adding cells directly to the bound phage, there is no backup available of eluted phage to repeat titrations or output amplification.

19. For optimal titration and infection, prepare phage dilutions in 2×TY medium, alternatively use PBS.
20. Phage dilutions are infected for 20 min and are spotted promptly on selective agar plates (e.g., containing ampicillin) in order to be representative for actual phage numbers eluted. Also include glucose at a final concentration of 2% for phage display systems under control of the lac operon.
21. The volume of neutralized eluted phage should not exceed 10% of the end volume.
22. The remainder of neutralized phage eluates can be used to repeat infections (and not the selection itself) in case of experimental problems. When it turns out that contaminated *E. coli* was used for titrations, use the stored eluted phage for a new infection of freshly grown *E. coli* TG1. Also use the stored phage eluates for infections and plating infected cells on LB agar plates with appropriate supplements such as the right antibiotic and glucose for phage display systems utilizing expression via the lac operon. Pick loose colonies and screen these individual clones for antigen binding.
23. In biopanning selections, typically low background binding is observed. Phage particles are preincubated in blocking solution before selection for 30 min to 2 h. After a typical binding phase of approximately 2 h with the antigen, nonbound phage are removed by extensive washing. Phage output numbers from blank wells are normally $\leq 10^5$. Typically, 10–100-fold enrichments are observed in first or second round selections, respectively.
24. Incubation of phage antibodies with biotinylated antigen is typically long (>1 h) to reach binding equilibrium; capturing of phage antibody with biotinylated antigen complexes on streptavidin is short (<15 min, <5 min, or ≤1 min). The capturing is short to avoid creating a high-density coating of antigen and consequently binding of lower affinity but avidly binding clones to the high-density antigen coating. Short capturing of complexes is still efficient due to high affinity binding of biotin to streptavidin.
25. Do not add neutralization buffer to the tubes containing the beads and the eluted phage as rebinding may occur upon neutralization.

26. Selecting for complementary epitopes. Antigens can be directly coated to a micro plate, but also be captured using a monoclonal antibody (or a single domain antibody). The epitope to which the capturing antibody binds is then shielded off for phage binding and selection to complementary epitopes occurs. Coat wells of a 96-well Maxisorp plate with capturing antibody in PBS. Fill the wells with 100 μL/well capturing antibody at 10 μg/mL. Seal the plate to avoid evaporation and perform coating overnight at 4°C without shaking. Proceed with the protocol as described for biopanning selections for washes and blocking (see Subheading 3.1, step 3). Include an additional antigen capture step to saturate the capturing antibody with the antigen. Fill the wells with 100 μL/well excess antigen. Use wells with only capturing antibody as blanks. Seal the plate to avoid evaporation and perform coating for 2 h at room temperature on an ELISA shaking platform at 450–900 rpm. Wash away excess noncaptured antigen by washing three to five times with ≥ 200 μL/well PBST. Proceed with the protocol as described for biopanning selections (see Subheading 3.1, steps 4–13). When using a capturing antibody, it is advised to include 10% serum in the phage preincubation solution to avoid selecting binders to the capturing antibody; i.e., when a mouse monoclonal antibody is used as the capturing antibody it includes 10% mouse serum in the phage premix solution. This inclusion of 10% serum is crucial when selecting naïve or synthetic libraries. As alternative for serum, i.e., when the antigen is naturally present in serum, use purified IgG from the same species. Preferably use IgG of the same isotype as the capturing antibody. Additional advantages of using a capturing antibody are (1) that at the same time of capturing the antigen in the well, an additional affinity purification takes place (impurities that may disturb biopanning selections are lost in this capturing step) and (2) epitopes that are prone to conformational change by passive adsorption to solid surfaces remain available for selection.
27. To select for species cross-reactive single domain antibodies, use alternated coating of antigen orthologs originating from different species in subsequent rounds of selection. Take along nonalternating selection conditions to compare and evaluate selection results.
28. To select for single domain antibodies that block protein–protein interactions (i.e., that block ligand binding to a receptor) perform selections as described for biopanning selections (see Subheading 3.1, steps 1–7) or in solution selections (see Subheading 3.2, steps 1–6). Use an excess of ligand in solution in the elution step to displace phage antibodies from the ligand binding site. Use one elution condition with excess ligand for

competitive elution and two control elution conditions. The control conditions comprise a total elution (i.e., by high pH or with trypsin) and a control elution with a molecule that resembles the ligand but does not interact with the receptor. The concentration of ligand to use for competitive elution depends on the affinity of the ligand for the antigen (i.e., use a tenfold excess over the affinity of the ligand for the binding site). Add 100 μL/well or 1 mL/tube with excess of ligand in PBS and incubate for 1–2 h at room temperature on an ELISA shaking platform at 450–900 rpm for micro plates or with head-over-head rotation at 20 rpm for tubes. It was found that even high affinity binders can be eluted with this competitive elution method in only 1 or 2 h. Continue with the biopanning selections (see Subheading 3.1, steps 9–13) or in solution selections as described (see Subheading 3.2, steps 8–9).

29. To select for single domain antibodies with high affinity so-called off-rate selections can be performed (8). Perform selections as described for biopanning selections (see Subheading 3.1, steps 1–13) or in solution selections (see Subheading 3.2, steps 1–9) with the following modifications. Add antigen in solution in the wash steps for biopanning selections or nonbiotinylated antigen for in-solution selections and increase washing times to minutes or even hours. The antigen in solution will capture quickly dissociating low affinity phage antibodies, and slowly dissociating clones and thus high affinity remain bound to the antigen.

30. So-called competition selections can be performed to select for single domain antibodies specific to one out of a panel of closely related antigens that differ at least in one epitope. The antigen to which selective binding is desired can be biotinylated and mixed with the closely related nonbiotinylated antigen(s). A suitable ratio can be 100-fold excess of nonbiotinylated antigen over biotinylated antigen or can be experimentally determined. Phage antibodies are added to the mixture of biotinylated antigen and closely related nonbiotinylated antigen(s). Depending on the chosen excess of nonbiotinylated antigens, strong enrichment may be achieved for antigens or epitopes of interest.

31. Keeping the cells on ice avoids target removal from cell surface via internalization.

32. Assess functional expression of the selection cell aliquot using the natural ligand(s) of the target protein or an appropriate monoclonal antibody to detect the target of interest on the cell surface via flow cytometry. Selection cells should maintain the receptor's native conformation throughout the whole selection procedure. Analyze this by a simple experiment in which

the cells are treated exactly as described in the selection protocol after which functional receptor expression is evaluated.

33. Pellet cells by centrifugation at 200 ×*g* for 5 min at 4°C.

34. Immediately before selections are started, harvest subconfluently grown cells via appropriate methods (e.g., trypsinization for adhering cells or centrifugation for suspension cells) without affecting the native conformation of the target of interest. Wash cells with PBS to remove all traces of compounds used for cell harvesting (e.g., trypsin), resuspend in PBS, 10% FCS and count cells. Do not use dead cells as these are permeable and allow phage binding to intracellular epitopes.

35. Wash in PBS to remove FCS or milk. FCS or milk will inhibit trypsin activity and reduce elution efficiency.

36. An alternative elution method using 0.2 M TEA can also be applied. Resuspend cells in 0.2 mL of H_2O, add 0.2 mL of 0.2 M TEA and pipette cell solution up and down (solution gets viscous). Spin 10 min at maximal speed and neutralize by adding 0.1 mL of 1 M Tris–HCl, pH 7.5.

37. To elute phage bound to a specific epitope on the target, a competitive reagent for that epitope such as a target-specific mAb, a receptor ligand, or (ant)agonist can be used. Do not use PBS only as cell lysis may occur. An example of this elution method has been described by Roovers et al. (9).

38. To decide whether monoclonal eluted phage should be screened for target specificity, target-specific phage enrichments are calculated. To calculate target-specific phage enrichments, an appropriate control selection needs to be performed in parallel. When choosing for an elution of total cell-bound phage, use 10^6 of the parental nontarget transfected cells or a parental cell line transfected with a nonrelated target (null cells) as suitable selection control. When epitope-specific elution is used, a suitable control selection is the elution with a similar but noncompeting agent on the same cell line (e.g., a nontarget-specific mAb of the same isotype, a nontarget interacting protein of the same molecular weight). Typically, a target-specific phage enrichment factor >5 is often a strong indication for enrichment of antigen-specific phage population and suggests that target-specific binders will likely be identified in the eluted phage population.

39. The conformation of the membrane protein on VLPs compared to conformation on a whole cell might not necessarily be identical for membrane proteins that require essential intracellular components to retain the membrane protein in its native conformation.

40. To determine the optimal amount of VLPs to immobilize, coat dilution series of the target presenting VLP and null

VLP and detect via ELISA the presence of target typically using ≥1 μg (approximately 15 nM) of a suitable detection reagent (mAb or ligand recognizing conformational epitopes of the target). For a first selection round and those where no enrichment is detected, use the quantity corresponding to that coating concentration where highest signal is detected. Use ten or more units of VLPs per well. Use an identical number of null VLPs, not presenting the target protein of interest and derived from the same cell background as control well to calculate enrichments. Units are proportional to the number of lipoparticles.

41. Avoid excessive vortexing to retain full stability of the particle. Avoid using detergents that can disrupt VLPs. Detergents typically used for washing procedures such as Tween-20 should be omitted from all wash solutions.

42. To calculate target-specific phage enrichments during selections, a control selection should be performed in parallel using null VLPs (prepared via budding from a nontransfected cell line or the parental cell line expressing a nonrelated target). Typically, an enrichment factor >10 is often a strong indicator for enrichment of antigen-specific phage population.

43. MEs contain 10–100 fold less of target protein compared to VLPs. Determine the optimal amount of MEs to immobilize similarly as for VLPs (see Note 40). Use the quantity corresponding to that coating concentration where the highest target-specific signal is detected. Coat with 100 μL/well of a≥10 μg/mL MEs diluted in PBS. For coating of the null MEs, use an identical amount (in mg total protein) as for the target expressing MEs.

44. Avoid excessive vortexing and the use of detergents that might disrupt MEs. Detergents typically used for washing procedures such as Tween-20 should be omitted from all wash solutions.

45. To calculate target-specific phage enrichments during selections, a control selection should be performed in parallel using null MEs (MEs derived from a nontransfected cell line or MEs presenting a nonrelated target). Typically, an enrichment factor >10 is often a strong indication for enrichment of antigen-specific phage population.

46. Coincubate parental background cells for depletion of non target binding phage.

47. During selection, keep adhering cells bound to plastic surface until cells are stripped.

48. Do not use FCS in washing solution as this will inactivate trypsin and decreases cell stripping efficiency.

References

1. Kay BK, Winter J, McCafferty J (1996) Phage display of peptides and proteins: a laboratory manual. Academic, San Diego
2. O'Brien PM, Aitken R (2001) Antibody phage display: methods and protocols. Humana Press, New Jersey
3. Barbas CF et al (2000) Phage display: a laboratory manual. Cold Spring Harbor Laboratory Press, New York
4. Koch-Nolte F et al (2008) Single domain antibodies from llama effectively and specifically block T cell ecto-ADP-ribosyltransferase ART2.2 in vivo. FASEB J 21:3490–3498
5. Patent WO/2010/070145. Genetic immunization for producing immunoglobulins against cell-associated antigen such as P2X7, CXCR7 or CXCR4
6. Hoffman TL et al (2000) A biosensor assay for studying ligand-membrane receptor interctaions. Binding of antibodies and HIV-1 Env to chemokine receptors. PNAS 97: 11215–11220
7. Poul M-A et al (2000) Selection of tumor-specific internalizing human antibodies from phage libraries. J Mol Biol 301: 1149–1161
8. Chen Y et al (1999) Selection and analysis of an optimized anti-VEGF antibody: crystal structure of an affinity-matured Fab in complex with antigen. J Mol Biol 293:865–881
9. Roovers RC et al (2006) Efficient inhibition of EGFR signaling and of tumor growth by antagonistic anti-EGFR Nanobodies. Cancer Immunol Immunother 56:303–317

Chapter 7

Semiautomated Panning of Naive *Camelidae* Libraries and Selection of Single-Domain Antibodies Against Peptide Antigens*

Jyothi Kumaran, C. Roger MacKenzie, and Mehdi Arbabi-Ghahroudi

Abstract

With the identification of vast numbers of novel proteins through genomic and proteomic initiatives, the need for efficient processes to characterize and target them has increased. Antibodies are naturally designed molecules that can fulfill this need, and in vitro methodologies for isolating them from either immune or naïve sources have been extensively developed. However, access to pure protein antigens for screening purposes is a major hurdle due to the limitations associated with recombinant production of eukaryotic proteins. Consequently, rational peptide design based on proteomic methodologies such as protein modeling, secondary sequence prediction, and hydrophobicity/hydrophilicity prediction, in combination with other bioinformatics data, is being explored as a viable solution to isolate specific antibodies against difficult antigens. Single-domain antibodies are becoming the ideal antibody format due to their structural advantages and ease of production compared to conventional antibodies and antibody fragments derived from conventional antibodies. For screening purposes, phage display technology is a well-established technique. With this technique, a repertoire of antibody fragments can be displayed on the surface of filamentous phages (f1, fd, M13) followed by screening against various antigenic targets. Furthermore, the technique can be expanded to a high-throughput scale using a magnetic-based, in-solution panning protocol which allows for the screening of multiple target antigens simultaneously. In this chapter, we describe a semiautomated panning method to screen a naïve *Camelidae* library against rationally designed peptide antigens, followed by preliminary characterization of isolated binders.

Key words: Single-domain antibody, *Camelidae*, Phage library, Peptide antigens, Manual panning, Semiautomated panning, Surface plasmon resonance, Binding affinity

1. Introduction

In the postgenomic era, the requirement of specific binders for use in molecular targeting in biotechnology and biomedical science fields has increased. The essential element for screening of binder

* This is National Research Council Canada Publication number: 50019.

Dirk Saerens and Serge Muyldermans (eds.), *Single Domain Antibodies: Methods and Protocols*,
Methods in Molecular Biology, vol. 911, DOI 10.1007/978-1-61779-968-6_7, © Springer Science+Business Media, LLC 2012

libraries is the availability of target antigens in sufficient quantities and in relative purities. This often requires recombinant production of the target protein(s) in either eukaryotic or prokaryotic hosts followed by a lengthy, costly, and labor-intensive purification, and sometimes in vitro refolding. If limitations such as the inability to express stable, purified target and to extract usable amounts of the target are also factored in, the task of developing specific binders becomes virtually impossible. In such cases, rational peptide design based on proteomic methodologies and bioinformatics data is being explored as a viable solution to isolate specific antibodies against difficult antigens, since peptides can be chemically synthesized in reasonably large quantities and tagged simultaneously with recognition markers such as biotin. Biotinylated peptides are well-suited for in-solution streptavidin magnetic bead-based panning. The isolated binders can then be screened for affinity to parental protein depending on antigen availability in either purified form or displayed on the cell surface.

The discovery and characterization of heavy chain antibodies from *Camelidae* (1, 2) have revitalized the original idea of Ward et al. (3) in which the variable domains (VH or VL) of antibodies can potentially be used as independent binding units. It was shown that the variable heavy domains (VHHs) of *Camelidae* heavy chain antibodies mediate antigen recognition through three complementarity determining region (CDR) loops, since the heavy chain is not paired with light chain, as is the case with conventional antibodies (2, 4, 5). In addition to the advantages associated with in vitro antibody generation (see Chapter 16), the VHH is a stable and soluble structure which, due to its relatively small, compact size with three CDR loops, allows for relative ease of genetic manipulations paired with the possibility of sampling close to maximal in vivo CDR loop diversity where randomization of loop residues is required (6).

Filamentous phages such as M13, F1, and fd are used to display peptides or proteins as fusion products of, most commonly, the pIII or the pVIII viral coat proteins (7, 8). For multidisplay purposes, fd or fd-tet-based vectors are prevalently used for construction of antibody phage libraries. The addition of a tetracycline resistance cassette within the fd-tet phage genome allows for a more stable library format resulting in an unlimited access to the phage library stock. This is not the characteristic of, for example, an fd phage library because the one-time prepared stock of plaque-based phage library cannot be reamplified due to lack of any selective pressure in the phage vector, and therefore, the antibody genes can easily be lost.

In screening phage antibody libraries, solid-phase manual panning against selected antigens has traditionally been the protocol of choice. Though effective, the methodology is a labor-intensive task and not time-effective, especially when screening of multiple target antigens is required. Alternatively, panning of multiple targets can be performed in solution using streptavidin magnetic beads coupled with an automated bead processor and washer (multipin method), followed by standard phage ELISA or bead-based ELISA screening—for a detailed review see (9). One main advantage of this technique is the increased surface area on beads compared to plates, allowing for more efficient panning compared to solid-phase manual panning. In addition, transferring magnetic beads between microtitre plates for incubation and washing reduces background binding to surfaces and transfers minimal volumes. Furthermore, bead-based ELISA screening can allow for detection of antigens normally difficult to assess using conventional ELISA (9). A fully automated panning methodology includes multiple automated modules for panning (multipin method), for colony picking followed by induction by a robotic arm (Qpix), and for ELISA screening by a robotic system (Biomek 2000) (10).

The goal of in vitro antibody-display libraries is to mimic as closely as possible an in vivo repertoire. Methods which maximize in vitro library diversity are essential to allow for successful retrieval of binders against targets. In constructing the naïve library used in this chapter, the VHH genes from three Camelid species, llama, alpaca, and camel, are represented in one phage library. This approach theoretically allows for increased diversity by combining the repertoires of three different but related animals, whose history of antigenic exposure and antibody repertoires is likely nonredundant, with high variability in the library repertoire to increase the success rate of selecting good binders. We, therefore, describe methodologies for semiautomated panning of this naive, *Camelidae* library against peptide targets to isolate Single-domain antibodies (sdAbs) having affinity for the antigens. We also present preliminary data on the characterization of sdAbs for binding to both the peptide targets and their parental proteins.

In conclusion, combining the advantages of large repertoire pooling from individual *Camelidae* family members, a semiautomated panning approach, and rational ELISA screening against the target antigen resulted in successful isolation of VHH binders recognizing peptide antigens as well as their parental proteins. This approach has the added value of simultaneous epitope mapping of the target antigen which may have important implications in functional studies of protein–protein interactions.

2. Materials

Prepare all solutions using ultrapure water (prepared by purifying deionized water to attain a sensitivity of 18 MΩ cm at 25°C) and analytical grade reagents. Prepare and store all reagents at room temperature (unless indicated otherwise). Diligently follow all waste disposal regulations when disposing waste materials.

2.1. Library Construction

See Subheading 3.1.

2.2. Selection of Peptide Antigen

See Subheading 3.2.

2.3. Manual Panning: Phage Rescue from the Library

1. LAC-M Naïve library (single-domain antibody group, Institute for Biological Science, National Research Council of Canada, Ottawa, Canada).
2. 2× YT-Tet (per liter): 16 g Bacto tryptone, 10 g Bacto yeast extract, 5 g NaCl, deionized H_2O, 12.5 μg/mL Tetracycline (final concentration).
3. 2× YT-Tet/agar plates: 16 g Bacto tryptone, 10 g Bacto yeast extract, 5 g NaCl, 15 g Bacto-agar, deionized H_2O, 12.5 μg/mL Tetracycline (final concentration).
4. Shaker flask.
5. 30°C incubator shaker.
6. 0.2 μm GP Express™ *Plus* Membrane filtration system (MILLIPORE Corporate, Billerica, MA, USA).
7. Sterile PEG solution: 20% (w/v) polyethylene glycol 6000 or 8000, 2.5 M NaCl. Autoclave to sterilize. (Note: the solution foams when heated and requires about a day to settle).
8. Sorvall high speed (RC5B Plus) and swinging bucket bench-top (RT6000B Refrigerated) centrifuges (Thermo Scientific, Asheville, NC, USA) or their equivalents.
9. Centrifuge tubes.
10. 50 mL Falcon tubes (if using a bucket bench-top centrifuge).
11. 10× phosphate-buffered saline stock (PBS): Dissolve the following in 800 mL of MilliQ H_2O: 80 g NaCl, 2 g KCl, 14.4 g Na_2HPO_4, 2.4 g KH_2PO_4, and adjust pH to 7.4 using 6 N HCl. Adjust volume to 1 L with additional MilliQ H_2O. Sterilize by autoclaving. Dilute ten times to prepare PBS. Make PBS-T by adding 0.05% (v/v) Tween-20 to PBS.
12. TG1 *Escherichia coli* cells (Stratagene, La Jolla, CA, USA).
13. 1.5 mL Eppendorf tubes.

2.4. Manual Panning: Panning Procedure

1. NUNC MaxiSorp™ plates (VWR Scientific).
2. Parafilm.
3. Streptavidin (ThermoFisher Scientific, Rockford, IL, USA).
4. Paper towels.
5. StartingBlock (Thermo Scientific-Pierce Protein Research Products, Rockford, IL, USA).
6. Phage library.

7. Biotinylated peptide(s).
8. PBS: Prepare 1× PBS using the 10× PBS stock solution (see Subheading 2.3, item 11).
9. Wash buffer (PBS-T): Make PBS-T by adding 0.05% (v/v) Tween-20 to 1× PBS.
10. 0.22 μm syringe filters (MILLIPORE Corporate).
11. 10 mL syringe(s).
12. Sterile PEG solution (see Subheading 2.3, item 7).
13. 50 mL Falcon tubes.
14. 1.5 mL Eppendorf tubes.
15. 100 mM triethylamine: 35 μL of 7.18 M triethylamine in 2.5 mL of MilliQ H_2O, made fresh daily.
16. 1 M Tris–HCl pH 7.4.
17. 2× YT-Tet/agar plates (see Subheading 2.3, item 3).
18. 2× YT-Tet broth (see Subheading 2.3, item 2).
19. Big and small diameter plates for agar.
20. TG1 *E. coli* cells (Stratagene).
21. Shaker incubator.
22. Vortex.
23. 37 and 32°C incubator.
24. Refrigerated centrifuge (4°C).

2.5. Semiautomated Panning Using KingFisher Flex

1. KingFisher 96 magnetic particle processor (KingFisher, ThermoElectron Corporation, Vantaa, Finland).
2. CELLection Dynabeads (Invitrogen Dynal AS, Oslo, Norway).
3. Sterile 1.5 mL Eppendorf tubes.
4. StartingBlock (Thermo Scientific-Pierce).
5. Biotinylated peptides (see Subheading 3.2).
6. Buffer 1: PBS without Ca^{2+} and Mg^{2+}, 0.1% BSA, pH 7.4.
7. Shaker for gentle mixing.
8. Phage library.
9. Microfuge.
10. 4°C fridge.
11. M9 agar plates: M9 minimal medium: 100 mL of 10× M9 salts, 1 mL of 1 M $MgCl_2$, 0.1 mL of 1 M $CaCl_2$, 5 mL of 1 mg/mL vitamin B1, 10 mL of 20% w/v glucose, 20 mL of 20% w/v Casamino acids. Add each sterilized solution to 900 mL of cooled, autoclaved MilliQ H_2O.
12. 10× M9 salts: 60 g Na_2HPO_4, 30 g KH_2PO_4, 10 g NH_4Cl, 5 g NaCl. Dissolve in 1 L of MilliQ H_2O and autoclave. 10× induction

media (per 100 mL): 12 g Bacto tryptone, 24 g Bacto yeast extract, 4 mL glycerol (11).

13. Luria-Bertani broth (per liter): 10 g Bacto tryptone, 5 g Bacto yeast extract, 10 g NaCl, deionized H_2O.
14. TG1 *E. coli* cells (Stratagene).
15. Cell culture incubator with shaker.
16. 3% w/v bovine serum albumin (BSA).
17. PBS: Prepare 1× PBS using the 10× PBS stock solution (see Subheading 2.3, item 11).
18. Wash buffer (PBS-T): Make PBS-T by adding 0.05% (v/v) Tween-20 to 1× PBS.
19. 100 mM triethylamine: 35 μL of 7.18 M triethylamine in 2.5 mL of MilliQ H_2O, made fresh daily.
20. 1 M Tris–HCl pH 7.4.
21. Biotinylated and nonbiotinylated peptide(s).
22. Magnetic separator (Promega Corporation, 2800 Woods Hollow Road, Madison, WI, USA).
23. 2× YT-Tet/agar plates (see Subheading 2.3, item 3).
24. 2× YT-Tet broth (see Subheading 2.3, item 2).
25. Big and small diameter plates for agar.
26. Refrigerated centrifuge (4°C).
27. 0.22 μm syringe filters (MILLIPORE Corporate).
28. PEG solution (see Subheading 2.3, item 7).

2.6. Large-Scale Screening: Polyclonal Phage ELISA

1. NUNC MaxiSorp™ plates.
2. Streptavidin (ThermoFisher Scientific).
3. Protein antigen(s).
4. PBS: Prepare 1× PBS using the 10× PBS stock solution (see Subheading 2.3, item 11).
5. Wash buffer (PBS-T): Make PBS-T by adding 0.05% (v/v) Tween-20 to 1× PBS.
6. Paper towels.
7. Biotinylated peptide(s).
8. 37°C incubator.
9. StartingBlock (Thermo Scientific-Pierce).
10. Phage library (see Subheading 3.5, steps 25 and 26).
11. HRP substrate: TMB peroxidase substrate and H_2O_2 (KPL, Gaithersburg, MD, USA).
12. 1 M phosphoric acid.
13. Multiskan FC microplate photometer (ELISA reader) (Thermo Scientific-Pierce Protein Research Products, Rockford, IL, USA).

2.7. Large-Scale Screening: Monoclonal Phage ELISA Screening

1. 2× YT-Tet broth (see Subheading 2.3, item 2).
2. 96-well U-bottom Microtest™ microtiter plates (Becton Dickinson and Company, Franklin lakes, NJ, USA).
3. 37°C humid chamber with shaker.
4. NUNC MaxiSorp™ plates.
5. Streptavidin (ThermoFisher Scientific).
6. StartingBlock (Thermo Scientific-Pierce).
7. Biotinylated peptides (see Subheading 3.2).
8. 4°C fridge.
9. PBS: Prepare 1× PBS using the 10× PBS stock solution (see Subheading 2.3, item 11).
10. Wash buffer (PBS-T): Make PBS-T by adding 0.05% (v/v) Tween-20 to 1× PBS.
11. Paper towels.
12. 1.5 mL Eppendorf tubes.
13. Microfuge.
14. Biotinylated peptide(s).
15. 2× YT-Tet broth (see Subheading 2.3, item 2).
16. 37°C incubator.
17. TMB peroxidase substrate and H_2O_2 (KPL, Gaithersburg, MD, USA).
18. 1 M phosphoric acid.
19. Multiskan FC microplate photometer (ELISA reader) (Thermo Scientific).

2.8. Subcloning, Expression, and Purification

1. pVT2 expression vector (12).
2. Pure Proteome Nickel Magnetic Beads (Millipore) for small-scale purification.
3. 5 mL HiTrap Chelating HP column (GE Healthcare) for large-scale purification.

2.9. Characterization of Binders: Affinity Measurements

1. Biacore 3000 instrument with BIAevaluation software 4.1 (GE Healthcare).
2. Superdex 200 gel filtration column (GE Healthcare).
3. ÄKTA FPLC purification system (GE Healthcare).
4. ND-1000 spectrophotometer (NanoDrop Technologies, Wilmington, DE, USA) or a similar instrument.
5. HBS-E containing 0.005% v/v P20.
6. CM5 sensor chip (GE Healthcare).
7. 50 mM NHS.
8. 200 mM EDC.

9. Streptavidin (Thermofisher).
10. 10 mM acetate buffer pH 4.5.
11. 1 M ethanolamine pH 8.5.
12. Biotinylated peptide(s).
13. Purified pentamer protein.

2.10. Characterization of Binders: Binding to Parental Proteins

1. NUNC MaxiSorp™ plates.
2. Protein antigen(s).
3. StartingBlock (Thermo Scientific).
4. 4°C fridge.
5. PBS: Prepare 1× PBS using the 10× PBS stock solution (see Subheading 2.3, item 11).
6. Paper towels.
7. Purified pentamer.
8. TMB peroxidase substrate and H_2O_2 (KPL, Gaithersburg, MD, USA).
9. 1 M phosphoric acid.
10. Multiskan FC microplate photometer (ELISA reader) (Thermo Scientific-Pierce Protein Research Products, Rockford, IL, USA).
11. 37°C incubator.
12. Wash buffer (PBS-T): Make PBS-T by adding 0.05% (v/v) Tween-20 to 1× PBS.

3. Methods

3.1. Library Construction

A naïve, *Camelidae* sdAb library was constructed in fd-tet-M vector using the methodology described by Arbabi-Ghahroudi et al. (13). This nonimmune library is composed of only VHH genes derived from a healthy llama, a healthy alpaca, and a healthy camel (LAC-M). The original fd-tet vector (14) was modified to introduce two *Sfi*I restriction sites in the multiple cloning sites (unpublished data). The VHH fragments were amplified and cloned as described before (15).

3.2. Selection of Peptide Antigen

Peptide targets were rationally chosen based on a combination of proteomics, glycomics, and bioinformatics approaches. A list of putative cell surface and secreted proteins from the human genome was created through mining of bioinformatics data. Secreted targets were further narrowed using subcellular fractionation and DNA microarray methods. Targets from this pool were chosen based on further evaluation, i.e., occurrence in disease.

Parallel approaches were pursued to maximize the success of retrieving a set of useful antibodies which bind to chosen peptide regions. First, peptides were chosen based on their occurrence in so-called intrinsically unstructured regions of the parental protein. These regions were identified by bioinformatics sequence analysis. Second, small structured regions from the parental protein were also identified through structural analysis and used as antigens to increase the range of potential epitopes.

3.3. Manual Panning: Phage Rescue from the Library

1. Grow 5×10^{10} cells of LAC-M phage library in 500 mL of 2× YT-Tet (12.5 μg/mL) at 220 rpm, 30°C overnight.
2. Next morning, centrifuge the culture at 4,400×*g* 4°C for 15 min.
3. Filter the supernatant through a 0.22 μm filter.
4. Precipitate phage supernatant with 1/5 the supernatant volume of PEG (8000)-NaCl. Incubate on ice for 1 h and centrifuge either at 14,000×*g* 4°C for 15 min using a *SORVALL RC 5B Plus* centrifuge or in Falcon tubes at 3,600×*g*, 4°C for 30 min using a bucket bench-top centrifuge.
5. Remove any traces of PEG and resuspend the phage pellet in 1 mL of PBS. Perform serial dilutions of the resuspension (from 10^{-2} to 10^{-12}) and infect *E. coli* TG1 with the diluted phage, spread them on 2× YT-Tet plates, and incubate at 37°C overnight (see Note 1).
6. Aliquot 100 μL of phage preparation into sterile 1.5 mL microtubes and store at −20°C for short-term storage and at −80°C for long-term use (see Note 2).

3.4. Manual Panning: Panning Procedure

1. Add 100 μL of 100 μg/mL streptavidin in PBS to two wells of a Maxisorp™ plate. Seal the wells with parafilm and incubate overnight at 4°C. Use one well as the subtraction well and the other one as the antigen well (see Note 3).
2. The next morning, discard the streptavidin solution and blot the wells on a paper towel. Add 200 μL StartingBlock™ to both wells and seal them. Incubate the wells at 37°C for 2 h.
3. Discard the blocking solution. Add 100 μL 10^{12} cfu phage in 100 μL of StartingBlock™ to the subtraction well and 100 μL of 5 μg/mL biotinylated peptide in PBS to the antigen well. Seal and incubate both wells at room temperature for 1.5 h.
4. Empty the antigen well and wash it three times with PBS. Transfer the phage from the subtraction well to the antigen well. Seal and incubate at room temperature for 1.5 h. Start the *E. coli* TG1 cell culture as described below (see Subheading 3.4, step 8).
5. Discard the unbound phage. Rinse the wells five times with 300 μL wash buffer and discard the wash solution. Wash five

times with PBS. After the last wash, blot the well on a paper towel to remove any remaining liquid.

6. Elute the bound phage by adding 100 μL of 100 mM triethylamine. Pipette the content of the well up and down several times and incubate at room temperature for exactly 10 min.
7. Following the incubation, pipette the contents of the well up and down several times, transfer the eluted phage to a sterile microfuge tube containing 50 μL of 1 M Tris–HCl, pH 7.4, and vortex to neutralize the triethylamine. Keep the tube on ice.
8. Prepare 10 mL of exponentially growing TG1 cells in a sterile 50 mL Falcon tube. Keep 100 μL of the exponentially growing TG1 cells for the negative control titer (see Subheading 3.4, step 9) and infect the remaining cells with 150 μL of the eluted phage by incubating the mixture of cells and phage at 37°C for 30 min without shaking followed by 30 min with slow shaking at 220 rpm (see Note 4).
9. Make serial dilutions (10^{-2}–10^{-6}) of the infected cells in 2× YT-Tet and spread 100 μL of each dilution on 2× YT-Tet plates. Also plate 100 μL of the uninfected cells as a negative control (see Note 5). Incubate at 32°C overnight. Keep the plates parafilm-sealed and stored at 4°C for clonal analysis.
10. Spin down the infected TG1 cells at 2,000 × *g* for 12 min at 4°C. Resuspend the pellet in 500 μL of 2× YT-Tet. Plate the cells on 2× YT-Tet plate (15 mm). Incubate at 37°C overnight.
11. The next morning, scrape colonies from the plate into 50 mL of 2× YT-Tet. Mix 5 mL of cell suspension and 5 mL fresh 2× YT-Tet broth and incubate for 5 h at 230 rpm, 30°C.
12. Centrifuge the phage at 3,600 × *g*, 4°C, for 30 min. Pass phage supernatant through a 0.22 μm filter. Precipitate phage supernatant with 1/5 volume of PEG-NaCl and incubate on ice for 1 h. Centrifuge the phage at 3,600 rpm, 4°C, for 30 min.
13. Resuspend phage pellet in 200 μL of sterile PBS. Use 100 μL of the phage for the second round of panning. Keep the remainder at −20°C. Make serial dilutions (10^{-2}–10^{-12}) of the phage solution in PBS and infect TG1 cells with 10 μL of each dilution (see Note 1).
14. Repeat Subheading 3.4, steps 1–13 for the second, third, and fourth rounds of panning.

3.5. Semiautomated Panning Using KingFisher Flex (See Note 6)

Biopannings of the phage library against 24 peptide antigens are performed simultaneously. An overview of the operational steps of KingFisher system to pan is shown in Fig. 1.

1. In order to prepare antigen for the first day of panning procedure, aliquot 50 μL of CELLection™ Dynabeads in 24 sterile microfuge tubes, one for each peptide.

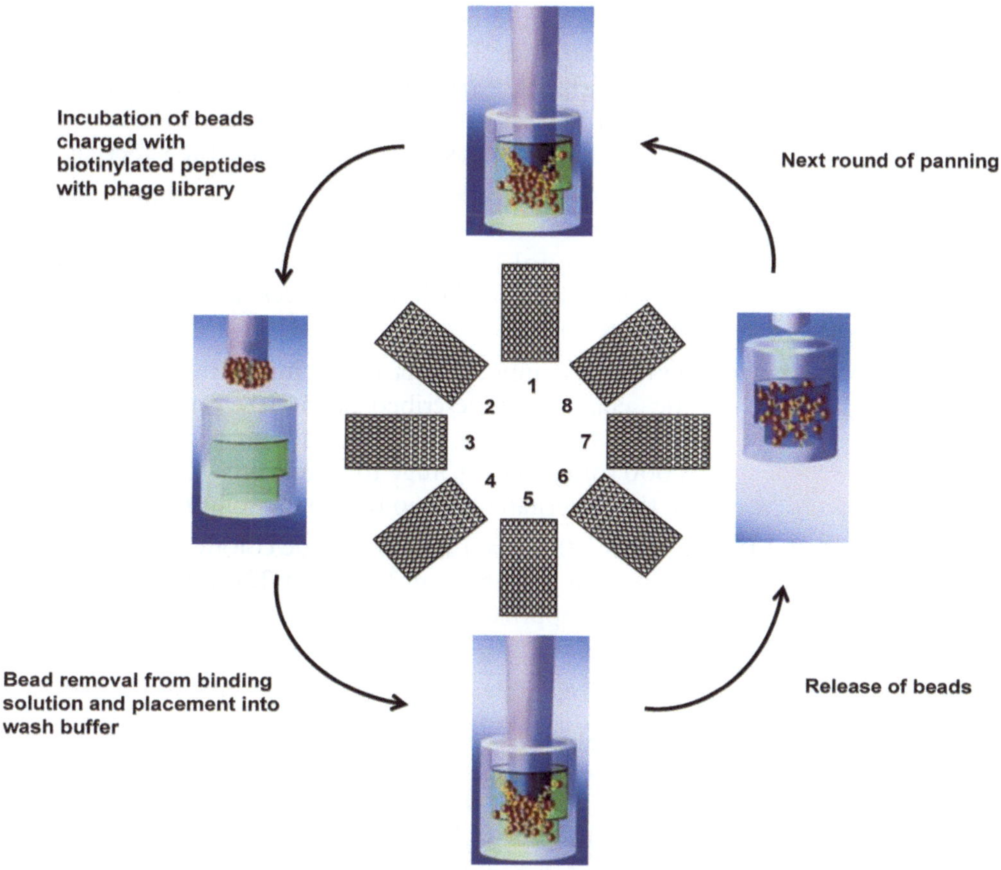

Fig. 1. Schematic representation of the KingFisher semiautomated panning setup. Eight 96-well plates filled with appropriate targets and buffers are placed on the turntable, which rotates clockwise to bring the plate in-line with the magnets. *Arrows* mark the order of the stages of panning depicted by the single well magnifications. (The single well magnifications were taken from http://www.thermo.com/eThermo/CMA/PDFs/Various/File_24142.pdf with permission).

2. Wash the beads twice with 500 μL of buffer 1. Place the tube in a magnetic separator for 1 min, aspirate, and discard the supernatant.
3. After washing the beads, remove the tube from the magnet and resuspend the Dynabeads in 198 μL of StartingBlock™ buffer and 2 μL of each respective peptide (10 mg/mL) (2 μL for round 2, 1.5 μL for round 3, and 1.0 μL for round 4 (see Note 7).
4. Incubate overnight at 4°C with gentle mixing (see Note 8).
5. To prepare the phage library, aliquot 50 μL of CELLection™ Dynabeads to a sterile microfuge tubes one for each peptide.
6. Wash the beads twice with 500 μL of buffer 1. Place the tube in a magnetic separator for 1 min, aspirate, and discard the supernatant.

7. After washing the beads, remove the tube from the magnet and resuspend the Dynabeads in the original volume (50 μL) of StartingBlock™ (see Note 9). Incubate at room temperature for 1 h with gentle mixing. Place the tube in a magnetic separator for 1 min, aspirate, and discard the supernatant.
8. Resuspend the blocked beads in 100 μL of appropriate blocking buffer (refer to table below) and 100 μL of phage library (6×10^{12} cfu/mL) for each target. Incubate overnight at 4°C with gentle mixing. This step reduces the background binders (see Note 8).
9. The next morning, collect phage in solution by using a magnetic separator as described previously (see Subheading 3.5, step 2). Spin down the collected phage and centrifuge at 13,000 rpm in a microfuge for 4 min at 4°C and carefully aspirate the supernatant. Keep the phage solution on ice.
10. Inoculate 10 mL of LB with a single colony of TG1 cells plated on M9 agar. Incubate at 37°C and 220 rpm until $OD_{600\ nm}$ is about 0.4 (approximately 3 h) (see Note 10).
11. Prepare and label KingFisher flex 96 well plates as described in the following table:

Plate number	Plate type	Components
1	Antigen/ bead	Biotinylated antigen and beads
2	Wash	Buffer 1
3	Blocking buffer	StartingBlock (rounds 1 and 3) 3% (w/v) BSA (rounds 2 and 4)
4	Incubation	Phage
5	Wash	PBS containing 0.05% (v/v) Tween-20
6	Wash	PBS containing 0.05% (v/v) Tween-20
7	Elution	100 mM triethylamine or nonbiotinylated peptide/ protein solution (see Note 12)
8	Tip/Wash	PBS-T (0.05% (v/v) Tween 20) for rounds 2–4 (see Note 11)

12. Pick up the tips from plate 8.
13. Mix beads-biotinylated peptide/protein (plate no. 1).
14. Wash beads three times with 300 μL of buffer 1 (plate no. 2). For round 1, mix for 20 s at slow speed. For rounds 2–4, mix for 1 min at medium speed.
15. Block the beads with 300 μL of StartingBlock™ buffer or 3% (w/v) BSA PBS for 30 min at room temperature (plate no. 3).

For each round, mix for 5 s at low speed and pause for 3 min with loop count set at 10.

16. Release the beads into 300 μL of the phage library and incubate for 60 min with gentle mixing at room temperature (plate no. 4). Mix for 5 s at low speed and pause for 5 min with loop count set at 12 for each round.
17. Wash beads two or three times with 300 μL wash buffer (plates 5 and 6 for round 1, and plates 5, 6, and 8 for subsequent rounds). For round 1, wash for 10 s at low speed. For rounds 2, 3, and 4, wash for 1 min at medium speed (see Note 11).
18. Elute phage particles with either 100 mM triethylamine or 0.1 mg/mL of nonbiotinylated peptide (plate no. 7) (see Note 12). Mix for 25 min for round 1 and 20 min for rounds 2–4 at medium speed. Collect beads and release them into a wash buffer plate.
19. Transfer the contents of the wells (100 μL) from KingFisher plate into sterile microfuge tubes containing 50 μL 1 M Tris–HCl pH 7.4 if eluted with TEA. Keep the tubes on ice.
20. Infect 2 mL exponentially growing TG1 cells with the eluted phage by incubating the mixture at 37°C for 15 min without shaking.
21. For phage titration, make a series of 100-fold dilutions using 10 μL of phage in 990 μL of PBS from 10^{-2} to 10^{-6}, then use 10 μL of the dilutions to infect 150 μL of exponentially growing cells. Spread 150 μL of the infected cells on 2× YT-Tet plates. Also plate 100 μL of the uninfected cells as a negative control.
22. Spin down the infected TG1 cells at 2,000 × *g* for 12 min at 4°C. Resuspend the pellet in 500 μL of 2× YT-Tet. Plate the cells on a 2× YT-Tet plate (15 mm). Incubate at 37°C overnight.
23. On day 3, scrape colonies from the plates into 50 mL of 2× YT-Tet. Use 5 mL of cell suspension and 5 mL fresh 2× YT-Tet broth and incubate for 5 h at 230 rpm, 30°C.
24. Centrifuge the phage at 3,600 × *g* 4°C, for 30 min. Pass phage supernatant through a 0.22 μm filter. Precipitate phage supernatant with 1/5 volume of PEG-NaCl and incubate on ice for 1 h. Centrifuge the phage at 3,600 × *g*, 4°C for 30 min.
25. Resuspend phage pellet in 200 μL of sterile PBS. Use 100 μL of the phage for the next round of panning. Keep the remaining phage at −20°C (see Note 13). Determine the phage titer by making serial dilutions of phage as described previously (see Subheading 3.4, step 9) (see also Note 1).
26. For subsequent rounds of panning, repeat steps 1–26 using the amplified phage eluted from the previous round.

3.6. Large-Scale Screening: Polyclonal Phage ELISA

Polyclonal phage ELISA is performed on amplified phage obtained from each round of panning (see Subheading 3.4, steps 1–14). The selection is performed for up to 12 peptide antigens in one microtitre plate and phage from rounds 1 to 4 are used along with an appropriate negative control.

1. For each 12 peptide antigen set, coat a full 96-well ELISA plate (A1–H12) with 100 μL of streptavidin (2–5 μg/mL) and incubate at 4°C overnight. Number the plate with each peptide antigen on the top so that each column (wells from A to H) represents one peptide. If screening against the parental protein antigen is desired, coat the ELISA wells overnight with the respective protein at a concentration of 5 μg/mL and proceed to step 4 the next day.
2. The next morning, remove streptavidin solution from ELISA plate and rinse the wells twice with PBS. Tap the plate on a paper towel to remove excess liquid.
3. Dilute each biotinylated peptide in PBS to 1–5 μg/mL and aliquot 100 μL of the diluted sample into each ELISA well (from A1 to D12). Add 100 μL PBS as a blank control to the rest of the wells (E1–H12). Incubate the plate at room temperature for 30 min.
4. Remove the contents of the wells and rinse them twice with PBS. Tap the plate on a paper towel to remove excess liquid.
5. Block the ELISA wells (A1–H12) with 200 μL per well of StartingBlock™ and incubate for 2 h at 37°C.
6. Add 100 μL of diluted phage (10^9–10^{10}/mL in PBS) of the stock phage (see Subheading 3.4, step 25) from rounds 1 to 4 to the respective peptide wells (A1–H1 for peptide 1, A2–H2 for peptide 2, and so on). Incubate the plate at 37°C for 1.5 h.
7. Wash five times with 250 μL of wash buffer. Tap the plate on a paper towel after the last wash to remove excess liquid.
8. Add 100 μL of HRP substrate to each well (from A1 to H12).
9. Stop the reaction after 5–10 min with 100 μL per well of 1 M phosphoric acid. Measure the absorbance at 450 nm (see Fig. 2a).

3.7. Large-Scale Screening: Monoclonal Phage ELISA Screening

1. At day 1 of the procedure, inoculate 96 colonies from each peptide target antigen in 200 μL of 2× YT containing 12.5 μg/mL tetracycline into a 96-well U-bottom microtitre plates. Incubate at 37°C in a humid chamber, shaking at 120 rpm overnight.
2. Coat one full ELISA plate (A1–H12) for each peptide antigen with 100 μL of streptavidin (2–5 μg/mL). At the same time, coat the second plate (A1–H12) with 100 μL of blocking

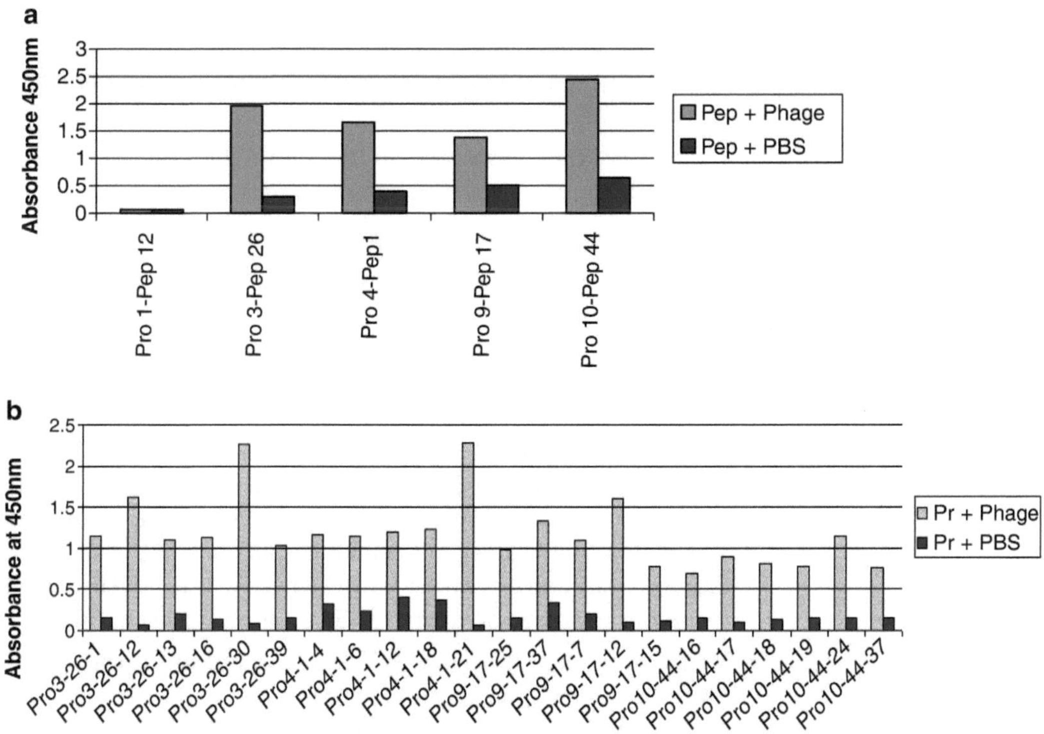

Fig. 2. Representative examples of (**a**) polyclonal phage ELISA and (**b**) monoclonal phage ELISA. (**a**) Pooled phage obtained from round four of panning against peptide were added to ELISA wells coated with the parental proteins (Pro 1, Pro 3, Pro 4, Pro 9, and Pro 10) from which the peptide targets (Pep 12, Pep 26, Pep 1, Pep 17, and Pep 44, respectively) were derived. The majority of the pools contain phage displaying variable heavy domains (VHHs) which bind to the protein target. (**b**) Individual phage clones (number before hyphens refers to parental protein and number between hyphens refers to peptide) chosen from fourth round pooled phage (see (**a**)) were tested for binding to the parental protein (Pro 3, Pro 4, Pro 9, and Pro 10). Several clones from each pooled phage sample demonstrate significant affinity toward their respective protein antigens.

buffer (StartingBlock™) as negative control and store at 4°C overnight.

3. At day 2 of the procedure, discard streptavidin solution from ELISA plate and rinse the wells twice with PBS. Tap the plate on a paper towel to remove excess liquid.
4. Dilute each biotinylated peptide in PBS to 1–5 μg/mL and aliquot 100 μL of the diluted sample into each ELISA well. Include 100 μL of PBS as a blank control for each sample and two negative control wells which do not get phage. Incubate the plate at room temperature for 30 min.
5. Remove the contents of the wells and rinse them twice with PBS. Tap the plate on a paper towel to remove excess liquid.
6. Block the ELISA wells with 200 μL per well of StartingBlock™ buffer. Incubate for 2 h at room temperature.
7. Transfer each overnight culture to 1.5 mL microfuge tubes and spin them at 14,000 rpm in a microfuge for 6 min at 4°C.

8. Add 100 μL of the supernatant from each culture to the corresponding wells on the ELISA plate. For blank wells, use the same supernatants. For the negative control wells, use 100 μL of 2× YT-Tet. Incubate the plate at 37°C for 1.5 h.
9. Wash five times with wash buffer. Tap the plate on a paper towel after the last wash to remove excess liquid.
10. Add 100 μL of HRP substrate to each well.
11. Stop the reaction after 5–10 min with 100 μL per well of 1 M phosphoric acid. Measure the absorbance at 450 nm.

3.8. Subcloning, Expression, and Purification

All the cloning steps were performed as described in Sambrook et al. (11). For specific subcloning of VHHs, see ref. (13) and Chapter 27.

1. Positive clones from phage ELISA screening are subcloned into the pVT2 expression vector in order to produce a pentameric format of VHHs (see Chapter 27). The pentameric VHH closely imitates pentavalent display of sdAbs on the surface of filamentous phage. Alternatively, the VHH can be cloned in monomeric format (13) or as an Fc-fusion (16, 17).
2. VHH genes are cloned in pVT2 vector and in fusion with the OmpA leader sequence for expression and export to the bacterial periplasm. For detailed protocols of protein expression and extraction, see Chapter 16.
3. The C-terminal His tag in the sdAbs makes it possible to do one-step protein purification by performing immobilized metal affinity chromatography (IMAC). This can be done by using Pure Proteome™ Nickel Magnetic Beads (Millipore) for small-scale purification or a 5 mL HiTrap™ Chelating HP column for large-scale purification. For a detailed protocol, see Chapter 16.

3.9. Characterization of Binders: Affinity Measurements

Accurate binding affinities and kinetics of binding are derived from surface plasmon resonance (SPR) analyses performed with a Biacore instrument.

1. Isolate monomeric fraction of the pentamer (see Note 15) prior to SPR analysis using size exclusion column chromatography. Determine the protein concentration.
2. Carry out SPR experiments at 25°C using a Biacore 3000 instrument with HBS-E containing 0.005% (v/v) surfactant P20 as the running buffer.
3. Immobilize streptavidin on a CM5 sensor chip to give maximum surface density which is approximately 2,500 response units (RUs). Activate CM-dextran surface with a 7 min injection of a mixture of 50 mM NHS and 200 mM EDC at a flow rate of 5 μL/min. Inject 50 μg/mL streptavidin, diluted in 10 mM acetate buffer, pH 4.5, for 7 min at a flow rate of 5 μL/min and block the surface with a 7 min injection of 1 M ethanolamine, pH 8.5.

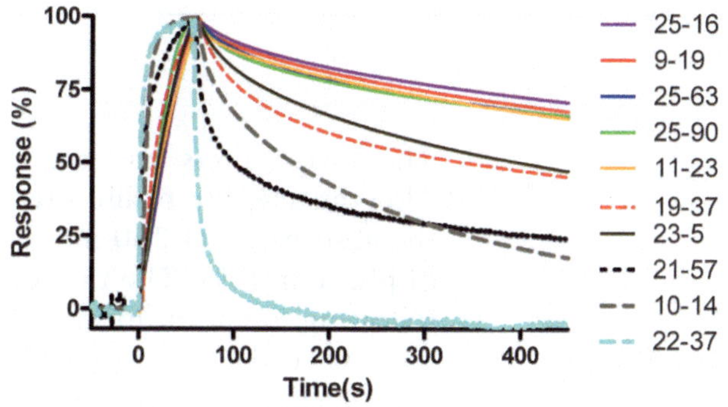

Fig. 3. Sensorgram overlays showing the binding of anti-peptide pentamers (9–19, 10–14, 11–23, 19–37, 21–57, 22–37, 23–5, 25–16, 25–63, and 25–90) to corresponding peptides 9, 10, 11, 19, 21, 22, 23 25. The amount of immobilized streptavidin was 2,700 RUs. The data are normalized with the maximum RUs bound for each peptide set at 100%.

4. Saturate the streptavidin surface with biotinylated peptide (range = 300–500 RUs) by injecting 35 μL of 200 nM biotinylated peptide at a flow rate of 5 μL/min.
5. Analyze pentameric VHH interaction with the peptide using a streptavidin surface as a reference. Inject 10 or 40 μL of 200 nM pentamer over both the streptavidin and streptavidin-antigen surfaces at a flow rate of 40 μL/min.
6. Analyze the data using BIAevaluation software 4.1 (Biacore Inc.) (see Fig. 3).

3.10. Characterization of Binders: Binding to Parental Proteins

1. For screening of 96 colonies, coat one full ELISA plate (A1–H12) with 100 μL of protein antigen (1–5 μg/mL). At the same time, coat a second plate (A1–H12) with 100 μL of blocking buffer (StartingBlock™) as negative control and store at 4°C overnight.
2. The next morning, remove the protein solution from ELISA plate and rinse the wells twice with PBS. Tap the plate on a paper towel to remove excess liquid.
3. Block the ELISA wells with 200 μL per well of protein-free blocking buffer (StartingBlock™). Incubate for 2 h at room temperature.
4. Add 100 μL of the purified pentamer (10–100 mg/mL) to the corresponding wells on the ELISA plate. For blank wells, use the same pentamer concentration. Incubate the plate at 37°C for 1.5 h.
5. Wash five times with wash buffer. Tap the plate on a paper towel after the last wash to remove excess liquid.
6. Add 100 μL of HRP substrate to each well.
7. Stop the reaction after 5–10 min with 100 μL per well of 1 M phosphoric acid. Read the plate at 450 nm (see Fig. 2b).

4. Notes

1. The phage titers are generally around 10^{12}–10^{13} cfu/mL. Alternatively, the phage titer can be estimated by measuring the absorbance at 260 nm. For this, prepare a 1:100 dilution of phage in PBS. The titer can be estimated according to the following empirical formula: phage/mL = $OD_{260\ nm} \times 100 \times 22.14 \times 10^{10}$ (18).
2. It is recommended that the phage be stored in PBS containing 1% (w/v) EDTA and 0.1 μM BSA to reduce proteolysis. The phage can be stored at 4°C for a few days.
3. In order to reduce phage binding to streptavidin, the phage library can be preadsorbed overnight with 100 μg/mL streptavidin solution or with streptavidin magnetic beads at 4°C with slow shaking. Subsequently, the phage solution is centrifuged at top speed in a microfuge at 4°C and the phage supernatant is used for panning.
4. It is advised to store some of the eluted phage after each round of panning at −80°C for future reference or to recover a round of panning in case of errors or mishaps.
5. It is recommended to include the noninfected or blank TG1 throughout the panning experiment since phage cross-contamination can occur easily. Generally, pipettors are a main source of cross-contamination and must be cleaned with appropriate reagents frequently. Moreover, all solutions used in panning must be prepared in small aliquots and discarded after the panning experiment.
6. All reagents, buffers, and solutions used for panning must be *free of biotin*. It is important to ensure that the blocking buffers used are free of biotin.
7. The required amount of peptide may vary depending on the peptide's solubility. Generally, peptide concentrations ranging from 5 to 100 μg/mL can be used or be determined experimentally. We have observed that using peptide concentrations at the higher end of the required concentration range led to better panning results.
8. It is necessary to carry out incubations in U-shaped bottom tubes to ensure thorough mixing of the biotinylated peptides and beads.
9. For naïve library panning, the blocking buffer is alternated from StartingBlock™ to 3% (w/v) BSA in PBS during panning rounds, in order to effectively reduce the blocking reagent phage binders.
10. Make sure that the TG1 cells are able to grow on M9 minimal medium plate. To start a new panning, streak the TG1 cells and

incubate at 37°C for 36 h. To start a fresh culture for panning, pick up a single colony and culture in 2–10 mL of LB medium.

11. The stringency conditions are increased during the subsequent rounds of panning by increasing the time and duration of the washes.
12. Alternatively, specific phage elution can be performed by using either nonbiotinylated free peptide solution in PBS (0.1 mg/mL) or its parental protein in PBS (0.1–0.15 mg/mL).
13. Make sure to preserve and store the amplified phage after each round of panning since they are required for polyclonal phage ELISA screening.
14. Decisions regarding the number of rounds of panning very much depend on the sequence heterogeneity of individual colonies after third or fourth round of panning. Panning may be stopped when sequencing of randomly picked clones reveals that many have the same sequence and when there is good enrichment in terms of the ratio of output to input phage (more than 1,000).
15. It is important to pass the pentameric antibodies through Superdex G200 column (GE Healthcare) to eliminate any possible aggregates prior to Biacore analysis.

Acknowledgments

We thank Shalini Katary and Hong Tong-Sevinc for preparing and reviewing the KingFisher protocol and Henk van Faassen for performing the SPR experiments. We also thank the NRC Genomics and Health Initiative and Sentinel, The Canadian Network for the Development and Use of Bioactive Paper, for financial support. The authors declare no competing interests.

References

1. Hamers-Casterman C et al (1993) Naturally occurring antibodies devoid of light chains. Nature 363:446–448
2. Arbabi Ghahroudi M et al (1997) Selection and identification of single domain antibody fragments from camel heavy-chain antibodies. FEBS Lett 414:521–526
3. Ward ES et al (1989) Binding activities of a repertoire of single immunoglobulin variable domains secreted from *Escherichia coli*. Nature 341:544–546
4. Muyldermans S (2001) Single domain camel antibodies: current status. J Biotechnol 74: 277–302
5. Muyldermans S, Cambillau C, Wyns L (2001) Recognition of antigens by single-domain antibody fragments: the superfluous luxury of paired domains. Trends Biochem Sci 26:230–235
6. Tanha J et al (2002) Selection by phage display of llama conventional V(H) fragments with heavy chain antibody V(H)H properties. J Immunol Methods 263:97–109
7. Kehoe JW, Kay BK (2005) Filamentous phage display in the new millennium. Chem Rev 105: 4056–4072
8. Pande J, Szewczyk MM, Grover AK (2010) Phage display: concept, innovations, applications and future. Biotechnol Adv 28:849–858

9. Konthur Z, Wilde J, Lim TS (2010) Semi-automated magnetic bead-based antibody selection from phage display libraries. In: Kontermann R, Dubel S (eds) Antibody engineering, 2nd edn. Springer-Verlag, Berlin Heidelberg, pp 267–287
10. Turunen L et al (2009) Automated panning and screening procedure on microplates for antibody generation from phage display libraries. J Biomol Screen 14:282–293
11. Sambrook J, Russell D (2001) Molecular cloning: a laboratory manual, 3rd edn. Cold Spring Harbor Laboratory Press, Cold Spring Harbor, New York
12. Stone E et al (2007) The assembly of single domain antibodies into bispecific decavalent molecules. J Immunol Methods 318:88–94
13. Arbabi-Ghahroudi M, Tanha J, MacKenzie R (2009) Isolation of monoclonal antibody fragments from phage display libraries. Methods Mol Biol 502:341–364
14. Zacher AN et al (1980) A new filamentous phage cloning vector: fd-tet. Gene 9: 127–140
15. Doyle PJ et al (2008) Cloning, expression, and characterization of a single-domain antibody fragment with affinity for 15-acetyl-deoxynivalenol. Mol Immunol 45:3703–3713
16. Zhang J et al (2009) Transient expression and purification of chimeric heavy chain antibodies. Protein Expr Purif 65:77–82
17. Zhang J, MacKenzie R, Durocher Y (2009) Production of chimeric heavy-chain antibodies. Methods Mol Biol 525:323–336
18. Lee CM et al (2007) Selection of human antibody fragments by phage display. Nat Protoc 2:3001–3008

Chapter 8

Pichia Surface Display: A Tool for Screening Single Domain Antibodies

Kristof De Schutter and Nico Callewaert

Abstract

Yeast surface display is being employed as an efficient tool for the isolation and engineering of traditional antibody fragments, both scFv and Fab, as well as single domain antibodies. Here we describe the protocols for a yeast surface display system developed in the methylothrophic yeast *Pichia pastoris*, the most commonly used yeast species for protein production. In this system the immune or maturated library of single domain antibodies is fused to the C-terminal domain of the *Saccharomyces cerevisiae* alpha-agglutinin gene (*SAG1*) and expressed on the surface of *P. pastoris* cells. Labeling with ligands enables rapid and quantitative analysis in conjunction with isolation of single domain antibodies with the desired characteristics.

Key words: *Pichia pastoris*, Surface display, Immune library, Matured library

1. Introduction

Ever since the introduction of yeast surface display (1), this powerful platform has been used for engineering, screening, and isolation of a variety of proteins. In particular, yeast surface display has evolved as a valuable tool for engineering and isolation of antibodies and antibody fragments. A significant advantage of the yeast display tool is that it uses an expression and processing pathway similar to that of higher eukaryotes. Proteins are folded in the endoplasmic reticulum, where they benefit from the presence of chaperones, foldases, and of quality control mechanisms and can have eukaryotic posttranslational modifications. Additional advantages include the possibility to rapidly and quantitatively screen on antibody affinity and display level through fluorescent-activated cell sorting (FACS). Up to now, the yeast display method has yielded the highest affinity (48 fM) for any antibody (2).

Dirk Saerens and Serge Muyldermans (eds.), *Single Domain Antibodies: Methods and Protocols*, Methods in Molecular Biology, vol. 911, DOI 10.1007/978-1-61779-968-6_8, © Springer Science+Business Media, LLC 2012

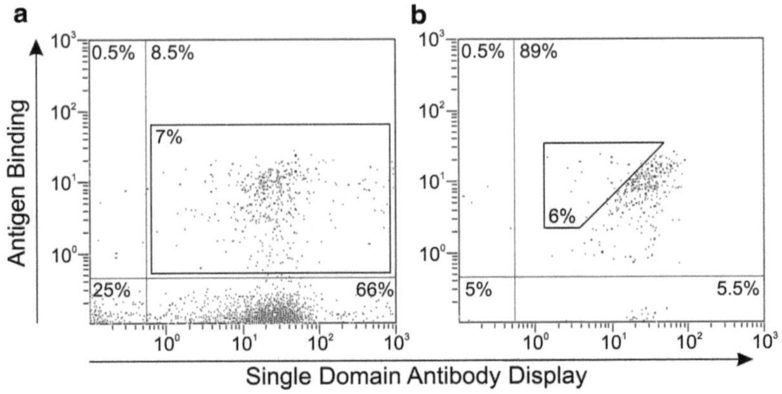

Fig. 1. Flow cytometric screening of an immune library. Dot plots of antigen binding and single domain antibody expression before sorting (**a**) and after a single sorting (**b**). After one round of sorting, about 90% of the cells were double positive (antigen binding and expression). The sorting gate used is depicted in (**a**). In a second sort on the enriched population, a more stringent sorting gate and lower concentrations of the biotinylated-antigen can sort out the clones with high affinity for the antigen.

Here we describe the methodology for displaying single domain antibodies on the cell surface of *Pichia pastoris*. Therefore, a library of single domain antibody sequences is cloned into the *Pichia* surface display vector, pPSDalpha (3). Cloned in this vector, the antibody sequences are N-terminally fused to the pre-pro-sequence of the *Saccharomyces cerevisiae* alpha mating factor and C-terminally fused to the sequence encoding the last 320 amino acids (containing the GPI anchor attachment site) of the *S. cerevisiae* alpha-agglutinin. The obtained library is transformed into a *P. pastoris* strain through a highly efficient transformation protocol (4). A minimum *Pichia* library size of 1×10^7 individual clones is desired. In *S. cerevisiae*, typically 40–80% of the cells do not express the surface protein, but this is not observed when displaying proteins in *P. pastoris* (3). This difference could be attributed to the integration of the expression cassettes in the *P. pastoris* genome compared to the episomal plasmids in *S. cerevisiae* which can be lost or of which the copy number can be reduced, in a significant fraction of the culture.

The *Pichia* library is screened by high-speed flow cytometric sorting. Expression of the antibody in the surface display format is detected through indirect immunostaining using the V5-epitope tag in the system. Antigen-binding activity is detected using a specific biotinylated-antigen and fluorophore-labeled streptavidin. Isolation of the antigen-binding clones is done by sorting out the double-stained cells (expression and antigen binding) on the FACS. From an immune library, we generally obtain about 5–8% double-stained cells, after one round of sorting we obtained an enrichment of the double-stained population to 90% (see Fig. 1). Consecutive rounds of sorting with adjusted sorting gates and lower concentrations of ligand will allow the sorting of clones with high affinity for the antigen.

Identification of the sorted clones is achieved through sequencing the single domain antibody genes, either by classical sequencing of individual clones or next-generation sequencing of pooled clones. To this effect, the antibody genes are amplified from the clones using universal primers for the single domain antibodies.

2. Materials

Prepare all media, buffers, and solutions using ultrapure deionized water (18 MΩ cm at 25°C).

All reagents, buffers, and media are prepared and stored at room temperature unless indicated otherwise. Shelf life of the media is approximately 1 month.

2.1. Transformation and Selection of *P. pastoris*

1. pPSDalpha vector: This vector allows N-terminal fusion of the single domain antibody genes to the *S. cerevisiae* pre-pro signal sequence of the alpha mating factor and C-terminal fusion to the sequence coding for the last 320 amino acids of the *S. cerevisiae* alpha-agglutinin (see Note 1).
2. YPD medium: 1% yeast extract, 2% peptone, 2% glucose monohydrate. Dissolve 10 g of yeast extract, 20 g of peptone, and 20 g of glucose monohydrate in 1 L deionized water. Autoclave for 15 min at 121°C.
3. LiAc/DTT solution: 100 mM LiAc, 10 mM DTT, 0.6 M sorbitol, 10 mM Tris-HCl, pH 7.5. Mix 20 mL of a 1 M LiAc stock, 2 mL of 1 M DTT, 120 mL of 1 M sorbitol, 2 mL of 1 M Tris-HCl, pH 7.5 and add deionized water to 200 mL. Sterilize by filter sterilization (see Note 2).
4. 1 M sorbitol. Dissolve 182.17 g sorbitol in 1 L deionized water. Autoclave for 15 min at 121°C and store refrigerated after cooling down.
5. MM-His medium: 2% dextrose, 0.62% yeast nitrogen base (YNB) without amino acids, 0.08% CSM-His, pH 7.0. Dissolve 20 g dextrose, 6.7 g yeast nitrogen base without amino acids (see Note 3), and 0.8 g Complete Supplement Mixture minus Histidine (CSM-His) (see Note 4) in 1 L deionized water and set pH to 7.0 using 1 M KOH. Autoclave at 121 C for 15 min.
6. Baffled shake flask. Sterilized by autoclaving.
7. Incubator set at 28°C with an agitation of 250 rpm
8. 50× TAE: 2 M Tris-acetate, 50 mM EDTA. Dissolve 242 g Tris in 750 mL deionized water, add 57,1 mL glacial acetic acid and 100 mL 0.5 M Na_2EDTA (pH 8.0), adjust the volume to 1 L.

9. 1% Agarose gel: 1% Agarose in 1× TAE buffer. Suspend 1 g agarose in 100 mL 1× TAE buffer and boil the suspension in the microwave until the agarose is dissolved. After cooling down to 60 C, pour the gel in the tank and insert comb. Run the gel in 1× TAE in a electrophoresis device.
10. Concentrator (see Note 5).
11. Ultracentrifuge (see Note 6).
12. Benchtop centrifuge (see Note 7).
13. *Pme*I restriction enzyme and reaction buffer (see Note 8).
14. PCR purification kit (see Note 9).
15. Electroporator device and electroporation cuvettes (see Note 10).
16. Glycerol.

2.2. Induction of Surface Display

1. 1 M potassium phosphate buffer: Dissolve 23 g of K_2HPO_4 and 118 g of KH_2PO_4 in 1 L of deionized water and confirm pH is 6.0. Autoclave at 121°C for 15 min.
2. 13.4% (wt/vol) YNB without Amino Acids: Dissolve 67 g of yeast nitrogen base without amino acids (see Note 3) in deionized water to a final volume of 500 mL. Filter sterilize and store refrigerated.
3. BMGY medium: 1% yeast extract, 2% peptone, 1.34% YNB without amino acids, 100 mM potassium phosphate buffer (pH 6.0), 1% glycerol. Dissolve 10 g of yeast extract and 20 g of peptone in 800 mL of deionized water and autoclave at 121°C for 15 min. After cooling down, add 100 mL of sterile 1 M potassium phosphate buffer (pH 6.0), 100 mL of sterile 13.4% YNB without Amino Acids, and 10 mL of sterile 100% glycerol.
4. BMMY medium: 1% yeast extract, 2% peptone, 1.34% YNB without amino acids, 100 mM potassium phosphate buffer (pH 6.0), 1% methanol. Dissolve 10 g of yeast extract and 20 g of peptone in 800 mL of deionized water and autoclave at 121°C for 15 min. After cooling down, add 100 mL of sterile 1 M potassium phosphate buffer (pH 6.0), 100 mL of sterile 13.4% YNB without Amino Acids, and 10 mL of 100% methanol.
5. Baffled shake flask. Sterilized by autoclaving.
6. Incubator set at 28°C with agitation of 250 rpm.
7. Benchtop centrifuge (see Note 7).

2.3. Staining and Sorting of the Yeast

Antibodies and PE-labeled streptavidin are stored at 4°C, unless indicated otherwise by the supplier.

1. Phosphate buffered saline (PBS; ×10): 8% NaCl, 0.2% KCl, 1.44% Na_2HPO_4, 0.24% KH_2PO_4, pH 7.4. Dissolve 80 g of NaCl, 2 g of KCl, 14.4 g of Na_2HPO_4, and 2.4 g of KH_2PO_4

in 800 mL of deionized water. Set the pH to 7.4 with 1 M HCl or 1 M NaOH. Sterilize by autoclaving at 121°C for 15 min. For 1× PBS, dilute 50 mL 10× PBS in 450 mL deionized water.

2. PBS containing 0.1% BSA (PBSB): 0.1% BSA in 1× PBS (see Note 11).
3. Mouse antiV5-tag monoclonal antibody (see Note 12).
4. Goat anti mouse antibody labeled with Alexa 647 (see Note 13).
5. Biotinylated-antigen specific for the antibody of interest (see Note 14).
6. Streptavidin labeled with PE (see Note 15).
7. Benchtop centrifuge (see Note 7).
8. Microcentrifuge (see Note 16).
9. YPD plates: 1% yeast extract, 2% peptone, 2% glucose monohydrate, 1.5% agar. Dissolve 10 g of yeast extract, 20 g of peptone, 20 g of glucose monohydrate, and 15 g of agar in 1 L deionized water. Autoclave for 15 min at 121 C.

3. Methods

3.1. Transformation and Selection of *P. pastoris*

The transformation protocol is adapted from Wu and Letchworth (4). Carry out all procedures in sterile conditions. The following steps contain (1) the preparation of the plasmid library, (2) the preparation of *P. pastoris* cells competent for electroporation, and (3) the transformation of the library by electroporation.

1. Digest 2 μg of the plasmid library with *Pme*I for linearization of the plasmid library in the *AOX1* promotor (see Note 17).
2. Check a small aliquot of the digest by agarose gel electrophoresis for complete linearization of the vector.
3. When the vector is completely linearized, stop the reaction and clean-up (desalt) by a PCR purification kit (see Note 18).
4. Evaporate the elution mix in a Concentrator and resuspend the DNA in 20 μL of ultrapure water.
5. Store the DNA refrigerated until use or at −20°C for longer storage.
6. Inoculate 5 mL of YPD medium with a fresh colony of wild-type *P. pastoris* cells, grow overnight at 28°C under agitation of 250 rpm.
7. Use the overnight preculture to inoculate a culture in 250 mL of YPD in a baffled shake flask. Grow this culture overnight at 28°C and 250 rpm to an $OD_{600\ nm}$ of about 1, 5 (see Note 19).

8. When the culture is grown to 1.5 $OD_{600\ nm}$ (approximately 7.5×10^7 cells/mL), cells are harvested by centrifugation at $1,519 \times g$ for 5 min at 4°C using an ultracentrifuge. Gently remove the supernatant.
9. Resuspend cells in LiAc/DTT solution at approximately 10^8 cells/mL; this is about 200 mL of LiAc/DTT solution for 250 mL ($OD_{600\ nm}$ 1.5) culture.
10. Incubate for 30 min at room temperature while gently shaking at 100 rpm (see Note 20).
11. Collect the cells by centrifugation at $1,519 \times g$ for 5 min at 4°C using an ultracentrifuge.
12. Remove the supernatant and resuspend the cells in 1.5 mL of ice-cold 1 M sorbitol per approximately 5×10^8 cells (37.5 mL for 250 mL culture). Keep the cells during this step and subsequent manipulations on ice (see Note 21). Collect the cells by centrifugation at $1,811 \times g$ for 5 min at 4°C using a benchtop centrifuge.
13. Repeat step 12 two more times.
14. Remove the supernatant and resuspend cells at approximately 10^{10} cells/mL in one ice-cold sorbitol (in total 1.875×10^{10} cells, resuspend in 1.875 mL) and store the cells on ice (see Note 22).
15. Add 80 μL of competent cells with 100 ng of linearized plasmid DNA in a prechilled 2 mm electroporation cuvette (see Note 23).
16. Incubate the cuvette with the cells and DNA on ice for 5 min.
17. Pulse cells according to the parameters for yeast as indicated by the manufacturer of the electroporation device (see Note 24).
18. Immediately after pulsing the cells, add 1 mL of 1 M ice-cold sorbitol.
19. Each transformation will give about 1×10^5 colony forming units, so that 100 transformations will give the required 10^7 size of the *Pichia* library (see Note 25).
20. Pool the transformations and inoculate cells in 50 mL MM-his medium
21. Incubate culture at 28°C and 250 rpm.
22. Make frozen stocks of the *Pichia* library. Harvest cells by centrifugation and suspend in YPD medium containing 15% glycerol. Freeze in liquid nitrogen and store at –80°C

3.2. Induction of Surface Display

Carry out all procedures in sterile conditions

1. Inoculate 10^8 cells in 50 mL of BMGY medium for 24 h at 28°C and 250 rpm in a 250 mL baffled shake flask.

2. Harvest cells by centrifugation at 1,811 ×*g* for 5 min at 4°C using a benchtop centrifuge. Gently remove the supernatant.
3. Wash cells in 50 mL of BMMY, centrifuge as in previous step, and remove the supernatant.
4. Resuspend cells in 50 mL of BMMY medium and grow them for 24 h at 28°C and 250 rpm in a 250 mL baffled shake flask.
5. To maintain induction, spike 1% methanol in the cultures every 12 h.

3.3. Staining and Sorting of the Yeast

1. Measure the $OD_{600\ nm}$ and harvest cells by centrifugation at 1,811 ×*g* for 5 min at 4°C using a benchtop centrifuge. Gently remove the supernatant.
2. Resuspend cells at 10^8 cells/mL (2 $OD_{600\ nm}$) in PBSB buffer (see Note 26).
3. Add 2 μg/mL mouse anti V5-tag antibody. The anti V5-tag antibody will bind the V5-epitope in the *Pichia* Surface Display system and will be used for the detection of expression (see Note 27).
4. Add 1.5 μg/mL biotinylated-antigen (see Note 28). The biotinylated-antigen will be bound by the single domain antibodies with specificity to this antigen and used to sort out the specific antibodies from the library.
5. Incubate the cells with the biotynylated-antigen and anti V5-antibody for 45 min at 4°C.
6. Add 500 μL PBSB and centrifuge for 3 min at 3,000 rpm in a microcentrifuge. Gently remove the supernatant.
7. Repeat previous step.
8. Resuspend the cells at 10^8 cells/mL in PBSB.
9. Add 4 μg/mL Alexa 647-labeled goat anti mouse IgG to label the cells for expression.
10. Add 4 μg/mL phytoerythrin (PE)-labeled streptavidin to label the cells for binding (see Note 29).
11. Incubate cells with the streptavidin and antibody for 45 min on ice.
12. Add 500 μL of PBSB and centrifuge for 3 min at 3,000 rpm in a microcentrifuge. Gently remove the supernatant.
13. Repeat previous step.
14. Resuspend the cells in PBSB buffer at a density suitable for FACS analysis and sorting.
15. Run cells on the FACS according to the manufacturer's instructions. Set gate on scatter plot to measure only single cells and set sorting gate to select for double positive cells.

16. Sorted cells are collected in tubes coated with PBS or medium (see Note 30).
17. Collected cells are pooled in YPD medium and grown overnight, plated on YPD plates for analysis of individual clones or pooled for analysis. The cells grown in liquid culture are harvested by centrifugation, suspended in YPD medium containing 15% glycerol, and frozen in liquid nitrogen to be stored at −80°C for a consecutive round of sorting.

4. Notes

1. The pPSDalpha vector and the generation of single domain antibody plasmid libraries are described by Ryckaert et al. (3).
2. We find it is best to prepare the 1 M DTT stock fresh each time or limit the number of refreezing cycles.
3. We use Yeast Nitrogen Base without Amino Acids from BD, Catalog number 291920 (BD, Franklin Lakes, NJ, USA).
4. We use CSM—His from Qbiogene Catalog number 4510-322 (Qbiogene, Montreal, QC, Canada).
5. We use the Thermo SpeedVac SPD111V (Thermo Scientific, Waltham, MA, USA).
6. We use a Sorvall RC5C plus with a SLA3000 rotor (Thermo Scientific, Waltham, MA, USA).
7. We use a Eppendorf 5810R (Eppendorf, Hamburg, Germany).
8. We use *Pme*I restriction enzyme from New England Biolabs (NEB, Ipswich, MA, USA) or *Mss*I (*Pme*I) from Fermentas (Thermo Fisher Scientific, Waltham, MA, USA) in the supplied buffer according to the manufacturer's instructions.
9. We use QIAquick Gel Extraction kit (QIAGEN, Hilden, Germany).
10. We use a BioRad Gene Pulser electroporation device with BioRad Gene Pulser Cuvettes 0.2 cm electrode gap, Catalog number 165-2086 (BioRad, Hercules, CA, USA).
11. Add 0.1% BSA fresh to 1× PBS buffer before use.
12. We use mouse monoclonal antibody from Invitrogen (46-0705) (Invitrogen, Carlsbad, CA, USA) or AbD Serotec (MCA2892) (AbD Serotec, Kidlington, UK).
13. We use Alexa Fluor 647 F(ab′)2 fragment of goat anti mouse IgG (A21237) (Invitrogen Molecular Probes, Eugene, OR, USA).
14. Will most likely have to be custom made using, for example, the amine biotinylation kit from Pierce (Thermo Fisher Scientific, Rockford, IL, USA).

15. We use PE Streptavidin from BD Pharmingen (Cat 554061) (BD Bioscience, San Diego, CA, USA).
16. We use a Eppendorf 5417C (Eppendorf, Hamburg, Germany).
17. Targeting the integration of the surface display vector to the *AOX1* promotor gives a higher number of transformants compared to targeting integration to, for example, the *HIS4* locus or targeting for random integration ((4) and personal experience). In addition, the *AOX1* locus is a highly transcribed locus (when promoter is induced) and will therefore not negatively influence the expression of the surface display system. If a *Pme*I restriction site is present in the sequence of your single domain antibodies, another restriction enzyme should be selected for linearization.
18. It is essential that the DNA mixture is desalted, as salt causes arching during the electroporation.
19. Calculate the amount of overnight preculture (in mL) to be added to the 250 mL medium using following formula: $((250 \times 1.5) / 2^n) / \mathrm{OD}$, where 250 is the volume of the culture (250 mL), 1.5 is the desired $\mathrm{OD}_{600\ \mathrm{nm}}$ of the culture, OD is the $\mathrm{OD}_{600\ \mathrm{nm}}$ of the preculture, and n is the number of generations −1 (to allow the cells to recover from stationary phase).
20. The agitation is to keep the cells suspended. If no shaker is available, cells can be incubated at RT without agitation; cells can be kept suspended by gently shaking the culture manually every 5–10 min.
21. It is essential to keep the cells from this step on cooled on ice; all buffers and instruments (centrifuge) should be precooled.
22. The purpose of the washing steps is to ensure the cells are "salt-free" (salt causes arching during electroporation) while suspending them in an osmotically stabilizing solution.
23. Transformation with 10 ng DNA is most efficient (most CFU/μg DNA), but more DNA can be added to obtain more CFU per transformation
24. We use following conditions on a GenePulser (BioRad, Hercules, CA, USA): 1.5 kV, capacitance of 25 μFD, extended capacitance of 125 μFD, and resistance of 200 Ω.
25. We use a 96-well High Throughput Electroporation Plate Handler (HT-100) with 2 mm gap size 96 well High Throughput Electroporation Plates (HT-P96-2) (BTX Instrument division, Harvard Apparatus, Holliston, MA, USA) connected to a GenePulser generator (BioRad, Hercules, CA, USA).
26. We perform stainings in volumes of 500 μL.
27. This staining can be performed without the staining for binding as a control of the single domain antibody expression in the

surface display system in the *Pichia* library. To this effect, expression of the surface display system is tested in 50 independent clones (therefore one of the transformations is plated instead of inoculated into liquid culture) by indirect immunostaining of the V5 epitope tag. On average, 70% should show expression of the V5 tag.

28. Optimization of the antigen concentration will be required for each antigen. In a first sorting round, a high concentration of antigen is used to obtain a maximal diversity of binding clones. In consecutive rounds, antigen concentration is lowered to sort out the clones with high binding affinity.
29. Optimization of the concentration of PE-labeled streptavidin will be required for each antigen.
30. Sterile FACS tubes are filled with PBS or medium (YPD or minimal medium) and stored overnight at 4°C. Before use, the buffer or medium is removed. This will protect the cells when being collected in the tube during sorting.

References

1. Boder ET, Wittrup KD (1997) Yeast surface display for screening combinatorial polypeptide libraries. Nat Biotech 15:553–557
2. Boder ET, Wittrup KD (2000) Yeast surface display for directed evolution of protein expression, affinity, and stability. Methods Enzymol 328:430–444
3. Ryckaert S et al (2010) Isolation of antigen-binding camelid heavy chain antibody fragments (nanobodies) from an immune library displayed on the surface of *Pichia pastoris*. J Biotech 145:93–98
4. Wu S, Letchworth GJ (2004) High efficiency transformation by electroporation of *Pichia pastoris* pretreated with lithium acetate and dithiothreitol. Biotechniques 36:152–154

Chapter 9

Bacterial Two Hybrid: A Versatile One-Step Intracellular Selection Method

Mireille Pellis, Serge Muyldermans, and Cécile Vincke

Abstract

Many antibody fragments, selected ex vivo by phage display, fail to form functional antigen-binding entities when expressed and used intracellularly (i.e., as intrabodies) because the interior of the cell poses significant challenges on the folding of antibodies. Such dropout can be avoided by employing intracellular selection methods like yeast or bacterial two hybrid systems. These involve four facile steps: construction of plasmids, transformation of microbial cells, intracellular expression of fusion proteins, and selection for reporter activity. Using *E. coli* as host instead of yeast offers the advantages of a faster growth and a higher transformation efficiency allowing to screen larger repertoires. This chapter describes the protocol, optimized to identify antigen-specific single domain antibodies (sdAbs), by bacterial two hybrid selection.

Key words: Intrabody, In vivo selection, Nanobody, Bacterial two hybrid, Single domain antibody

1. Introduction

The most frequently used methods to select antigen-specific antibodies are ex vivo techniques, such as phage display (1–3) and ribosome display (4–6). The employment of these selected, highly specific reagents for use as intrabodies, i.e., intracellular functional antibodies, holds a great promise for functional genomics, proteomics, and gene therapy (7, 8). However, the interior of the cell poses significant challenges regarding antibody folding, assembly, and functionality as the reducing conditions prevailing within the cell prevent the formation of the conserved intradomain disulfide bonds and will often result in reduced efficacy of intrabodies. It is clear that the ex vivo selections do not guarantee the identification of antibodies suitable for intrabody applications.

Therefore, it would be preferable to develop an efficient, fast, and easy to handle intracellular selection system if the final application requires intrabodies. Several different intracellular

Dirk Saerens and Serge Muyldermans (eds.), *Single Domain Antibodies: Methods and Protocols*, Methods in Molecular Biology, vol. 911, DOI 10.1007/978-1-61779-968-6_9, © Springer Science+Business Media, LLC 2012

selection systems have been reported: the yeast two hybrid (Y2H) selection; the intracellular antigen capture technology (IACT), and the protein fragment complementation assay (PCA) or bimolecular fluorescence complementation assay (BiFC). In the first approach, the Y2H system (9), two fusion proteins are expressed in a yeast cell. One, known as the bait, encodes a site-specific DNA binding domain (DBD) from LexA or GAL4 fused to the protein of interest. This hybrid binds by itself to an operator adjacent to a promoter. The second, called the target, contains a transcriptional activation domain fused to a second protein of interest. If the fused proteins interact with each other, the bait hybrid bound to the operator recruits the target hybrid with its activation domain stimulating the expression of a suitable reporter gene and generating an easily detectable phenotype. Unfortunately, the application of Y2H for antibody selection is rather limited because of its inability to handle large diverse libraries (over 10^6–10^7 individual clones). To overcome this problem, Visintin et al. (10) introduced the IACT whereby they used first a round of phage display selection(s) to enrich a large library for potential binders, followed by subsequent in vivo selections in a Y2H system.

The third strategy, the BiFC or PCA, is based on the possibility to heterodimerize two half proteins restoring a function. In case of PCA (11–13), it was shown that mouse dihydrofolate reductase (mDHFR) can be split into two polypeptide fragments that complement each other (like RNAse A, β-lactamase, or β-galactosidase). The affinity of the mDHFR fragments is too low to associate in *E. coli* into a functional enzyme rendering the host cell resistant against the trimethoprim antibiotic. Conjugation of two interacting partner proteins to each of the mDHFR fragments manages to keep the mDHFR fragments together and conferring resistance and survival of the cell in presence of trimethoprim. The Achilles heel of such systems is the spontaneous self-assembly of the protein parts into functional proteins contributing to a background, and the lack of a second reporter system to validate the interaction between bait and target.

In 1997, Dove et al. (14) designed vectors and host cells for a bacterial two hybrid (B2H) strategy (Fig. 1). Similarly to the Y2H, this method is based on reconstituting the activity of a protein from its separate domains. In this approach, the bait is fused to the full-length bacteriophage λcI repressor protein, containing the DNA binding and the dimerization domains, whereas the target is fused to the α-subunit of RNA polymerase, a transcriptional activation domain. Interaction of the fusion partners within the cell will lead to expression of the *HIS3-aad3* reporter cassette (under control of the phage λ operator) (Fig. 1), which results in survival of the cells on selective medium (14–16). Expression of the *HIS3* reporter gene allows the cells to grow in presence of 3-AT (3-amino-1,2,4-triazole), a competitive inhibitor of the *His3* enzyme. Surviving cells are subsequently tested using the *aadA* gene as a

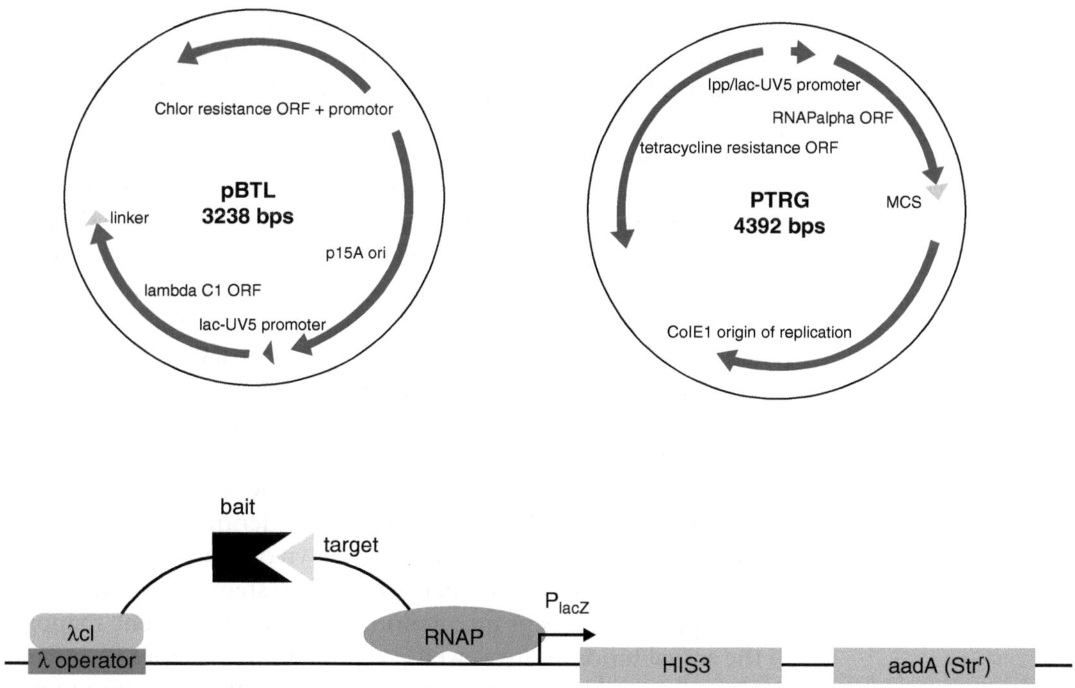

Fig. 1. Schematic representation of the two plasmids used for the B2H selection screening (*top*) and the principle of the reporter gene activation (*bottom*). The pBTL vector at the left is an adapted pBT vector from Stratagene containing a modified cloning site to accommodate the VHH genes of HCAbs (see Note 1) from camelid. The plasmid confers chloramphenicol resistance and the sdAb is cloned in the multiple cloning site (MCS) at the 3′ end of the λcI gene encoding a DNA binding domain recognizing the λ operator sequence. The pTRG plasmid (*right*) is taken from the Stratagene Bacterial Two Hybrid kit. The gene for tetracycline resistance, the colE1 origin of replication, and the gene for the α fragment of the RNA polymerase (RNAPalpha) are indicated. The cDNA of the target antigen is cloned downstream the latter gene (see Note 4). Expressions of the λcI and RNAP alpha fusion genes are under the control of the lac UV5 promotor. Presence of both plasmids and expression of the fusion proteins inside the BMII reporter cells will lead to the binding of the λcI DNA binding domain to the λ operator. The fused sdAb might interact with the target antigen fused to the RNAPalpha so that the reporter genes *HIS3* and *aadA* are expressed (*bottom*), allowing the formation of baterial colonies on plates in the presence of 3-AT and streptomycin.

secondary reporter, which confers streptomycin resistance. The major advantages of bacteria vs. yeasts as host comprise faster growth and higher transformation efficiency, allowing better coverage in library-based screenings.

To identify antigen-specific sdAbs, we routinely immunize a camel or llama. During the immunization, the B-cells expressing antigen-specific heavy-chain antibodies in these animals are stimulated to proliferate so that the ratio of affinity matured, antigen-specific versus non-specific heavy-chain antibodies increase to well above $1/10^6$. Since the antigen-binding fragment of these heavy-chain-only antibodies is comprised in one single domain, the cloning of this gene fragment maintains the integrity of the in vivo affinity matured paratope. Consequently, the construction of an immune sdAb library in the B2H vector of some 10^6 individual transformants should contain sufficient high affinity binders that can be retrieved after a single round of selection. The procedure to construct an immune library is similar as for phage display, except that the pBTL vector (Fig. 1) replaces the phage display vector and specific reporter cells are used as host. In this chapter, we describe how a representative aliquot of cells of this library is made electro-competent and transformed by a pTRG plasmid harboring the gene of the antigen of interest. All transformants are plated on selective medium so that only cells with a faithfull interaction between sdAb and antigen will grow. Since the selection of the sdAb occurred inside bacterial cells, it is expected that all these sdAb will also be functional as intrabody in the cytoplasm of eukaryotic cells.

An additional benefit of two hybrid systems is that the availability of antigen as a purified protein is not required, since cloning cDNA or the gene fragment encoding the target protein of interest in the pTRG vector is sufficient to initiate the selection. Thus, this intracellular selection offers a solution to identify binders to proteins or domains, which are unstable ex vivo, difficult to purify, or expensive to purchase. Furthermore, this system allows the detection of protein–protein interactions and the subsequent mapping of the actual binding site as well (i.e., an epitope mapping). Indeed, the site-directed mutagenesis or randomly cloning of subfragments in the target vector provides valuable information on the interaction site between both partners, e.g., to map the epitope targeted by selected antigen-specific sdAbs.

2. Materials

2.1. Preparation of Selective Medium Plates

Plates with various media are required for selection, these are referred to as Non Selective Medium (NSM), Single Selective Medium (SSM), and Dual Selective Screening Medium (DSSM)

1. Micro-agar (Duchefa Biochemie, Haarlem, The Netherlands)
2. 10× M9 salts (1 L): 74.76 g $Na_2HPO_4.H_2O$; 30 g KH_2PO_4; 5 g NaCl, 10 g NH_4Cl; bring to 1 L in H_2O and autoclave
3. M9 Medium additives (prepare this six times for 500 mL M9+ medium: 1× for NSM, 3× for SSM, 1× for DSSM, and once for the M9+ His-dropout broth)

   Prepare solution I and solution II separately by mixing the individual components. Add solution I to solution II and mix well. This mixture may then be added to the different M9+ medium variants.

   Solution I: 10 mL 20% (w/v) glucose (autoclaved or filter-sterilized), 5 mL of 20 mM adenine-HCl (Sigma, St. Louis, MO) (filter-sterilized), 50 mL of 10× His-dropout amino acid supplement (BD/Clontech, Mountain View, USA) (sterilized by autoclaving at 121°C, not longer than 15 min).

Solution II: 0.5 mL of 1 M $MgSO_4$ (autoclaved), 0.5 mL of 1 M Thiamine-HCl (filter-sterilized), 0.5 mL of 10 mM $ZnSO_4$ (autoclaved), 0.5 mL of 100 mM $CaCl_2$ (autoclaved), 0.5 mL of 50 mM IPTG (Isopropyl-β-D-thiogalactopyranoside, filter-sterilized).

4. 1 M 3-AT stock solution (15 mL): 1261.2 mg 3-AT (3-amino-1,2,4-triazole, Sigma) in 15 mL of DMSO (dimethyl sulfoxide). Make aliquots of 2.5 mL (six tubes) and store at −20°C for up to 1 month.
5. Chloramphenicol: 25 mg/mL, prepared in 100% ethanol.
6. Tetracycline: 12.5 mg/mL, prepared in 50% ethanol.
7. Streptomycin: 12.5 mg/mL, prepared in H_2O
8. Round Petri dishes (90 mm in diameter, referred to as "small" Petri dishes).
9. Square Petri plates (24.5 cm ×24.5 cm, referred to as "large" Petri dishes).

2.2. Preparation of Electrocompetent E. coli Cells

1. Immune library of sdAb cloned in the pBTL vector and hosted in BMII cells (see Note 1).
2. LB medium (1 L): dissolve 25 g of LB Broth High Salt (Duchefa Biochemie, Haarlem, The Netherlands) in 1 L of H_2O, distribute 3×330 mL in 3 baffled shake flasks (1 L) and autoclave.
3. 1 mM Hepes-HCl pH 7.0 (at least 300 mL); autoclave.
4. 10% glycerol in H_2O (at least 200 mL).
5. Sterile Falcon tubes (50 mL) (6–8 in total).
6. Sterile microcentrifuge tubes (1.5 mL) (approximately 30 in total).

2.3. Transformation of Electrocompetent Cells

1. Electroporation cuvettes (0.1 cm), electroporation apparatus (Bio-Rad, Hercules, CA)
2. pTRG-antigen plasmid, at 10 ng/μL in 1 mM EDTA, 10 mM Tris-HCl pH 8.0. An "empty" pTRG plasmid at the same concentration in the same buffer is used as control (A pTRG plasmid with an "irrelevant" antigen can also be included but is not discussed here).
3. SOB (100 mL): 2 g of peptone, 0.5 g of yeast extract, 0.5 mL of 2 M NaCl, 1 mL of 250 mM KCl; bring to 100 mL and autoclave.
4. SOC (this medium should be prepared fresh and used immediately): 25 mL SOB, 500 μL of 20% (w/v) glucose (autoclaved or filter-sterilized), 250 μL of 1 M $MgSO_4$ (autoclaved), 125 μL of 2 M $MgCl_2$ (autoclaved).

5. M9+ His-dropout broth (500 mL): 380 mL of sterile H_2O, 50 mL of 10× M9 salts (autoclaved), 67.5 mL of the M9 medium additives (see Subheading 2.1, item 3). Store at 4°C, use within 1 month. Bring at room temperature prior to use.
6. Falcon tubes (50 mL).

2.4. Plating the Transformed Cell Suspensions

1. M9+ His-dropout broth (500 mL): 380 mL of sterile H_2O, 50 mL of 10× M9 salts (autoclaved), 67.5 mL of the M9 medium additives (see Subheading 2.3, item 5). Bring at room temperature prior to use.
2. NSM plates (15 small Petri dishes).
3. SSM plates (10 small and 5 large Petri dishes).
4. LB-Tet agar plates containing 12.5 μg tetracycline/mL (15 small plates).
5. LB-Cm agar plates, containing 25 μg chloramphenicol/mL (5 small plates).
6. Glass beads: 0.25–0.35 cm diameter, autoclaved.

2.5. Transfer of Colonies from SSM to LB-Cm Agar Plates and DSSM Plates

1. LB-Cm agar plates, containing 25 μg chloramphenicol/mL (5 small Petri dishes).
2. DSSM plates (5 small Petri dishes).

3. Methods

3.1. Preparation of Selective Medium Plates

Always use fresh components to make the selective medium plates. Plates older than 1 month should never be used as essential components might become less effective.

1. For each specific medium (once for NSM, 3 times for SSM, and once for DSSM), add 7.5 g Micro-agar to 380 mL of H_2O in a 500 mL flask. Autoclave at 121°C, allow to cool to 70°C before adding 50 mL of 10× M9 salts. Cool the agar mixtures further to 50°C and add the M9 Medium additives. Proceed immediately to next steps.
2. For NSM, take 1 bottle previously prepared (see Subheading 3.1, step 1) and add 0.5 mL of 25 mg/mL chloramphenicol and 0.5 mL of 12.5 mg/mL tetracycline, mix well and pour in approximately 20 small Petri dishes.
3. For SSM, take 3 bottles previously prepared (see Subheading 3.1, step 1) and add to each 0.5 mL of 25 mg/mL chloramphenicol, 0.5 mL of 12.5 mg/mL tetracycline, and 2.5 mL 1 M 3-AT. Mix well and pour a total of 10 small Petri dishes and 5 large square Petri dishes.

4. For DSSM, take 1 bottle previously prepared (see Subheading 3.1, step 1) and add 0.5 mL of 25 mg/mL chloramphenicol, 0.5 mL of 12.5 mg/mL tetracycline, 2.5 mL 1 M 3-AT, and 0.5 mL 12.5 mg/mL streptomycin. Mix well and pour in ~20 small Petri dishes.
5. The plates can be stored at 4°C, wrapped in aluminum foil, for maximum 1 month.

3.2. Preparation of Electrocompetent E. coli Cells

Since the efficiency of cotransforming pTRG and pBTL derived vectors simultaneous in one cell is too low to screen a library, we first make an immune library of the sdAb in the pBTL vector and transform the BMII host cells (see Note 1). The cells within a representative aliquot of this library are then made electrocompetent to transform the pTRG-antigen vector into these cells so that each sdAb is tested against the antigen.

1. Take an aliquot of the sdAb library in the pBTL vector (see Note 2) and inoculate 300 mL of LB medium (1 L baffled shake flask) and shake at 200–250 rpm/min at 37°C until an $OD_{600\ nm}$ of 0.5–0.6 is reached.
2. Cool the culture by incubating the shake flask for at least 1 h on ice in the cold room.
3. Cool 50 mL Falcon tubes, 1 mM Hepes-HCl pH 7.0, and 10% glycerol on ice in cold room. Precool centrifuge at 4°C.
4. Transfer culture to cooled Falcon tubes and centrifuge for 7 min at 2,200 × *g*.
5. From now everything is performed in the cold room!
6. Decant supernatant, and invert tubes on paper tissue.
7. Add 20 mL of ice-cold 1 mM Hepes-HCl pH 7.0 per tube and resuspend the cell pellet very carefully, preferably by very gently pipetting in and out with a micropipet.
8. Add ice-cold 1 mM Hepes-HCl pH 7.0 until the original volume of the culture (i.e., 300 mL) is reached.
9. Centrifuge for 7 min at 2,100 × *g* in a cooled centrifuge.
10. Remove supernatant. Resuspend the cell pellet in each tube in 10 mL of ice-cold 10% glycerol, again very carefully, and add ice-cold 10% glycerol till half of the original culture volume is reached (i.e., 150 mL).
11. Centrifuge 7 min at 2,100 × *g* in cooled centrifuge.
12. Decant the supernatant. Add 20 mL of ice-cold 10% glycerol to the cell pellet of the first tube, resuspend cells (by swirling, without pipetting) and pour content in the next tube, resuspend and continue till last tube contains all pooled cells.
13. Use 20 mL of ice-cold 10% glycerol to rinse all tubes (again transfer liquid from one tube to the other) so that finally, a single tube contains all cells in 40 mL of 10% glycerol.

14. Centrifuge for 6 min at 2,100 × *g* in cooled centrifuge.
15. Decant supernatant promptly. Resuspend the pellet with a 1 mL micropipet with a precooled tip (cut off the end of the tip to reduce shearing of cells) in ice-cold 10% glycerol to a final volume of 2 mL. Dispense the cell suspension in 75 μL aliquots in ice-cold microcentrifuge tubes (approximately 25 tubes).

3.3. Transformation of Electrocompetent Cells

Perform the transformation directly after making the cells electrocompetent (see Note 3). Transform the pTRG-antigen plasmid (see Note 4) into the freshly made electrocompetent BMII cells harboring the pBTL-sdAb library. Controls are included for testing the transformation efficiency, the absence of antigen toxicity on the cells, the absence of reporter gene self-activation triggered by presence of sdAb or antigen alone, the absence of unwanted plasmid contamination with chloramphenicol or tetracycline resistence, etc.

1. Keep two aliquots of 75 μL electrocompetent cells (see Subheading 3.2, step 15) for the controls.
2. Add 75 ng of pure pTRG-antigen plasmid DNA per remaining tube with 75 μL electrocompetent cells (see Subheading 3.2, step 15). Place on ice for 1 min.
3. Transfer the mixture of one tube to an ice-chilled 0.1 cm electroporation cuvette. Dry the exterior of the cuvette with paper tissue, place the cuvette in the electroporation chamber, and apply a pulse of 1.8 kV/cm to electroporate the cells.
4. Immediately after the pulse, add 500 μL of SOC medium, and transfer to a 50 mL Falcon tube. Rinse the cuvette with an additional 500 μL of SOC medium. Pool the cell suspensions in the Falcon tube.
5. Repeat previous steps (see Subheading 3.3, step 2–4) until approximately 20 transformations are performed (use 2 Falcon tubes to contain all cell suspensions of the approximately 20 transformations with pTRG-antigen).
6. Shake the cell suspensions at 220–250 rpm for 90 min at 37 C.
7. Use one tube of electrocompetent cells (see Subheading 3.3, step 1) for transformation with 75 ng "empty" pTRG vector to check the absence of self-activation of reporter genes by the pBTL-sdAb. Use one tube (see Subheading 3.3, step 1) and add 7.5 μL of H_2O for a "mock" transformation. Incubate both tubes for 1 min on ice. For both samples follow the protocol outlined in previous steps (see Subheading 3.3, step 3–6, except step 5).
8. Spin down the cells in the Falcon tubes at 2,100 × *g* for 10 min.
9. Aspirate the supernatant, taking care not to disturb the cell pellet.

10. Wash the cells by resuspending the cell pellet in 7.5 mL of M9+ His-dropout broth (room temperature) (do this for the two pTRG-antigen transformed samples and for the two control tubes). Spin down the cells at 2,100 × *g* for 10 min and aspirate the supernatant.
11. Resuspend the pTRG-antigen transformed cells in fresh M9+ His-dropout broth, combine the cell suspension into one tube and bring to a final volume of 15 mL. Resuspend the pTRG and the mock-transformed cells, each in 0.75 mL of M9+ His-dropout broth.
12. Incubate the cell suspension at 37°C for 2 h, shaking at 225 rpm. This allows the cells to adapt to minimal medium, prior to plating.

3.4. Plating the Transformed Cell Suspensions

Take plates stored at 4°C and bring to room temperature (see Note 5)

1. Take an aliquot of the 15 mL transformed cell suspension (see Subheading 3.3, step 12) to make 1/10 (350 μL), $1/10^2$ (350 μL), $1/10^3$ (350 μL), $1/10^4$ (350 μL), and $1/10^5$ (350 μL) dilutions in M9+ His-dropout broth and plate 100 μL of each dilution of the cell suspension, separately on 5 small NSM plates. Use 100 μL of the same samples to spread on 5 small SSM plates and 100 μL to spread on LB-Tet agar plates.
2. Plate the rest of the library transformed with pTRG-antigen on large square SSM plates (24.5 cm × 24.5 cm). Use 3 mL/large square plate.
3. Make dilutions of the mock-transformed cells as previously explained (see Subheading 3.4, step 1) and plate 100 μL of the diluted cell suspensions on 5 small LB-Cm agar plates. Put also 100 μL of the diluted cell suspensions on 5 LB-Tet-agar plates.
4. Make dilutions of the "empty" pTRG transformed cells as previously explained (see Subheading 3.4, step 1) and plate 100 μL of the diluted cell suspensions on 5 small LB-Tet agar plates. Put also 100 μL of the diluted cell suspensions on 5 small NSM plates and on 5 small SSM plates.
5. Add glass beads to the plates, close the lid and shake so that glass beads roll over the total surface of agar and that the liquid (i.e., the cell suspension) is spread evenly. Turn the plates upside down so that glass beads fall into the lid of the Petri dish and incubate the plates at 37°C for 24 h (see Note 6).
6. Take the LB-Cm plates with the mock-transformed electrocompetent BMII cells harboring the pBTL-sdAb library (see Subheading 3.4, step 3). The number of colonies, taking into account the dilution and volumes used to plate, allows to

calculate the number of cells that survived the electroshock and handlings (see Note 7).

7. Take the LB-Tet agar plates with the mock-transformed electrocompetent BMII cells harboring the pBTL-sdAb library (see Subheading 3.4, step 3). There should be no colonies growing on these plates as the cells should not be resistant to tetracycline (Tetracycline resistance gene is only on the pTRG vector) (see Note 8).
8. Take the LB-Tet agar plates containing the "empty" pTRG transformed cells (see Subheading 3.4, step 4). The number of colonies, taking into account the dilution and volumes used to plate, allows to calculate the transformation efficiency of the electrocompetent cells (see Note 9).
9. Take the LB-Tet agar plates containing the pTRG-antigen transformed cells (see Subheading 3.4, step 1). The number of colonies, taking into account the dilution and volumes used to plate, allows to calculate the efficiency of the electrocompetent cells to be transformed with the pTRG-antigen vector (see Note 9). This transformation efficiency should approach that of the "empty" pTRG vector (see Subheading 3.4, step 8). Any deviation indicates a lack of purity of the pTRG-antigen plasmid or a toxicity of the antigen gene in the host cells.
10. Take the LB-Tet agar plates and the NSM plates (containing the "empty" pTRG transformed cells (see Subheading 3.4, step 4)) and put them side by side according to the dilution. The same number of colonies should be present. Any deviation indicates a toxicity from the plasmid vector preparation in the host cell.
11. Take the LB-Tet agar plates and the NSM plates containing the pTRG-antigen transformed cells (see Subheading 3.4, step 1) and put them side by side according to the dilution. The same number of colonies should be present. Any deviation indicates a toxicity of the recombinant vector in the host cell. In addition, any difference in number of colonies between the NSM plates of the pTRG-antigen (see Subheading 3.4, step 1) and of the "empty" pTRG vector (see Subheading 3.4, step 4) reflects a toxicity of the expressed antigen fusion in the host cells, possibly masked by a possible difference in purity (transformation efficiency) of the plasmid preparations as noted from the difference of colonies between plates checked in previous steps (see Subheading 3.4, steps 8 and 9) (see Note 9).
12. Put the NSM and the SSM small plates from the cells transformed with the "empty" pTRG vector (see Subheading 3.4, step 4) side by side according to the dilution. From the number of colonies on the SSM plate, taking into account the dilution and volumes used to plate allows to calculate the number of sdAb-fusions in the library that are able to activate the

reporter gene in absence of an antigen fused to the α-subunit of RNA polymerase (see Note 10). Normally, there should be no (or any) colonies on the SSM plates.

13. Put the SSM small plates from the cells transformed with the pTRG-antigen vector (see Subheading 3.4, step 1) and those transformed with the "empty" pTRG vector (see Subheading 3.4, step 4) side by side according to the dilution. Any increase in colonies in favor of the pTRG-antigen plates reflects the number of sdAb proteins that interact with the antigen to trigger the reporter gene. The actual number is possibly masked by the difference in purity (transformation efficiency) of the plasmid preparations as noted from the difference of colonies between plates checked in previous steps (see Subheading 3.4, step 8 and 9).
14. The comparison of the number of colonies on the NSM and SSM plates of the pTRG-antigen transformed cells allows to calculate the percentage of cells where a productive recognition between the sdAb and the antigen occurred resulting in a reporter gene activation (see Note 11).

3.5. Transfer of Colonies from SSM to LB-Cm Agar Plates and DSSM Plates

1. Pick single colonies (see Note 12) from the large SSM selection plates using a sterile tip, and streak them on a DSSM plate and on an LB-Cm agar plate. Make sure that cells forming one colony on SSM are streaked at equivalent positions on the DSSM plate and the LB-Cm agar plates. Incubate the plates for 24 h at 37°C to allow cells to grow.
2. Put the DSSM and LB-Cm plates side by side. The cells of all streaks on LB-Cm should have grown if cells have not lost their pBTL-sdAb plasmid (see Note 12). Cells from streaks that grow on DSSM plates indicate that the sdAb and antigen from the pBTL-sdAb and pTRG-antigen plasmids, respectively, interact to express the two reporter genes. Monitor the survival of the colonies on the DSSM plate (see Note 13). Purify the pBTL-sdAb plasmid from cells of each streak on the LB-Cm plate that was also growing on the DSSM plate. The sdAb gene is amplifed by PCR and the amplicon is send for DNA sequence analysis (see Note 14).

Finally, the intracellular interaction between the sdAb and antigen needs to be confirmed by transforming the segregated pBTL-sdAb plasmids inside the BMII host cell containing the pTRG-antigen or "empty" pTRG vector and plating on all possible NSM, SSM, and DSSM plates (see Note 15).

The B2H selection is also employed to identify the targeted epitope on the antigen of the sdAb (i.e., an epitope mapping experiment explained in Note 16).

4. Notes

1. To generate the pBTL vector we introduced a double stranded oligonucleotide with the coding sequence (5′-GGCCGCATC GGTCCAGGTGCAGCTGCAGGGTCTAGATG-3′) to introduce a *PstI* site (underlined) in the pBT vector (Stratagene, La Jolla, USA) between the *NotI* and *EcoRI* sites. The sdAb genes were amplified with specific primers, from the cDNA of blood lymphocytes of an immunized dromedary or llama (as described in other chapters in this book) and used as a template in a nested PCR with the A6E (5′-GATGTGCAGCTGCAGGAG TCTGGA/GGGAGG-3′) and MP023 (5′-ACCGGAATTCT GAGGAGACGGTGACCTGGGTC-3′) primers (*PstI* and *EcoRI* restriction enzymes sites are underlined), that are annealing at the 5′ end and 3′ end, respectively, of the VHH gene fragment of camelid heavy-chain antibodies. These PCR fragments are cut with *PstI* and *EcoRI* and ligated into the pBTL vector, restricted with the same enzymes. Thereby the VHH sequences are in frame with the bacteriophage λ repressor protein (λcI). The ligated material is then transformed into BMII *Escherichia coli* cells (*XL1-Blue MRF' KanR*, Stratagene) and plated on LB-agar plates containing 25 μg/mL chloramphenicol. The sdAb library size should contain preferably around 10^7 individual transformants (as counted from a properly diluted fraction of the transformed cells plated LB-agar plates supplemented with chloramphenicol). Minimal 50% of these transformants should contain an insert of the proper size of a sdAb gene (as estimated from a colony PCR to amplify a cloned sdAb insert and an agarose gelelectorphoresis of the amplicon). The colonies of the immune library are scraped from the plates in LB medium, and the cell suspension transferred to sterile centrifuge tubes or 50 mL Falcon tubes. The cell suspension is centrifuged at low speed (e.g., 2,100 × *g*, 10 min) and the cell pellet is resuspended in 10 mL of LB medium and brought to 20 ml with sterile 100% glycerol to reach a final concentration of 25% glycerol. The 1 mL aliquots of the library are stored at −80°C. An aliquot of the library as stored in glycerol is diluted in LB medium and plated on LB-agar containing 25 μm/mL chloramphenicol. After overnight incubation at 37°C, we count the number of colonies growing on the plate that was appropriately diluted. From this number, we can calculate the total amount of bacterial cells in the library. The total number of cells divided by the number of transformants corresponds to the average number of cells within every colony (i.e., the library amplification).
2. The aliquot should cover at least ten times the number of individual transformants of the primary library to have a reasonable chance that all sdAbs of the library are represented. The initial

$OD_{600\,nm}$ of the cell suspension in LB medium should be below 0.2. If higher, dilute the suspension with LB medium and distribute over more than 1 culture flask (1 L).

3. In our hands, storage of electrocompetent cells reduces dramatically their transformation efficiency. Since we envisage to test every sdAb in the library for its possible interaction with the antigen, we require a maximal transformation efficiency, therefore these electrocompetent cells of the library are not stored.
4. The gene of the antigen is amplified by PCR to contain appropriate restriction enzyme sites at the extremity of the gene. The amplicon is digested with the restriction enzymes and ligated into the multiple cloning site of the pTRG vector (Stratagene), in frame with the N-terminal domain of the α-subunit of RNA polymerase. We commonly use restriction enzymes *NotI* and *EcoRI*. The ligated material is transformed in *E. coli* cells (e.g., WK6) from where the plasmid is purified with Qiagen plasmid mini kit and stored in 1 mM EDTA, 10 mM Tris-HCl, pH 8.0 at a concentration of 10 ng/mL. The insert is sequenced to confirm the presence of the correct antigen gene. The purity of the plasmid preparation is checked by inspection of its UV absorption spectrum and by agarose gelelectrophoresis.
5. Be certain of the adequate humidity of your plates before plating. If the plates are too dry (too old), the cells will have difficulties to grow. If the plates are too wet (liquid minidroplets on plate), it may result in false positives.
6. Cells grow much slower on minimal NSM, SSM, or DSSM plates compared to LB-agar plates. If the cells are yet too small on the former plates after 24 h at 37°C, incubate the plates for maximally an additional 12 h at 37°C or room temperature. The persistent lack of colonies may indicate that no sdAb in the library binds to the antigen or that the selection procedure failed.
7. To ensure that a full coverage of the sdAb library will be transformed with pTRG-antigen (see later), we expect that 10^7–10^8 electrocompetent cells survive the mock electrotransformation.
8. If colonies are growing on the LB-Tet plates after mock transformation, either the electrocompetent cells or any solution used were contaminated with cells or plasmids conferring tetracycline resistance (such as pTRG) or the tertracycline antibiotic is not active. You should start over again.
9. Assessing the electrocompetence of the BMII cells prepared according to Subheading 3.2: With the parental "empty" pTRG vector, and the pTRG-antigen vector as well, the transformation efficiency should be at least 10^6 transformants/μg pTRG. If this efficiency is not approached, it is advisable to repeat the experiments and to make fresh electrocompetent cells.

If the quality of the pTRG and pTRG-antigen plasmid is equivalent (according to UV spectrophotometry and gelelectrophoresis revealing no evidence of DNA plasmid degradation) and you noticed a reduced number of colonies for the pTRG-antigen transformed cells compared to the "empty" pTRG transformed cells on the NSM plates (and possibly also on LB-Tet agar plates), then it probably indicates that the presence of antigen is toxic for the host cells. In that case, you might clone the sdAb library in the pTRG plasmid and the antigen gene in the pBTL vector, since the pBTL plasmid has a lower copy number compared to the pTRG plasmid.

10. Evaluating the number of sdAb in the immune library with the capacity to self-activate the reporter genes with the "empty" pTRG plasmid. After overnight incubation at 37°C, there should be no colonies on the SSM plates as these arise when the sdAb-fusion encoded in the pBTL vector is recruiting the activation domain RNA polymerase and triggers the reporter gene. Of course it cannot be excluded that a single sdAb might self-activate the reporter gene; however, this should be an extremely low number. The self-activation can also be tested by transforming the electrocompetent host cells with the pBTL-sdAb library with a pTRG plasmid with a cloned gene of an irrelevant antigen.
11. Compare the number of colonies on SSM plates with the number on NSM plates. The percentage of colonies growing on the SSM plates will depend on the quality of your library and the antigen-specific binders it harbors.
12. The size of the colonies is not correlated necessarily to the equilibrium association constant between the sdAb and its cognate antigen. In our experience, the same binder can produce small as well as larger colonies, i.e., slow or faster growing cells. Therefore, all colonies from large SSM plates are picked irrespective of the colony size.
13. If none of the streaked cells growing on SSM proliferate on DSSM, then it is advisable to reduce the amount of streptomycin to 10 μg/mL in the DSSM plates and restreak the cells (from the SSM plate).
14. Colonies growing on DSSM plates contain DNA of both the pBTL and pTRG plasmid. So using the cells from such plates to perform a colony PCR yields sufficient material to determine the DNA sequence of the insert sdAb gene. Alternatively, inocculating the cells surviving on the dual selection medium in rich medium such as LB might result in a loss of the pTRG plasmids. Therefore, you need to grow the cells in LB medium supplemented with chloramphenicol if you intend to purify the pBTL-sdAb plasmid for sequence analysis.

15. Confirm the intracellular interaction between the antigen and each sdAb that was identified by the sequence analysis (see Subheading 3.5, step 2). Take electrocompetent cells prepared according to the protocols outlined in Subheading 3.2 but starting from BMII host cells containing either the "empty" pTRG or the pTRG-antigen-derived plasmid. Mix the pBTL-sdAb plasmid (see Note 14) with these electrocompetent BMII cells and transform. Plate dilutions (made as explained in Subheading 3.4, step 1) of the transformation mixture on NSM, SSM, and DSSM plates. Incubate the plates at 37°C for 24 h. A positive interaction is validated if cells with the "empty" pTRG are not growing and those with pTRG-antigen are growing on SSM and DSSM plates.
16. For epitope mapping, start from a 3 mL overnight culture of BMII cells containing recombinant pBTL harboring the sdAb of interest. In order to characterize the region targeted by the investigated sdAb, clone different subdomains, overlapping subfragments, or randomly mutated variants of the antigen gene in the pTRG vector by standard cloning techniques. Transform 50 ng of each variant/subfragment of the antigen ligated in the pTRG vector in different 60 μL aliquots of electrocompetent sdAb-pBTL BMII cells. Plate all the different transformations individually on separate small NSM and SSM plates. Growth on selective medium will confer evidence on the targeted region of the antigen by reconstituting a consensus sequence from the individual positively scoring interacting partners.

References

1. Smith GP (1985) Filamentous fusion phage: novel expression vectors that display cloned antigens on the virion surface. Science 228: 1315–1317
2. Barbas CF 3rd, Kang AS, Lerner RA et al (1991) Assembly of combinatorial antibody libraries on phage surfaces: the gene III site. Proc Natl Acad Sci USA 88:7978–7982
3. Griffiths AD, Malmqvist M, Marks JD et al (1993) Human anti-self antibodies with high specificity from phage display libraries. EMBO J 12:725–734
4. Mattheakis LC, Bhatt RR, Dower WJ (1994) An in vitro polysome display system for identifying ligands from very large peptide libraries. Proc Natl Acad Sci USA 91:9022–9026
5. Hanes J, Plückthun A (1997) In vitro selection and evolution of functional proteins by ribosome display. Proc Natl Acad Sci USA 94:4937–4942
6. Zahnd C, Amstutz P, Pluckthun A (2007) Ribosome display: selecting and evolving proteins in vitro that specifically bind to a target. Nat Methods 4:269–279
7. Lo AS, Zhu Q, Marasco WA (2008) Intracellular antibodies (intrabodies) and their therapeutic potential. In: Chernajovsky Y, Nissim A (eds) Therapeutic antibodies. Handbook of experimental pharmacology, vol 181. Springer, UK, pp 343–373
8. Messer A, Lynch SM, Butle DC (2009) Developing intrabodies for the therapeutic suppression of neurodegenerative pathology. Expert Opin Biol Ther 9:1189–1197
9. Fields S, Song O (1989) A novel genetic system to detect protein-protein interactions. Nature 340:245–246
10. Visintin M, Settanni G, Maritan A et al (2002) The intracellular antibody capture technology (IACT): towards a consensus sequence for intracellular antibodies. J Mol Biol 317:73–83
11. Mossner E, Koch H, Pluckthun A (2001) Fast selection of antibodies without antigen

purification: adaptation of the protein fragment complementation assay to select antigen-antibody pairs. J Mol Biol 308:115–122

12. Pelletier JN, Arndt KM, Pluckthun A et al (1999) An in vivo library-versus-library selection of optimized protein-protein interactions. Nat Biotechnol 17:683–690
13. Pelletier JN, Campbell-Valois FX, Michnick SW (1998) Oligomerization domain-directed reassembly of active dihydrofolate reductase from rationally designed fragments. Proc Natl Acad Sci USA 95:12141–12146
14. Dove SL, Joung JK, Hochschild A (1997) Activation of prokaryotic transcription through arbitrary protein-protein contacts. Nature 386:627–630
15. Joung JK, Ramm EI, Pabo CO (2000) A bacterial two hybrid selection system for studying protein-DNA and protein-protein interactions. Proc Natl Acad Sci USA 97:7382–7387
16. Dove SL, Hochschild A (1998) Conversion of the omega subunit of *Escherichia coli* RNA polymerase into a transcriptional activator or an activation target. Genes Dev 12:745–754

Chapter 10

Intracellular Antibody Capture (IAC) Methods for Single Domain Antibodies

Tomoyuki Tanaka and Terence H. Rabbitts

Abstract

Intracellular single domain antibodies are recombinant proteins, comprising one variable region domain fragment, that bind specifically to intracellular molecules and can interfere with their particular functions within various cellular compartments. They are valuable tools in bioscience and potential macrodrugs in biotherapeutics; however, their application is still limited because of the difficulty and inefficiency of acquisition of functional intracellular antibodies. We describe here the new generation protocol for intracellular antibody capture to facilitate selection of functional single domains. This protocol uses a series of optimized single domain libraries, based on designed intracellular variable (VH or VL) region scaffolds, for direct in vivo isolation of single domains that bind to target proteins and interaction and for affinity maturation to develop sub-nM affinity antibody fragments. The method has advantages over other methods in that specific single domains are isolated directly within the reducing cellular environment and can be selected without in vitro antigen protein preparation.

In an accompanying methods paper, we describe a simple extension of the methodology to isolate subsets of IAC-captured single domains that interfere with protein–protein interactions.

Key words: Single domains, Intracellular antibody, Intrabody Intracellular antibody capture, Yeast, Two-hybrid, Protein–protein interactions, Dab, iDab

1. Introduction

There is now no doubt that monoclonal antibodies are indispensable reagents for widespread bioscience research and medical fields (1, 2); however, their usage is always restricted in vitro or for extracellular molecules on viable cells. The idea of intracellular antibodies (intrabodies) is to use recombinant antibody fragments inside viable cells and modify/interfere with protein functions (3, 4). There are two main reasons. Intracellular antibodies can be utilized as powerful laboratory reagents in bioscience studies, such as functional genomics or the investigation of the components of protein complexes, or

Dirk Saerens and Serge Muyldermans (eds.), *Single Domain Antibodies: Methods and Protocols*, Methods in Molecular Biology, vol. 911, DOI 10.1007/978-1-61779-968-6_10, © Springer Science+Business Media, LLC 2012

as progenitors of drug-like molecules in medical applications. However, until recently acquiring functional intracellular antibodies has been problematic, despite progress in recombinant antibody and protein engineering technologies, because most antibodies or fragments obtained using general methods (e.g., hybridomas and phage display) do not necessarily work when expressed inside cells because the reducing environment precludes protein folding. The intracellular antibody capture (IAC) technology was originally developed to circumvent this drawback (5) but in itself it was hampered by the inclusion of an initial phage single chain Fv (scFv) selection prior to an in vivo yeast IAC step. This was improved by the next stages of IAC which used in vivo scFv selections in yeast based in VH and VL frameworks designed from comparison of a set of functional intracellular scFv isolated by IAC (6–8). Finally, we found that single domain antibodies (designated *I*ntracellular single *D*omain *a*nti*b*odies, iDabs), rather than scFv, were the most effective intracellular antibody fragments (9) and that the intra-chain disulphide bond-forming cysteine residues in VH and VL were not required for single domain protein folding (10). This led to the development of the third generation of IAC (IAC^3) (11).

The IAC^3 method, described here, facilitates the acquisition of intracellular antibodies against any protein antigen. The methodology is based on yeast two-hybrid (Y2H) selections (12), which is an in vivo genetic method that allows detection of the binding partners in bait and prey interactions. In this Y2H, two proteins to be tested are expressed in yeast nuclei fused either to a DNA binding domain (DBD) (bait) or to a transcriptional activation domain (AD) (prey). If the bait and prey interact, a reporter gene(s) is activated which affects a particular phenotype of the yeast. In IAC^3, target proteins or protein domains are expressed as baits and iDabs as preys. The iDab has only three antigen binding regions called complementarity determining regions (CDRs) which are flexible peptide loops which directly contact antigen but exhibit specificity. The use of single domain antibodies thus simplifies the construction of high diversity libraries and facile manipulation of the antibody binding site (CDRs) for affinity manipulation.

The IAC^3 protocol comprises (1) preparation of bait antigen; (2) screening initial single domain library; (3) generation of sublibrary(ies) from first round selected clones; and (4) confirmation of positive clones. The IAC^3 has several practical benefits: (1) An ability to isolate intracellular antibodies with high performance (high affinity and specificity) by direct genetic selection; (2) Obviation of the need for in vitro preparation of native antigens, some of which are very difficult to prepare as recombinant proteins; (3) Critical isolation of iDabs binding native antigens; (4) Low false positive since two different bait systems are used in screening; (5) Large scale screening after CDR randomization from the first round selected iDabs.

2. Materials

Prepare all solutions using ultrapure water (prepared by purifying deionized water to attain a sensitivity of 18 MΩ cm at 25°C) and analytical grade reagents. Prepare and store all reagents at room temperature (unless indicated otherwise). Diligently follow all waste disposal regulations when disposing waste materials.

2.1. Preparation of the Yeast Bait Lines and Yeast Transformation

1. Bait plasmid: pBTM116 (13) and pBD-GAL4 (see Fig. 1). The two bait plasmids contain the *TRP1* gene for yeast selectable marker and either the ampicillin resistant gene (pBTM116) or chloramphenicol acetyltransferase gene (pBD-GAL4) respectively for bacterial selection.
2. Yeast reporter strains: L40 (*MATa*, *leu2-3112*, *his3Δ200*, *trp1Δ1*, *ade2*, *LYS2::(LexA-op)$_4$-HIS3*, *URA3::(LexA-op)$_8$-lacZ*), MaV203 (*MATα*, *leu2-3,112*, *trp1-901*, *his3Δ200*, *ade2-101*, *gal4Δ*, *gal80Δ*, *SPAL10::URA3*, *GAL1::lacZ*, *HIS3$_{UAS\ GAL1::}$HIS3@LYS2*, *can1^R*, *cyh2^R*), AH109 (*MATa*, *trp1-901*, *leu2-3*, *112*, *ura3-52*, *his3-200*, *gal4Δ*, *gal80Δ*, *LYS2::GAL1$_{UAS}$-GAL1$_{TATA}$-HIS3*, *MEL1*, *GAL2$_{UAS}$-GAL2$_{TATA}$-ADE2*, *URA3::MEL1$_{UAS}$-MEL1$_{TATA}$-lacZ*).
3. YPD medium and plates: dissolve 10 g yeast extract and 20 g peptone (and 20 g agar for plates) in 900 mL of water and autoclave. Cool down to 55°C and add 100 mL of filter-sterile 20% glucose (and pour into sterile dishes.). Store at room temperature (RT).
4. 20% glucose solution: sterilize by passing through a 0.22 μm filter. Store at RT.
5. 1× TE: 10 mM Tris–HCl, 1 mM EDTA, pH 7.5. Store at RT.
6. Lithium acetate (LiAc)/TE: 100 mM LiAc, 10 mM Tris–HCl, 1 mM EDTA, pH 7.5 (see Note 1). Prepare prior to use.
7. LiAc/TE/polyethylene glycol (PEG) solution: 100 mM LiAc, 10 mM Tris–HCl, 1 mM EDTA, pH 7.5, 40% PEG 3350 (see Note 1). Prepare prior to use.
8. Salmon sperm DNA (ssDNA): 20 mg/mL, dissolve ssDNA in 1× TE by stirring at 4°C until homogeneous. To reduce viscosity, sonicate for 30 s using a large probe at 20–30% power. Dispense 2 mL aliquots and store at −20°C. Boil the ssDNA for 10 min prior to use.
9. Dimethyl sulfoxide (DMSO). Store at RT.
10. Yeast complete (YC)—4 amino acid dropout (YC-4aa) supplement: stocks as 100× solution at 4°C. Dissolve 1 g phenylalanine,

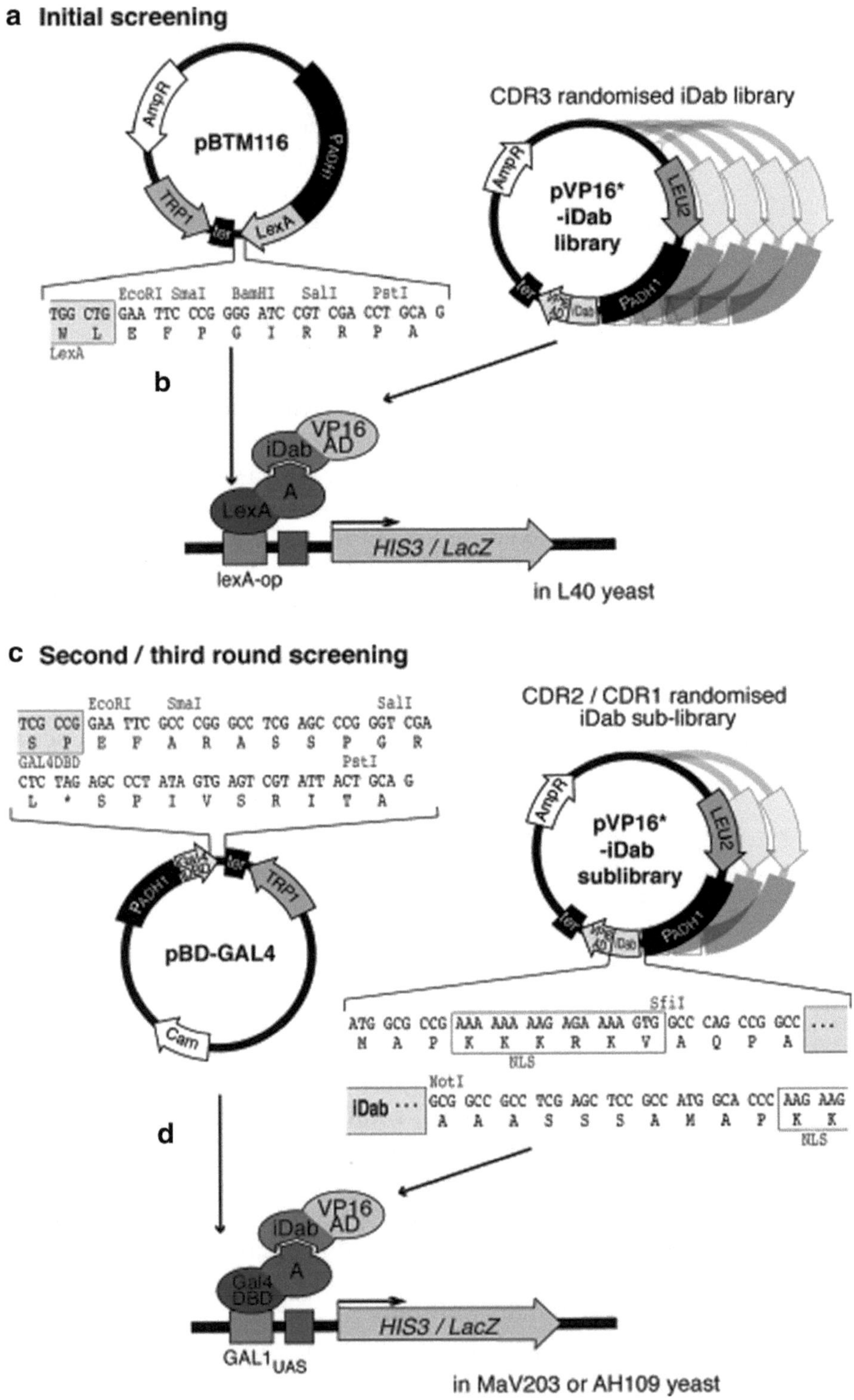
a Initial screening
pBTM116
AmpR
TRP1
ter
LexA
PADH1
EcoRI SmaI BamHI SalI PstI
TGG CTG GAA TTC CCG GGG ATC CGT CGA CCT GCA G
W L E F P G I R R P A
LexA
CDR3 randomised iDab library
pVP16*
-iDab
library
AmpR
LEU2
ter
VP16 AD
iDab
PADH1
b
VP16 AD
iDab
A
LexA
HIS3 / LacZ
lexA-op
in L40 yeast
c Second / third round screening
EcoRI SmaI SalI
TCG CCG GAA TTC GCC CGG GCC TCG AGC CCG GGT CGA
S P E F A R A S S P G R
GAL4DBD
PstI
CTC TAG AGC CCT ATA GTG AGT CGT ATT ACT GCA G
L * S P I V S R I T A
PADH1
GAL4 DBD
ter
TRP1
pBD-GAL4
Cam
CDR2 / CDR1 randomised
iDab sub-library
pVP16*
-iDab
sublibrary
AmpR
LEU2
ter
VP16 AD
iDab
PADH1
SfiI
ATG GCG CCG AAA AAA AAG AGA AAA GTG GCC CAG CCG GCC ...
M A P K K K R K V A Q P A
NLS
NotI
iDab ... GCG GCC GCC TCG AGC TCC GCC ATG GCA CCC AAG AAG
A A A S S S A M A P K K
NLS
d
VP16 AD
iDab
A
Gal4 DBD
HIS3 / LacZ
GAL1UAS
in MaV203 or AH109 yeast

1 g isoleucine, 2 g arginine, 1 g valine, 1 g aspartic acid, 1 g proline, 1 g serine, 2 g lysine, 0.2 g adenine, 1 g methionine, and 2 g threonine in 200 mL of water and filter sterilize. Make 10 mL aliquots and store at 4°C.

11. Amino acid supplements: stocks as 100× solution (except uracil). Dissolve either 1 g tryptophan, 1 g histidine, or 2 g leucine in 200 mL of water and filter sterilize. Make 10 mL aliquots and store at 4°C (except leucine, store at RT). For 10× uracil stock, dissolve 1 g uracil in 1 L water and filter sterilize. Make 100 mL aliquots and store at 4°C.

12. YC dropout medium and plate (for 1 L): dissolve 1.2 g yeast nitrogen base (YNB) (without amino acids or ammonium sulphate), 5 g $(NH_4)_2SO_4$, 10 g succinic acid, 0.05 g tyrosine, and 6 g NaOH in 600 mL of water and adjust pH to 7.0 by adding additional NaOH pellets (and add 20 g agar if making plates). Autoclave and then cool down to 55°C. Add 100 mL of sterile 20% glucose, 10 mL of YC–4aa, 100 mL of 10× uracil solution, and 10 mL of each amino acid supplement except dropout amino acid (i.e., YC-W, tryptophan dropout). If 3-amino-1,2,4-triazole (3-AT) is needed (see below), add appropriate amount of 3-AT stock at this point. Make up 1 L solution by adding autoclaved water. If making plates, pour the media into sterile large square dishes (25×25 cm, approximately 250 mL per dish), 14 cm small round dishes (approximately 65 mL per dish) or 9 cm small round dishes (approximately 25 mL per dish) in sterile hood. Leave the plates at RT to solidify and dry. Store the plate upside down at 4°C (storage may be for up to 3 months but check the plates before use for contamination).

Fig. 1. The principle of yeast single domain intracellular antibody capture (IAC) screening. (**a**) The maps of plasmid vectors for initial screening. pBTM116 (*left*) is LexA DBD bait vector, carrying the ampicillin resistant gene (*AmpR*) and *TRP1* for selectable marker for bacteria and yeast, respectively. The cDNA of the target of interest should be cloned in-frame with the LexA DBD using the multiple cloning site (MCS) show and the LexADBD-target fusion protein is expressed from the yeast alcohol dehydrogenase 1 promoter (P_{ADH1}) (*left hand panel*). The pVP16* (*right hand panel*) is the yeast prey vector, carrying *AmpR* and *LEU2* genes for selection and expression. The single domain antibody fragment (iDab) is fused to VP16 activation domain (AD); iDabs are expressed with initially CDR3 randomized (iDab libraries). (**b**) The plasmid vectors are transformed in L40 yeast strain, carrying *HIS3* and *LacZ* reporter genes regulated by the LexA operator (*LexA-op*). When an iDab from a library, fused with the VP16AD of pVP16*, interacts with the target of interest (fused to LexA from pBTM116) a transcriptional complex is reconstructed, which results in the expression of the *HIS3* auxotrophic maker, which allows yeast growth on histidine drop-out yeast plates. Alternatively, the complex activates the *LacZ* gene causing blue coloration of yeast colonies. (**c**) The maps of the plasmid vectors for second and third rounds IAC^3 screening. pBD-GAL4 (left) is used as the Gal4-DBD bait vector (rather than the LexA-DBD vector) carrying chloramphenicol resistant gene (*Cam*) and *TRP1* for selectable markers. The cDNA of target of interest is cloned in-frame with Gal4-DBD using the MCS show and the GAL4DBD-target fusion protein is expressed driving by P_{ADH1} (*left hand panel*). The iDabs selected from initial library screens are cloned in-frame with the VP16AD in the *SfiI*/*NotI* sites of pVP16* (*right hand panel*). The interactive CDR2 and then CDR1 randomization is carried out in pVP16* as before (*right hand panel*) (**d**). The pBD-GAL4 and sub-libraries pVP16* vectors are transformed in MaV203 or AH109 yeast strains, carrying *HIS3* and *LacZ* reporter genes regulated by *GAL1* upstream activating sequence (UAS).

2.2. Validation of DBD-Antigen Fusion Expression in Yeast Bait Line

1. Y-PER protein extraction reagent (PIERCE, Rockford, IL, USA) (see Note 2).
2. SDS-PAGE buffer, 2×: 60 mM Tris–HCl, pH 6.8, 3% SDS, 10% glycerol, 0.05% bromophenol blue, 10% β-mercaptoethanol.
3. Antibodies: anti-lexA (clone 2–12, Santa Cruz Biotechnology, Santa Cruz, CA, USA), anti-Gal4DBD (clone RK5C1, Santa Cruz Biotechnology), or antibodies for your target.

2.3. Assessing Possible Auto-activation by the DBD-Antigen Fusion Protein

1. 3-AT stock: 2 M 3-AT in water and filter sterilize. Store at 4°C (see Note 3).

2.4. First Round Single Domain Antibody Screening

See Subheadings 2.1, 2.7, 2.14, and 2.15.

2.5. Large-Scale Yeast Transformation for Library Screening

See Subheading 2.1.

2.6. Preparation of Yeast Plasmid DNA for Second Sub-library Construction

See Subheading 2.7.

2.7. Preparation of Prey Plasmid DNA from Yeast

1. Phenol/chloroform/isoamyl alcohol: 25 mL of TE-saturated phenol, 24 mL of chloroform, and 1 mL of isoamyl alcohol. Mix and store at 4°C in dark.
2. Glass beads (425–600 μm).
3. Yeast lysis solution: 2% Triton x-100, 15% SDS, 100 mM NaCl, 10 mM Tris–HCl, pH 8.0, and 1 mM EDTA.
4. Absolute and 70% aqueous ethanol (v/v). Store at −20°C.
5. Sodium acetate (NaOAc) solution: 3 M in water, adjust pH 5.2 with glacial acetic acid. Store at RT.

2.8. Construction of the Single Domain Sub-library with CDR2 Randomization for Second Round Screening

1. PCR reagents: 10× PCR buffer, 25 mM $MgSO_4$, 2 mM dNTP, KOD DNA polymerase (Novagen Inc, Madison, WI, USA, see Note 4).
2. Restriction enzymes: SfiI, NotI-HF (New England Biolabs (NEB), Beverly, MA, USA, see Note 5).
3. Calf intestine alkaline phosphatase (CIAP).
4. T4 DNA ligase.

5. Yeast tRNA: 10 mg/mL in RNase-free water. Aliquot and store frozen at −20°C.
6. Competent bacterial cells: commercial or home-made.
7. Ampicillin stock (1,000×): 100 mg/mL in water. Aliquot and store frozen at −20°C.
8. SOC medium: 0.5% yeast extract, 2% tryptone, 10 mM NaCl, 2.5 mM KCl, 10 mM $MgCl_2$, 10 mM $MgSO_4$. After autoclaving, add filter-sterile 20% glucose (final 1%). Store at RT.
9. TYE plate: dissolve 1.5% agar, 1% tryptone, 0.5% yeast extract, and 135 mM NaCl. After autoclaving, cool to 55°C, add antibiotics (if necessary) with stirring and pour into sterile dishes. Store at 4°C.
10. 2× TY medium: 1.6% tryptone, 1% yeast extract, and 85 mM NaCl. Autoclave. Store at RT.

2.9. Second Round Screening

See Subheadings 2.1.

2.10. Preparation of Yeast Prey Plasmid DNA and Construction of Third Sub-library

See Subheadings 2.7 and 2.8.

2.11. Third Round Screening

See Subheadings 2.1.

2.12. Extraction of Yeast Prey Plasmid DNA from Individual Selected Yeast Colonies

See Subheading 2.7.

2.13. Re-testing the Single Domain VH or VL-VP16 Plasmids Using the Yeast Antibody–Antigen Interaction Assay

See Subheadings 2.1, 2.12, 2.14, and 2.15.

2.14. β-Galactosidase Filter Assay

1. Z buffer: 60 mM Na_2HPO_4, 60 mM NaH_2PO_4, 10 mM KCl, 1 mM $MgSO_4$, adjust pH 7.0 with NaOH. Store at RT.
2. Stock X-gal solution: 50 mM 5-bromo-4-chloro-3-indolyl-beta-D-galactopyranoside in *N*,*N*-dimethyl formamide. Store at −20°C.
3. Z buffer with X-gal: 0.8 mM X-gal (from stock solution) and 38 mM β-mercaptoethanol in Z buffer. Prepared fresh prior to use.

4. Whatmann filter paper.
5. Nylon membrane filter.

2.15. Replica Plating

1. Plate replicator stamp, for 10 cm diameter plates.
2. Velvets, sterilize by autoclaving.

3. Methods

3.1. Preparation of the Yeast Bait Lines and Yeast Transformation

1. Clone your target antigen cDNA as an in-frame fusion with a DBD in pBTM116 (see Fig. 1, LexADBD) and into pBD-GAL4 (see Fig. 1, Gal4DBD) using standard genetic cloning methods (14). Confirm the final construct by DNA sequencing with primers, BTM116F and BTM116R (for pBTM116) or Gal4F and T7F (for pBD-GAL4) (see Table 1).

Table 1
Oligonucleotides for PCR and sequencing

Primer names	Sequence (5′–3′)
sFvVP16F	TTGTTTCTTTTTCTGCACAAT
sFvVP16R	CAACATGTCCAGATCGAA
BTM116F	CAGAGCTTCACCATTGAAC
BTM116R	TCAATAAGAGCGACCTCATG
Gal4F	GTCACAGATAGATTGGCTTCAGTGG
T7F	TAATACGACTCACTATAGGG
rdmVHCDR2Rev	CAGAGTCTGCATAGTATATMNNMNNMN NMNNNMNNACTAATGTATGAAACCCAC
VHCDR2Fw	ATATACTATGCAGACTCTG
rdmVLCDR2Rev	AACCTTGATGGGACCCCACTMNNMNNMNN GGATGCMNNATAGATCAGGAGCTTAGGGG
VLCDR2Fw	TTGCAAAGTGGGGTCCCTTC
rdmHCDR1Rev	CCTGGAGCCTGGCGGACCCAMNNCATMN NMNNNMNNACTGAAGCTGAATCCAGAGG
HCDR1Fw	TGGGTCCGCCAGGCTCCAGG
rdmVLCDR1Rev	CCTGGTTTCTGCTGATACCAMNNTAAMNN GCTGCTAATMNNCTGACTTGCCCG GCAAGTGATG
VLCDR1Fw	TGGTATCAGCAGAAACCAGG

2. Inoculate a single colony of L40 and MaV203 (or AH109) respectively into 2 mL of YPD medium and culture overnight with shaking at 30°C (see Note 6).
3. Dilute 1 mL of overnight culture into 10 mL of YPD medium and culture at 30°C with shaking until the culture reaches $OD_{600\ nm}$ 0.6 (usually 3–4 h) (see Note 7).
4. Harvest the yeast by centrifuging at 1,000×*g* for 5 min at RT.
5. Wash the yeast pellet in 10 mL of sterile water and spin again at 1,000×*g* for 5 min at RT.
6. Resuspend washed yeast pellet in 100 μL of freshly made, sterile 1× LiAc/TE. These are the competent yeast cells.
7. Mix 200 ng of bait plasmid (see Subheading 3.1, step 1) and 100 μg of ssDNA in a sterile 1.5 mL microtube.
8. Add 100 μL of competent yeast cells to this mixture of DNA and vortex for approximately 30 s. Make sure of using the appropriate combination of bait plasmid and yeast strain, i.e., L40 for pBTM116 and MaV203 (or AH109) for pBD-Gal4, (see Note 6).
9. Add 600 μL of freshly prepared sterile LiAc/TE/PEG and vortex vigorously for approximately 30 s (see Note 1).
10. Incubate at 30°C for 30 min with shaking at 225 rpm, and then add 70 μL of DMSO and mix gently by inversion. Heat shock at 42°C for 15 min in a water bath.
11. Put on ice for 2 min, fill the microtube with sterile water, and pellet the cells by centrifuging at 3,000×*g*, RT for 5 min.
12. Resuspend the yeast pellet in 100 μL of 1× TE and plate 50 μL on a YC-W plate. Culture the plate at 30°C for 2–3 days.

3.2. Validation of DBD-Antigen Fusion Expression in Yeast Bait Line (See Note 8)

1. Inoculate a single yeast clone from the YC-W plate (prepared in Subheading 3.1, step 12) into 2 mL each of YC-W media and resuspend by vortexing until homogeneous. Culture overnight at 30°C with shaking at 225 rpm.
2. Dilute 1 mL of the overnight yeast culture into 10 mL of prewarmed YPD medium. Use the remaining overnight culture to make a glycerol and store at −80°C.
3. Incubate at 30°C with shaking until the $OD_{600\ nm}$ reaches 0.6 (see Note 9).
4. Quickly chill on ice for 2 min and pellet the cells by centrifuging at 3,000×*g* for 1 min at 4 C.
5. Resuspend cells (until homogeneous) in 20 μL of Y-PER protein extraction reagent (see Note 2) and transfer to a 1.5 mL microtube.
6. Incubate on ice for 20 min and pellet the cell debris by centrifuging at 13,000×*g* for 5 min at 4°C.

7. Transfer the supernatant to new 1.5 mL tube, add 20 μL of 2× SDS-PAGE buffer to the supernatant and boil for 5 min.
8. Use 20 μL of the supernatant for SDS-PAGE and Western blot. Detect DBD fusion antigen using antibody binding to the anti-LexA or the anti-Gal4DBD antibody as appropriate.

3.3. Assessing Possible Auto-activation by the DBD-Antigen Fusion Protein

1. Streak a single colony from an established bait line (from Subheading 3.1, step 12) on a new YC-W plate and culture at 30°C for 1–2 days.
2. Make replica onto a series of YC-WH plates containing various concentration of 3-AT (ranging 0–50 mM) (see Subheading 3.15).
3. Culture at 30°C for 2–3 days.
4. Assess yeast growth to determine the minimal concentration of 3-AT to prevent self-activation (see Note 3).

3.4. First Round Single Domain Antibody Screening

1. Perform first round screening of single domain initial libraries with an established L40 yeast bait strain using large scale yeast transformation method as described in Subheading 3.5.
2. Plate each 1.5 mL transformant from Subheading 3.5, step 17 onto 5 large square plates of YC-WLH + 3AT (using the minimal concentration preventing for self-activation in Subheading 3.3, step 4) (see Note 10).
3. Culture the plates at 30°C for 4–5 days.
4. Pick yeast growth colonies with 2–3 mm diameter and separately streak onto a new YC-WLH plate (as a master plate).
5. Culture at 30°C for 1–3 days until colony is visible.
6. Carry out a β-galactosidase filter assay (see Subheading 3.14).

3.5. Large Scale Yeast Transformation for Library Screening (See Note 11)

1. Homogenously resuspend 5–20 colonies of the established bait strain from Subheading 3.1, step 12 in 1 mL of sterile water and inoculate into 200 mL of YC-W media.
2. Culture overnight at 30°C with shaking.
3. Inoculate 100–200 mL of overnight culture into 1 L of prewarmed YPD medium to produce an $OD_{600\ nm}$ between 0.2 and 0.3 (see Note 7).
4. Culture at 30°C with shaking until $OD_{600\ nm}$ reaches 0.6 (usually 3–4 h).
5. Harvest the yeast cells by centrifuging at 1,000 × *g* for 2 min at RT.
6. Resuspend pellet in 200 mL of sterile water.
7. Centrifuge the yeast cells at 1,000 × *g* for 5 min at RT. Repeat twice as in steps from Subheading 3.5, step 6.

8. Resuspend the pellet in 8 mL of freshly made, sterile 1× LiAc/TE (see Note 1).
9. Combine 300 μg of a yeast single domain library DNA and 10 mg ssDNA and mix well by pipetting.
10. Add the DNA mix to 8 mL of competent yeast cells and mix well by vortexing for 30 s.
11. Add 60 mL of freshly sterile LiAc/TE/PEG (see Note 1), vortex for 30 s. Incubate at 30°C for 30 min with shaking at 225 rpm.
12. Add 7 mL of DMSO and mix gently by inversion.
13. Heat shock at 42°C in a water bath for 15 min and swirl to mix every 2 min.
14. Put on ice for 2 min, then fill the tube with sterile water and spin at 2,500 ×*g* for 5 min (see Note 12).
15. Discard supernatant and resuspend the yeast pellet with 10 mL of sterile water, and then filling up with sterile water to 200 mL and centrifuging at 2,500 ×*g*.
16. Repeat steps from Subheading 3.5, step 15.
17. Resuspend washed yeast pellet in 10 mL of 1× TE. These are the transformed yeast for plating on large screening plates.
18. To determine the total number of transformants, make 100 μL serial dilutions of the yeast from the step in Subheading 3.5, step 17 (the equivalent of 10 μL (dilution 1:10), 1 μL (dilution 1:100), 0.1 μL (dilution 1:1,000), and 0.01 μL (dilution 1:10,000)) in 1× TE and plate on 9 cm YC-WL plates. Culture at 30°C for 2–3 days.
19. Calculate transformation efficiency in the total 10 mL of yeast from Subheading 3.5, step 17 (see Note 13).

3.6. Preparation of Yeast Plasmid DNA for Second Sub-library Construction

1. Inoculate all (or groups of) positive yeast colonies from master plates (i.e., from -His growth and β-galactosidase expressors) into 5 mL of YC-L medium in a 50 mL sterile tube. Culture overnight at 30°C with shaking.
2. Extract plasmid DNA from the yeast cultures as in Subheading 3.7 (see Note 14).

3.7. Preparation of Prey Plasmid DNA from Yeast

1. Culture yeast in 5 mL of YC-L media overnight at 30°C with shaking at 225 rpm.
2. Harvest the yeast cells by centrifuging at 2,000 ×*g* for 5 min at RT.
3. Resuspend pellet in 200 μL of yeast lysis solution.
4. Add 200 μL of phenol/chloroform/isoamyl alcohol (25:24:1) and 0.3 g of acid-washed glass beads. Vortex for 5 min.
5. Centrifuge at 15,000 ×*g*, RT for 5 min.

6. Carefully pipette the upper layer without disturbing the interphase and transfer to 1.5 mL microtubes.
7. Add 20 μL of 3 M NaOAc (pH 5.2), mix well and then 500 μL of cold 100% ethanol.
8. Centrifuge again at 15,000 × *g*, RT for 10 min.
9. Wash the DNA pellet once with 500 μL of 70% ethanol.
10. Re-spin at 15,000 × *g*, RT for 10 min and remove supernatant.
11. Dry the pellet at RT for 10–15 min and dissolve in 20 μL of 1× TE.

3.8. Construction of the Single Domain Sub-library with CDR2 Randomization for Second Round Screening (Fig. 2)

1. Set up two 50 μL PCR reactions with primers pair A (sFvVP16F plus rdmVHCDR2Rev, see Table 1) or B (VHCDR2Fw plus sFvVP16R) to randomize CDR2 of VH (template sources from VH library screenings). Use primer pair C (sFvVP16F plus rdmVLCDR2Rev) and D (VLCDR2Fw plus sFvVP16R) for VL (from VL library screening) as in Table 2.
2. Put the tubes into a thermocycler and run the following PCR programme as in Table 3.
3. Take 10 μL of each PCR reaction and run on a 1.5% agarose gel.
4. Cut out the correct sized band from the gel (see Note 15) and extract DNA using commercial gel extraction kit according to manufacturer's instruction or use general extraction methods. Final DNA volume should be 50 μL.
5. For assembly of the two PCR products from Subheading 3.8, step 4, set up a second 50 μL PCR reactions as in Subheading 3.8, step 1 but using primers pair sFvVP16F and sFvVP16R plus 1 μL of each DNA product from primers pair A and B or from C and D and extracted as in Subheading 3.8, step 4.
6. Carry out the PCR using the same thermocycling conditions as in Subheading 3.8, step 2.
7. Take 2 μL of the PCR reactions and run on a 1.5% agarose gel.
8. If the analytical gel shows the correct size PCR product (see Note 16), purify the remaining PCR reaction. Final DNA should be 50 μL.
9. Add 6 μL of 10× NE buffer 4, 0.5 μL of 100× BSA, and 20 U of *Sfi*I restriction enzyme to the eluted PCR fragment and mix well (see Note 5). Incubate at 50°C until complete digestion (at least for 1 h).
10. At the same time, also set up a digestion of 5 μg pVP16* yeast plasmid with 50 U of *Sfi*I enzyme in 50 μL total reaction and mix well. Incubate at 50°C until digested completely (1 h at least).

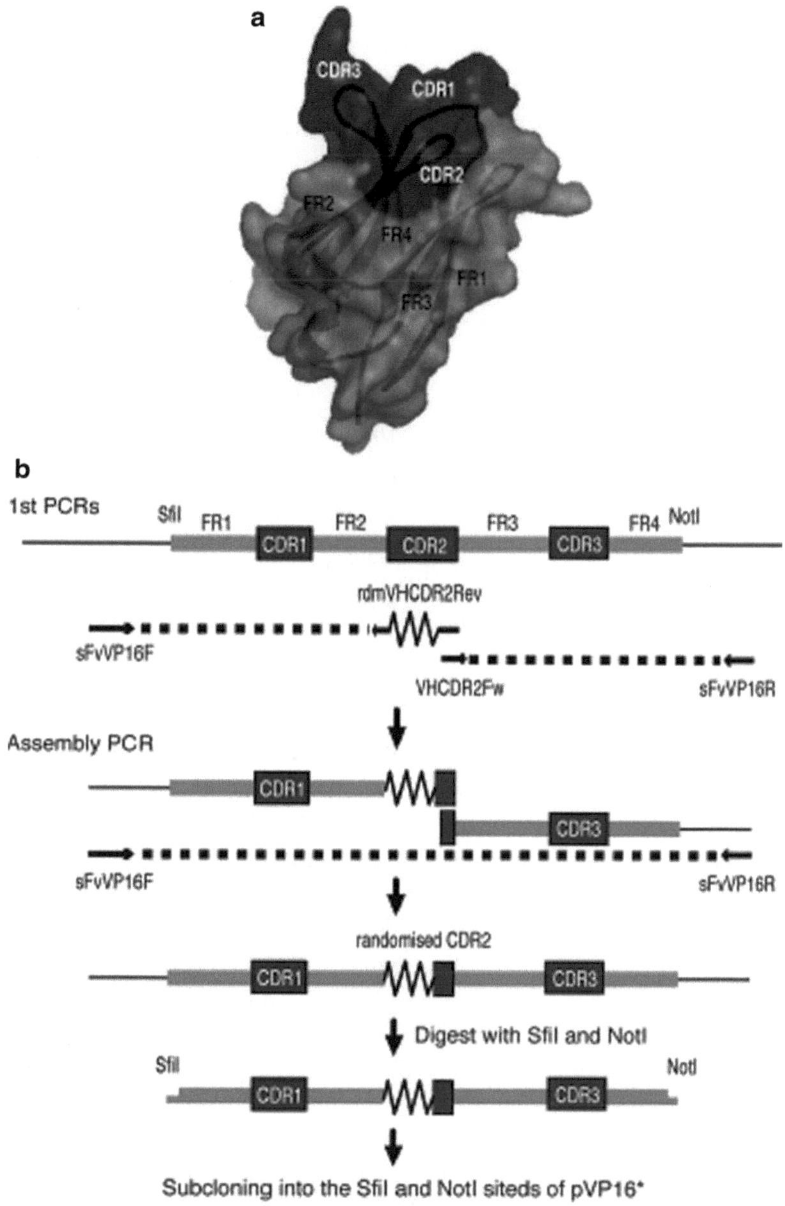

Fig. 2. Single domain intracellular antibodies and sub-library construction. (**a**) The protein structure of a single VH domain is shown in ribbon form with surface image. Three complementarity determining regions (CDR1, CDR2, and CDR3) are shown in *dark gray* and framework scaffold regions (FR) in *light gray*. (**b**) Diagrammatic representation of CDR randomization of single domain sub-libraries generation by assembly PCR (17). As exemplar, the construction of single domain VH sub-library with CDR2 randomization is shown. The *top line* illustrates the organization of the single VH domain (where FR = framework regions 1–4) with the flanking *SfiI* and *NotI* restriction sites. In iDabs, isolated from an initial library screen (in pVP16*), the mixed set of iDabs would be used as the PCR template for two PCR reactions carried out with either sFvVP16F + rdmVHCDR2Rev or VHCDR2Fw + sFvVP16R (*line 2*). The two PCR products are used as templates for assembly PCR using sFvVP16F + sFvVP16R primers, to yield an assembled iDab with CDR2 randomization (*lines 3 and 4*). The assembled PCR fragment is digested with *SfiI* and *NotI* restriction enzymes and re-cloned into pVP16* yeast prey vector for the next round of screening. A similar final round of CDR1 randomization can be done if needed using the PCR primers shown in Table 1.

Table 2
PCR mixture

Reagents	Amount (μL)
10× PCR buffer	5
25 mM $MgSO_4$	4
2 mM each dNTP	5
10 μM forward primer	1.5
10 μM back primer	1.5
Plasmid DNA from Subheading 3.6, step 2 (20–50 ng)	1
Water	31
KOD DNA polymerase	1

Table 3
PCR amplification programme (see Note 4)

Temperature (°C)	Time	Cycle
95	2 min	
95	20 s	
60	10 s	40 cycles
70	20 s	
70	5 min	

11. After each *Sfi*I digestion, add 20 U (or 50 U) of *Not*I-HF enzyme, mix well, and incubate at 37°C until digested completely for 1 h at least.
12. Add 1 μL of CIAP to the *Sfi*I-*Not*I digested pVP16* reaction and incubate at 37°C for a further 30 min.
13. Run the digested DNAs on a preparative 2% agarose gel (for *Sfi*I-*Not*I digested PCR products) or 0.8% gel (for CIAP-treated linearized pVP16* plasmid).
14. Cut out the appropriate band (see Note 17) from the gel and extract the DNA. Elute DNAs with 50 μL of elution buffer.
15. Set up set of 30 μL ligations in sterile microtubes as in Table 4, mix briefly, and incubate at 4°C overnight.
16. Add 59 μL of water, 1 μL of yeast tRNA (10 mg/mL), and 10 μL of 3 M NaOAc and mix well.

Table 4
Ligation reactions

Reagents	Amount (μL)
Purified *Sfi*I-*Not*I linear pVP16* plasmid	3
Purified *Sfi*I-*Not*I PCR fragment	1–23
10× ligation buffer	3
T4 DNA ligase (10 U/μL)	1
Water	Up to 30

17. Add 250 μL of ice-cold absolute ethanol, vortex and incubate on dry ice (or −80°C) for 10 min (or −20°C for 2–3 h).
18. Centrifuge at 15,000 ×*g*, RT for 10 min.
19. Wash the DNA pellet once with 500 μL of 70% ethanol and re-spin at 15,000 ×*g*, RT. Dry the pellet at RT for 10–15 min and then re-dissolve in 10 μL water.
20. Use 2 μL of ligation reactions for bacterial transformation by electroporation with commercially available or home-made competent cells, according to manufacturer's instructions or general methods (see Note 18).
21. After transformation, add SOC medium (at RT) made up to 10 mL in sterile 50 mL Falcon tube and culture at 37°C for 60 min.
22. Plate 1 mL each of the transformation mix on each of 10 large square plates (25 cm × 25 cm) of TYE plates containing 100 μg/mL ampicillin. Culture overnight at 37°C.
23. To determine the transformation efficiency/size of sub-library, make 100 μL of tenfold serial dilutions (from 1: 100 to 1: 100,000) from 10 mL transformant from Subheading 3.8, step 21 and plate on 9 cm TYE + ampicillin (100 μg/mL) plates. Culture all the plates overnight at 37°C (see Note 13)
24. Inoculate total 10–20 individual colonies selected randomly from titration plates in 2 mL of 2× TY containing 100 μg/mL ampicillin, culture overnight at 37°C with shaking at 225 rpm.
25. Harvest the bacteria from each culture and prepare the plasmid DNA using commercial plasmid mini-prep kits according to manufacturer's instruction or general methods.
26. Digest 0.5 μg of each plasmid DNA with *Sfi*I (at 50°C for 1 h at least) and *Not*I-HF (at 37°C for 1 h at least) and run on 1.5% agarose gel as in Subheading 3.8 steps 9 and 11.
27. Sequence the plasmids from Subheading 3.8, step 25 (first confirm the correct size of inserts from Subheading 3.8, step 26)

using either sFvVP16F or sFvVP16R primers. You can estimate the size of sub-library from the total number of transformants (see Subheading 3.8, step 23) and the percentage of plasmids with inserts (see Subheading 3.8, step 26) and the sequence data (see Subheading 3.8, step 27).

28. After overnight growth on the large plates (see Subheading 3.8, step 22), add 5 mL of 2× TY+100 μg/mL ampicillin onto each plate and scrape off all bacterial colonies using a sterile glass spreader.
29. Transfer the scraped bacteria suspension into 50 mL tubes and make bacterial pellets by centrifuging at 2,500×*g*, 30 min at 4°C.
30. Extract the plasmid DNA from the recovered cells using commercial large-scale plasmid prep kit according to manufacturer's instruction or general methods (15). The extracted plasmid DNA is the CDR2 randomized sub-library.
31. Measure the quality and concentration of plasmid DNA by a UV spectrometer.

3.9. Second Round Screening

1. Prepare a stable MaV203 (or AH109) yeast bait line expressing Gal4DBD-antigen as in Subheading 3.1, step 12. Determine the minimum concentration of 3-AT that can be used to prevent auto-activation of the MaV203 (or AH109) bait line as in Subheading 3.3. The CDR2 sub-library DNA is prepared as in Subheading 3.8, step 31.
2. Screen the CDR2 sub-library following the procedure in Subheading 3.4, using the MaV203 (or AH109) bait line.
3. Plate 1.5 mL each of transformed yeast onto 5 large YC-WLH plates containing either the minimum 3-AT to stop auto-activation or with 25, 50, 75, or 100 mM 3-AT (this will allow iDabs with increased in vivo binding affinity to be selected on the higher concentrations of 3-AT). Save the remainder of the transformants at 4°C as a backup. Culture at 30°C for 4–7 days.
4. Pick yeast colonies and separately streak onto a new YC-WLH plate (as your master plate). Culture the plates at 30°C until yeast growth is visible (1–2 days).

3.10. Preparation of Yeast Prey Plasmid DNA and Construction of Third Sub-library

1. Inoculate the yeast colonies from the YC-WLH plate (*see* Subheading 3.9, step 4) into 5 mL of YC-L medium and culture overnight at 37°C.
2. Extract plasmid DNA from yeast cultures as described in Subheading 3.7.
3. Construct a CDR1-randomized sub-library as described in Subheading 3.8 for third round screening.

4. Set up two 50 μL PCR reactions as in Subheading 3.8, step 1 using primer pairs A (sFvVP16F plus rdmVHCDR1Rev, see Table 1) and B (VHCDR1Fw plus sFvVP16R) to randomize CDR1 of VH (template sources from VH library screenings) or primer pair C (sFvVP16F plus rdmVLCDR1Rev) and D (VLCDR1Fw plus sFvVP16R) for VL (from VL library screening).
5. Template DNA: plasmid DNA from Subheading 3.10, step 2 (20–50 ng).
6. Perform the PCR reaction as in Subheading 3.8, step 2.
7. Extract and purify the amplified PCR fragments as in Subheading 3.8, step 4 (see Note 19).
8. Perform the PCR assembly as in Subheading 3.8, steps 5–8 and digest the assembled PCR fragment with *Sfi*I and *Not*I-*HF* as in Subheading 3.8, steps 9 and 11.
9. Construct the third sub-library by sub-cloning the PCR fragment from step 8 into *Sfi*I and *Not*I-*HF* sites of pVP16* DNA (see Subheading 3.8, step 13) as in Subheading 3.8, steps 15–31.

3.11. Third Round Screening

1. Follow the same protocol as in Subheading 3.9 except using the library constructed in Subheading 3.10, step 9. Screening is done with YC-WLH plates containing higher concentrations of 3-AT than with the second round screening.
2. After screening, pick yeast colonies and separately streak onto a new YC-WLH plate (as your master plate). Culture the plates at 30°C until yeast growth is visible (1–2 days).

3.12. Extraction of Yeast Prey Plasmid DNA from Individual Selected Yeast Colonies

1. Inoculate the yeast colonies from the YC-WLH plate into 5 mL of YC-L medium and culture overnight at 30°C and then harvest yeast.
2. Extract plasmid DNA from yeast cultures as described in Subheading 3.7 (see Note 20).
3. Transform 1–5 μL of the DNA stock into bacteria using electroporation or chemical transformation and plate on TYE + ampicillin (100 μg/mL). Culture the plate overnight at 37°C.
4. Inoculate several bacterial colonies individually into 2 mL of 2× TY containing 100 μg/mL ampicillin and culture overnight at 37°C (see Note 21).
5. Harvest bacteria by centrifuging and extract plasmid DNA as in Subheading 3.8, step 25. Final DNA volume is 50 μL.
6. To check for the identity of yeast single domain-VP16 plasmid, digest 5 μL of DNA with *Sfi*I and *Not*I-*HF* enzymes and separate on a 1.5% agarose gel as in Subheading 3.8, step 26.

3.13. Re-testing the Single Domain VH or VL-VP16 Plasmids Using the Yeast Antibody–Antigen Interaction Assay

1. Using both yeast baits (L40 and MaV203 (or AH109)) in Subheading 3.1, step 12, prepare small volumes of competent cells yeast bait strains as described in Subheading 3.1, steps 2–6.
2. Prepare two DNA mixtures of 200 ng of the isolated yeast single domain-VP16 plasmid DNAs as prepared in Subheading 3.12 and 100 μg of ssDNA. Add 100 μL each of the appropriate competent yeast bait strain to each DNA mixture and mix well.
3. Follow the same procedure as in Subheading 3.1, steps 9–11.
4. Resuspend the pellet in 100 μL. Plate the transformants by spreading 10 μL resuspended yeast onto one 10 cm YC-WL plate. Culture at 30°C for 1–3 days until yeast growth is visible.
5. Replica (see Subheading 3.15) plates from step 4 onto YC-WLH plates with 3-AT (using several concentrations of 3-AT as determined for minimum to maximum in the screening).
6. Culture the plate at 30°C for 2–3 days. True positive prey clones will make grow as histidine-independent growth on both LexA-bait (L40) and Gal4-bait (MaV203 or AH109) colonies. These plates can be used for β-galactosidase filter assay as described in Subheading 3.14. These true positive iDab clones should be verified by sequencing the isolated plasmid DNA with the primer sFvVP16F or sFvVP16R.

3.14. β-Galactosidase Filter Assay

1. Make replica plates (see Subheading 3.15) on new YC-WLH using the master plates from Subheading 3.11, step 2.
2. Culture the plates at 30°C for 1–2 days.
3. Place a nylon membrane filter directly onto the surface of the yeast plates.
4. During Subheading 3.14, step 3, drop 2 mL of Z buffer/X-gal solution onto a petri dish lid, and carefully overlay on a Whatmann filter onto this solution and remove any bubbles between the filter and the lid.
5. Take the nylon filter carefully from the yeast replica plates and float it on a pool of liquid nitrogen for approximately 30 s (colony side upwards).
6. After the 30 s, immerse the filter for 5 s in the liquid nitrogen.
7. Remove the filter from the liquid N_2 and leave to thaw at RT for 2 min.
8. Place the nylon filter on the top of the wet Whatmann paper containing Z buffer/X-gal solution (see Subheading 3.14, step 4) with the yeast colonies facing upwards.
9. Cover with the bottom of the petri dish, incubate at 30°C, and check periodically for appearance of blue colonies (see Note 22).

3.15. Replica Plating

1. Place sterile velvet over a replicator (see Note 23).
2. Gently press the surface of the master plate (with yeast growth) onto the velvet and remove carefully from a replicator.
3. Gently press the velvet onto the surface of a new plate and remove carefully.
4. Be sure there is some transfer of yeast onto replica plates. It should show faint white marks.
5. Repeat Subheading 3.15, steps 3 and 4 to generate up to 5 replica plates.
6. Change to a new sterile velvet on the replicator and remove excess yeast from replica plates by pressing the surface of plates onto the clean velvet.
7. Be sure to clean the plates which should only have shadowy yeast colonies (see Note 24).

4. Notes

1. 1× LiAc/TE and LiAc/TE/PEG should always be freshly prepared to maximize the efficiency of yeast transformation. You can usually keep the following stock solutions and make up mixtures as needed: 1 M LiAc: adjusted pH to 7.5 by acetic acid, autoclave; 10× TE: 100 mM Tris, 1 mM EDTA adjusted pH to 7.5 with HCl, autoclave; 50% PEG3350: filter sterilized. If transformation efficiency is getting low, it may be necessary to make up a new stock solution.
2. We are using the reagent for protein extraction from yeast. Alternatively you can use a general glass bead disruption method (16).
3. 3-AT is the inhibitor of imidazole glycerol phosphate dehydratase encoded by the *HIS3* gene. Addition of 3-AT to histidine dropout plates can reduce auto-activation effects by bait strains (in a dose-dependent manner) and also can decrease the occurrence of nonspecific or low affinity iDabs in screening. If your bait lines grow on YC-WH containing more than 30 mM 3-AT, this bait line is not suitable for use in IAC^3 screening because almost all initial iDabs have binding affinities that will not allow growth at the 3-AT concentration. In this case, you will need to consider if your target construct design can be modified (e.g., elongate or shorten the cDNA fused to LexA and Gal4DBD).
4. In our hands, KOD polymerase shows good amplification using the PCR amplification programme shown in Table 3. Other DNA polymerases can be used for PCR, but must be

with high polymerization fidelity. (Taq polymerase is not recommended for this purpose.) If using other DNA polymerases, you may need to follow the suitable PCR programmes for each enzymes.

5. We have used restriction enzymes from NEB and their buffer systems for DNA digestions. Enzymes from other manufacturers can be used, following their instructions.

6. The combination of the yeast reporter stains and the bait vector is crucial. L40 yeast have to be used for the pBTM116 LexA vector and MaV203 or AH109 for pBD-Gal4. When you use a yeast reporter strain from a long-term frozen stock, it is strongly recommended that yeast phenotype is checked by culturing on selective YC-dropout plate lacking the appropriate amino acid. It is not recommended to use yeast that have been maintained on plates for any length of time.

7. Yeast transformation efficiency will dramatically decrease when a yeast is over-grown (i.e., if the $OD_{600\ nm}$ of the culture exceeds 0.7). The $OD_{600\ nm}$ of yeast cultures from the start and end points should be monitored periodically. The $OD_{600\ nm}$ of initial cultures should be no more than 0.2 and at the end about 0.6. This usually takes 3–4 h of growth. If cultures require more than 5 h to reach $OD_{600\ nm}$ 0.6, this culture should not be used for yeast competent cell preparation.

8. The protocol here describes Western blotting for verifying DBD-antigen expression in yeast baits using antibodies against either DBD or antigen itself. Alternatively, if a protein partner that binds to your target intracellularly is known, and is available, you may be able to validate bait expression in your yeast clones by yeast two-hybrid interaction phenotype with its partner protein. The prey plasmid pVP16* with partner protein cDNA sub-cloned can be transformed into the bait by using same protocol as in Subheading 3.2 and tested by growth on YC-WLH. This alternative is more comprehensive than the Western blot method, but note that this approach will depend on the intracellular properties (e.g., stability, affinity) of both the target and its partner.

9. The $OD_{600\ nm}$ should not be allowed to exceed 0.6 as the *ADH1* promoter driving the bait protein expression shuts down during late log growth phase and the level of endogenous yeast protease increases.

10. The remainder of the yeast transformants can be saved at 4°C as a backup for about a week.

11. You would expect 10^4–10^5 transformants/μg DNA for yeast large-scale transformation. For library screening, each screening (i.e., total number of transformants grown on—WL dropout plates) should be at least greater than the initial library size.

12. The yeast pellet after centrifugation may not be solid because of remaining high concentrations of PEG. The supernatant should be removed carefully by decanting or by pipetting.
13. For calculation of the transformation efficiency, count the number of colonies on each plate and multiply by the dilution ratio (e.g., if 20 colonies are on the plate seeded with the equivalent 0.1 μL (dilution 1:1,000) and 180 colonies on 1 μL (1:100), the average is 190 colonies per μL (1:100)). This makes $190 \times 100 \times 10 = 1.9 \times 10^6$ transformants per mL yeast/bacteria suspension.
14. The DNA from yeast will be a mixture of bait and prey plasmids at this point; however this can be used as the PCR template for the second sub-library construction without any further purification steps (i.e., ignore any carryover of the LexA bait plasmid as the second library screening will be carried out under Gal4DBD system).
15. The expected size of amplified PCR fragments are: 328 bp for primer pair A, 360–399 bp for B, 320 bp for C, and 345 bp for D, respectively.
16. The expected size of amplified PCR fragments are: 669–708 bp for VH (using PCR products amplified from primer pair A and B), 645 bp for VL (using from C and D), respectively.
17. The expected sizes of DNA fragments which should be extracted from the gel are: 359–396 bp for VH and 333 bp for VL, respectively.
18. Electomax DH10B competent cells (Invitrogen, Carlsbad, CA, USA) show sufficient transformation efficiency to establish high diversity sub-libraries. Other commercial or home-made competent cells can be used for bacterial transformation, but should have high transformation efficiency (at least 10^9 transformants/μg plasmid DNA) to achieve the 10^6 size of sub-library.
19. The expected size of amplified PCR fragments are: 263 bp for primer pair A, 426–465 bp for B, 257 bp for C, and 408 bp for D, respectively.
20. At this point, extracted plasmid DNAs from yeast are a mixture of bait and prey vectors, but only the prey will be selected by bacterial transformation by growth on ampicillin antibiotic plates.
21. It is preferable to prepare prey plasmid DNA from several bacterial colonies for each yeast clone because the latter are isolated by library screening and may sometimes have more than one prey vector present.
22. Blue staining by X-gal depends on the quantification of interaction of your target and any isolated iDab. With those iDabs

that have high affinity and specificity against your target (e.g., true clones after third round screening), yeast with either DBD-bait or prey (L40 and MaV203 or AH109) would turn strong blue within a couple of hours. On the other hand, yeast with bait and prey isolated from first round screening may only be pale blue after overnight staining, since the prey clones are very likely to have low affinity and/or be false positives.

23. If a colony replicator is not available in your lab, you can use an alternative method for replica plating. Prepare 1:10 serial dilution (from 1:10 to 1:10,000) of yeast suspension in 1× TE. Pipette 10 μL each of the serial diluted yeast onto a plate in a small spot. Dry the spots completely at RT and culture at 30°C.
24. The step to remove excess yeast from the master plate is important for preventing misinterpretation of results caused by biomass effects. This cleaning should be repeated until the white yeast shadow is no longer visible.

Acknowledgements

This work was supported by the Leeds Institute of Molecular Medicine, University of Leeds, by grants from the Medical Research Council, UK and Leukaemia and Lymphoma Research, UK.

Disclaimer

1. Any person following this method/protocol should adhere to approved health and safety regulations and apply only good laboratory practice guidelines.
2. As far as we are aware at the time of writing this article, there is no other copyrightable article and that our article does not infringe upon any copyright, trademark, or patent, that it does not invade the right of privacy or publicity of any person or entity.

References

1. Reichert JM, Rosensweig CJ, Faden LB, Dewitz MC (2005) Monoclonal antibody successes in the clinic. Nat Biotechnol 23: 1073–1078
2. Holliger P, Hudson PJ (2005) Engineered antibody fragments and the rise of single domains. Nat Biotechnol 23:1126–1136
3. Lobato MN, Rabbitts TH (2003) Intracellular antibodies and challenges facing their use as therapeutic agents. Trends Mol Med 9: 390–396
4. Perez-Martinez D, Tanaka T, Rabbitts TH (2010) Intracellular antibodies and cancer: new technologies offer therapeutic opportunities. Bioessays 32:589–598
5. Visintin M, Tse E, Axelson H, Rabbitts TH, Cattaneo A (1999) Selection of antibodies for intracellular function using a two-hybrid *in vivo*

system. Proc Natl Acad Sci U S A 96: 11723–11728

6. Tse E, Lobato MN, Forster A, Tanaka T, Chung GTY, Rabbitts TH (2002) Intracellular antibody capture technology: application to selection of single chain Fv recognising the BCR-ABL oncogenic protein. J Mol Biol 317: 85–94
7. Visintin M, Settanni G, Maritan A, Graziosi S, Marks JD, Cattaneo A (2002) The intracellular antibody capture technology (IACT): towards a consensus sequence for intracellular antibodies. J Mol Biol 317:73–83
8. Tanaka T, Rabbitts TH (2003) Intrabodies based on intracellular capture frameworks that bind the RAS protein with high affinity and impair oncogenic transformation. EMBO J 22:1025–1035
9. Tanaka T, Lobato MN, Rabbitts TH (2003) Single domain intracellular antibodies: a minimal fragment for direct *in vivo* selection of antigen-specific intrabodies. J Mol Biol 331: 1109–1120
10. Tanaka T, Rabbitts TH (2008) Functional intracellular antibody fragments do not require invariant intra-domain disulfide bonds. J Mol Biol 376:749–757
11. Tanaka T, Rabbitts TH (2010) Protocol for the selection of single-domain antibody fragments by third generation intracellular antibody capture. Nat Protoc 5:67–92
12. Fields S, Song O (1989) A novel genetic system to detect protein-protein interactions. Nature 340:245–246
13. Bartel PL, Chien C, Sternglanz R, Fields S (1993) Using the two-hybrid system to detect protein-protein interaction. In: Hartley DA (ed) Cellular interaction in development: a practical approach. IRL Press, Oxford, pp 153–179
14. Sambrook J, Russell PW (2001) Molecular cloning: a laboratory manual. Cold Spring Harbor Laboratory Press, New York
15. Engebrecht J, Brent R, Kaderbhai MA (1992) *Escherichia coli*, Plasmids, and Bacteriophages. In: Ausubel FM et al (eds) Short protocols in molecular biology, 3rd edn. Wiley, New York
16. Lundblad V (1992) *Saccharomyces Cerevisiae*. In: Ausubel FM et al (eds) Short protocols in molecular biology, 3rd edn. Wiley, New York
17. Tanaka T, Chung GTY, Forster A, Lobato MN, Rabbitts TH (2003) *De novo* production of diverse intracellular antibody libraries. Nucleic Acids Res 31:e23

Chapter 11

Selection of Functional Single Domain Antibody Fragments for Interfering with Protein–Protein Interactions Inside Cells: A "One Plasmid" Mammalian Two-Hybrid System

Tomoyuki Tanaka and Terence H. Rabbitts

Abstract

As a complement to the intracellular antibody capture method to isolate intracellular single domain antibody fragments (iDabs) from high diverse libraries, we describe here a simple mammalian two-hybrid (M2H) protocol using a "bait-prey hybrid single plasmid" to assess those interfering iDabs that will block protein–protein interactions of a target with its natural partner proteins. This rapid method identifies interfering iDabs in one step and improves the reproducibility of the results between experiments and samples (e.g., different single domain antibody clones) compared to traditional M2H. This method yields functional, interfering iDabs and can be applied to any interfering molecule for use as a research tool or template for clinical inhibitor production.

Key words: Protein–protein interaction, Mammalian two hybrid, Single domains, Intrabodies, Intracellular antibodies, IAC, M2H, Competition, iDab

1. Introduction

Protein–protein interactions (PPIs) are involved in the control of such indispensable processes as transcription, protein transport, or signaling and are key components in biological functions. In addition, human diseases such as cancer, viral infections, and inflammatory disorders are mediated in large part by intracellular PPIs that can be a target for molecules that can interfere with these vital biochemical events. One such class of interfering molecules are single domain intracellular antibodies which are single antibody variable segments that bind to specific target molecules (e.g., protein, DNA, RNA) inside cells (1–3).

In the previous chapter (see Chapter 10), we described a protocol called intracellular antibody capture (IAC) (4, 5) to isolate intracellular antibody binders against any native protein using optimized

Dirk Saerens and Serge Muyldermans (eds.), *Single Domain Antibodies: Methods and Protocols*, Methods in Molecular Biology, vol. 911, DOI 10.1007/978-1-61779-968-6_11, © Springer Science+Business Media, LLC 2012

single domain libraries (3, 5). After the intracellular single domain antibodies (designated iDabs for intracellular domains antibodies) are selected as specific binders using IAC in yeast cells, the ability of these single domains must be tested for their ability to bind the target antigens in mammalian cells and of specific relevance is selecting iDabs affect biological functions of target molecule through interfering with their PPIs (1, 6). Here we described a simple mammalian two-hybrid (M2H) protocol, using a simple "bait-prey hybrid single plasmid," to assess those iDabs in any panel of selected iDabs that can block PPI of target with natural partner proteins.

The triplex M2H vector (see Fig. 1a) used here comprises a dual promoter plasmid from which a bait and prey (Gal4 DNA binding domain (DBD)-bait and prey-VP16 activator domain (AD) fusions) are expressed in mammalian cells. Our triplex vector has compatible multi-cloning sites for shuttling from the yeast bait vector pBTM116 (7) and the library plasmid pVP16* (8, 9) used in IAC. In addition, the Renilla luciferase reporter gene and the DBD-bait are controlled by same *SV40* early promoter, thus normalizing not only copy number of transfected triplex plasmids but also expression level of the DBD-bait fusion. The vector can be co-transfected with a plasmid (e.g., pEF/myc/nuc, see Fig. 1b) expressing the potential competitor single domains and their effects are monitored by reporter activity. Generally M2H assays require multiple plasmids (e.g., bait, prey, reporter, and a further reporter for normalization) to be transfected into mammalian cells giving deviations in data and poor reproducibility. The method we describe here improves data reproducibility and facilitates the comparison of inhibition ability of a series of functional single domain antibody fragments made from IAC screening or other means of isolation.

2. Materials

Prepare all solutions using ultrapure water (prepared by purifying deionized water to attain a sensitivity of 18 MΩ cm at 25°C) and analytical grade reagents. Prepare and store all reagents at room

Fig. 1. (continued) are co-transfected into a CHO-Luc reporter cell line (5) which has a reporter gene, stably integrated, comprising the Firefly luciferase (*Fluc*) gene with minimal adenovirus E1b promoter linked to five copies of *Gal4* binding site (bs) (CHO-luc cells are puromycin-resistant). (**d**) A histogram showing a theoretical result of dual-luciferase assay with and without competitor. The *y*-axis indicates a Fluc reporter activity normalized with Rluc activity. Supposing there is an interaction between proteins XX with YY, the interaction of Gal4DBD-XX fusion and YY-VP16AD in CHO-luc cells would give defined, normalized Fluc reporter activity. If a competitor protein ZZ (e.g., single domain against a protein XX) were co-expressed, proteins ZZ and YY-VP16AD would compete for binding to protein XX and the Fluc reporter activity would consequently be reduced as there would be lower amounts of Gal4DBD-XX/YY-VP16AD activation complex in transfected cells.

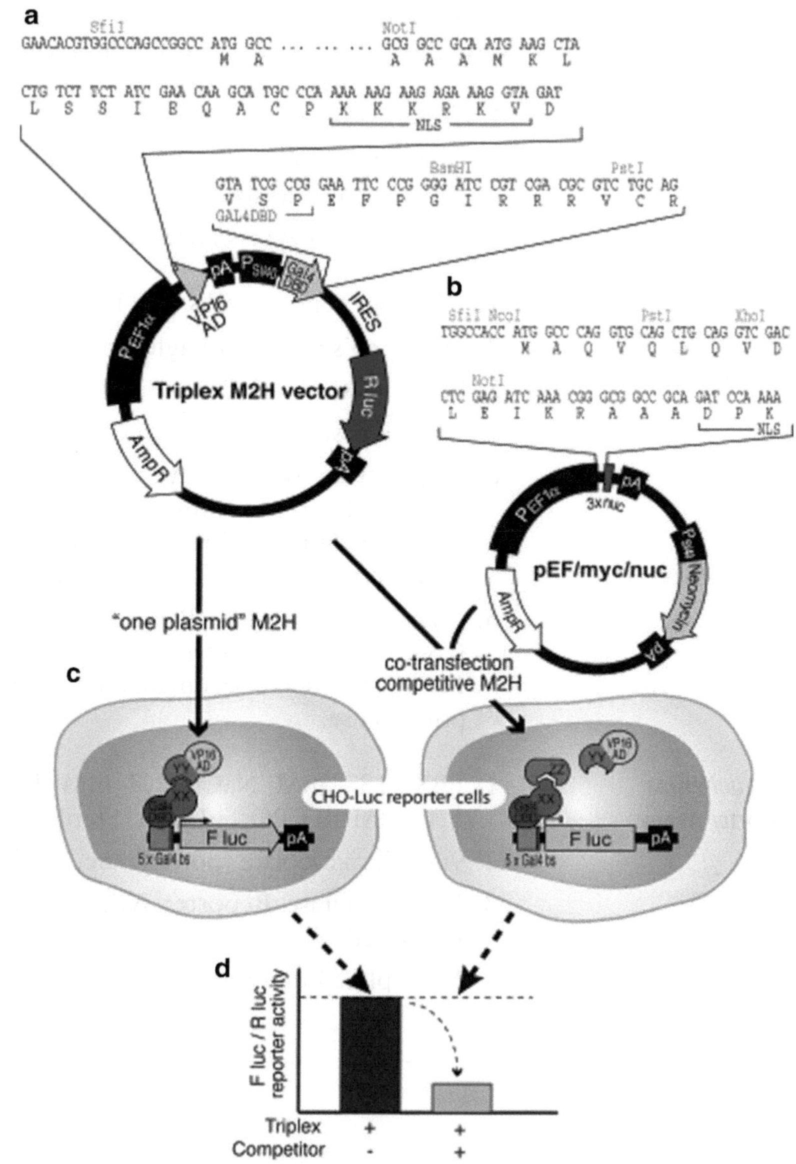

Fig. 1. Determination of single domain inhibitors of protein–protein interaction in mammalian cells using one-plasmid: two-hybrid assay.(**a**) The plasmid vector (Triplex M2H vector (5)) is used to co-express a Gal4 DBD-protein antigen fusion protein (bait) controlled by the *SV40* early promoter and the interacting protein (prey) which can be a protein known to bind to the antigen, or a single domain, fused to the VP16 activator domain (AD); this expression is controlled by the strong elongation factor-1 alpha (EF1α) promoter. Additionally, the Gal4 DBD-antigen mRNA has an internal ribosome entry site (IRES) sequence followed by Renilla luciferase (*Rluc*). The Rluc expression is used as internal transfection control. The nucleotide sequences shown code for the amino acids (and unique restriction enzyme sites of the multiple cloning site (MCS)) of Gal4DBD and VP16AD fusions. (**b**) The map of pEF/myc/nuc for expressing a competitor protein (e.g., a single domain to potentially inhibit the protein–protein interaction of antigen and a natural partner protein). This vector has a compatible MCS with the pVP16* yeast vector used in IAC screening (5). (**c**) The Triplex M2H vector (from **a**) and competitor vector (from **b**)

temperature (unless indicated otherwise). Diligently follow all waste disposal regulations when disposing waste materials

2.1. Plasmid Construction

1. Triplex plasmid (see Fig. 1) (5).
2. Competitive plasmid: pEF/myc/nuc (see Fig. 1, see Note 1) (Invitrogen, Carlsbad, CA, USA).
3. Restriction enzymes (*BamHI, PstI, SfiI, NotI, NcoI, XhoI*).

2.2. Transfection into CHO Reporter Cell Lines

1. CHO-luc reporter cells (see Fig. 1, Note 2) (5).
2. Dulbecco's modified Eagle's medium (DMEM).
3. Fetal calf serum (FCS).
4. 12-well tissue culture plate.
5. Transfection solution A: 4 μL of LipofectAMINE 2000™ reagent (Invitrogen) into 100 μL of Opti-MEM®-I Reduced serum medium (Invitrogen) per sample. Incubate for 5 min at room temperature (RT). Prepare prior to use.
6. Transfection solution B: 0.5 μg of Triplex M2H vector and 0.5–2 μg of pEF/myc/nuc-competitor into 100 μL Opti-MEM®-I Reduced serum medium per sample. Mix well. Prepare prior to use.

2.3. Luciferase Reporter Assay

1. PBS: 137 mM NaCl, 2.7 mM KCl, 4.3 mM Na_2HPO_4, 1.47 mM KH_2PO_4, pH 7.4. Sterile by autoclaving.
2. 96-well microplate (polystyrene, black or white).
3. Dual-luciferase Reporter Assay System (Promega, Madison, WI, USA).
4. Microplate Luminometer.

3. Methods

3.1. Plasmid Construction

1. Using standard genetic cloning methods (10), sub-clone cDNA of the protein antigen, single domain iDab, or a protein you wish to study into the BamHI/PstI sites of triplex M2H vector (5) as in-frame fusions with a Gal4DBD (see Notes 3 and 4).
2. Following the first cloning, sub-clone a cDNA of the protein antigen, single domain iDab, or a known protein interaction partner, to use as target, in the SfiI/NotI sites of triplex M2H vector as in-frame fusions with a VP16AD (see Notes 4 and 5).
3. Sub-clone the cDNA of single domain antibodies or a known protein interaction partner you wish to study in SfiI, PstI, XhoI, or NotI sites of pEF/myc/nuc vector as in-frame fusions with the nuclear localization signal (nls; see Note 5).

Table 1
Oligonucleotides for DNA sequencing

Primers	Sequence (5'–3')	Note
Gal4F	GTCACAGATAGATT GGCTTCAGTGG	Forward primer for Gal4DBD fusion
PMRev	ATGTTTCAGGTT CAGGGGAGGTG	Reverse primer for Gal4DBD fusion
EFFP2	GGAGGGGTTTT ATGCGATGG	Forward primer for VP16AD fusion and for pEF/myc/nuc
sFvVP16R	CAACATGTCC AGATCGAA	Reverse primer for VP16AD fusion
BGH rev	TAGAAGGCACAG TCGAGG	Reverse primer for pEF/myc/nuc

4. Confirm clones by DNA sequencing using oligonucleotide primers (see Table 1).
5. Prepare the plasmid DNA using large-scale methods (11).

3.2. Transfection into CHO Reporter Cell Lines (See Note 6)

1. Seed 5×10^4 CHO-luc cells (see Note 2) per well of a 12-well tissue culture plate (see Note 7) in 1 mL of the DMEM with 10% FCS without antibiotics (see Note 8).
2. Incubate the cells at 37° C overnight in a 5% CO_2 incubator until the cells are about 90% confluent.
3. Combine the solutions A and solution B, mix gently, and incubate at RT for 20 min to generate DNA-lipofectamine complexes (see Note 9).
4. Add the DNA-Lipofectamine complexes to each well containing cells and medium. Mix gently by rocking by hand.
5. Incubate the plates at 37° C in a 5% CO_2 for 48 h.
6. At 48 h from the start of transfection, perform a reporter assay by using a Dual-Luciferase Reporter Assay System as in Subheading 3.3.

3.3. Luciferase Reporter Assay (See Note 10)

1. Wash transfected cells 3 times with PBS and remove PBS completely.
2. Dispense 250 μL of 1× passive lysis buffer (PLB from the manufacturer's kit).
3. Gently rock the culture plates for 15 min at RT.
4. Transfer 20 μL to 96-well white/black assay plate.
5. Set the plate in a luminometer.
6. Add 50 μL of luciferase assay reagent (LAR II from the kit) to each well.

7. Measure firefly luciferase activity (use 2 s delay and 10 s read time).
8. Add 50 μL of Stop & Glo® Reagent to each well.
9. Measure Renilla luciferase activity (use 2 s delay and 10 s read time).

4. Notes

1. We have used the pEF/myc/nuc vector (Invitrogen) for expression of competitor protein in mammalian cells. The plasmid has same *EF1alpha* promoter as prey in triplex M2H vector and we expect equal transcript levels of VP16 fusion and competitor when the cell has the same copy number of plasmids. Alternatively, you can use other mammalian expression vectors driven by other promoters (e.g., *SV40, CMV, CAGG*), but it is important to introduce nuclear localization signals (nls) with your competitor cDNA.
2. A Chinese hamster ovary (CHO) cell line has been developed with multiple copies of the firefly luciferase reporter gene with a minimal adenovirus E1b promoter linked to five-repeat consensus *GAL4* binding sites (12). We established this stable line by co-transfecting CHO cells with linearized *pG5-Fluc* (1) and *PGK-puro* (13) plasmids. Stably transfected cells were selected for 7 days using 10 μg/mL puromycin. The cells are usually cultured in DMEM with FCS and penicillin and streptomycin plus 5–10 μg/mL puromycin.
3. The stop codon needs to be introduced at 3′ end of cDNA when part of your protein (i.e., a domain or domains) is/are used at the C-terminus of a Gal4DBD fusion.
4. You should change the sub-cloning order (i.e., bait and prey or prey and bait) depending on the unique restriction enzyme recognitions of your gene.
5. A translation initiation codon (ATG) needs to be introduced at the 5′ end of the cDNA when part of your protein (e.g., a domain or domains) is/are used at the N-terminus the VP16 fusion. The *SfiI-NotI* cloning sites of the triplex M2H have the same protein translation reading frame as that of the yeast pVP16* vector (i.e., candidate single domain antibody fragments from IAC can be directly shuttled from pVP16* into triplex M2H vector).
6. Currently, several transfection methods including chemical-based (e.g., calcium phosphate, liposome, cationic polymer) and non-chemical-mediated (e.g., electroporation) are established and many eukaryotic transfection kits are now available. Here we

have used a method to use stable firefly reporter cell lines with LipofectAMINE 2000™ (Invitrogen) transfection reagent as we have confirmed high transfection efficiency for CHO cells.

7. You can scale up or down for transfection. Follow manufacturer's instruction, but we recommend you use 6-well or 12-well culture vessel format for transfection as deviations of luciferase reporter assays are much lower than with smaller scale cultures (e.g., 24-well and 96-well format).
8. Do not add antibiotics because this will affect viability.
9. Do not leave more than 30 min as this may decrease its activity.
10. Many reporter assay kits for luciferase are now also available. Here we use the Dual-Luciferase Assay System (Promega) transfection reagent. The method allows simultaneous measurement of both Firefly luciferase activity (from reporter activity by two-hybrid interaction) and Renilla luciferase (from the triplex vector using normalization of transfection efficiency between each assay).

Acknowledgments

This work was supported by the Leeds Institute of Molecular Medicine, University of Leeds, by grants from the Medical Research Council, UK, and Leukaemia and Lymphoma Research, UK.

Disclaimer

1. Any person following this method/protocol should adhere to the standard health and safety regulations and apply only good laboratory practice guidelines.
2. As far as we are aware at the time of writing this article, there is no other copyrightable article and that our article does not infringe upon any copyright, trademark, or patent, that it does not invade the right of privacy or publicity of any person or entity.

References

1. Tanaka T, Lobato MN, Rabbitts TH (2003) Single domain intracellular antibodies: a minimal fragment for direct in vivo selection of antigen-specific intrabodies. J Mol Biol 331:1109–1120
2. Colby DW, Chu Y, Cassady JP, Duennwald M, Zazulak H, Webster JM, Messer A, Lindquist S, Ingram VM, Wittrup KD (2004) Potent inhibition of huntingtin aggregation and cytotoxicity by a disulfide bond-free single-domain

intracellular antibody. Proc Natl Acad Sci U S A 101:17616–17621
3. Tanaka T, Sewell H, Waters S, Philips S, Rabbitts TH (2011) Single domain intracellular antibodies from diverse libraries: emphasizing dual functions of LMO2 protein interactions using a VH single domain. J Biol Chem 286:3707–3716
4. Tse E, Lobato MN, Forster A, Tanaka T, Chung GTY, Rabbitts TH (2002) Intracellular antibody capture technology: application to selection of single chain Fv recognising the BCR-ABL oncogenic protein. J Mol Biol 317:85–94
5. Tanaka T, Rabbitts TH (2010) Protocol for the selection of single-domain antibody fragments by third generation intracellular antibody capture. Nat Protoc 5:67–92
6. Tanaka T, Williams RL, Rabbitts TH (2007) Tumour prevention by a single antibody domain inhibiting binding of signal transduction molecules to activated RAS. EMBO J 26:3250–3259
7. Bartel PL, Chien C, Sternglanz R, Fields S (1993) Using the two-hybrid system to detect protein-protein interaction. In: Hartley DA (ed) Cellular interaction in development: a practical approach. IRL Press, Oxford, pp 153–179
8. Visintin M, Tse E, Axelson H, Rabbitts TH, Cattaneo A (1999) Selection of antibodies for intracellular function using a two-hybrid in vivo system. Proc Natl Acad Sci USA 96:11723–11728
9. Vojtek AB, Hollenberg SM, Cooper JA (1993) Mammalian Ras interacts directly with the serine/threonine kinase Raf. Cell 74:205–214
10. Sambrook J, Russell PW (2001) Molecular cloning: a laboratory manual. Cold Spring Harbor Laboratory Press, New York
11. Engebrecht JBR, Kaderbhai MA (1992) *Escherichia coli*, plasmids, and bacteriophages. Wiley, New York
12. Sadowski I, Bell B, Broad P, Hollis M (1992) *GAL4* fusion vectors for expression in yeast or mammalian cells. Gene 118:137–141
13. Tucker KL, Beard C, Dausmann J, Jackson-Grusby L, Laird PW, Lei H, Li E, Jaenisch R (1996) Germ-line passage is required for establishment of methylation and expression patterns of imprinted but not of nonimprinted genes. Genes Dev 10:1008–1020

Chapter 12

Cell-Free Selection of Domain Antibodies by In Vitro Compartmentalization

Armin Sepp and Andrew Griffiths

Abstract

Efficient identification of antibodies, or any fragments thereof, displaying desired specificity and affinity is critical for the development of novel immunotherapeutics. Here we describe the adaptation of in vitro compartmentalization for the cell-free selection of Vκ and VH domain antibodies (dAbs™) from large combinatorial libraries. The dAbs™ are in vitro expressed in fusion to the N-terminus of single-chain variant of phage P22 Arc repressor DNA-binding domain that links the compartmentally expressed protein molecules to their encoding PCR fragment-based genes via cognate operator sites present on the DNA. Libraries of up to 10^{10} in size can be rapidly assembled and selected for improved affinity in equilibrium and off-rate conditions.

Key words: Domain antibodies, Therapeutic antibodies, Antibody engineering, In vitro selection, In vitro expression, DNA-binding protein, Single chain Arc repressor, Tus *E. coli* replication factor

1. Introduction

Although most of the approved immunotherapeutics are full IgGs, there is an increasing interest in smaller antibody fragments that retain full affinity and specificity (1). Until recently, phage display has been the method of choice for the cloning of antibody fragments and improvement of their affinity (2), but completely in vitro approaches like ribosome display appear to have an edge if sub-nanomolar affinities are required (3).

This chapter describes the application of in vitro compartmentalization (IVC) (4) for the affinity maturation of domain antibodies (dAbs™)—the smallest units of immunoglobulins that retain antigen-binding activity (see Fig. 1) (5). In IVC, large libraries of

---

Dirk Saerens and Serge Muyldermans (eds.), *Single Domain Antibodies: Methods and Protocols*, Methods in Molecular Biology, vol. 911, DOI 10.1007/978-1-61779-968-6_12, © Springer Science+Business Media, LLC 2012

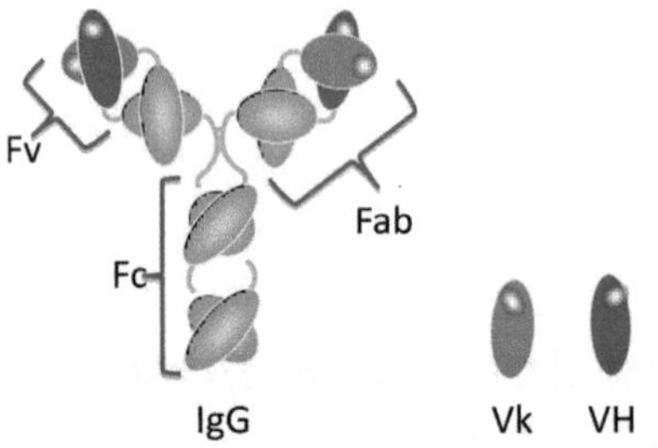

Fig. 1. Vκ and VH domain antibodies (dAbs™) are derived from the Fv variable fragment of IgG light and heavy chains respectively. Both Vκ and VH dAbs™ are comprised of a single polypeptide chain, contain one disulphide bond and are the smallest units of immunoglobulins that can independently retain antigen-binding activity located in their three complementarity-determining regions (CDRs).

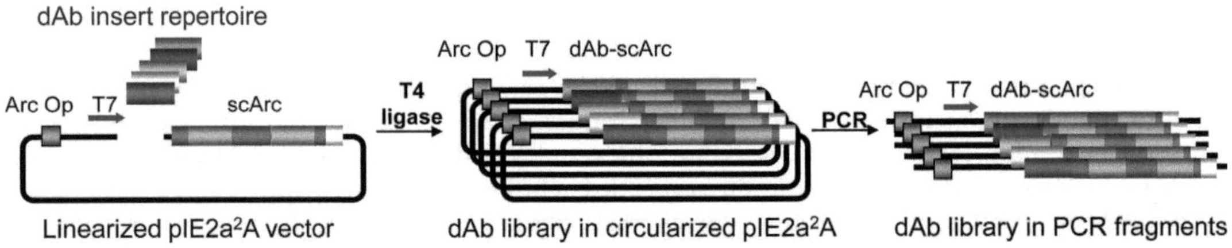

Fig. 2. PCR-based library assembly for antibody selection in emulsion. dAb™ library is first ligated into linearized pIE2a²A vector using T4 DNA ligase and then recovered from the vector by PCR already in fusion with scArc encoding sequence. The final linear construct contains the Arc operator, T7 promoter and terminator, and the dAb–scArc expression cassette.

genes comprised of linear DNA fragments can be rapidly generated by PCR without any need to transform bacteria at any stage (see Fig. 2). During selection, an aliquot of 10^9–10^{10} genes from a PCR fragment-based library is added to 50 μL of *E. coli* coupled transcription–translation extract which is rapidly dispersed by stirring in mineral oil (see Fig. 3a). A typical water-in-oil emulsion formed contains about 10^{10} droplets of 2.5 μm diameter on average. The distribution of genes into the droplets upon emulsification of the in vitro translation mix is a stochastic process that is expected to follow Poisson distribution, as was demonstrated during dispersal of cells in a microfluidic experiment (6). In these conditions the highest number of correct protein–DNA complexes are formed (about 50% of input genes) when the number of genes equals to the number of uniform droplets. At gene-to-droplet ratio of 1:10, about 90% of the library will be segregated at one gene per droplet (7), albeit at the expense of the number of smaller number of genes entered into selection.

The dAbs are expressed within these droplets in fusion with single-chain Arc repressor DNA-binding domain that has 3.2 pM affinity for the cognate Arc operator and dissociation half-life of about 5 h from the operator (see Fig. 3b) (8). The fusion protein molecules expressed within the droplets of the emulsion bind to their encoding genes via one or more Arc operators present on the DNA, thus creating genotype–phenotype linkage (see Fig. 3c).

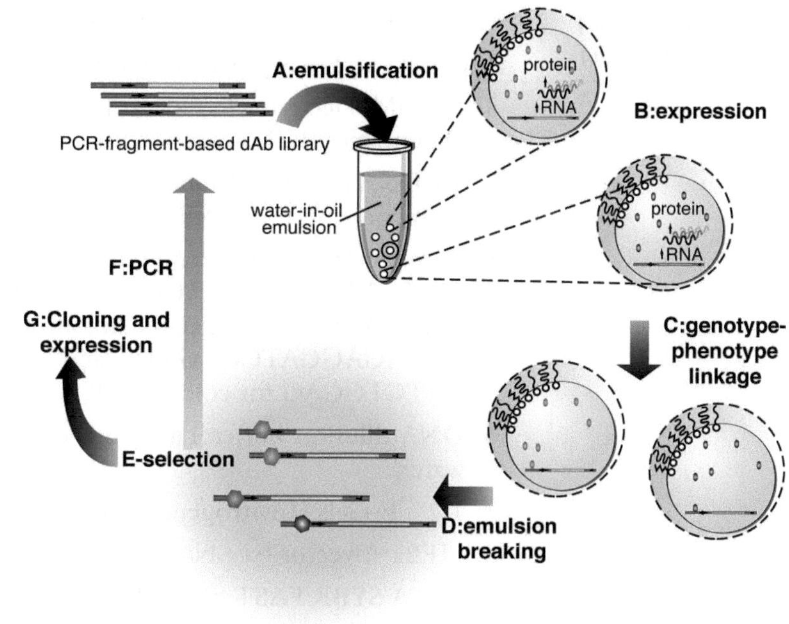

Fig. 3. The emulsion-based selection of antibody fragments is a Darwinian process. (**a**) PCR fragment based linear genes are randomly encapsulated in the microscopic droplets of in vitro coupled transcription–translation extract dispersed in mineral oil. (**b**) Compartmentalized expression of dAbs™ takes place during the expression phase. The reaction products and the encoded genes are oil-insoluble and hence do not equilibrate between droplets. (**c**) As long as there is no more than one gene present per droplet, correct of genotype–phenotype linkage is formed between a gene and its encoded protein. (**d**) The emulsion is broken and extracted to remove the detergents. (**e**) Biopanning is used to recover dAb™–scArc complexes with the highest antigen-binding activity. (**f**) PCR is used to amplify the genes that were corecovered with the highest-affinity dAb™ clones. (**g**) After the final round of selection, the remaining dAb™ repertoire is cloned for functional analysis.

The dAb™–DNA complexes are recovered by breaking the emulsion (see Fig. 3d) and fractionated according to their affinity for the target or the dissociation rate (see Fig. 3e). The genes that copurify with the captured dAbs of are amplified by PCR for the next round of selection (see Fig. 3f) using a series of nested primers until clones with desired affinity are obtained and cloned for functional screening (see Fig. 3g).

2. Materials

All solutions should be prepared using ultrapure deionized water at 18 MΩ cm at 25°C sensitivity, autoclaved and passed through 0.22 μm filter before use. All solutions are stored at room temperature unless stated otherwise. Filter tips should be used throughout to avoid sample cross-contamination.

2.1. Library Assembly and Characterization

1. Pfu Ultra DNA polymerase (Stratagene, UK).
2. SuperTaq DNA polymerase (HT Biotechnology Ltd., UK).
3. 10 mM Deoxynucleoside triphosphate (dNTP) mix (Roche Diagnostics, UK).
4. T4 DNA ligase, *Sal* I and *Not* I restriction enzymes, preferably high concentration (NEB, UK).
5. Primers: Any primers required to randomize the dAb sequence, AS11: TTCGCTATTACGCCAGCTGG and AS17: CAGTC AGGCACCGTGTATG for library amplification, AS79 5′GG CGTAGAGGATCGAGATC and AS80 5′TTGTTACCGGA TCTCTCGAG for colony PCR.
6. DNA dilution buffer 1 mg/mL of BSA (NEB) in autoclaved water.
7. 1.2% E-Gels (Invitrogen, UK).
8. pIE2a^{2}A vector (see Note 1).
9. KAPA SYBR FAST qPCR Kit (KAPA Biosystems, USA).
10. LB carbenicillin plates: 10 g Bacto-tryptone (Sigma), 5 g yeast extract (Sigma), 10 g NaCl (Sigma), 15 g agar (Sigma), 100 μg/mL carbenicillin (Sigma).
11. XL10 Gold Supercompetent *E. coli* cells (Agilent, USA).
12. Bio-Rad Mini Opticon (Bio-Rad, USA).

2.2. Preparation of dAb Display Library in Emulsion

1. Oil-detergent mix for emulsions: Light white mineral oil (Sigma, UK) + 4.5% Span-80 (Fluka, UK) + 0.5% Triton X100 (Sigma) (see Note 2).
2. Disposable 5 mL glass vials (GE Healthcare, UK).
3. High-speed 2,000 rpm magnetic stirrer (Variomag Multipoint, USA).
4. Stir bars (3 × 8 mm, pivot rings, polytetrafluoroethylene; VWR International, UK) (see Note 3).
5. 100 mM oxidized glutathione (Sigma) in water (see Note 4).
6. Expressway Cell-Free Expression system (Invitrogen) (see Note 5).
7. 3F10 anti-HA rat monoclonal antibody (Roche Diagnostics) at 100 μg/mL in water (see Note 6).
8. Hexane (Sigma).
9. Buffer C: 0.1 M KCl, 0.05% Tween-20, 5 mM $MgCl_2$, 0.1 mM EDTA, 10 mM Tris–HCl (All Sigma), pH 7.4.
10. Microcentrifuge tubes (MaxyClear, 1.7 mL; Axygen Scientific, USA).

2.3. Biopanning

1. Biotinylated antigen.
2. Nonbiotinylated antigen (for off-rate selection).
3. MyOne C1 Streptavidin Dynabeads (Invitrogen) (see Note 7).
4. 1.2% E-Gels (Invitrogen).
5. 96-Well polypropylene PCR plates (ABgene, UK).
6. Microcentrifuge tubes (MaxyClear, 1.7 mL; Axygen Scientific, USA).
7. Magnetic stand for microcentrifuge tubes (see Note 8).
8. Refrigerated microcentrifuge, e.g., Eppendorf 5415R.
9. Emulsion Breaking Solution: *n*-Hexane (Sigma).
10. Buffer C: 0.1 M KCl, 0.05% Tween-20, 5 mM $MgCl_2$, 0.1 mM EDTA, 10 mM Tris–HCl (All Sigma), pH 7.4.
11. Primers: Round 1-AS12 5′AAAGGGGGATGTGCTGCAAG and AS18 5′AACAATGCGCTCATCGTCATC, Round 2-AS13 5′ AAGGCGATTAAGTTGGGTAAC and AS19 5′TCGGC ACCGTCACCCTGG,Round3-AS145′CCAGGGTTTTCCC AGTCAC AS20 5′TGCTGTAGGCATAGGCTTGG, Round 4-AS15 5′GAGATGGCGCCCAACAGTC and AS21 ′CCTCT TGCGGGATATCGTC, Round 5-AS16 5′CTGCCACCATAC CCACGCC and 5′TCCATTCCGACAGCATCGC, Round 6-AS29 5′GAAACAAGCGCTCATGAGCC and AS153 5′CA GTCACTATGGCGTGCTGC, Round 7-AS98 5′CCAGCA ACCGCACCTGTG and AS154 5′TAGCGCTATATGCGTT GATGC, Round 8-AS97 5′TGCCGGCCACGATGCGTC and AS155 5′TTCTATGCGCACCCGTTCTC, Round 9-AS79 5′GGCGTAGAGGATCGAGATC AS156 5′AGCACTGTCC GACCGCTTTG, Round 10-AS267 5′AGATCTCGATCCC GCGAAATTAATAC and AS254 5′CCAGTCCTGCTCGCT TCG, sequencing primers AS9 5′CAGGAAACAGCTATG ACCATG and AS65 5′TTGTAAAACGACGGCCAGTG.

2.4. Assessment of Library Fitness

1. Biotinylated antigen.
2. Biotinylated BSA (Sigma).
3. Real-time PCR cyler, e.g., Mini-Opticon (Bio-Rad, UK).
4. Disposable agarose gel electrophoresis cells (E-Gel, Invitrogen).
5. PCR and agarose gel DNA purification kits (Qiagen, UK).
6. 96-Well streptavidin-coated PCR plates (ABgene).
7. Buffer C: 0.1 M KCl, 0.05% Tween-20, 5 mM $MgCl_2$, 0.1 mM EDTA, 10 mM Tris–HCl (All Sigma), pH 7.4.

2.5. Cloning and Screening of Library Selection Output

1. 2xTY: 16 g Bacto-tryptone (Sigma), 10 g Bacto-yeast extract (Sigma), 5 g NaCl (Sigma), deionized water to 1 L. Autoclave.
2. Carbenicillin (Sigma), 100 mg/mL in water.

3. SalI and NotI restriction enzymes (NEB).
4. Bacterial expression vector, e.g., pDOM5 (see Note 9).
5. T4 DNA ligase (NEB).
6. 2% E-gel (Invitrogen).
7. Gel extraction kit (Qiagen).
8. OnEx autoinduction system for bacterial expression (Invitrogen).
9. Heraeus Biofuge 15R.
10. High-speed orbital shaker.

3. Methods

In vitro selection of dAbs in emulsion includes library assembly, selection, and screening. All procedures are carried out at room temperature unless stated otherwise.

3.1. Library Assembly and Characterization

A number of different methods can be used to introduce diversity into antibody sequence. These include error-prone PCR, oligonucleotide-directed codon randomization and others, depending on the type of library required (9).

The rest of the sequence components required for the IVC selection of dAbs, namely, Arc operators, translation start codon ATG, scArc encoding sequence, T7 promoter and terminator motifs, are added by temporary subcloning of the dAb™ fragment library into pIE2a^{2}A vector.

1. Ligation of dAb library into pIE2a^{2}A in vitro expression vector.

Amount	Reagent
≈50 ng	Sal I/Not I-cut pIE2a^{2}A vector (≈10^{10} molecules)
≈15 ng	Sal I/Not I-cut dAb™ insert (≈4×10^{10} molecules)
2.5 μL	10× T4 DNA ligase buffer
x μL	H_2O (to 24 μL final volume)
1 μL	400 U/μL T4 DNA ligase

Incubate for 30 min at room temperature or overnight at 16°C for better yield.

2. Verification of library diversity
Transform 1 μL of ligation mix into XL10 Gold chemically competent *E. coli* cells (Agilent, USA) and plate onto LB/carbenicillin plates for overnight growth. The next day amplify the expression cassettes of at least 20–30 colonies using SuperTaq DNA polymerase with primers AS79 and AS80.

Cycle number	Denaturation	Annealing	Extension
1	2 min at 95°C		
2–35	15 s at 95°C	30 s at 60°C	1 min at 72°C
36	5 min at 72°C		

3. Sequence the PCR reaction products with T7 primer to verify the diversity (see Note 10).
4. Assemble the library amplification reactions without adding Pfu DNA polymerase

Amount	Reagent
24 μL	dAb library ligation mix from Subheading 3.1, step 1
20 μL	10× Pfu Buffer
0.6 μL	100 μM primer AS11
0.6 μL	100 μM primer AS17
4 μL	10 mM dNTP
150 μL	H_2O

5. Remove and save 1 μL of the PCR amplification mix for library size quantification by qPCR.
6. Add 2 μL of Pfu polymerase to the remaining 199 μL of PCR mix and split into 4 × 50 μL aliquots for amplification using the following profile:

Cycle number	Denaturation	Annealing	Extension
1	2 min at 95°C		
2–26	15 s at 95°C	30 s at 60°C	1 min at 72°C
27			5 min at 72°C

7. Gel-purify each 1.68 kb library PCR product on a separate 1.2% EGel, quantify spectrophotometrically, and dilute to 1.7 nM concentration in 1 mg/mL BSA (NEB) in water. Store at −20 C.
8. The expression cassettes for IVC selection are formed in circularized vectors only and these can be quantified by qPCR using a flanking primer set AS79 and AS80. Add the 1 μL aliquot of the ligation mix without Pfu polymerase (step 5 in Subheading 3.1) to a qPCR reaction solution comprised of:

Amount	Reagent
12.5 μL	SYBR FAST qPCR 2× master mix (KAPA Biosystems)
1.5 μL	10 μM primer AS79
1.5 μL	10 μM primer AS80
9.5 μL	H_2O

9. Run the qPCR reaction on a Mini Opticon (Bio-Rad) real-time PCR cycler whilst recording the SYBR green fluorescence channel. Include a standard curve to cover 500-5 × 10^8 copies per reaction range (see Note 11)

Cycle number	Denaturation	Annealing	Polymerization
1	2 min at 95°C		
2–41	15 s at 95°C	30 s at 60°C	1 min at 72°C
42			Melting curve 72–95°C

10. Use Opticon Monitor software (Bio-Rad Laboratories) to quantify the number of template molecules in each qPCR and multiply the result by 200 to get the number of circularized vector molecules in the library (see Note 12).

3.2. Preparation of dAb Display Library in Emulsion

1. Place a sterile 2.5 × 8 mm-magnetic bar in a 5 mL BIAcore glass vial using sterile forceps and add 600 μL of the mineral oil–detergent mixture, and stir at 2,000 rpm.
2. Each in vitro expression reaction in emulsion contains 50 μL of modified Expressway in vitro translation mix:

Amount	Reagent
10 μL	SlyD extract
10 μL	2.5× reaction buffer
12.5 μL	2× feed buffer
1.0 μL	Methionine (75 mM)
1.25 μL	Amino Acid mix (50 mM)
15 μL	H_2O
0.5 μL	T7 Polymerase
0.25 μL	50 μg/mL anti-HA mAb 3F10 (see Note 6)
1.5 μL	100 mM Oxidized glutathione (Sigma)

3. Keep on ice until required.
4. Add 0.5 μL of 1.7 nM library DNA to each 50 μL translation mix aliquot, mix by pipetting up and down, and transfer the entire solution immediately to the vial with stirred oil. Stir for another 5 min and cover the vial with a piece of tape to prevent any evaporation during incubation.
5. Incubate the vials at 25–30°C for 2–3 h.

6. Towards the end of the incubation, prepare one 1.7 mL Axygen microcentrifuge tube for each emulsion reaction containing:

Amount	Reagent
200 μL	Buffer C
0.4 mL	*n*-Hexane

7. Add the contents of an Axyxen tube to a vial with emulsion, mix by pipetting up and down, and transfer everything back to the tube. Repeat for all samples.
8. Spin the Axygen tubes at maximal speed for 1 min in a refrigerated microcentrifuge at 20°C.
9. Remove and discard the top layer (approximately 1.2 mL) and add 1 mL of fresh *n*-hexane to the aqueous phase that was left in the tube. Mix carefully by pipetting and repeat the extraction for four more times.
10. After final extraction, remove carefully all of the organic phase and any debris left in the interface with a 20 μL pipette (see Note 13). The dAb™–DNA complexes are now ready for selection on target antigen.

3.3. Biopanning

The dAb™–scArc complexes with their encoding DNA are fractionated according to the antigen-binding affinity of the dAb™ moiety. The DNA molecules that copurify in complex with the dAb™–scArc fusion proteins are amplified by PCR for the next round of selection. It is beneficial to carry out 1–2 rounds of selection using biotinylated antigen at 50–100 nM concentration in order to capture and enrich the binding population of dAbs™.

In subsequent rounds the stringency of selection is increased either by reducing the concentration of the antigen (down to about 5 nM) or off-rate competition with unlabelled ligand, whilst trying to keep the fraction of genes recovered at each round in 0.5–5% bracket. The total number of selection cycles can vary from five in naïve selection (10) to ten or more in affinity maturation (11) (see Note 14)

1. Add biotinylated antigen to each reaction to reach the desired concentration in solution (see Note 15).
2. Incubate the reactions for 15 min at room temperature.
3. In off-rate condition selections, add 10–100-fold excess of unlabelled antigen to saturate any free dAb™ binding sites as they dissociate from their complex with biotinylated antigen (see Note 16).
4. Wash 1.5×10^8 streptavidin or neutravidin-coated C1 MyOne beads per selection into buffer C and add to the dAb™–antigen complexes (see Note 17).
5. Incubate for 15 min at room temperature.

6. Place the tubes into a magnetic rack, remove the supernatant, and resuspend the beads gently in 400 μL of Buffer C. Recapture the beads and repeat twice. After the final wash carefully remove any remaining buffer with a 20 μL pipette.
7. Use the next pair of nested primers to prepare 200 μL of Pfu PCR mix without adding DNA polymerase for the amplification of the captured gene population (see Note 18).
8. Add the PCR mix to the washed beads, resuspend, and remove 1 μL of the suspension for qPCR to measure the fraction of library captured on the beads as in Subheading 3.1, step 8 (see Note 19).
9. Add Pfu enzyme to the remaining suspension of beads, split into 4 × 50 μL aliquots, and PCR-amplify, as in Subheading 3.1, step 3 (see Note 20).
10. Purify, quantify, and dilute the amplified library for the next round of selection as in Subheading 3.1, step 4.

3.4. Assessment of Library Fitness

Library fitness characterizes the average affinity of the clones at a given stage of selection. Improvement in the library fitness from round to round of selection suggests that enrichment for improved binders has taken place. Library fitness can be assayed by in vitro expression of aliquots of polyclonal library in solution and then measuring the amount of DNA cocaptured on antigen-coated PCR plates by qPCR (see Note 21).

1. Coat one well of Strep ThermoFast plate with 3 fmol of biotinylated target antigen and one with 3 fmol of biotinylated BSA in buffer C for each polyclonal library sample to be assayed (include the unselected library as well).
2. Incubate for 1 h at room temperature, followed by three washes with buffer C.
3. Assemble 10 μL in vitro expression reactions, one per each library sample:

Amount	Reagent
0.5 μL	1.7 nM DNA template
2.0 μL	SlyD extract
2.0 μL	2.5× reaction buffer
2.5 μL	2× feed buffer
0.2 μL	75 mM methionine
0.25 μL	50 mM amino acid mix
2.5 μL	H_2O
0.05 μL	Anti-HA mAb 3F10
0.3 μL	100 mM oxidized glutathione
0.1 μL	T7 enzyme mix

4. Incubate 3 h at 25°C
5. Dilute the expression reactions to 90 μL in buffer C and split into two 50 μL aliquots.
6. Add one aliquot to the Strep ThermoFast well previously coated with biotinylated antigen and the other to the well coated with BSA.
7. Incubate the reactions for 1 h at room temperature and wash three times with 100 μL of buffer C to remove any unbound protein–DNA complexes.
8. Assemble 50 μL of qPCR master mix with primers AS79 and AS80 per well used and eight for the standard curve and perform qPCR, as in Subheading 3.1, step 8.
9. For each library, plot the amount of DNA retained on antigen-coated wells against the round of selections performed. The amount of DNA retained should increase from round to round, indicating that the fitness of the library is improving and selection is taking place.

3.5. Cloning and Screening of Library Selection Output

As a rule, there is significant diversity left in the libraries even after ten rounds of selection, although sequence convergence should be obvious by that stage. It is therefore necessary to assay the clones for binding activity in order to identify the most improved ones.

1. Take 250 ng of in vitro selection library PCR product and cut with *Sal*I and *Not*I restriction enzymes
2. Run the reaction products on a 2% E-gel, cut out the 330 bp band with dAb genes, purify using Qiagen Gel Extraction kit, and elute the DNA in 20 μL of water.
3. Ligate the dAb inserts into *Sal*I and *Not*I-digested pDOM5 bacterial expression vector and transform into *E. coli.*
4. Plate the transformed cells on a Carbenicillin–Glucose agar plate and incubate overnight at 37°C.
5. The next day pick 96 colonies using a pipette tip to inoculate in turns: (A) a 96-well PCR sequencing plate set up using oligonucleotides AS9 and AS65 (see Subheading 3.1, step 2) (for sequencing with M13 reverse primer), (B) a 96-well storage plate containing 100 μL of 2xTY carbenicillin well and (C) 96-well expression deepwell plate containing 500 μL of 2xTY carbenicillin/OnEx (Invitrogen) per well.
6. Run the PCR plate on a thermal cycler using the protocol detailed in Subheading 3.1, step 2.
7. Incubate the 2xTY master plate at 30°C overnight, from then on at 4°C.
8. Grow the expression plate at 30°C in a high-speed shaker for 48–60 h.

9. Spin down the cells from the expression plate at 4,500 × *g* in a Heraeus 15R benchtop centrifuge and screen for dAb activity in supernatant using your assay of choice, e.g., by surface plasmon resonance or ELISA.

4. Notes

1. pIE2a²A vector is based on pIVEX2.2b Nde (Roche) with the following modifications: (1) a tandem Arc operator site has been cloned into *Bgl* II site upstream of the T7 promoter (sequence 5′ AGATCCATAGTAGAGTGCTTCTATCATAGATCCTCCGTTTCGTGATGAGTATAGTAGAGTGCTTCTATCATAGATCT), with Arc operators underlined and separated by two helical turns of the DNA, (2) the expression cassette of pIVEX2.2b Nde has been replaced with a construct that encodes a single-chain Arc with a *Nco*I-*Sal*I-*Not*I-based dAb cloning site at its 5′ end: 5′CCATGGGGTCGACCGGCGGCGCGGCCGCAGGATCTGGTGGCGGATCAGGCGGTGGACATATGAAAGGAATGAGCAAAATGCCGCAGTTCAATTTGCGGTGGCCTAGAGAAGTATTGGATTTGGTACGCAAGGTAGCGGAAGAGAATGGTCGGTCTGTTAATTCTGAGATTTATCAGCGAGTAATGGAAAGCTTTAAGAAGGAAGGGCGCATTGGCGCCGGTGGCGGATCAGGCGGTGGATCTGGTGGCGGATCAGGCGGTGGACATATGAAAGGAATGAGCAAAATGCCGCAGTTCAATTTGCGGTGGCCTAGAGAAGTATTGGATTTGGTACGCAAGGTAGCGGAAGAGAATGGTCGGTCTGTTAATTCTGAGATTTATCAGCGAGTAATGGAAAGCTTTAAGAAGGAAGGGCGCATTGGCGCCGGTGGCGGATCAGGCGGTGGATCCTATCCGTATGATGTGCCGGATTATGCGTAACTCGAG

   Protein sequence: MGSTGGAAAGSGGGSGGGHMKGMSKMPQFNLRWPREVLDLVRKVAEENGRSVNSEIYQRVMESFKKEGRIGAGGGSGGGSGGGSGGGHMKGMSKMPQFNLRWPREVLDLVRKVAEENGRSVNSEIYQRVMESFKKEGRIGAGGGSGGGSYPYDVPDYA*

   pIE2a²A vector carries two Arc operators for tetravalent display of dAbs and has been found suitable for selection of dAbs with K_D values ranging from subnanomolar to micromolar, although the number of valency can be adjusted by changing the number of Arc operators, if desired. Although the single-chain Arc DNA-binding protein gene in pIE2a²A was assembled from synthetic oligonucleotides (10), direct gene synthesis is also possible. In addition to pIVEX2.2b Nde vector, (Roche), T7-driven expression vector pET23d (Merck,

UK) has also been used to provide the elements required for in vitro expression (12, 13). In addition to scArc repressor, *E. coli* Tus replication factor (14, 15), an engineered Zn-finger protein (13), and streptavidin (16) have also been used to create genotype–phenotype linkages in emulsified in vitro translation reactions.

2. Use positive displacement technique or a multistepper to add correct volume of 4.5 mL of Span-80 and 0.5 mL of Triton X-100 to 100 mL of mineral oil whilst stirring. Continue for 30 min. The oil-detergent mix can be stored at room temperature in dark for at least a month.
3. These can be recycled. Rinse the stirrers three times in hexane and once in acetone. Add 0.5 M NaOH and autoclave. Rinse in sterile water until pH drops below 7.0 and air dry in drying cabinet. Store in a sterile container for use.
4. Filter sterilized and stored in 50 μL aliquots at −20°C. Use one aliquot at a time, mix and make sure that the solution is clear before adding to the in vitro expression solution. Oxidized glutathione is applied at an empirically determined concentration that promotes intra-dAb disulphide bond formation whilst not interfering with T7 RNA polymerase or extract activity.
5. Split Expressway SlyD extract into small aliquots upon first use to minimize freeze-thaw cycles. Store at −80°C, alongside with other components of the kit. Promega S30 T7 and EcoPro T7 from Merck have also been used successfully for IVC.
6. 3F10 mAb is a very high affinity rat anti-HA monoclonal antibody. Its role is to cross-link Arc operator-bound dAb–scArc molecules via their C-terminal HA tags and thus to stabilize the protein-DNA complex via avidity effect. Split the reconstituted mAb solution into aliquots and store at −20°C. Working aliquot is stored at 4°C.
7. C1 MyOne beads are preferred over T1 type as the residual carboxyl groups reduce nonspecific adsorption of library DNA. If naïve selection with biotinylated antigen is attempted, it is recommended to alternate neutravidin- and streptavidin-coated beads to avoid selecting dAbs to either of those. C1-COOH MyOne Dynabeads can be coated with neutravidin by using carbodiimide-catalyzed coupling
8. Invitrogen MagnaRack is convenient for rapid parallel processing of larger number of samples. Up to ten can be processed in about 45 min.
9. pDOM5 vector is bacterial expression vector with a proprietary GAS universal leader (17) but any bacterial expression vector compatible with OnEx autoinduction system can be used. XL10-Gold (Agilent) and Mach1 (Merck) are among *E. coli* strains suitable for bacterial expression of dAbs.

10. Successful selections require optimal mutation frequencies. In our hands, about three protein sequence mutations per gene are optimal in error-prone PCR libraries prepared using GeneMorph II kit from Agilent. In parsimonious libraries, 91% of parent base and 3% each of the remaining three bases has proven useful for randomizing the targeted codons.
11. The PCR product generated and detected with primers AS79 and AS80 is about 900 bp long and not all qPCR master mixes are compatible with that kind of length.
12. A typical ligation reaction yields about 10% recircularized vectors and a library of about 10^9 in size. The fraction of vectors with no insert can also be assessed by a control transformation of a small aliquot of the ligation reaction (see Subheading 3.1, step 2).
13. The aqueous phase left in the tube contains the PCR fragments added to the in vitro translation reaction (now at about 5 pM concentration) in complex with their encoded dAbs, as well as an excess of in vitro expressed dAb–scArc fusion protein molecules (about 0.5–1 nM concentration).
14. In naïve selection conditions the aim is to recover the entire binding repertoire by removing the nonbinding fraction and the level of enrichment is dictated by the nonspecific recovery level of the library (about 0.1% input DNA). In affinity maturation conditions, following the initial rapid removal of nonbinding clones, the aim is to enrich those clones that are improved over the parent clones. Depending on the spread of differences in the antigen-binding dAb repertoire, off-rate selections can still be expected to be more effective for enriching even marginally improved clones from the rest.
15. The optimal concentration of the capturing antigen allows for the best enrichment of the highest affinity clone in the library. This can be expected to be around or below the K_D value of the best binder which in practice is an unknown value. We have been using 50–100 nM antigen concentrations during the first round of, followed by decrease to 5–10 nM in twofold steps, whilst monitoring the library recovery from the selection by qPCR (see Subheading 3.1, step 8).
16. Competition times up to 2 h at room temperature can be used with scArc-based constructs. This is sufficient to select clones with k_{off} values 0.0001 per seconds and less. The competition time is limited by the dissociation rate constant of the protein-DNA complex and the nuclease activity of the extract. Theoretical analysis of selecting optimal off-rate competition conditions has been published and can serve as a useful guide (18).
17. A wide selection of streptavidin-coated microbeads of different sizes, uniformity and binding capacity are commercially available

from various sources. For emulsion selection, smaller sizes may be preferable because they will settle more slowly, thus eliminating the need for rather rigorous mixing on or rotator platform and they also have higher specific surface area. Second, weak residual negative charge on C1 MyOne beads helps to suppress nonspecific binding of library DNA by an order of magnitude, compared with T1 MyOne uncharged beads.

18. Pfu DNA polymerase interferes with qPCR.
19. In qPCR with SYBR Green dye, C1 MyOne microbeads partially quench the fluorescence without affecting the $C(t)$ value.
20. It is highly recommended to use proofreading DNA polymerase to carry out amplifications of captured DNA and we have used successfully also Hot Start KOD (Merck), Pwo and HiFi Taq (Roche), among others. After ten rounds of selection, some of the clones will have been through close to 400 cycles of PCR (with assembly steps included), without accumulation of PCR-mediated mutations! In addition, we have noticed extensive PCR cycling occasionally to give rise to in vitro recombination in the form of CDR shuffling and hence access to true Darwinian in vitro sexual recombination in addition to the selection aspect.
21. In our hands, library fitness often improves throughout ten-round series of selection and can jump significantly upon making the selection conditions more stringent.

Acknowledgements

The authors would like to thank Dr. Allart Stoop and Dr. Peter Ertl for helpful advice and suggestions. Dr. A. Sepp was an employee of Domantis Ltd. at the time this work was carried out.

References

1. Enever C et al (2009) Next generation immunotherapeutics-honing the magic bullet. Curr Opin Biotechnol 20:405–411
2. Griffiths AD, Duncan AR (1998) Strategies for selection of antibodies by phage display. Curr Opin Biotechnol 9:102–108
3. Dufner P, Jermutus L, Minter RR (2006) Harnessing phage and ribosome display for antibody optimisation. Trends Biotechnol 24:523–529
4. Tawfik DS, Griffiths AD (1998) Man-made cell-like compartments for molecular evolution. Nat Biotechnol 16:652–656
5. Holt LJ et al (2003) Domain antibodies: proteins for therapy. Trends Biotechnol 21: 484–490
6. Baret JC et al (2009) Fluorescence-activated droplet sorting (FADS): efficient microfluidic cell sorting based on enzymatic activity. Lab Chip 9:1850–1858
7. Sepp A, Ghadessy F, Choo Y (2007) Cell-Free Protein-Evolution Systems for Engineering of Novel Sequence-Specific DNA-Binding and -Modifying Activities. In: Progress in Gene Therapy. R. Bertolotti (ed) World Scientific 3:116–132

8. Robinson CR, Sauer RT (1996) Equilibrium stability and sub-millisecond refolding of a designed single-chain Arc repressor. Biochemistry 35:13878–13884
9. Neylon C (2004) Chemical and biochemical strategies for the randomization of protein encoding DNA sequences: library construction methods for directed evolution. Nucleic Acids Res 32:1448–1459
10. Sepp A, Griffiths AD (2009) Selection US2009176209 (A1)
11. Duffield S et al (2010) Improved anti-TNFR1 polypeptides, antibody variable domains and antagonists. WO2010094720
12. Sepp A, Tawfik DS, Griffiths AD (2002) Microbead display by in vitro compartmentalisation: selection for binding using flow cytometry. FEBS Lett 532:455–458
13. Sepp A, Choo Y (2005) Cell-free selection of zinc finger DNA-binding proteins using in vitro compartmentalization. J Mol Biol 354: 212–219
14. Coskun-Ari FF, Hill TM (1997) Sequence-specific interactions in the Tus-Ter complex and the effect of base pair substitutions on arrest of DNA replication in *Escherichia coli.* J Biol Chem 272:26448–26456
15. Stoop A, Sepp A (2007) Tus DNA binding domains. US Patent 11728574
16. Yonezawa M et al (2004) DNA display of biologically active proteins for in vitro protein selection. J Biochem (Tokyo) 135: 285–288
17. De Wildt R (2007) Universal GAS 1 leader. US Patent 11494965
18. Zahnd C, Sarkar CA, Pluckthun A (2010) Computational analysis of off-rate selection experiments to optimize affinity maturation by directed evolution. Protein Eng Des Sel 23: 175–184

Chapter 13

Selection of VHHs Under Application Conditions

Edward Dolk, Theo Verrips, and Hans de Haard

Abstract

The successful application of antibody fragments such as VHHs in diagnostic assays, affinity purification, imaging, or therapy is not determined by the specificity and affinity of the antibody fragment alone. The ability to bind the target protein in the environment in which the antibody fragment is intended to functionally perform determines to a great extent its success. To identify antibodies with the required stability profile selection of naturally occurring variants from an immune library or mutants from an engineered library should be performed via phage display. The conditions under which the designed antibodies displayed on phage bind to the target ideally should mimic the environment in which the antibody should be effective. After selection individual antibodies need to be tested in appropriate screening assays, again taking into account the conditions under which the antibody should bind to the target and induce the desired effect.

Key words: Phage display, Application conditions, Stability, Selection, Screening

1. Introduction

The functional stability of a protein is determined by its capacity to maintain the native conformation and remain functional despite the presence of extreme conditions such as high concentrations of salts, extreme pH, or elevated temperatures. Even upon complete denaturation the high probability of refolding correctly into the native conformation contributes to a large extend to their functional stability. VHHs consist of only a single domain unit, a feature which favors their stability as compared to fragments derived from multidomain antibodies. The refolding of a single-domain antibody is a more efficient process, because to regain antigen binding properties only a single fragment is involved, whereas for other antibody formats, derived from conventional antibodies, at least two fragments have to refold individually and on top the two domains have to associate to form the antigen binding unit. Several studies demonstrated the unusual high stability of VHH upon unfolding

Dirk Saerens and Serge Muyldermans (eds.), *Single Domain Antibodies: Methods and Protocols*,
Methods in Molecular Biology, vol. 911, DOI 10.1007/978-1-61779-968-6_13, © Springer Science+Business Media, LLC 2012

induced by temperature (1–3), by chemicals (4), or by pressure (5). The publication from Dumoulin et al. (5), suggest the refolding of VHHs in particular is more efficient as compared to the unfolding of conventional antibody derived fragments. During unfolding hydrophobic interfaces of both the heavy and light chain are exposed to the solvent, which causes aggregation and precipitation resulting in lower or even nonfunctional molecules.

Display on bacteriophage M13 aids in the identification of stable antibody fragments due to the extreme stability of the phage (6). It is extremely difficult to find conditions for inactivation of the phage, which sometimes can be a serious handicap of the system leading to isolation of "contaminations" of high affinity antibodies previously picked up in a lab. The phage particle resists denaturation under extreme temperatures, pH extremes, high concentration of detergents, and even chemical denaturants such as urea. When doing selections under application conditions the only limiting factor is the stability of the displayed antibody fragment, since the infectivity of the phage will not be affected or only marginally.

The combination of the ability to refold to its native conformation under extreme conditions (possibly induced by its antigen) and the extreme stability of the phage form the basis of a unique technique to identify stable VHH variants, i.e., phage display of VHHs under application conditions. It was shown that a library of human VH domain antibodies (dAbs) with synthetic CDRs when preincubated for 10 min at 80°C and subsequently cooled down for 10 min at 4°C yielded more thermostable fragments after selection on protein A, which ensured the isolation of correctly folded dAbs (7). Analysis of individual dAbs obtained after selection revealed improved expression levels and better solubility properties consistent with the finding that the formation of periplasmic aggregates limits the expression yields of recombinant antibody fragments in *Escherichia coli*. Finally the elution profiles obtained during size exclusion chromatography suggested the absence of interactions with the column matrix frequently observed for non-engineered dAbs. The selection of thermostable dAbs by phage display delivered fragments with improved biophysical properties. Other groups have shown that a screening method including a heat treatment can results in VH or VHH domains with higher recombinant expression. Furthermore, the heating step combined with refolding could even be used to purify these fragments from bacterial periplasm (8).

VHHs with appropriate stability profiles have been selected under different application conditions. These conditions were necessary for application in a wide range of products from consumer goods, therapeutics, prophylactic products to affinity chromatography products. Here a few examples are presented on how to adjust the selection strategy which affects the (increase in) applicability of the selected antibodies.

VHHs neutralizing Rotavirus should preferably interact with the virus in the intestine, where it replicates and infects host cells. The orally applied antibody fragments should survive the passage through the stomach; therefore, it should be inherently stable against the acidic conditions and resistant against proteases present in the stomach (9). Even more relevant, the antibody fragments should bind virus despite the high concentrations of bile salts present in the intestine and preferably to an epitope, which achieves virus neutralization.

Antibodies targeting the fungus *Malassezia furfur* intended to be included in shampoo should recognize the target protein in the presence of high concentrations of detergents (4). Selections of an immune library generated from a llama immunized with the cell surface protein Malf1 from the fungus in the presence of high concentrations of detergent yielded VHHs capable of binding the target under these extreme conditions. In contrast, selections under physiological conditions resulted in VHHs which were not able to bind in the presence of detergent. Remarkably, sequence analysis revealed that the stable VHHs only differed in a few amino acid residues from VHHs selected under physiological conditions.

A comparable method was used for selecting VHH against human pancreatic lipase (HPL) and human gastric lipase (HGL) (10). VHHs should inhibit dietary enzymes in order to prevent the uptake of fatty acids by inhibiting the digestion of triglycerides in the stomach. In order to do so, VHHs stable at low pH should be selected in order to survive the proteases present in the stomach. For this reason selections were performed whereby binding occurs at pH 4.5 with sodium acetate buffer in the presence of pepsin. Subsequent, a screening assay was set up to measure the inhibition of lipase activity in intestinal juices. Hereto, periplasmic fractions from clones derived from the selection procedure were incubated in the presence of intestinal juice from pigs and tested in ELISA for their capacity to bind to captured lipase.

Antibodies used for depletion of abundant serum proteins or for the purification of serum components in affinity chromatography applications should bind the soluble form of the protein and not the coated protein, which often adopts a different conformation during immobilization or binds preferentially at a certain side of the protein to the plastic surface (11). The antibody should recognize the target protein in the presence of other serum proteins including proteases. The selection conditions were adapted by using biotinylated target protein spiked in full serum for incubation with antibodies displayed on phage, subsequently complexes of target and phage antibodies were captured by immobilized streptavidin. Screening was performed by preparing small affinity chromatography columns from individual antibody fragments and the capability to purify the serum protein was tested by incubation of the matrices with serum (Personal communication Hans de Haard).

Alternatively, His-tagged fragments were captured by TALON beads that served as matrices for affinity purification (12).

While describing the methods we briefly discuss the setup of pilot experiments to examine the stability of the bacteriophage under the intended application conditions, i.e., to analyze its infectivity after incubation under these circumstances. Also the stability of the target protein needs to be verified in an ELISA based assay before the selection experiment is performed. The screening assay should demonstrate the desired function of the antibody under application conditions. Finally, the leads obtained from the selections and identified in the screens have to produced and purified and tested in *in vitro* and *in vivo* models for establishing their efficacy.

2. Materials

2.1. Checking the Stability of the Antigen Under Application Conditions

1. Phosphate Buffered Saline (PBS): Weigh 10 g NaCl, 0.3 g $NaH_2PO_4 \cdot H_2O$, and 7.2 g $Na_2HPO_4 \cdot 2H_2O$ and dissolve in 1 L of H_2O.
2. Nunc MaxiSorp 96-well U bottom plates (Nunc 442404) or Nunc immunotubes (Nunc 444202) are used for immobilizing proteins.
3. Blocking buffer: PBS containing 4% Marvel. Weigh 2 g of dried skimmed milk Marvel (Britstore, UK) and dissolve in 50 mL of PBS by incubating head over head for 30 min. Store at 4°C, but not for longer than 2 days.
4. Application buffer: buffer containing the conditions necessary for the application the VHH are going to be used in. For the acidic environment of the gut, diluted HCl (pH 2.3) was used as a preincubation buffer. For the shampoo selection up to 40% of shampoo in PBS with 0.1% Marvel was used (see Note 1).
5. Washing buffer: PBST. Add 5 mL of a 10% Tween-20 solution to 1 L of PBS (see Note 2).

2.2. Checking the Stability of Phage Under Application Conditions

1. TG1 cells: The *E. coli* strain used in these studies was *E. coli* TG1 (F′ traD36 lacI^q Δ[lacZ]M15 proA$^+$B$^+$/supE Δ[hsdM-mcrB]5 [$r_k^-m_k^-$McrB$^-$] thi Δ[lac-proAB]).
2. LB medium: Weigh 10 g tryptone, 5 g yeast extract, and 5 g NaCl and dissolve in 1 L of H_2O. Sterilize by autoclavation.
3. 2TY medium: Weigh 16 g tryptone, 10 g yeast extract, and 5 g NaCl and dissolve in 1 L of H_2O. Sterilize by autoclavation.
4. Application buffer: buffer containing the conditions necessary for the application the VHH are going to be used in. For the acidic environment of the gut, diluted HCl (pH 2.3) was used

as a preincubation buffer. For the shampoo selection up to 40% of shampoo in PBS with 0.1% Marvel was used (see Note 1).

5. Detergents to mimic application conditions used are 2–40% (v/v) Andrelon® and 2–20% (v/v) Organics®. Dilutions are made in deionized water and 0.1% (w/v) Marvel and 0.05% (v/v) Tween-20.
6. Ampicillin 100 μg/mL: Weigh 1 g ampicillin (art. Nr. 10835269001, Roche) and dissolve in 10 mL of deionized water. This results in a 1,000× stock solution which can be stored at −20°C.
7. PBS: Weigh 10 g NaCl, 0.3 g $NaH_2PO_4 \cdot H_2O$, and 7.2 g $Na_2HPO_4 \cdot 2H_2O$ and dissolve in 1 L of H_2O.
8. Phage are made using standard protocols (see Chapter 6) and stored in a concentration of approximately 10^{12} phages/mL.
9. LB agar plates: Warm up 200 mL of water agar (15% agar in water) and add 200 mL of 2× concentrated LB medium. Cool down to hand-warm temperature and add antibiotics when necessary.

2.3. Phage Display Selection Under Atypical Conditions

1. TG1 cells: The *E. coli* strain used in these studies was *E. coli* TG1 (F′ traD36 $lacI^q$ Δ[lacZ]M15 $proA^+B^+$/supE Δ[hsdM-mcrB]5 [$r_k^- m_k^-$ $McrB^-$] thi Δ[lac-proAB]).
2. LB medium: Weigh 10 g tryptone, 5 g yeast extract, and 5 g NaCl and dissolve in 1 L of H_2O. Sterilize by autoclavation.
3. Ampicillin 100 μg/mL: Weigh 1 g ampicillin (art. Nr. 10835269001, Roche) and dissolve in 10 mL of deionized water. This results in a 1,000× stock solution which can be stores at −20°C.
4. PBS: Weigh 10 g NaCl, 0.3 g $NaH_2PO_4 \cdot H_2O$, and 7.2 g $Na_2HPO_4 \cdot 2H_2O$ and dissolve in 1 L of H_2O.
5. Nunc MaxiSorp 96-well U bottom plates (Nunc 442404) or Nunc immunotubes (Nunc 444202) are used for immobilizing proteins.
6. Blocking buffer: PBS containing 4% Marvel. Weigh 2 g of dried skimmed milk Marvel (Britstore, UK) and dissolve in 50 mL of PBS by incubating head over head for 30 min. Store at 4°C, but not for longer than 2 days.
7. Phage are made using standard protocols (see Chapter 6) and stored in a concentration of approximately 10^{12} phages/mL.
8. Incubation buffer: PBS containing 2% Marvel and 0.05% Tween-20. Weigh 1 g of Marvel and dissolve in 50 mL of PBS by incubating head over head for 30 min. Add 250 μL of a 10% Tween-20 solution. Store at 4°C, but not for longer than 2 days.

9. Application buffer: buffer containing the conditions necessary for the application the VHH are going to be used in. For the acidic environment of the gut, diluted HCl (pH 2.3) was used as a preincubation buffer. For the shampoo selection up to 40% of shampoo in PBS with 0.1% Marvel was used (see Note 1).
10. Washing buffer: PBST. Add 5 mL of a 10% Tween-20 solution to 1 L of PBS (see Note 2).
11. Elution buffer: 1 mg/mL trypsin in PBS buffer. Weigh 10 mg of trypsin and dissolve in 10 mL of PBS. Aliquot in tubes with 1 mL and use fresh or store at −20°C.
12. Trypsin inhibition: Soy bean trypsin inhibitor (SBTI) (T9128, sigma Aldrich) is used. Weigh 10 mg of SBTI and dissolve in 5 mL of deionized water. Add 50 μL of this stock solution to 100 μL of 1 mg/mL trypsin.

2.4. Screening

1. LB medium: Weigh 10 g tryptone, 5 g yeast extract, and 5 g NaCl and dissolve in 1 L of H_2O. Sterilize by autoclavation.
2. Ampicillin 100 μg/mL: Weigh 1 g ampicillin (art. Nr. 10835269001, Roche) and dissolve in 10 mL of deionized water. This results in a 1,000× stock solution which can be stores at −20°C.
3. Microtiter plates: 96-well v-bottom plates (sterile) (cat nr. 651161, Greiner) are used for growing bacteria in small volumes.
4. 2TY medium: Weigh 16 g tryptone, 10 g yeast extract, and 5 g NaCl and dissolve in 1 L of H_2O. Sterilize by autoclavation.
5. PBS: Weigh 10 g NaCl, 0.3 g $NaH_2PO_4 \cdot H_2O$, and 7.2 g $Na_2HPO_4 \cdot 2H_2O$ and dissolve in 1 L of H_2O.

3. Methods

3.1. Checking the Stability of the Antigen Under Application Conditions

1. Coat MaxiSorp plates with antigen overnight at 4°C, typically between 1 and 5 μg/mL in PBS (see Note 3). Control wells remain empty.
2. Empty the plate by tapping it onto tissue and wash once with PBS (see Note 4).
3. Block the plate with 250 μL of blocking buffer for 30 min at room temperature on a shaking platform at 600 rpm.
4. Empty the plate by removing the blocking buffer and subsequent tapping of the plate onto a tissue to carefully remove all liquid.
5. Incubate the coated antigen for 2 h in application buffer on a shaking platform at 600 rpm.

6. Wash the plate twice with 300 μL of washing buffer.
7. Check the immunoreactivity of the antigen with a (commercially) available antibody specific for your protein of interest.

3.2. Checking the Stability of Phage Under Application Conditions

1. Inoculate a colony of TG1 bacteria from a minimal medium plate into 50 mL of LB medium and grow overnight at 37°C.
2. Dilute the overnight culture 1:100 in LB medium and grow the TG1 bacterial cells at 37°C to the logarithmic phase ($OD_{600\ nm}$ between 0.6 and 0.9) and store on ice for later use or use immediately.
3. Prepare a 2× concentrated application buffer. For shampoo application conditions a 50% shampoo solution was made by mixing 25 mL of shampoo with 25 mL of PBS. From this stock, the desired shampoo concentration was reached by dilution with PBS. For selections mimicking gut conditions diluted HCl pH 2.3 was used.
4. Dilute 2×10^{11} phages in 50 μL of PBS or H_2O.
5. Add 50 μL of 2× concentrated application buffer to the 50 μL of phage and mix well. As a control add 50 μL of PBS to 50 μL of phage and treat them similarly.
6. Incubate the phage for 2 h in application conditions.
7. Make serial dilutions of the phage with steps of 10.
8. Add 5 μL of phage dilution to 95 μL of TG1 bacterial cells in logarithmic phase ($OD_{600\ nm}$ between 0.6 and 0.9) and incubate for 30 min without shaking at 37°C.
9. Spot 5 μL of infected TG1 bacteria dropwise on a LB agar plate with appropriate antibiotics and let it dry for 10 min. The LB agar plates should preferably be prewarmed at 37°C and should be dried carefully.
10. Incubate overnight at 37°C
11. Transducing units can be determined from the spot dilutions and can be compared with phage incubation in physiological conditions.

3.3. Phage Display Selection Under Atypical Conditions

1. Inoculate a colony of TG1 bacteria from a minimal medium plate into 50 mL of LB medium and grow overnight at 37°C.
2. Dilute the overnight culture 1:100 in LB medium and grow the TG1 bacterial cells at 37°C to the logarithmic phase ($OD_{600\ nm}$ between 0.6 and 0.9) and store on ice for later use or use immediately.
3. Coat MaxiSorp plates with the desired antigen concentrations overnight at 4°C, typically between 1 and 5 μg/mL for first round of selection and typically between 0.1 and 2 μg/mL for second round of selection.

4. Empty the plate by tapping it onto tissue and wash once with PBS.
5. Block the plate with 250 μL of blocking buffer for 30 min at room temperature on a shaking platform at 600 rpm.
6. Preincubate phages in application buffer for 15 min. Save at least 10 μL of the preincubated input phages for titration.
7. Empty the plate by removing the blocking buffer and subsequent tapping of the plate onto a tissue to carefully removing all liquid. Do not wash after this step, because this will increase aspecific binding of phages (see Note 5).
8. 100 μL of preincubated phages are incubated on the antigen for 2 h on a shaking platform at 600 rpm (see Notes 6 and 7).
9. Wash nonbound phages from the plate with 300 μL of washing buffer, repeat washing five times. At the fifth washing step, the plate is incubated on a shaking platform for 10 min. This procedure is repeated four times. The last two of the 20 washes are performed with washing buffer without Tween-20.
10. Phages are typically eluted by trypsin elution. Elution buffer is incubated for 25 min where after trypsin is inactivated by addition of equimolar amounts of SBTI (see Notes 8 and 9).
11. Make serial dilutions of the output phages and the input phages.
12. Add 5 μL of phage dilution to 95 μL of TG1 bacterial cells in logarithmic phase ($OD_{600\ nm}$ between 0.6 and 0.9) and incubate for 30 min without shaking at 37°C.
13. Spot 5 μL of infected TG1 cells on a LB agar plate containing ampicillin and let it dry for 10 min. The LB agar plates should preferably be prewarmed at 37°C and should be dried carefully.
14. Incubate overnight at 37°C
15. Transducing units can be determined from the spot dilutions and can be compared with phage incubation in physiological conditions.

3.4. Screening

1. Make a selection of phage outputs to be screened based on transducing units determined from the selection outputs.
2. Bacteria expressing monoclonal VHHs are picked by inoculating 94 different clones in 100 μL LB/2% glucose/AMP in a 96-well microtiter plate and are grown overnight at 37°C (see Note 10).
3. The bacterial cultures are diluted 1:100 in 2TY/AMP/0.1% glucose in 96-deepwell plates and grown at 37°C to the logarithmic phase ($OD_{600\ nm}$ between 0.6 and 0.9).
4. Protein expression is induced by addition of 1 mM IPTG and production is continued for 4 h at 37°C.

5. The microtiter plate is spun down at 4,600 × *g* for 10 min and the bacterial pellets are resuspended in 100 μL PBS and are frozen at −20°C.
6. The plates are slowly defrosted and the spheroplasts are pelleted by spinning at 4,600 × *g* for 10 min. Subsequently, periplasmic fractions are transferred to a new plate and stored at −20°C for later use.
7. The screening method should be adjusted to the application. This can include ELISA assays, immunofluorescence, immunoprecipitation, etc. (see Notes 11–13).

4. Notes

1. The application buffer should preferably contain a (low) concentration of Marvel or BSA to avoid aspecific binding. However, it should be taken into account that the blocking agent should also be stable at the application condition. For this reason there was no Marvel or BSA added to the low pH HCl buffer pH 2.3 mimicking the gastric environment.
2. The washing buffer contains Tween-20 to wash away aspecific binding phages more efficiently. In the last two steps of the procedure Tween-20 should be emitted since remnants of Tween-20 could hinder the elution process.
3. Other coating buffers like carbonate buffers or elevated temperatures can be applied to optimize coating of the antigen.
4. It was demonstrated that firm tapping of the plate onto tissue removes small amounts of liquid remaining inside the wells after removal by inverting the plate or removal with a pipette. Since there are 20 washing steps in the protocol, the consequent firm tapping significantly reduces the number of aspecific phages.
5. Washing after the blocking step might wash away blocking agent from the plate, thereby inducing spots for aspecific binding of phages. In this light washing of the plate after blocking should be avoided.
6. In the case of an antigen stable in application conditions, this step should be performed under these conditions. In the case that the antigen is not stable under the application conditions only a preincubation in application conditions can be sufficient to achieve desired antibody stability or capability of correct refolding in these conditions.
7. A heat shock of 15 min at 70°C can be applied to select for antibodies which have a higher probability of correct refolding, which was shown to be in relationship with higher production levels.

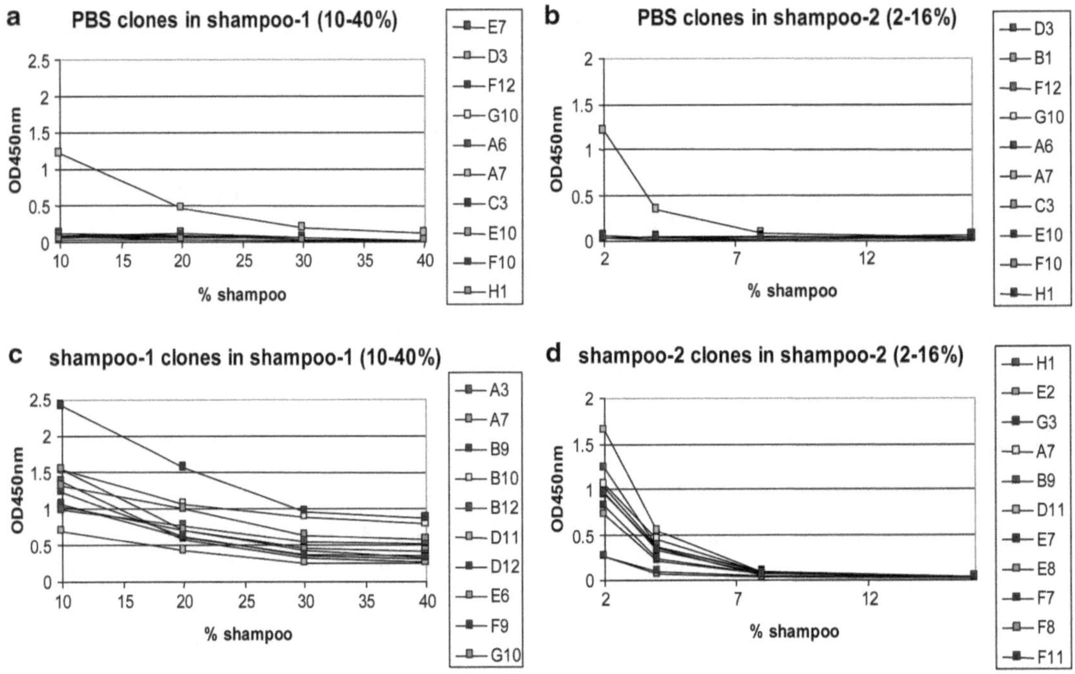

Fig. 1. Binding ELISA of anti-Malf1 VHH obtained by selection in PBS (**a**, **b**) or in shampoo (**c**, **d**) and tested in the presence of shampoo-1 (**a**, **c**) or shampoo-2 (**b**, **d**). Reprinted from ref. (4) with permission.

8. Phages can also be eluted specifically by competition, for instance a monoclonal antibody which has the desired epitope recognition, the ligand of a receptor to target the ligand binding site. Specific elution is carried out by incubating with one of the above mentioned proteins in PBS for 2–4 h.
9. Specific elution is sometimes performed by discarding the eluate of the first half hour, where it is believed that the low affinity clones are preferentially being eluted. Specific elution is then continued for 4 h where it is believed that the high affinity clones will be eluted.
10. Monoclonal VHHs are picked and grown in a 96-well microtiter plate. Two wells are kept empty to allow for controls in subsequent assays.
11. The screening procedure should be adapted to the application in mind. In the case of VHHs against Malf1 both the clones selected in PBS and the clones selected in the presence of shampoo were tested for binding in shampoo (see Fig. 1). This showed that the selection in application conditions was successful and delivered VHHs stable in the application condition.
12. The screening procedure should be fit to be carried out in high throughput fashion. If it is not possible to screen more than

ten clones in the screening assay, it is recommendable to first screen for one parameter, for instance binding capacity and subsequently screen a smaller group of binders for stability under application conditions.

13. Individual characterization of the selected clones can lead to good understanding of the criteria which are needed for stability in certain application conditions (see Chapters 22 and 23).

Acknowledgements

This work has mainly been performed at Unilever Research Vlaardingen.

References

1. van der Linden RH, Frenken LG, de Geus B, Harmsen MM, Ruuls RC, Stok W, de Ron L, Wilson S, Davis P, Verrips CT (1999) Comparison of physical chemical properties of llama VHH antibody fragments and mouse monoclonal antibodies. Biochim Biophys Acta 1431:37–46
2. Pérez JM, Renisio JG, Prompers JJ, van Platerink CJ, Cambillau C, Darbon H, Frenken LG (2001) Thermal unfolding of a llama antibody fragment: a two-state reversible process. Biochemistry 40:74–83
3. Dolk E, van Vliet C, Perez JM, Vriend G, Darbon H, Ferrat G, Cambillau C, Frenken LG, Verrips T (2005) Induced refolding of a temperature denatured llama heavy-chain antibody fragment by its antigen. Proteins 59: 555–564
4. Dolk E, van der Vaart M, Lutje Hulsik D, Vriend G, de Haard H, Spinelli S, Cambillau C, Frenken L, Verrips T (2005) Isolation of llama antibody fragments for prevention of dandruff by phage display in shampoo. Appl Environ Microbiol 71:442–450
5. Dumoulin M, Conrath K, Van Meirhaeghe A, Meersman F, Heremans K, Frenken LG, Muyldermans S, Wyns L, Matagne A (2002) Single-domain antibody fragments with high conformational stability. Protein Sci 11:500–515
6. Jung S, Honegger A, Plückthun A (1999) Selection for improved protein stability by phage display. J Mol Biol 294:163–180
7. Jespers L, Schon O, Famm K, Winter G (2004) Aggregation-resistant domain antibodies selected on phage by heat denaturation. Nat Biotechnol 22:1161–1165
8. Olichon A, Schweizer D, Muyldermans S, de Marco A (2007) Heating as a rapid purification method for recovering correctly-folded thermotolerant VH and VHH domains. BMC Biotechnol 26:7
9. van der Vaart JM, Pant N, Wolvers D, Bezemer S, Hermans PW, Bellamy K, Sarker SA, van der Logt CP, Svensson L, Verrips CT, Hammarstrom L, van Klinken BJ (2006) Reduction in morbidity of rotavirus induced diarrhoea in mice by yeast produced monovalent llama-derived antibody fragments. Vaccine 24:4130–4137
10. Bezemer S, van de Burg M, de Haard HJ, Tareilus E (2001) Antibody heavy chain variable domains against human dietary lipases, and their uses. Patent Application, EP1134231
11. Klooster R, Maassen BT, Stam JC, Hermans PW, Ten Haaft MR, Detmers FJ, de Haard HJ, Post JA, Verrips TC (2007) Improved anti-IgG and HSA affinity ligands: clinical application of VHH antibody technology. J Immunol Methods 324:1–12
12. Verheesen P, ten Haaft MR, Lindner N, Verrips CT, de Haard JJ (2003) Beneficial properties of single-domain antibody fragments for application in immunoaffinity purification and immuno-perfusion chromatography. Biochim Biophys Acta 1624:21–28

Chapter 14

Isolation and Characterization of *Clostridium difficile* Toxin-Specific Single-Domain Antibodies*

Greg Hussack, Mehdi Arbabi-Ghahroudi, C. Roger MacKenzie, and Jamshid Tanha

Abstract

Camelidae single-domain antibodies (VHHs) are a unique class of small binding proteins that are promising inhibitors of targets relevant to infection and immunity. With VHH selection from hyperimmunized phage display libraries now routine and the fact that VHHs possess long, extended complementarity-determining region (CDR3) loop structures that can access traditionally immunosilent epitopes, VHH-based inhibition of targets such as bacterial toxins are being explored. Toxin A and toxin B are high molecular weight exotoxins (308 kDa and 269 kDa, respectively) secreted by *Clostridium difficile* that are the causative agents of *C. difficile*-associated diseases in humans and in animals. Here, we provide protocols for the rapid generation of *C. difficile* toxin A- and toxin B-specific VHHs by llama immunization and recombinant antibody/phage display technology approaches and for further characterization of the VHHs with respect to toxin-binding affinity and specificity and the conformational nature of their epitopes.

Key words: Single-domain antibody, VHH, *Clostridium difficile*, Toxin, Infectious disease, Immunotherapy

1. Introduction

An increasing number of single-domain antibodies (VHHs) have been isolated against targets relevant to infection, immunity, and toxicology (1). For example, several proteinaceous toxins have been targeted by VHHs including: alpha-cobrotoxin (2), verotoxin (3), AahI′ scorpion toxin (4, 5), botulinum toxins (6–8), staphylococcal toxins (9, 10), *Escherichia coli* heat-labile toxin (11), ART2.2 ecto-enzyme (12), *Salmonella* SpvB toxin (13), ricin (9, 14), cholera toxin (9), and *Clostridium difficile* toxin A and toxin B (15). Many of these antitoxin antibodies possessed high target affinities and several were

*This is National Research Council Canada Publication 50017.

Dirk Saerens and Serge Muyldermans (eds.), *Single Domain Antibodies: Methods and Protocols*, Methods in Molecular Biology, vol. 911, DOI 10.1007/978-1-61779-968-6_14, © Springer Science+Business Media, LLC 2012

potent neutralizers of biological toxin function. With their long CDR3 loops capable of binding into deep cavities and enzymatic clefts that are normally immunosilent and inaccessible epitopes with conventional antibodies, VHHs are establishing themselves as a class of antibodies with great potential as anti-infective, toxin-neutralizing therapeutics. Their high affinity towards protein targets, cost-effective production, amenability to multivalent display formats (e.g., bispecific, pentameric, Fc fusions), and overall stability suggests exploration of VHH-based anti-infective binding agents is warranted.

C. difficile is a Gram-positive, gastrointestinal pathogen that can cause chronic episodes of diarrhea and death in some patients (16). The bacterium is one of the most common nosocomial infections in developed nations and is a significant challenge to health care providers with respect to infection control and associated financial costs. *C. difficile* relies on the secretion of two high molecular weight toxins that bind intestinal epithelial cells, leading to the disruption of gastrointestinal tract membrane integrity and ultimately causing massive fluid loss and inflammation (16). While numerous antibiotics and toxin-binding compounds are in various stages of development, toxin-binding monoclonal antibodies have shown promise as effective therapeutics (17–19).

Here we present protocols for the isolation and characterization of *C. difficile* toxin A- and B-specific VHHs. Specifically, we describe methods for: (1) llama immunization with recombinant fragments of the C-terminal cell receptor binding domain, (2) construction of a VHH phage display library from the immunized llama, (3) isolation of toxin-specific VHHs from the phage display library by panning and phage-binding assays, (4) production of the isolated antitoxin VHHs in *E. coli* by recombinant antibody cloning techniques, and (5) characterization of the antitoxin VHHs in terms of specificity, toxin-binding affinity, and the conformational nature of the epitopes. These protocols should be expandable to other proteinaceous toxin targets.

2. Materials

All solutions and media were prepared with distilled and deionized water (ddH_2O). Autoclaving (sterilizing) of solutions and media were performed on liquid cycle at 121°C, 15 lb/in.^{2}, and 20 min. Filter-sterilized solutions were prepared using 0.2 μm filter units (see Note 1). Media were supplemented with antibiotics when their temperatures were below 55°C.

2.1. Llama Immunization and Serum Response Monitoring

1. Recombinant *C. difficile* toxin (rTcd) A and B fragments (see Note 2).
2. Purified *C. difficile* toxin A and toxin B from strain 10463 (see Note 3).

3. Male llama (*Lama glama*, see Note 4).
4. Phosphate-buffered saline (PBS): 8 g NaCl, 0.2 g KCl, 1.4 g Na_2HPO_4, 0.24 g KH_2PO_4, pH 7.3, in 1 L of ddH_2O. Sterilize by autoclaving, store at room temperature.
5. Freund's complete and incomplete adjuvants (Sigma, Mississauga, ON, Canada).
6. 20 mM NaPi buffer: 8.46 mL of 1 M NaH_2PO_4, 11.54 mL of 1 M Na_2HPO_4, pH 7.0, in 1 L of ddH_2O.
7. 100 mM citrate buffer: 3.11 g citric acid, 1.53 g sodium citrate, pH 3.5, in 200 mL of ddH_2O. Adjust to pH 3.5 with 1 M NaOH, filter-sterilize, store at 4°C.
8. 100 mM glycine buffer: 1.5 g glycine, in 200 mL of ddH_2O. Adjust to pH 2.7 with 3 M HCl, filter-sterilize, store at 4°C.
9. 100 mM sodium acetate buffer: 2.7 g sodium acetate, in 200 mL of ddH_2O. Adjust to pH 4.5 with acetic acid, filter-sterilize, store at 4°C.
10. 1 M Tris–HCl buffer: 24.1 g Tris-base, in 200 mL of ddH_2O. Adjust to pH 8.8 with 3 M HCl, filter-sterilize, store at 4°C.
11. SDS-PAGE (sodium dodecyl sulfate-polyacrylamide gel electrophoresis) reagents and equipment.
12. 1 M dithiothreitol (DTT).
13. Syringes and needles for llama immunization and blood collection.
14. Heparin-coated tubes.
15. HiTrap™ Protein G HP and HiTrap™ Protein A HP columns (GE Healthcare, Baie-d'Urfé, QC, Canada).
16. ÄKTA™ FPLC purification system (GE Healthcare).
17. BSA: 5 mg/mL in PBS. Filter-sterilize, store at 4°C.
18. PBS-T: PBS + 0.05% (v/v) Tween 20.
19. Buffer A: 5% (w/v) BSA in PBS-T.
20. Goat anti-llama IgG and swine anti-goat IgG labeled with horse radish peroxidase (HRP) (Cedarlane, Burlington, ON, Canada).
21. HRP substrate solutions for enzyme-linked immunosorbent assay (ELISA).
22. 1 M H_3PO_4.
23. 96-well microtiter plates.
24. Microtiter plate reader.

2.2. VHH Phage Display Library Construction

1. QIAamp RNA Blood Mini™ kit (Qiagen, Mississauga, ON, Canada).
2. First-Strand cDNA Synthesis™ kit (GE Healthcare).

Table 1
Primers used in this work

Name	Sequence 5′→3′	Purpose
MJ1[a]	GCC CAG CCG GCC ATG GCC SMK GTG CAG CTG GTG GAK TCT GGG GGA	Library construction
MJ2	GCC CAG CCG GCC ATG GCC CAG GTA AAG CTG GAG GAG TCT GGG GGA	Library construction
MJ3	GCC CAG CCG GCC ATG GCC CAG GCT CAG GTA CAG CTG GTG GAG TCT	Library construction
CH2FORTA4[b]	CGC CAT CAA GGT ACC AGT TGA	Library construction
CH2B3-F	GGG GTA CCT GTC ATC CAC GGA CCA GCT GA	Library construction
MJ7	CAT GTG TAG ACT CGC GGC CCA GCC GGC CAT GGC C	Library construction
MJ8	CAT GTG TAG ATT CCT GGC CGG CCT GGC CTG AGG AGA CGG TGA CCT GG	Library construction
BbsI-VHH	TAT GAA GAC ACC AGG CCC AGG TAA AGC TGG AGG AGT CT	Subcloning
BbsI2-VHH	TAT GAA GAC ACC AGG CCC AGG TGC AGC TGG TGG AGT CT	Subcloning
BamHI-VHH	TTG TTC GGA TCC TGA GGA GAC GGT GAC CTG	Subcloning
-96gIII	CCC TCA TAG TTA GCG TAA CGA TCT	Colony-PCR, sequencing
M13FP	GTA AAA CGA CGG CCA GT	Colony-PCR, sequencing
M13RP	CAG GAA ACA GCT ATG AC	Colony-PCR, sequencing

[a]See Note 35
[b]See Ref. (29)

3. Primers (10 pmol/μL): CH2FORTA4, CH2B3-F, MJ1, MJ2, MJ3, MJ7, MJ8, -96gIII, M13RP (see Table 1 and Note 5).
4. 10× PCR buffer and *Taq* DNA polymerase (5 units/μL).
5. dNTPs: 10 mM each of dTTP, dATP, dCTP, and dGTP.

6. *Sfi*I, *Xho*I and *Pst*I restriction endonucleases and their respective 10× buffers.
7. pMED1 phagemid vector (20).[1]
8. LigaFast™ Rapid DNA Ligation System (Promega, Madison, WI).
9. Electrocompetent TG1 *E. coli* cells (Stratagene, La Jolla, CA).
10. Ampicillin: 100 mg/mL, filter-sterilize, store at −20°C in 1 mL aliquots.
11. Kanamycin: 50 mg/mL, filter-sterilize, store at −20°C in 1 mL aliquots.
12. SOC medium: 20 g tryptone, 5 g yeast extract, 0.58 g NaCl, 0.19 g KCl, in 1 L of ddH_2O. Autoclave, cool, and add 0.4% filter-sterilized glucose, 10 mM filter-sterilized $MgCl_2$. Store at −20°C in 1 mL aliquots.
13. 2xYT medium: 16 g tryptone, 10 g yeast extract, 5 g NaCl, in 1 L of ddH_2O. Autoclave to sterilize.
14. 2xYT-Amp-Kan medium: 2xYT + 100 μg/mL ampicillin + 50 μg/mL kanamycin.
15. 2xYT-Amp-Glu medium: 2xYT + 100 μg/mL ampicillin + 2% (w/v) filter-sterilized glucose.
16. 2xYT-Amp plates: 2xYT medium, 15 g agar, in 1 L of ddH_2O. Autoclave, cool to ~55°C, add ampicillin to a final concentration of 100 μg/mL, pour plates, store at 4°C for up to a month.
17. PBS (see Subheading 2.1, item 4).
18. 70% (v/v) glycerol. Autoclave to sterilize.
19. M13KO7 helper phage.
20. PEG/NaCl: 20% (v/v) PEG 8000, 146.1 g NaCl, in 1 L of ddH_2O. Autoclave, store at room temperature.
21. QIAquick Gel Extraction™ and QIAquick PCR Purification™ kits (Qiagen) (see Note 6).
22. Agarose gel electrophoresis reagents and equipment.
23. Electroporation cuvettes.
24. MicroPulser™ electroporator (BioRad, Hercules, CA) or equivalent electroporation device.
25. ND-1000 spectrophotometer (Thermo Scientific, Wilmington, DE) or similar instrument (see Note 7).
26. Stock plate of *E. coli* TG1 cells (see Note 8).
27. DNA sequencing reagents and equipment.

[1]All phagemid and cloning vectors are freely available upon request.

2.3. VHH Phage Display Library Screening

1. Recombinant and whole *C. difficile* toxins (see Subheading 2.1, items 1 and 2).
2. BSA: 5 mg/mL in PBS. Filter-sterilize, store at 4°C.
3. PBS (see Subheading 2.1, item 4).
4. Stock plate of *E. coli* TG1 cells (see Note 8).
5. M13KO7 helper phage.
6. PEG/NaCl (see Subheading 2.2, item 20).
7. Growth media (see Subheading 2.2, items 11, 13, 15, and 16).
8. Spectrophotometer (see Subheading 2.2, item 25).
9. PBS-T (see Subheading 2.1, item 18).
10. Primers (10 pmol/μL): –96gIII, M13RP (see Table 1).
11. DNA amplification and sequencing supplies (see Subheading 2.2, items 4, 5, 22, and 27).
12. Buffer B: PBS + 1% (w/v) casein. Autoclave to sterilize.
13. 100 mM Triethylamine, prepared fresh daily.
14. 1 M Tris–HCl buffer: 121.4 g Tris-base, in 1 L of ddH_2O. Adjust to pH 7.4 with 3 M HCl, filter-sterilize, store at 4°C.
15. Anti-M13 IgG conjugated to HRP (GE Healthcare).
16. ELISA supplies (see Subheading 2.1, items 21–24).

2.4. VHH Subcloning, Soluble Expression, and Purification

1. Primers (10 pmol/μL): BbsI-VHH, BbsI2-VHH, BamHI-VHH, M13FP, M13RP (see Table 1).
2. DNA amplification, purification, and sequencing supplies (see Subheading 2.2, items 4, 5, 21, 22, 25, and 27).
3. *E. coli* transformation supplies (see Subheading 2.2, items 9, 12, 23, and 24).
4. pSJF2H expression vector (20) (see Footnote 1).
5. *Bbs*I and *Bam*HI restriction endonucleases and respective 10× buffers.
6. T4 DNA ligase and 10× ligase buffer (Invitrogen, Burlington, ON, Canada).
7. LB-Amp: 10 g tryptone, 5 g yeast extract, 10 g NaCl, in 1 L of ddH_2O. Autoclave, cool to ~55°C, add to 100 μg/mL ampicillin final.
8. LB-Amp plates: 10 g tryptone, 5 g yeast extract, 10 g NaCl, 15 g agar, in 1 L of ddH_2O. Autoclave, cool to ~55°C, add ampicillin to 100 μg/mL final, pour plates, store at 4°C for up to a month.

2.5. VHH Specificity and Affinity Profiling by Soluble ELISA and Surface Plasmon Resonance Measurements

1. Coating antigens: Native *C. difficile* toxins, recombinant *C. difficile* toxin fragments (rTcd), and BSA (5 mg/mL in PBS).
2. Buffer C: PBS + 3% (w/v) skim milk powder.
3. Rabbit anti-His_6 IgG conjugated with HRP (Cedarlane).
4. ELISA supplies (see Subheading 2.1, items 4, 18, and 21–24).
5. Superdex™ 75 10/300 GL size exclusion column (bed volume: 24 mL; bed dimensions: 10 × 300 mm) (GE Healthcare).
6. Filtered and degassed ddH_2O. Degas the filtered water with a conventional water aspirator.
7. Filtered and degassed PBS (see Subheading 2.1, item 4). Degas the filtered PBS with a conventional water aspirator.
8. Appropriate control (reference) protein for Biacore.
9. HBS-E buffer: 10 mM HEPES, 150 mM NaCl, 3 mM EDTA, pH 7.4. This buffer can be purchased from GE Healthcare. If not purchased from GE Healthcare, it should be thoroughly degassed before use.
10. Surfactant P20 (GE Healthcare).
11. Amine coupling kit containing *N*-hydroxysccinimide (NHS), *N*-ethyl-*N*′-(3-dimethylaminopropyl)carbodiimide hydrochloride (EDC), and ethanolamine (GE Healthcare).
12. 10 mM acetate buffer, pH 4.0.
13. 1 M ethanolamine, pH 8.5.
14. CM5 sensorchips (GE Healthcare).
15. BIACORE 3000 (GE Healthcare) or other Surface Plasmon Resonance (SPR) instrument with similar capabilities.

2.6. Probing the Conformational Nature of VHH Epitopes

1. TcdA and TcdB (see Subheading 2.1, item 2).
2. Control anti-TcdA IgG PCG4 (Novus Biologicals, Littleton, CO).
3. SDS-PAGE and Western blotting reagents and equipment.
4. 1 M DTT.
5. Goat anti-mouse IgG (H + L) conjugated to alkaline phosphatase (AP) (Cedarlane).
6. HisDetector™ Nickel-AP Conjugate kit (Mandel Scientific, Guelph, ON, Canada).
7. Buffer A (see Subheading 2.1, item 19) and Buffer C (see Subheading 2.5, item 2).
8. AP substrate solutions for Western blotting.
9. 3× Native-PAGE sample buffer: 0.5 mL of 1% (w/v) Bromophenol Blue, 0.6 mL of 0.5 M Tris–HCl, pH 6.8, 2.9 mL of 50% glycerol, 1 mL of ddH_2O.

10. Native-PAGE running buffer: 4 g glycine, 3.03 g Tris-base, in 1 L of ddH_2O. Store at room temperature.
11. ELISA supplies (see Subheading 2.1, items 4, 18, and 21–24).
12. Rabbit anti-His_6 IgG conjugated with HRP (Cedarlane).

3. Methods

In this section, we provide detailed protocols for the isolation and characterization of anti-*C. difficile* toxin VHHs. Specifically, we describe the protocols for: (1) llama immunization and serum response monitoring, (2) VHH phage display library construction, (3) VHH phage display library screening, (4) VHH subcloning, soluble expression, and purification, (5) VHH specificity and affinity profiling by soluble ELISA and SPR measurements, and (6) probing the conformational nature of VHH epitopes.

3.1. Llama Immunization and Serum Response Monitoring

In this step, two recombinant fragments of *C. difficile* toxin A (TcdA) and toxin B (TcdB), referred to here as rTcdA and rTcdB, are used for llama immunization and injected simultaneously on all injection days. These fragments are a portion of the C-terminal cell receptor binding domain (RBD), a region of the toxin responsible for host-cell binding (see Fig. 1a). Following immunizations, llama antisera are monitored for toxin-specific heavy-chain antibody responses by ELISA.

1. Obtain regulatory approval. Follow all animal protocols within your jurisdiction and/or country.
2. Immunize one male llama by subcutaneous, lower-back injection with both recombinant toxin antigens simultaneously, using the schedule shown in Fig. 1b (see Note 9). On Day 1, immunize with 200 μg of each antigen (diluted in PBS to 1 mL total and filter-sterilized) and 1 mL of Freund's complete adjuvant (FCA) for a total immunization volume of 2 mL. On Days 22, 36, and 50, immunize with 100 μg of each antigen (diluted in PBS to 1 mL total) and 1 mL of Freund's incomplete adjuvant (FIA). On Day 77, immunize with 100 μg of each antigen (diluted in PBS to 1 mL total) with no adjuvant. Collect blood (10–15 mL) into heparin-coated tubes on Days 22, 43, 57, and 84. Immediately store the collected blood on ice. Conduct a pre-immune bleed on Day 1 as well (this serves as a nonimmunized control for a subsequent ELISA; see Subheading 3.1, steps 10–15).
3. Store the collected blood from each bleed overnight at 4°C. Prepare the serum the next day by centrifugation at 2,700 × *g* for 10 min at 4°C and store at 4°C.

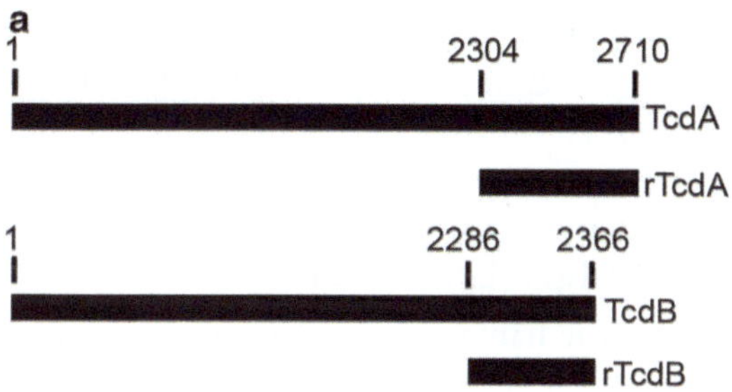

b

Day	Event
1	Pre-immune bleed
1	200 μg Ags + FCA
22	Bleed 1
22	100 μg Ags + FIA
36	100 μg Ags + FIA
43	Bleed 2
50	100 μg Ags + FIA
57	Bleed 3
77	100 μg Ags
84	Bleed 4

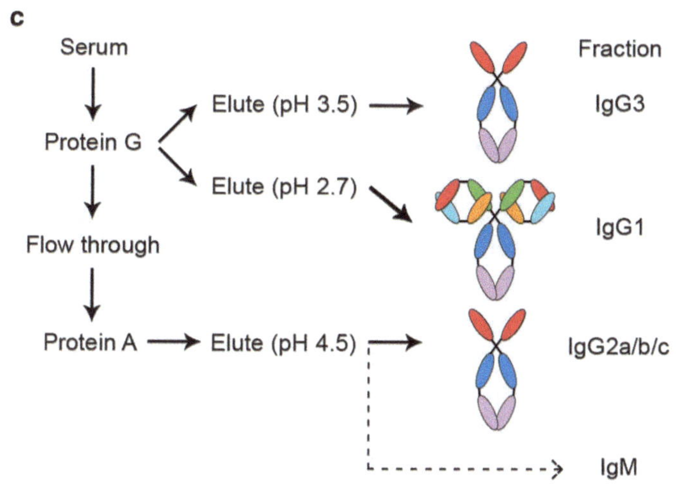

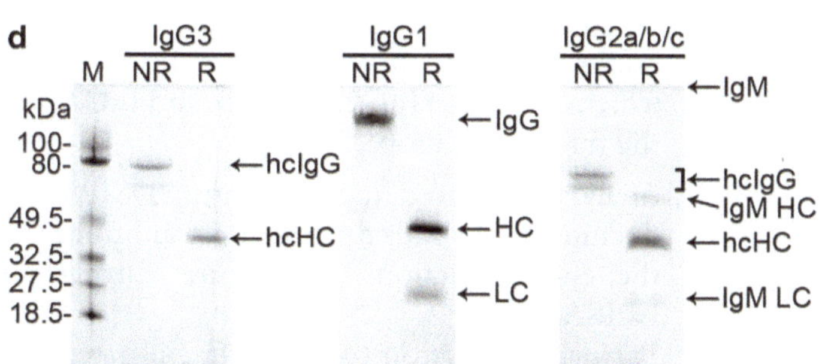

Fig. 1. Llama immunization and serum response. (**a**) Native *Clostridium difficile* toxins (TcdA and TcdB) from strain 10463 were purified as described (28). Recombinant fragments of the C-terminal cell receptor binding domain of the toxin (rTcdA and rTcdB) were produced recombinantly and used for llama immunization and library screening. (**b**) Immunization and bleed schedule for one male llama. Both rTcdA and rTcdB ("Ags") were injected simultaneously and the amount of Ag listed is the amount of each injected. *FCA* Freund's complete adjuvant; *FIA* Freund's incomplete adjuvant. (**c**) Overview of the serum fractionation procedure to separate conventional IgG (IgG1) and hcIgGs (IgG2a/b/c, IgG3) from serum using Protein G and Protein A affinity columns. Minor amounts of IgM may co-elute with the IgG2a/b/c fraction. (**d**) SDS-PAGE analysis of eluted fractions from the Protein G and Protein A columns in (**c**). Fractionated IgGs were analyzed under nonreducing (NR) or reducing (R) conditions. M: protein molecular weight marker; IgG3: heavy-chain IgG3 fraction eluted from Protein G; IgG1: conventional IgG1 fraction eluted from Protein G; IgG2a/b/c: heavy-chain IgG2a, IgG2b and IgG2c fraction eluted form Protein A; hcHC: IgG2/IgG3 heavy-chain; HC: IgG1 heavy chain; LC: light chain. Full-length IgM is difficult to visualize in the gel due to its high molecular weight.

4. Isolate the lymphocytes from blood collected on Day 84 and use for phage display library construction (see Subheading 3.2).

   Fractionate the sera prepared from blood on Day 57 and Day 84 bleeds (see Fig. 1c) in order to separate conventional IgG from heavy-chain IgG (hcIgG) (21, 22):

5. Load 1–2 mL of the llama serum (dialyzed against NaPi buffer and clarified by sterile filtration) onto a 1-mL HiTrap™ Protein G HP column previously equilibrated with 10 mL of filter-sterilized NaPi buffer, all under the control of an ÄKTA™ FPLC purification system.
6. Collect the flow-through and set aside at 4°C for a second round of purification (see Subheading 3.1, step 8). Wash the Protein G column with 10 mL of filter-sterilized NaPi buffer and apply 1–2 mL of citrate buffer (pH 3.5) to elute the hcIgG3 fraction (see Fig. 1c). Immediately neutralize the eluted fraction by adding 1 M Tris–HCl buffer (pH 8.8) until a pH of at least 6.0 is reached.
7. Perform a second elution with 2–4 mL of glycine buffer (pH 2.7) to elute the conventional IgG1 fraction (see Fig. 1c). Neutralize the fraction as above.
8. Next, load the flow-through from the Protein G column (see Subheading 3.1, step 6) onto a 1-mL HiTrap™ Protein A HP column previously equilibrated with 10 mL of filter-sterilized NaPi buffer. After loading, wash the Protein A column with 10 mL of NaPi buffer and apply 1–2 mL of sodium acetate buffer (pH 4.5) to elute the hcIgG2 fraction (see Fig. 1c), which consists of IgG2a, IgG2b, and IgG2c isotypes. Neutralize the fraction as above.
9. Analyze the eluted fractions on an SDS-PAGE gel under nonreducing (NR) and reducing (R) conditions (see Fig. 1d). Store the eluted fractions at 4°C for further analysis by serum ELISA.

   Perform ELISA on total and fractionated sera to determine if a toxin A/B-specific, heavy-chain antibody type immune response has been obtained.

10. Coat 96-well microtiter plates with rTcdA, rTcdB, and BSA control overnight at 4°C, all at 1–5 μg/well diluted in a total of 100 μL of PBS. Include another control well which contain PBS.
11. Block the wells with Buffer A (200 μL/well) for 2 h at 37°C.
12. Add serial dilutions of pre-immune total serum (collected on Day 1), post-immune total serum from various bleeds (collected on Days 22, 43, 57, and 84), and fractionated serum (IgG3, IgG1, and IgG2a/b/c fractions) from Day 57 and

Day 84 bleeds diluted in a total of 100 μL of PBS for 1.5 h at room temperature. The last well should contain PBS only.

13. Wash the wells with PBS-T (5 × 300 μL) and add 100 μL/well of goat anti-llama IgG (previously diluted 1:1,000 in PBS) for 1 h at 37°C.
14. Wash the wells as above and add 100 μL/well of swine anti-goat IgG-HRP (previously diluted 1:3,000 in PBS) for 1 h at 37°C.
15. Wash the wells again, add HRP substrate (100 μL/well), and incubate at room temperature for 5–10 min. Stop the reaction with 1 M H_3PO_4 (100 μL/well) and read at 450 nm with a microtiter plate reader (see Note 10).

A typical SDS-PAGE gel profile illustrating the successful separation of hcIgG and conventional IgG antibodies from the immune llama serum is shown in Fig. 1d. The expected molecular weight of conventional IgGs, IgG heavy chains, and IgG light chains is approximately 150 kDa, 55 kDa, and 25 kDa, respectively. The expected molecular weight of heavy-chain IgGs (hcIgG) and hcIgG heavy chains is approximately 85 kDa and 42 kDa, respectively. Faint bands appearing at approximately 75 kDa and 25 kDa in the reduced (R) "IgG2a/b/c" lane indicate the fraction contains minor amounts of IgM, due to the binding of IgM to protein A (23). The separated fractions are then tested by ELISA against the immunogen (rTcdA or rTcdB) and other nonspecific proteins to determine if a hcIgG immune response has been generated (data not shown). If a positive response is found within the heavy-chain IgG fractions, proceed with VHH phage display library construction (see Note 11).

3.2. VHH Phage Display Library Construction

In this step, leukocytes are isolated from the serum prepared from Day 84 blood and used as a source of mRNA for library construction. cDNA is synthesized from the mRNA and used to produce dsDNA. VHH dsDNA is inserted into a phagemid vector and transformed into *E. coli*, creating the phage display library.

1. Isolate total lymphocyte RNA from 2 mL of llama blood drawn on Day 84 (see Subheading 3.1, step 4) by using the QIAamp RNA Blood Mini™ kit according to the manufacturer's instructions. Measure the RNA concentration and purity at $A_{260\ \mathrm{nm}}$ and $A_{280\ \mathrm{nm}}$, respectively, with a spectrophotometer (24).
2. Use a total of 3–5 μg of RNA in 20 μL of ddH_2O to synthesize cDNA in a total reaction volume of 33 μL, using the First-Strand cDNA Synthesis™ kit and CH2-specific primers, CH2FORTA4 and CH2B3-F, according to the manufacturer's instructions (see Note 12).

3. Perform test polymerase chain reactions (PCRs) using various amounts of the cDNA reaction mix ranging in volume from 0.5 to 5 μL using an equimolar mix of framework 1-specific primers MJ1, MJ2, and MJ3 with either CH2FORTA4 or CH2B3-F primer. Set up the PCR reaction as follows:

10× buffer	5 μL
MJ1–3 primer mix (10 pmol/μL each)	0.5 μL
CH2FORTA4 or CH2B3-F primer	0.5 μL
dNTPs	1 μL
cDNA	0.5–5 μL
Taq DNA polymerase	0.5 μL
ddH_2O	Add to 50 μL

Perform a PCR using a program consisting of an initial step of 94°C for 3 min, 30 cycles of 94°C for 1 min, 55°C for 30 s, and 72°C for 30 s, and a final extension of 72°C for 7 min.

4. Analyze 5 μL of the PCR reaction on a 1% agarose gel (24). Identify the cDNA volume that gives the best yield in terms of amplifying the VHH genes and perform the PCR experiment for the remaining cDNA mixture under the same conditions. Gel-purify the VHH bands on a 1% agarose gel using the QIAquick Gel Extraction™ kit (see Note 13). Pool the DNA and measure the concentration (see Subheading 3.2, step 1).

5. Re-amplify the purified product (10–20 ng of the amplified cDNA/reaction tube) in a second PCR under the exact same conditions above, using sense and framework 4-specific primers MJ7 and MJ8, respectively. Perform a total of 20 PCR reactions. Analyze a small amount of the PCR reaction on a 1% agarose gel, expecting to see bands ranging from 400 to 450 bp, which corresponds to the VHH fragments. Desalt the PCR products with the QIAquick PCR Purification™ kit and determine the concentration.

6. Digest the PCR products with *Sfi*I (5 units/μg DNA) overnight at 50°C and subsequently analyze a few microliters on a 1% agarose gel to ensure that it is of the proper size. Repurify the digested DNA with QIAquick PCR Purification™ kit and measure its concentration.

7. Digest 30 μg of pMED1 phagemid vector with *Sfi*I (5 units/μg DNA) for 5 h at 50°C. The next day, add 1 μL (10 units) of each of *Xho*I and *Pst*I enzymes for an additional 2 h at 37°C to reduce self ligation of pMED1. Examine the digested pMED1 on a 1% agarose gel against the undigested control vector to

ensure that the vector is completely linearized. Purify the digested vector with QIAquick PCR Purification™ kit and measure its concentration.

8. Use the LigaFast™ Rapid DNA Ligation System to ligate the *Sfi*I-digested VHH DNA with *Sfi*I-digested pMED1 vector as follows:

Digested vector	20 μg
Digested VHH insert	3.5 μg
T4 DNA ligase buffer	50 μL
T4 DNA ligase	8 μL
Sterile ddH_2O	Add to 100 μL

Incubate at room temperature for 60 min (see Note 14).

9. Purify the ligated materials using a QIAquick PCR Purification™ kit using two spin columns and elute the DNA in a final volume of 35 μL of sterile ddH_2O per column. Pool the eluted material and measure its concentration.
10. Transform 50 μL of electrocompetent TG1 cells with 3 μL of the purified ligated material using a MicroPulser™ electroporator or an equivalent instrument (25). Transfer the electroporated cells into a tube containing 1 mL of SOC medium and incubate for 1 h at 37°C and 180 rpm. Repeat the transformation for the remaining DNA for a total of 20 transformations.
11. Pool the transformed cells, take a small aliquot and carry out 10^3-, 10^4- and 10^5-fold dilutions in 2xYT. Spread 100 μL of the diluted cells on 2xYT-Amp plates and incubate overnight at 32°C. In the morning, use the plates to determine the functional size of the library (see Subheading 3.2, steps 14–16).
12. Amplify the library by transferring the transformed cells into 500 mL of 2xYT-Amp-Glu and incubating overnight at 220 rpm and 37°C.
13. In the morning, centrifuge the cells at 5,000 × *g* for 20 min at 4°C. Discard the supernatant and resuspend the cells in 50 mL of 2xYT-Amp-Glu. Make dilutions of the cells in 2xYT, measure the absorbance at $A_{600\ nm}$ and use this value to calculate the cell density (# of cells/mL) in the stock solution ($1\ A_{600\ nm} \cong 10^9$ cells). Add 50 mL of sterile 70% glycerol to the cell stock, make several aliquots of 10^{10} bacterial cells/vial, and freeze the cells at −80°C (see Note 15).
14. Count the colonies on the titer plates (see Subheading 3.2, step 11) and determine the total library size.

15. Perform a colony-PCR on the colonies from the titer plates in a total volume of 15 μL. Prepare a master mix for 50 PCR reactions as follows:

10× PCR buffer	80 μL
dNTPs	16 μL
-96gIII primer	8 μL
M13RP primer	8 μL
Taq DNA polymerase	8 μL
ddH_2O	680 μL

Aliquot 15 μL volumes from the master mix in 50 PCR tubes. Touch single colonies from the titer plates with a P10 pipette tip and swirl in the PCR tubes. Place the reaction tubes in a thermal cycler and perform a PCR with a program consisting of a preheating step at 94°C for 5 min followed by 30 cycles of 94°C for 30 s, 55°C for 30 s, and 72°C for 1 min, and a final step of 72°C for 7 min.

16. Analyze a few microliters of each PCR reaction on a 1% agarose gel to identify the clones with full inserts (approximately 600 bp band). Use 0.5 μL of the PCR mixture and M13RP as primer to sequence the clones and identify those expressing VHH sequences (26, 27) (see Notes 16–18). Determine the functional library size by multiplying the percentage of the 50 clones with VHH sequences by the total library size.

17. To produce the phage library, thaw 1–2 mL of frozen library cells (see Subheading 3.2, step 13) and grow in 200 mL of 2xYT-Amp-Glu at 37°C and 220 rpm until the cell culture density reaches an $A_{600\ nm}$ of 0.5 (2–3 h). Infect the cells with a 20× excess of M13KO7 helper phage (2×10^{12} plaque-forming units, pfu) for 1 h at 37°C. Pellet the infected cells by centrifugation at 5,000 ×*g* for 10 min at 4°C. Resuspend the pellets in 200 mL of 2xYT-Amp-Kan and grow overnight at 37°C and 250 rpm.

18. To purify the phage, pellet the overnight culture (10,000 ×*g*, 15 min, 4°C), filter the supernatant through a 0.2 μm filter unit, then add 1/5 the volume of PEG/NaCl to the filtrate. Incubate for 1 h on ice, centrifuge as above and discard the supernatant. Resuspend the pelleted phage in 1.5 mL of sterile PBS, determine its titer (see Notes 19 and 20) and store at -80°C. Use the purified phage as the input phage for round 1 of library screening.

3.3. VHH Phage Display Library Screening

In this step, the library is screened for phage displaying VHHs with specificity to rTcdA or rTcdB. A phage ELISA is then performed to identify individual phage displaying VHHs specific to whole TcdA or TcdB toxins.

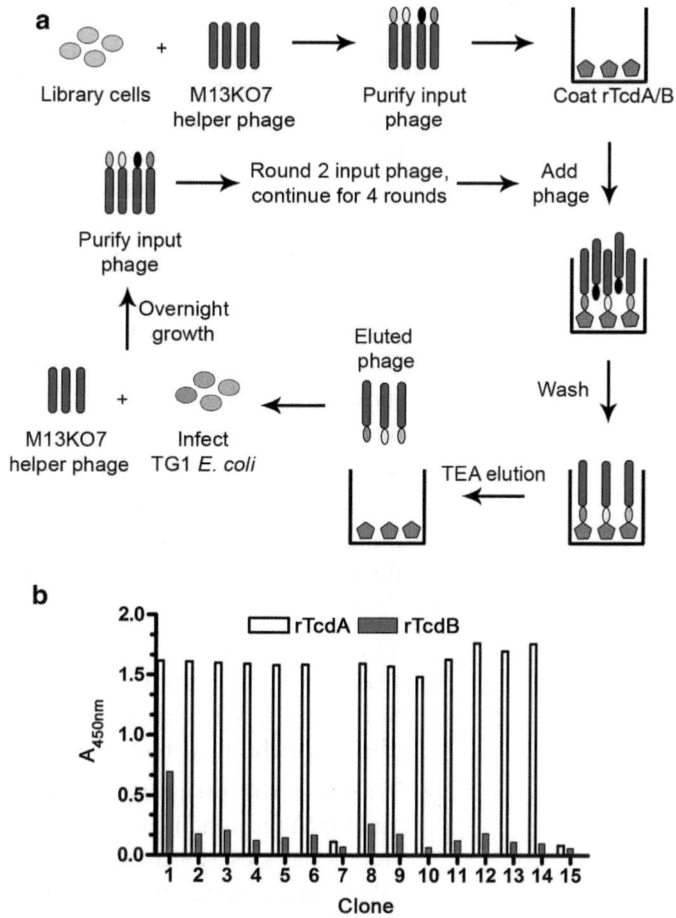

Fig. 2. Overview of the phage display library screening procedure. (**a**) Phage displaying VHHs were screened against rTcdA and rTcdB to isolate toxin-specific VHHs. By screening with the recombinant toxin fragments, selection was driven for binders that target the C-terminal cell receptor binding domains of the toxins. Four rounds of selection were performed in total. After selection, VHHs were screened by phage ELISA (**b**) with positive, unique binders subcloned into high-yielding expression vectors. *TEA* triethylamine. (**b**) The specificity of several VHH-displaying phages obtained by panning against rTcdA was evaluated by phage ELISA.

1. Begin panning (see Fig. 2a) by coating a 96-well microtiter plate with 20 μg of recombinant rTcdA or rTcdB fragments (100 μL/well diluted in PBS) overnight at 4°C.
2. Remove the contents of the coated wells the next day, wash with 300 μL of PBS and block for 2 h at 37°C with 200 μL/well of Buffer B. Start preparing 10 mL of exponentially growing TG1 cells in a sterile 50-mL Falcon tube (see Note 19).
3. Remove the blocking buffer and add ~10^{12} input phage (see Subheading 3.2, step 18) in 100 μL of PBS to the blocked wells for 2 h at 37°C. Remove unbound phage, wash 10× with

PBS-T (300 μL per wash), and elute the bound phage by incubating with 0.1 M triethylamine (100 μL/well) for exactly 10 min at room temperature. Pipette the elution solution up and down several times in the well, remove the contents and neutralize with 50 μL of 1 M Tris–HCl, pH 7.4, in a separate tube. Keep the tube on ice.

4. Keep 100 μL of the exponentially growing TG1 cells (see Subheading 3.3, step 2) for the negative control titer (see below) and infect the remaining with 100 μL of the eluted phage by incubating the mixture of the two at 37°C for 15 min without shaking and for 1 h with shaking at 220 rpm (store the remaining phage at −80°C for future reference). Titrate the infected cells (see Note 21).
5. Superinfect the infected bacterial cells (approximately 10 mL) with 10^{11} pfu of M13KO7 helper phage as described (see Subheading 3.3, step 4). Subsequently, add kanamycin at a final concentration of 50 μg/mL and incubate overnight at 37°C and 250 rpm.
6. The next day, purify the phage in a final volume of 200 μL of PBS and determine the phage titer as described (see Subheading 3.2, step 18). Use the purified phage as the input phage for the next round of panning.
7. To assess the progress of the panning, perform colony-PCR and DNA sequencing on titer plate colonies (see Subheading 3.3, step 4) as described (see Subheading 3.2, steps 15 and 16). (We usually sequence 15–20 clones in each of the first two rounds, 25 clones in the third round, and 50–100 clones in the fourth round).
8. Repeat the panning process (see Subheading 3.3, steps 1–7) for three more rounds using the amplified phage from the previous round (see Subheading 3.3, step 6) as the input phage for the next round and reduce the amount of coated antigen by 5 μg for each subsequent round (e.g., 15 μg of rTcdA or rTcdB in round 2).

   After four rounds of selection (see Fig. 2a), a phage ELISA (see Fig. 2b) is performed on colonies containing unique VHH DNA sequences (determined by colony-PCR and sequencing (see Subheading 3.3, step 7) to identify toxin-binding VHH phages. In the phage ELISA, the binding of VHH-displaying phages to toxins is detected colorimetrically by adding a secondary anti-phage antibody-HRP conjugate and HRP substrate.
9. Coat microtiter wells with toxin (TcdA or TcdB), recombinant fragments (rTcdA or rTcdB) and BSA as described (see Subheading 3.1, step 10).
10. Aliquot 1 mL of 2xYT-Amp-Glu into sterile 15-mL Falcon tubes. Add a small colony of TG1 cells containing the

VHH-phagemid (that was previously screened by colony-PCR and DNA sequencing). Grow the cell culture at 37°C and 250 rpm until the $A_{600\ nm}$ of the culture reaches 0.5. Next, infect the cells with 10^{10} pfu of M13KO7, add kanamycin and then grow overnight as described (see Subheading 3.3, step 5).

11. The next day, block each well with Buffer B as described (see Subheading 3.1, step 11).
12. While blocking, spin down the overnight cultures at 10,000 × *g* for 20 min in microtubes at 4°C. Carefully remove the supernatant which contains the VHH-displaying phage particles and decant into new microtubes. Keep on ice.
13. Remove the blocking agent, wash each well with PBS-T (5 × 300 μL) and pat dry. Add 100 μL/well of phage supernatants (see Subheading 3.3, step 12) to the appropriate wells. Include a negative control well in duplicate with 10^9 M13KO7 helper phage replacing the phage supernatant. Incubate the wells for 1.5 h at room temperature.
14. Remove unbound phage particles and wash with PBS-T (6 × 300 μL). Add 100 μL/well of anti-M13 IgG-HRP conjugate (previously diluted 1:5,000 in PBS) and incubate for 1 h at room temperature.
15. Discard the unbound anti-M13 IgG-HRP and proceed with 6× PBS-T washes and addition of HRP substrate (see Subheading 3.1, step 15).
16. Store the ELISA-positive phages (see Subheading 3.3, step 12) at −20°C for future reference.

A phage ELISA, shown in Fig. 2b, was conducted on 15 phage populations displaying unique VHHs that were isolated from rTcdA-based selection. Of the 15 phage populations analyzed, 12 recognized rTcdA specifically, 1 (clone 1) cross-reacted with rTcdB and 2 showed no binding to either target. A similar binding pattern was seen for these phages against whole TcdA and TcdB (data not shown).

3.4. VHH Subcloning, Soluble Expression, and Purification

Upon positive identification of TcdA- or TcdB-binding phages by phage ELISA, VHH fragments are subcloned into an expression vector, expressed, and purified for characterization. While it is an option to express VHHs in pMED1 phagemid vector in an amber non-suppressor *E. coli* strain, we prefer to subclone our VHHs in our dedicated expression vector for higher protein expression yields.

1. To subclone positive VHH binders for soluble expression, amplify the VHH gene directly from TG1 colonies containing the VHH gene in the pMED1 phagemid vector by colony-PCR (see Subheading 3.2, step 15) in a total volume of 50 μL

using either the BbsI-VHH or BbsI2-VHH framework 1-specific primer and BamHI-VHH framework 4-specific primer (see Note 22). Analyze a small amount of the PCR reaction by 1% agarose gel, looking for the correct size of 400–450 bp. Purify the PCR fragment with a QIAquick PCR Purification™ kit and determine its concentration.

2. Digest the purified VHH DNA and pSJF2H vector with *Bbs*I as follows (see Note 23):

VHH fragment or pSJF2H	80 ng or 500 ng, respectively
10× *Bbs*I buffer	10 μL
*Bbs*I (5 units/μL)	5 μL
ddH_2O	Add to 100 μL

Incubate the reactions at 37°C for 12 h. Purify the digested fragment or vector with a QIAquick PCR Purification™ kit and determine its concentration.

3. Digest the purified *Bbs*I-digested fragment or vector with *Bam*HI as follows:

VHH fragment or pSJF2H	60 ng or 400 ng, respectively
10× *Bam*HI buffer	10 μL
*Bam*HI (10 units/μL)	2 μL (fragment) or 6 μL (vector)
ddH_2O	Add to 100 μL

Incubate, purify, and determine the concentration as above (see Subheading 3.4, step 2).

4. Ligate the *Bbs*I/*Bam*HI digested insert (fragment) and vector as follows:

Digested pSJF2H	100 ng
Digested insert	20 ng
10× ligase buffer	0.5 μL
T4 DNA ligase (5 units/μL)	0.5 μL
ddH_2O	Add to 5 μL

Include a vector-only control reaction mixture where insert is replaced with ddH_2O. Incubate reaction mixtures at room temperature for 2 h.

5. Transform 50 μL of electrocompetent TG1 *E. coli* cells with 1.2 μL of ligation reaction (~30 ng DNA) as described (see Subheading 3.2, step 10). Following incubation in SOC medium, spread 50 μL of cells on prewarmed LB-Amp plates, and incubate overnight at 32°C (see Note 24).

6. The next day, count the number of colonies on LB-Amp plates, including control ligation/transformation reactions containing vector-only (see Note 25). Perform 5–10 colony-PCRs to screen for colonies with inserts as described (see Subheading 3.2, step 15) using the primer pair M13FP and M13RP. Use the same P10 pipette tip which was used to introduce colonies into the PCR reaction tubes to make a reference plate of the colonies being screened (see Note 26).
7. Analyze 5 μL of each PCR reaction on a 1% agarose gel to identify clones with insert (≅600 bp) or without insert (≅200 bp). Sequence as described (see Subheading 3.2, step 16).
8. After sequencing and identification of positive clones, refer to the reference plate (see Subheading 3.4, step 6) and prepare permanent stocks of the positive clones for long-term storage at −80°C (see Note 27). Regularly re-streak the clones on LB-Amp plates for short term storage at 4°C.
9. Express and purify the VHHs by immobilized metal-affinity chromatography (IMAC) (see Chapter 16).
10. Analyze purified VHHs by size exclusion chromatography (see Chapter 21).

Expressed VHHs were purified to homogeneity, as shown by SDS-PAGE and size exclusion chromatography analyses (see Fig. 3a, b), with yields as high as 105 mg/L of bacterial culture. Size exclusion chromatography analysis also reveals that the VHHs—as expected—are non-aggregating.

3.5. VHH Specificity and Affinity Profiling by Soluble ELISA and SPR Measurements

ELISA and SPR are used here to characterize the specificity and affinity of the isolated antitoxin VHHs. In the ELISA, purified VHHs are analyzed for their cross reactivity with nonspecific proteins (including the *C. difficile* toxin the antibodies were not raised against), as well as their specificity for the recombinant toxin fragments. The affinity of the VHHs binding to toxins A and B is then determined with SPR. Gel filtration is performed immediately prior to SPR to ensure only monomeric VHH species are used for SPR analysis.

As VHHs are fused to C-terminal His_6 tags, their binding to toxins is detected colorimetrically by adding a secondary anti-His_6 antibody-HRP conjugate and HRP substrate:

1. Coat 96-well microtiter plates with BSA, TcdA, rTcdA fragment, TcdB, and rTcdB fragment and subsequently block with Buffer C as described (see Subheading 3.1, steps 10 and 11).
2. Add the purified VHHs to the wells and serial dilute them in PBS from a starting concentration of 10 μg/mL (using 100 μL/well), leaving the last well with an equivalent volume of PBS. Incubate the VHHs for 1 h at 37°C.

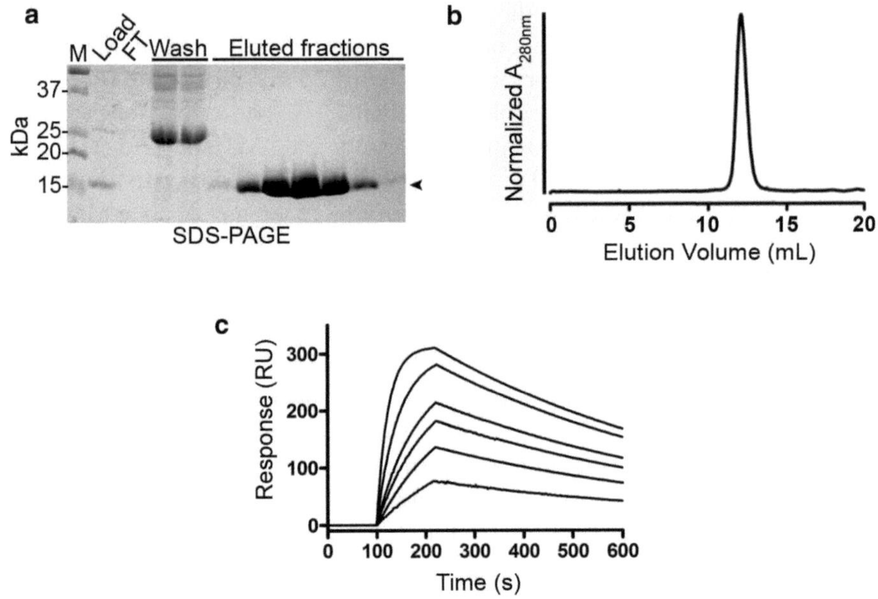

Fig. 3. Purification and activity profiling of antitoxin VHHs. (**a**) Non-reducing SDS-PAGE illustrating the IMAC purification profile of a TcdB-specific VHH that was expressed using the method described in the text. Soluble VHH expression is targeted to the *E.coli* periplasm in the pSJF2H expression vector. M: protein molecular weight marker; Load: sample of periplasmic extraction before loading onto the IMAC column; FT: sample of IMAC column flow-through after loading; Wash: sample wash fractions collected from the IMAC column; Eluted fractions: eluted VHH fractions from the IMAC column. The *arrow* indicates the purified VHH. (**b**) Size exclusion chromatography analysis of a TcdA-specific VHH reveals a single, monomeric peak indicating the VHH is non-aggregating. (**c**) SPR analysis illustrating the high affinity binding of a VHH to TcdA.

3. Wash the wells with PBS-T (5×300 μL) and incubate them with 100 μL of rabbit anti-His$_6$ IgG conjugated to HRP (previously diluted 1:2,500 in PBS) for 1 h at room temperature.
4. Proceed as described (see Subheading 3.1, step 15) (see Note 28).

   Since the selected VHHs have been raised against recombinant TcdA or TcdB fragments, this ELISA is critical to ensure the VHHs also recognize full-length native toxins from *C. difficile*. This indeed was the case, as all VHHs that bound the recombinant toxin fragments (i.e., rTcdA or rTcdB) also bound the corresponding whole toxin (i.e., TcdA or TcdB), indicating the toxin fragments were a good choice of antigen (data not shown).
5. Before SPR analysis, collect monomeric VHH peaks from a gel filtration column (see Fig. 3b). Protocols for size exclusion chromatography are described in another chapter in this volume (see Chapter 21).
6. Perform SPR affinity measurements at 25°C using a BIACORE 3000 or equivalent instrument. Begin by immobilizing approximately 10,000 response units (RUs) of purified *C. difficile*

TcdA on a CM5 sensorchip (see Fig. 3c, see Note 29). Protocols for the coupling of target proteins to CM5 dextran surfaces and SPR data collection are described in Chapter 27.

7. For TcdB, immobilize the anti-TcdB VHHs directly on sensorchips and flow purified TcdB over to collect affinity data (see Note 30).

SPR analysis illustrating the high affinity binding of a VHH to TcdA is shown in Fig. 3c. The SPR sensorgram was generated by injecting 50, 25, 12.5, 9.38, 6.25, and 3.13 nM concentrations of VHH over immobilized TcdA. At this point VHHs should be further characterized for toxin-neutralizing capacity (15) if the desired application is for *C. difficile* therapy.

3.6. Probing the Conformational Nature of VHH Epitopes

Western blotting and heat-denaturing ELISA are two relatively simple methods that can be used to determine if the isolated anti-toxin VHHs recognize linear or conformational epitopes.

To gain insight into the nature of the VHH epitopes, purified TcdA or TcdB are separated under native-PAGE or reducing SDS-PAGE conditions and probed with various VHHs in Western blotting. Binding of His_6-tagged VHHs to toxins is detected colorimetrically by adding the His_6 tag-specific Nickel-AP conjugate and AP substrate:

1. For denaturing SDS-PAGE, prepare a 12.5% SDS-PAGE gel and load the following samples: TcdA or TcdB (0.75 μg/lane), control VHH (1 μg/lane), PCG4 IgG control (1 μg/lane), and molecular weight marker (see Note 31). All samples are boiled for 10 min in 3× SDS-PAGE sample buffer containing DTT before loading.
2. Run the gel at 200 V for 1 h before transferring to a PVDF membrane at 100 V for 1 h. Block the PVDF membrane with Buffer A for 1 h at room temperature.
3. Probe the blots by incubating with purified VHH (25 μg/mL diluted in Buffer A) or PCG4 IgG (10 μg/mL diluted in Buffer A) for 1 h at room temperature.
4. Wash the blot with PBS-T for 5 min (3 × 25 mL) before adding either HisDetector™ Nickel-AP conjugate (diluted previously 1:5,000 in Buffer A) to blots probed with VHHs, or goat anti-mouse IgG-AP conjugate (diluted previously 1:10,000 in Buffer A) to blots probed with PCG4 for 1 h at room temperature.
5. Wash the blot as above and incubate with the AP substrate (10 mL/blot) for 10 min at room temperature (see Note 28).
6. For native-PAGE blots, prepare an 8% PAGE gel (without adding SDS) and load the same samples described above. Samples for native-PAGE analysis are diluted in 3× sample buffer (without SDS and DTT) and are not heated prior to loading.

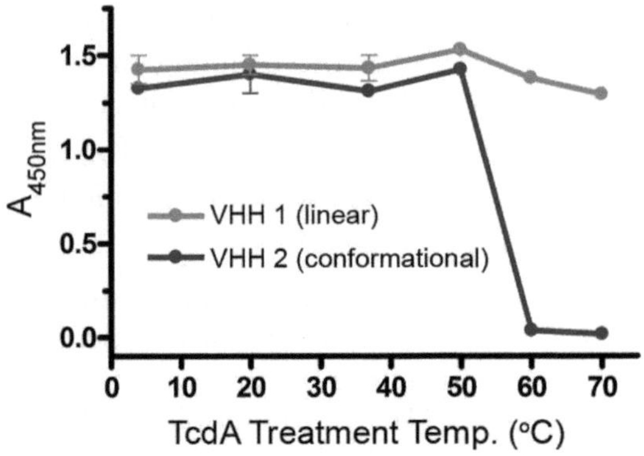

Fig. 4. Heat-denaturing ELISA demonstrating the binding profiles of two VHHs to differentially heat-treated TcdA. VHHs that retain binding to denatured TcdA (exposed to temperatures above 55°C, the T_m of TcdA) are considered to recognize a linear epitope on TcdA (e.g., VHH 1). VHHs that lose binding to denatured TcdA are considered to recognize a conformational epitope on TcdA (e.g., VHH 2).

7. Run the gel at 100 V for 2 h at 4°C. Transfer the gel to a PVDF membrane at 20 V for 14–16 h at 4°C.
8. Block and probe membranes in the exact same way as for reducing SDS-PAGE blots described above (see Note 32).

   Under denaturing Western blot conditions, VHHs that bind a linear TcdA epitope will produce a signal at approximately 300–310 kDa. No signal will be generated from antibodies recognizing conformational epitopes under denaturing conditions. Under native Western blot conditions, VHHs recognizing a conformational TcdA epitope will produce a positive signal. Linear epitope-binding VHHs should also produce a signal under native conditions.

   Another method to determine the nature of the VHH epitopes is to expose TcdA or TcdB to various temperatures above and below their thermal midpoint unfolding temperatures (T_ms) (see Note 33). Heated toxin samples are then coated on 96-well ELISA plates and probed with purified VHHs (see Note 34).
9. To perform the heat-denaturation ELISA (Fig. 4), aliquot TcdA or TcdB (5 μg/mL) into seven microtubes and expose the toxins to the following temperatures for 30 min: 4, 20, 37, 50, 60, 70, or 80°C.
10. After heating, add the heat-treated toxins to 96-well microtiter plates (100 μL/well) and coat overnight at 4°C.
11. The next day, remove the unbound toxin, block with Buffer C for 2 h at room temperature and probe with purified VHHs (0.05–1 μg/mL) for 1 h at room temperature.

12. Following PBS-T washes (5 × 300 μL), add rabbit anti-His_6 IgG-HRP (previously diluted 1:2,500 in PBS) for 1 h at room temperature.
13. Proceed as described (see Subheading 3.1, step 15) (see Note 28).

If VHHs recognize conformational epitopes, binding to TcdA or TcdB will be abolished above 55 or 70°C (the approximate T_ms of TcdA and TcdB, respectively). Conversely, VHHs capable of binding TcdA or TcdB above these temperatures suggests the VHH recognizes a linear epitope. The TcdA heat-denaturation ELISA in Fig. 4 illustrates two TcdA-binding VHHs that recognize either a linear or conformational epitope. Together with the native and denaturing Western blot analyses, the conformational nature of the TcdA or TcdB epitope can be determined. For example, the linear epitope-binding VHH 1 in Fig. 4 bound to heat-denatured TcdA and detected TcdA in a Western blot run under both denaturing and native conditions. On the other hand, the conformational epitope-binding VHH 2 did not bind heat-denatured TcdA by ELISA or chemically denatured TcdA by Western blot, but did bind to TcdA in a Western blot run under native conditions (data not shown).

4. Notes

1. We typically use Millipore's (Millipore, Cambridge, ON, Canada) 0.2 μm MILLEx®-GV filter units for sterilizing small volumes and 0.2 μm GP Express™ Plus Membrane filtration systems for sterilizing large volumes.
2. Recombinant toxins encompassing a fragment of the C-terminal cell receptor binding domain of each toxin were expressed with N-terminal His_6 tags, purified by immobilized metal-affinity chromatography and stored in PBS at 4°C (15). The rTcdA fragment is approximately 43 kDa in size spanning amino acid residues 2304–2710 of TcdA. The rTcdB fragment is approximately 10 kDa in size, spanning residues 2286–2366 of TcdB.
3. *C. difficile* toxin A and toxin B were purified from *C. difficile* strain 10463, according to the protocol described by Keel and Songer (28), and stored in 50 mM Tris–HCl, pH 7.5, at 4°C. Toxin A and toxin B should be treated as Biosafety Level 2 (BL2) agents and disposed of accordingly.
4. Before immunizing any animals, ensure animal-use permits are approved and followed. Immunization of the male llama used in this study was approved by the National Research Council

Canada Animal Care Committee. The male llama used for immunization was in good health, as determined by a veterinarian, and given food and water ad libitum.

5. Prepare the primer solutions in autoclaved ddH_2O and always store at −20°C to prevent their degradation. We typically prepare a 100× (100 pmol/μL) stock solution and 10× working solutions in 100 μL aliquots.
6. We always elute the bound DNA with sterile ddH_2O as opposed to the manufacturer's recommended elution buffer.
7. In contrast to a conventional spectrophotometer, the ND-1000 spectrophotometer (or instruments with similar technology) measures absorbance at very low volumes (1 μL) and without the use of cuvettes.
8. To make a stock plate of *E. coli* TG1 cells, streak out a frozen stock of TG1 on a minimal plate (24) supplemented with thiamine. Incubate at 37°C for at least 24 h. Seal the plate with parafilm and store at 4°C for up to a month. It is recommended to grow the TG1 cells on minimal media to ensure that the F pilus, which mediates phage infection, is maintained on the cells. Thiamine is added to the media since TG1 cells are auxotrophic for thiamine.
9. If feasible, use two llamas for immunization, as the quality of the immune response is individual dependent.
10. With proteins as immunogen we typically obtain both conventional IgG type and hcIgG type responses.
11. If a positive response is generated from the IgG2a/b/c fraction, but not from the hcIgG3 fraction, make sure that the response in the IgG2a/b/c fraction is not from contaminating IgM species.
12. It may sometimes be necessary to optimize the amount of input RNA, but generally 3–5 μg total RNA per cDNA synthesis reaction results in a good yield of synthesized DNA by RT-PCR.
13. Three bands are obtained following RT-PCR: one with a size of ≅850 bp, which correspond to conventional antibodies, and two intimately close bands with sizes in the range of 550–650 bp, which correspond to heavy-chain antibodies and contain the VHH genes. Others have reported similar banding patterns (29). We frequently observe that CH2B3-F primer gives a banding pattern which consists of an intense VHH band and a faint conventional antibody band. The aim of optimizing the PCR reaction is to increase the intensity of the VHH bands relative to the conventional antibody band. However, differential intensities of the two VHH bands with respect to each other are routinely observed on agarose gels.

Ideally, the PCR may be optimized in six separate reactions, each utilizing a unique primer pair.

14. With a ligation of this magnitude, library sizes of around 10^8 should be obtained. When larger size libraries are required, as in the case for synthetic and naïve libraries, it is advisable to first identify the ligation conditions which give the biggest library size. This can be done by performing small scale ligations with different total input DNA and molar ratios of insert to vector. Moreover, the scale of the ligation and the number of transformations needs to be significantly increased. In the case of naïve libraries, the amount of input blood, taken from several individuals, should also be increased as it is the number of antibody-displaying B cells that determines the actual library diversity.
15. One may additionally store the library as a purified library vector prep.
16. With typical PCR yields, a 0.5 μL aliquot can be used directly for DNA sequencing that will give clean sequencing profiles. In instances where the sequencing profile is not readable, purify the PCR product with a QIAquick PCR Purification™ kit before proceeding with DNA sequencing.
17. One primer gives enough sequencing read coverage and thus it is not necessary to use both reverse and forward primers for DNA sequencing.
18. VHHs can be distinguished from contaminating VHs by the nature of the amino acids at positions 37, 44, 45, and 47 (Kabat numbering system (30)). VHHs characteristically have Phe or Tyr, Glu or Gln, Arg or Cys and Gly, Ser, Leu or Phe at positions 37, 44, 45, and 47, respectively, whereas VHs have Val, Gly, Leu, and Trp at these four positions.
19. Prepare exponentially growing TG1 cells by inoculating a 2–3 mL of 2xYT medium in a sterile 15-mL Falcon tube with a single colony from a stock plate of *E. coli* TG1 cells (see Note 8). Incubate at 37°C in a rotary bacterial shaker at 220 rpm. Remove aliquots from the culture flask at different time intervals and measure the $A_{600\ nm}$ in a spectrophotometer in disposable cuvettes using 2xYT as the blank. Stop the incubation at $A_{600\ nm} = 0.4–0.5$ (2–3 h).
20. To determine the titer of the phage, make 10^6, 10^8, 10^{10}, and 10^{12} serial dilutions of phage in PBS, mix 10 μL of each dilution with 100 μL of the exponentially growing TG1 cells (see Note 19). Incubate the cells at room temperature for 15 min and subsequently plate them on 2xYT-Amp medium. In the morning count the colonies and determine the titer. Phage titers are typically $1 \times 10^{13}–5 \times 10^{13}$ colony-forming units/mL.

21. To titrate the infected cells, make serial dilutions (10^{-2}–10^{-6}) of the infected cells in 2xYT in 500 μL volumes. Spread 100 μL of each dilution on 2xYT-Amp plates. Also plate 100 μL of the uninfected cells as a negative control. Incubate at 32°C overnight and count the colonies in the morning to determine the titer. Keep the plates parafilm-sealed and stored at 4°C for clonal analysis (colony-PCR, sequencing and phage ELISA).
22. The choice of framework 1-specific primer, BbsI-VHH or BbsI2-VHH (see Table 1), depends on the nucleotide sequence of the VHH's 5′ end.
23. For subcloning into the expression vector pSJF2H, we routinely digest the vector and amplified VHH sequences with *Bbs*I and *Bam*HI. In some cases, we have found VHH sequences which contain internal *Bbs*I or *Bam*HI restriction sites. Instead of mutating these sites, cleavage of the VHH gene from the pMED1 phagemid with *Sfi*I restriction enzyme allows for subcloning into the pMED2 expression vector, which is a pSJF2H-based vector with *Sfi*I sites in the multiple cloning site. Digestion of pMED2 with *Sfi*I facilitates ligation of *Sfi*I-digested VHH fragments. In this case when the VHH contains *Bbs*I or *Bam*HI internal sites, the colony-PCR (see Subheading 3.4, step 1) is not required.
24. With TG1 *E. coli*, we incubate plates at 32°C as opposed to 37°C to avoid the formation of satellite colonies. As a result of a lower incubation temperature, a longer incubation time may be necessary for the appearance of visible colonies on the plate.
25. Plates of control transformants (vector-only) should yield fewer colonies than plates of transformants with ligated insert and vector. If the control plate contains as many colonies as the test plate, one or both of the restriction enzymes may not have cut the vector. Redigest the vector with each enzyme and perform a diagnostic DNA gel to confirm digestion. In addition, dephosphorylation of the vector will prevent self ligation.
26. To make a colony reference plate, touch the surface of an LB-Amp plate with sterile 10 μL micropipette tip containing a small amount of colony to form spots. Label the spots for each clone, and incubate the plate over night at 32°C. In the morning, seal the plate airtight with parafilm and store at 4°C for later reference.
27. To prepare a permanent stock of a clone, touch the respective colony on the reference plate with a disposable inoculation loop and swirl the loop in 2 mL of LB-Amp medium in a sterile 15-mL Falcon tube. Incubate the culture at 37°C and 230 rpm for 20 h. Add 0.7 mL of the bacterial culture and 0.3 mL of sterile 50% glycerol to a sterile cryogenic vial. Vortex briefly to mix and store at −80°C.

28. A false negative signal may be due to the absence of His_6 tag. Occasionally, VHHs lose their His_6 tags following a few months of storage at 4°C.
29. Approximately 10,000 RUs of *C. difficile* TcdA were immobilized on a CM5 dextran sensorchip by injecting 30 μL of TcdA (~1 mg/mL) at 5 μL/min diluted in 10 mM acetate buffer, pH 4.0. Before injection the chip is activated with 35 μL of EDC/NHS (5 μL/min flow rate) and following immobilization the chip was blocked with 35 μL of 1 M ethanolamine, pH 8.5, injected at 5 μL/min. For all buffer recipes and SPR immobilization and data-collection protocols, refer to Chapter 27.
30. Due to the low theoretical pI of TcdB, we have consistently had problems immobilizing this protein on CM5 dextran sensorchips. As a result, the VHH should be immobilized directly onto the sensorchip for all TcdB-binding studies.
31. The anti-TcdA IgG PCG4 is used as a control antibody in denaturing Western blots since it recognizes a linear TcdA epitope.
32. Under native-PAGE conditions, we have found a number of monoclonal antibodies, including mouse anti-His_6 IgG-AP and goat anti-mouse IgG-AP, to bind non-specifically to TcdA in Western blots (15), presumably through their glycosylated CH1 regions. To overcome this problem of nonspecific binding in native blots, probe VHH binding to TcdA with a Nickel-AP conjugate. The aforementioned nonspecific binding does not occur under denaturing SDS-PAGE conditions.
33. The reported melting temperatures of TcdA and TcdB at physiological pH are approximately 50–55°C and 65–70°C, respectively (31).
34. It is highly recommended to include a linear epitope-binding antibody, e.g., PCG4, which would recognize both linear and conformational epitopes.
35. The DNA degenerate alphabet. S: G or C; M: A or C; K: G or T.

Acknowledgments

We thank Glenn Songer and Hien Trinh (Iowa State University) for providing us with purified *C. difficile* toxins and preparing the recombinant toxin fragments. The authors declare no financial conflict of interest.

References

1. Wesolowski J et al (2009) Single domain antibodies: promising experimental and therapeutic tools in infection and immunity. Med Microbiol Immunol 198:157–174
2. Stewart CS, MacKenzie CR, Hall JC (2007) Isolation, characterization and pentamerization of alpha-cobrotoxin specific single-domain antibodies from a naïve phage display library: preliminary findings for antivenom development. Toxicon 49:699–709
3. Stone E et al (2007) A novel pentamer versus pentamer approach to generating neutralizers of verotoxin 1. Mol Immunol 44:2487–2491
4. Hmila I et al (2008) VHH, bivalent domains and chimeric heavy chain-only antibodies with high neutralizing efficacy for scorpion toxin AahI′. Mol Immunol 45:3847–3856
5. Hmila I et al (2010) A bispecific nanobody to provide full protection against lethal scorpion envenoming. FASEB J 24:3479–3489
6. Goldman ER et al (2008) Thermostable llama single domain antibodies for detection of botulinum A neurotoxin complex. Anal Chem 80:8583–8591
7. Conway JO et al (2010) Llama single domain antibodies specific for the 7 botulinum neurotoxin serotypes as heptaplex immunoreagents. PLoS One 5:e8818
8. Dong J et al (2010) A single-domain llama antibody potently inhibits the enzymatic activity of botulinum neurotoxin by binding to the non-catalytic alpha-exosite binding region. J Mol Biol 397:1106–1118
9. Goldman ER et al (2006) Facile generation of heat-stable antiviral and antitoxin single domain antibodies from a semisynthetic llama library. Anal Chem 78:8245–8255
10. Adams H et al (2009) Specific immuno capturing of the staphylococcal superantigen toxin-shock syndrome toxin-1 in plasma. Biotechnol Bioeng 104:143–151
11. Harmsen MM, van Solt CB, Fijten HP (2009) Enhancement of toxin- and virus-neutralizing capacity of single-domain antibody fragments by N-glycosylation. Appl Microbiol Biotechnol 84:1087–1094
12. Koch-Nolte F et al (2007) Single domain antibodies from llama effectively and specifically block T cell ecto-ADP-ribosyltransferase ART2.2 in vivo. FASEB J 21:3490–3498
13. Alzogaray V et al (2010) Single-domain llama antibodies as specific intracellular inhibitors of SpvB, the actin ADP-ribosylating toxin of *Salmonella typhimurium*. FASEB J 25:526–534
14. Anderson GP et al (2007) Multiplexed fluid array screening of phage displayed anti-ricin single domain antibodies for rapid assessment of specificity. Biotechniques 43: 806–811
15. Hussack G et al (2011) Neutralization of *Clostridium difficile* toxin A with single-domain antibodies targeting the cell receptor binding domain. J Biol Chem 286:8961–8976.
16. Rupnik M, Wilcox MH, Gerding DN (2009) *Clostridium difficile* infection: new developments in epidemiology and pathogenesis. Nat Rev Microbiol 7:526–536
17. Lowy I et al (2010) Treatment with monoclonal antibodies against *Clostridium difficile* toxins. N Engl J Med 362:197–205
18. Hussack G, Tanha J (2010) Toxin-specific antibodies for the treatment of *Clostridium difficile*: current status and future perspectives. Toxins 2:998–1018
19. Demarest SJ et al (2010) Neutralization of *Clostridium difficile* toxin A using antibody combinations. MAbs 2:1–9
20. Arbabi-Ghahroudi M, MacKenzie R, Tanha J (2009) Selection of non-aggregating V_H binders from synthetic V_H phage-display libraries. Methods Mol Biol 525:187–216
21. Nguyen VK, Desmyter A, Muyldermans S (2001) Functional heavy-chain antibodies in *Camelidae*. Adv Immunol 79:261–296
22. Doyle PJ et al (2008) Cloning, expression, and characterization of a single-domain antibody fragment with affinity for 15-acetyl-deoxynivalenol. Mol Immunol 45:3703–3713
23. De Simone E et al (2006) Immunochemical analysis of IgG subclasses and IgM in South American camelids. Small Ruminant Res 64:2–9
24. Sambrook J, Fritsch EF, Maniatis T (eds) (1989) Molecular cloning: a laboratory manual. Cold Spring Harbor Laboratory, Cold Spring Harbor, NY
25. Tung WL, Chow KC (1995) A modified medium for efficient electrotransformation of *E. coli*. Trends Genet 11:128–129
26. Muyldermans S, Cambillau C, Wyns L (2001) Recognition of antigens by single-domain antibody fragments: the superfluous luxury of paired domains. Trends Biochem Sci 26: 230–235
27. Harmsen MM et al (2000) Llama heavy-chain V regions consist of at least four distinct subfamilies revealing novel sequence features. Mol Immunol 37:579–590

28. Keel MK, Songer JG (2007) The distribution and density of *Clostridium difficile* toxin receptors on the intestinal mucosa of neonatal pigs. Vet Pathol 44:814–822
29. Arbabi Ghahroudi M et al (1997) Selection and identification of single domain antibody fragments from camel heavy-chain antibodies. FEBS Lett 414:521–526
30. Kabat EA et al (eds) (1991) Sequences of proteins of immunological interest. US Department of Health and Human Services, US Public Health Service, Bethesda, MD
31. Salnikova MS et al (2008) Physical characterization of *Clostridium difficile* toxins and toxoids: effect of the formaldehyde crosslinking on thermal stability. J Pharm Sci 97:3735–3752

Chapter 15

Selection of VHH Antibody Fragments That Recognize Different Aβ Depositions Using Complex Immune Libraries

Rinse Klooster, Kim S. Rutgers, and Silvère M. van der Maarel

Abstract

Phage display technology is frequently used to obtain antigen specific binders with predetermined characteristics. Phage display libraries are often constructed from animals immunized with the antigen of interest. An important point of consideration when making immune libraries is the availability of an appropriate antigen sources. When available, often either the amount is not sufficient for immunization or it is expensive to obtain. To overcome this problem, these antigens are typically obtained by over expression in prokaryotic or eukaryotic expression systems. While this could solve the problem of obtaining sufficient quantities of antigen for a reasonable price and effort, correct folding and differences in posttranslational modification could potentially lead to binders that recognize the recombinant, but not the endogenous protein. In addition, selection of binders against specific modifications or structural epitopes could be missed.

In this chapter we describe a particular selection of VHH antibody fragments from phage display libraries that were constructed from llamas immunized with different complex protein samples containing the antigen of interest. We show that this can result in binders that preferentially recognize the target of interest when present in specific structures depending on the antigen source.

Key words: Complex immune libraries, Amyloid beta, VHH, Alzheimer, Antibody, Histochemistry, Immunoreactivity, Cerebral amyloid angiopathy

1. Introduction

Antibody phage display technology is a very powerful technique to select for antigen specific affinity binders from a library containing millions of different clones. These libraries are either constructed from nonimmunized or immunized animals (1–4), so-called non-immune or immune libraries, respectively. Nonimmune libraries have the advantage that the time consuming immunization and library construction protocols can be omitted for every new target. However, selections from nonimmune libraries are laborious and

Dirk Saerens and Serge Muyldermans (eds.), *Single Domain Antibodies: Methods and Protocols*, Methods in Molecular Biology, vol. 911, DOI 10.1007/978-1-61779-968-6_15, © Springer Science+Business Media, LLC 2012

often do not yield binders with the required characteristics. In general, selection of binders from immune libraries is more straightforward and typically leads to binders with higher affinities because of somatic hypermutation of VH and VL genes in B-cells during the immunization process. Therefore, immune libraries are often the library of choice when there is sufficient time and resources. The limiting factor however in many cases is the availability of a good antigen source especially when dealing with antigens from eukaryotic origin. Often antigens are not commercially available or in insufficient amounts, or expensive when available. As an alternative, animals can be immunized with recombinant proteins. Although this can lead to appropriate binders, this approach has several drawbacks. As the recombinant proteins or fragments thereof are often expressed in expression systems such as *Escherichia coli* (5, 6), they can be incorrectly folded or can lack proper post-translational modifications (7). This might lead to binders that are very potent in recognizing the recombinant protein, but are less able to bind the endogenous protein. Furthermore, contamination with components of the expression host, which can be very immunodominant, is not uncommon complicating the selections. Additionally, proteins are mostly present in large protein complexes that can have an effect on epitope availability, and on the presentation of unique protein complex related epitopes, which will not be present when the protein is expressed in a different expression host. Therefore, triggering a B-cell related immune response using complex protein samples of endogenous origin instead of a purified recombinant protein could lead to the generation of better, more biologically and functionally relevant antibodies. This can vary from the use of whole tissue homogenates or cell lysates to the use of enriched fractions, such as membrane fractions during the immunization process (8–10). As this approach results in an immune response against a wide variety of proteins present in this complex sample, the use of phage display techniques is invaluable to select the relevant binders.

In this case study we describe the selection of Alzheimer disease (AD) relevant beta-amyloid (Aβ) binders from two VHH immune phage display libraries (11). These libraries were generated by the immunization of *Llama glama* with either tissue homogenates of affected blood vessels from a hereditary cerebral hemorrhage with amyloidosis-Dutch type (HCHWA-D) patient, or gray matter from a Down Syndrome patient with confirmed parenchymal Aβ deposits. HCHWA-D is a genetic condition in which a point mutation in the APP1 gene leads to Aβ deposits in the cerebral vessel wall, cerebral amyloid angiopathy (CAA), and diffuse plaques in the cerebral parenchyma (12). Selection with the two different libraries resulted in VHH antibody fragments that have different binding properties in immunohistochemistry (IH) for parenchymal and vascular beta amyloid deposits, suggesting that these deposits are distinct in structure and/or consistence. This exemplifies the relevance of using complex protein samples as an alternative for purified protein samples as antigen source for obtaining biologically and functionally relevant affinity binders.

2. Materials

2.1. Preparation of Samples for Immunization

1. Liquid nitrogen.
2. Postmortem tissue material, obtained in line with the Code of Good Conduct, from Aβ-affected blood vessels of a HCHWA-D patient (Blood vessel library), and gray matter of a Down Syndrome patient with confirmed parenchymal Aβ deposits (Gray matter library) (see Note 1).
3. Mortar and pestle.
4. Round bottom 15 mL tube.
5. Ultra-Turrax T25 (IKA labortechnik, Staufen, Germany). Note that other similar homogenizers can be used.
6. 19G needle.
7. BCA protein assay kit (Pierce, Rockford, USA).

2.2. Production of Polyclonal VHH Antibody Fragments for Library Assessment in IH

1. TG1 phage display library.
2. LB medium: 1% (w/v) Tryptone, 0.5% (w/v) yeast extract, 1% (w/v) NaCl, pH 7.0.
3. 20% D-glucose.
4. 100 mg/mL ampicillin.
5. 2TY medium: 1.6% (w/v) Tryptone, 1% (w/v) yeast extract, 0.5% (w/v) NaCl, pH 7.0.
6. 1 M Isopropyl β-D-1-thiogalactopyranoside (IPTG).
7. p-Shock buffer: 1 M NaCl, 1 mM EDTA in PBS, pH 7.4.
8. Extraction buffer: 50 mM Sodium phosphate, 0.3 M NaCl, pH 7.0.
9. TALON resin (Clontech, Mountain View, USA).
10. Gravity flow column (Biorad, Veenendaal, The Netherlands).
11. Imidazole elution buffer: 50 mM sodium phosphate, 0.3 M NaCl, 150 mM imidazole, pH 7.0.
12. T1 membrane (Interchim, Monluçon Cedex, France).

2.3. Assessment of Library Specificity in IH

1. 5 μm thick frozen tissue sections.
2. Ice-cold acetone.
3. Peroxidase blocking reagent (Dako, Glostrup, Denmark).

4. BlockA buffer: 1% BSA in PBS.
5. Mouse anti-Myc (Roche, Woerden, The Netherlands).
6. EnVision+® system labeled Polymer-Hrp anti-Mouse (Dako, Glostrup, Denmark).
7. LiquidDAB + Substrate Chromogen System (Dako, Glostrup, Denmark).
8. Micromount mounting medium (Leica, Rijswijk, The Netherlands).
9. Olympus Provis AX70TF light microscope. Note that other similar light microscopes can be used.
10. Olympus digital DP12 camera. Note that other similar digital cameras can be used.

2.4. Selection of Aβ Binders

1. Polysorp 96 well plates (Nunc., Roskilde, Denmark).
2. Aβ (1–42) (rPeptide, Bogart, USA).
3. BlockB buffer: 4% marvel (skimmed milk powder) in PBS.
4. Phage stock of phage display library.
5. BlockC buffer: 4% marvel, 1% BSA in PBS.
6. TG1 cells.
7. LB agar: LB medium with 1.4% (w/v) agar, 7.5% (v/v) glycerol.
8. 20% D-glucose.
9. 100 mg/mL ampicillin.
10. PBST: 0.05% Tween20 in PBS.
11. Elution buffer: 100 mM triethylamine (TEA).
12. Neutralization buffer: 1 M Tris–HCl pH 7.5.
13. LB medium: 1% (w/v) Tryptone, 0.5% (w/v) yeast extract, 1% (w/v) NaCl, pH 7.0.

2.5. Screening and Characterization of Positive Clones

1. U-bottom 96 well plates (Nunc., Roskilde, Denmark).
2. LB medium: 1% (w/v) Tryptone, 0.5% (w/v) yeast extract, 1% (w/v) NaCl, pH 7.0.
3. 20% D-glucose.
4. 100 mg/mL ampicillin.
5. Glycerol.
6. V-bottom 96 well plates (Nunc., Roskilde, Denmark).
7. 2TY medium: 1.6% (w/v) Tryptone, 1% (w/v) yeast extract, 0.5% (w/v) NaCl, pH 7.0.
8. VCS M13 helper phage.

9. 50 mg/mL kanamycin.
10. Polysorp 96 well plates (Nunc., Roskilde, Denmark).
11. Aβ (1–42) (rPeptide, Bogart, USA).
12. BlockB buffer: 4% marvel (skimmed milk powder) in PBS.
13. PBST: 0.05% Tween20 in PBS.
14. HRP conjugated anti-M13 (GE Healthcare, Diegem, Belgium).
15. OPD solution: 3.7 mM *o*-phenylenediamine, 50 mM Na_2HPO_4, 25 mM citric acid, 0.03% (v/v) H_2O_2.
16. 1 M H_2SO_4.
17. Synergy HT microplate reader (Biotek, Winooski, VT). Note that other similar readers can be used.

3. Methods

3.1. Preparation of Samples for Immunization

1. Snap-freeze the tissue in liquid nitrogen directly after extraction and store at −80°C till further use.
2. Pulverize the tissue in liquid nitrogen using a mortar and pestle that are prechilled in −80°C freezer.
3. Transfer the powdered material to an ice-cold round-bottom 15 mL tube (see Note 2) and resuspend in sterile ice-cold PBS (see Note 3). Homogenize the tissue further using an Ultra-Turrax T25 for five times 5 s (see Note 4).
4. Pull sample three times through a 19G needle and subsequently spin down at 10,000 × *g* and 4°C for 10 min to separate the soluble from the insoluble fraction. Resuspend the insoluble fraction in an equal volume sterile PBS.
5. Determine the protein content of the soluble fraction using a BCA protein assay kit (see Note 5).
6. Snap-freeze the sample in liquid nitrogen and store at −80°C until the immunizations start.
7. Use each sample to immunize two animals (*Llama glama*) (see Note 6) every week, with six boosts in total. Approximately 12 mg of soluble protein sample was injected per boost, with an equivalent amount of the insoluble fraction (see Note 7). Extract peripheral blood lymphocytes 1 week after the last boost for phage display library generation. For library generation we would like to refer to Chapters 4 and 5. The maximal library size of both complex immune libraries was approximately 1×10^7.

3.2. Production of Polyclonal VHH Antibody Fragments for Library Assessment in IH

1. Produce soluble polyclonal VHH antibody fragments from the TG1 phage display libraries by inoculating 1×10^9 cells (see Note 8) in 50 mL of LB containing 2% D-glucose and 100 μg/mL ampicillin and grow overnight shaking at 37°C and 200 rpm.
2. Dilute the overnight culture 100 times in 500 mL of 2TY containing 0.1% D-glucose and 100 μg/mL ampicillin, and grow shaking at 37°C and 200 rpm till the culture reaches an $OD_{600\,nm}$ of approximately 1.0.
3. Induce VHH production by adding IPTG to a final concentration of 1 mM. After 5 h, centrifuge the culture for 10 min at $4{,}000 \times g$ and 4°C to spin down the cells.
4. Freeze the cell pellet at −20°C for 30 min, subsequently thaw on ice, and resuspend in 1 mL p-shock buffer per 50 mL culture.
5. After an overnight incubation at 4°C centrifuge the suspension for 10 min at $3{,}000 \times g$ and 4°C, and discard the pellet. Repeat this step until no more pellet is obtained (see Note 9).
6. Equilibrate TALON resin in extraction buffer and add 100 μL to the supernatant of a 50 mL culture production. Incubate rotating for 20 min at room temperature (see Note 10).
7. Wash the TALON twice by spinning down the resin for 2 min at $700 \times g$ and at 4°C and subsequently incubate for 10 min in 15 bed volumes of extraction buffer.
8. Resuspend the resin in 15 bed volumes of extraction buffer and allow the resin to settle out of suspension in a 15 mL gravity-flow column with a closed end-cap.
9. Allow the buffer to drain, followed by two additional washes with 15 bed volumes of extraction buffer.
10. Elute bound VHHs with four half bed volumes imidazole elution buffer, and directly dialyze to PBS using a T1 membrane (see Note 11). This VHH sample can be used for IH.

3.3. Assessment of Library Specificity in IH

1. Rinse 5 μm thick frozen brain tissue sections of AD/CAA patients in PBS and fix with ice-cold acetone for 10 min.
2. Block sections with peroxidase blocking reagent for 20 min and subsequently wash in PBS, before incubation overnight in a wet chamber with 20 ng/μL of the purified VHH pools diluted in BlockA buffer.
3. Rinse sections with PBS and incubate with mouse anti-myc antibody (1:6,000) for 1 h.
4. Incubate sections subsequently with EnVision+® system labeled Polymer-Hrp anti-Mouse for 30 min.
5. Remove unbound antibodies by washing in PBS.

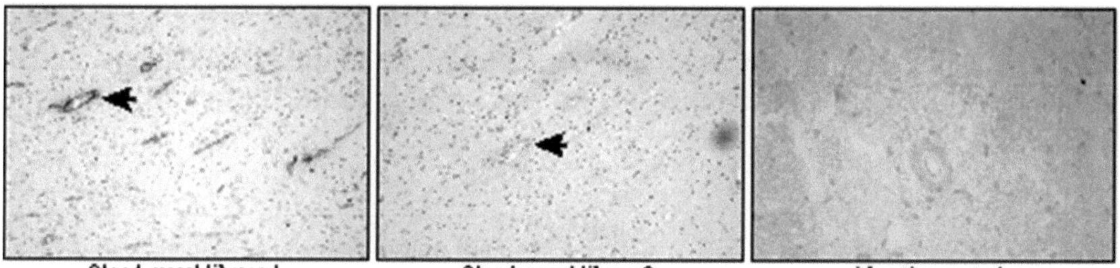

Fig. 1. Polyclonal VHH produced from both blood vessel libraries stain blood vessels (*solid arrow*) of an AD patient brain section, suggesting the presence of VHH antibody fragments specific for Aβ deposits in the library. Library 1 showed a more pronounced staining compared to library 2, with no apparent staining in the negative control without VHH.

6. Perform detection with LiquidDAB + Substrate Chromogen System as described by manufacturer.
7. Perform hemotoxylin counterstaining, dehydrate the sections, and mount in micromount mounting medium.
8. Analyze preparations with a light microscope (see Note 12) and obtain images using a digital camera. (For results of the VHH pools from the blood vessel libraries on brain tissue sections of an AD patient, see Fig. 1).

3.4. Selection of Aβ Binders

1. Coat 96 well polysorb plates with 10 μg Aβ in 100 μL of PBS for 1 h at 37°C (see Note 13) and incubate overnight at room temperature.
2. Wash coated wells twice with 200 μL/well of PBS and subsequently block for 1 h with BlockB buffer.
3. For each well, prepare a phage input mix by preincubating 10 μL of each library phage stock for 30 min with 90 μL blockC buffer.
4. Calculate phage input numbers by making serial dilutions (6, 8) of the phage input mix. Use 100 μL of each mix to infect 900 μL of exponentially growing TG1 cells during a 30 min incubation at 37°C. Plate 100 μL of the infected cells on LB agar plates containing 2% D-glucose and 100 μg/mL ampicillin, and incubate overnight at 37°C (see Table 1 for phage input numbers).
5. Add the phage input mix (see Note 14) subsequently to the Aβ containing wells and incubate shaking for 2 h at room temperature.
6. Remove nonbound phage by extensive washing with five times 200 μL of PBST with a 10 min incubation after the last wash. Repeat this washing procedure an additional two times, followed by two 200 μL washes with PBS (see Note 15).
7. Elute bound phage by incubation for 10 min in 100 μL per well of elution buffer. Neutralize the eluate subsequently in an eppendorf tube containing 50 μL of neutralization buffer.

Table 1
Phage input and output numbers of the Aβ selections using the blood vessel (A) and the gray matter library (B)

	CFU	
	First round 10 mg	Second round 1 mg
(A) Blood vessel library		
Input	4×10^{10}	4×10^{9}
Output Aβ	4×10^{6}	1×10^{6}
Output control	4×10^{2}	2×10^{3}
(B) Gray matter library		
Input	1×10^{11}	n.d.
Output Aβ	2×10^{3}	n.d.
Output control	60	n.d.

Only one round of selection was performed with the gray matter library as the phage output and thus the clone diversity herein was relatively low

8. Use half of the eluted phage (see Note 16) to infect 925 μL of exponentially growing TG1 cells during a 30 min incubation at 37°C. Plate 100 μL of the infected cells on LB agar plates containing 2% D-glucose and 100 μg/mL ampicillin (see Table 1 for phage output numbers).
9. Add the rest of the infected cells to 5 mL of LB containing 2% D-glucose and 100 μg/mL ampicillin and grow overnight at 37°C shaking at 200 rpm. Use this stock for phage rescue at the second round of selection.

3.5. Screening and Characterization of Positive Clones

1. Grow single colonies from the selection outputs in U-bottom 96 well plates containing 100 μL per well of LB with 2% D-glucose and 100 μg/mL ampicillin for 3 h (see Note 17). This is the master plate, which will be stored at −80°C after addition of glycerol to a final concentration of 20%.
2. Transfer 5 μL of each well of the master plate to a V-bottom 96 well plate containing 95 μL of 2TY with 0.1% D-glucose and 100 μg/mL ampicillin and grow shaking for an additional 3 h. This is the induction plate (see Note 18).
3. Prepare a mix of 2xTY containing 100 μg/mL ampicillin and 1×10^{9} pfu VCS M13 helper phage. Add 25 μL of this mix to each well and incubate for 30 min at 37°C.
4. Prepare a mix of 2xTY containing 100 μg/mL ampicillin and 300 μg/mL kanamycin. Add 25 μL of this mix to each well and incubate overnight at 37°C shaking at 200 rpm. The next day, centrifuge this plate for 15 min at $1,200 \times g$ at 4°C to separate the TG1 cells from the phage containing medium.

5. Additionally, coat a polysorb 96 well plate (see Subheading 3.4) with 200 ng Aβ (see Note 19). The next day, wash this plate twice with 200 μL per well of PBS and subsequently block with 200 μL per well of blockB buffer for 1 h.
6. Incubate the blocked plate with 80 μL per well of blockB buffer with 20 μL of medium of the phage induction plate, and incubate for 2 h at room temperature.
7. Wash wells with 200 μL of PBST and incubate for 1 h with 100 μL per well of a 1:10,000 dilution in blockB buffer of the HRP conjugated anti-M13 antibody.
8. Wash the wells three times with 200 μL of PBST and twice with PBS.
9. Visualize bound HRP-conjugated antibodies by adding 100 μL of OPD solution to which the H_2O_2 was added freshly prior to use. Stop the reaction with 50 μL per well of 1 M H_2SO_4 and measure absorption at 490 nm on a microplate reader.
10. Determine the DNA sequence of each positive clone (13). Compare clones according to their amino acid sequence. Produce unique clones and purify as described (see Subheading 3.2). These VHH antibody fragments can be used for IH to compare the performance of the selected binders from the different complex immune libraries similarly as described previously (see Subheading 3.3) (see Fig. 2 for one representative selected binder from each library).

4. Notes

1. The success of using complex protein samples for obtaining binders against a single protein present in this mixture depends largely on the immune response generated during the immunization process. This will depend on the abundance and availability of the target protein in this sample, and on the immunodominance of the epitopes that are presented by the target. Although the immunodominance of a target cannot be changed, the abundance and availability of the target in the complex protein sample can be increased in some cases, which could lead to a better immune response against the protein of interest. This can be achieved (1) by overexpression of the target using eukaryotic expression constructs containing the open reading frame of the target protein or (2) by fractionation of the biological sample to separate antigen containing fractions from non-antigen-containing fractions. A possible disadvantage of applying these techniques when preparing a sample for immunization could be that the composition or folding of the

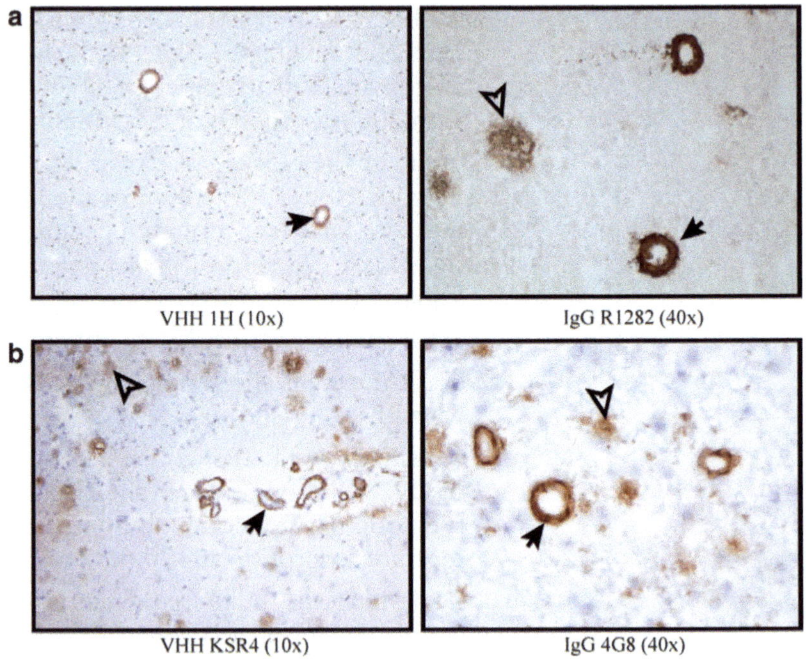

Fig. 2. Representative staining patterns of binders from the blood vessel library (**a**) and gray matter library (**b**). VHH 1H selected from the blood vessel library stains primarily Aβ deposits in blood vessels (*solid arrow*) of a HCHWAD patient, while staining with the commercial anti-Aβ antibody R1282 stains both parenchymal (*open arrowhead*) and vascular deposits in the same patient. In contrast, VHH KSR4 selected from the gray matter library can recognize both vascular and parenchymal Aβ deposits as shown here with a brain section of an AD patient. This staining pattern is comparable to results obtained with the commercial anti-Aβ antibody 4G8. This indicates that these VHH antibody fragments that are obtained from different complex immune libraries have different structure dependent binding characteristics for Aβ depending on the antigen source used for immunization.

antigen containing protein complex is changed (e.g., the antigen becomes incorrectly folded or forms complexes that do not normally occur).

2. Powdered tissue can be best transferred by pouring the liquid nitrogen containing the pulverized tissue into the tube.
3. We prepared the tissue homogenates in PBS. Other buffers can be used as well, as long as the used chemicals comply with immunization of life animals. Be aware that use of chemicals can have an effect on antigen extraction efficiency, stability and presentation. When a commercial antibody against the target is available, the sample should be checked for presence of the target.
4. When using an Ultra-Turrax, homogenization should be performed on ice to avoid heat buildup.
5. The protein content of the complex protein sample should be high enough to inject sufficient material upon each boost. The volume of buffer that is used to homogenize the sample should therefore be determined experimentally when possible.

6. For each project, we typically immunize two animals to overcome potential problems of inter-individual variation in antibody response. In practice, generating two independent libraries for the same antigen yields sufficient binders of good quality.
7. The llamas were immunized with both the soluble and insoluble fraction of the tissue homogenates as there was no prior information on the distribution of the target between the different fractions. These fractions were injected at either side of the animal, with the rationale to stimulate the lymph system on each side of the animal differently. With prior knowledge of target distribution, immunization protocols could be simplified using only the target containing subfractions for immunization.
8. The amount of cells should at least be 10 times the library size to ensure that the entire complexity of the library is represented.
9. All cell debri should be removed from the sample before adding TALON as remaining cell debri will clog the resin at later steps during the purification.
10. The EDTA present in the p-shock buffer can sometimes strip the cobalt ions from the TALON resin resulting in a low protein yield in the purified sample. When this is a problem, the EDTA should be removed prior to use by dialysis or by using spin-columns.
11. The imidazole present in the elution buffer can affect antibody fragment stability and should therefore be removed.
12. Characterization of the VHH pools obtained from the whole phage display library provides information on the specificity and functionality of the binders present in the library. A negative result does not mean that there are no binders present in the library with the required characteristics, as these binders could be enriched in successive selection rounds. Polyclonal VHHs produced from these selection outputs can be applied to monitor whether the selection has resulted in the enrichment of relevant binders.
13. When using a 96 well plate for selection, always try to avoid using neighboring wells to avoid contamination.
14. When using a complex immune library the selection strategy should be adapted to avoid selecting for binders that recognize proteins or epitopes in the complex sample other than the target of interest. Therefore, the antigen used in the selection should be either as pure as possible or the antigen should be produced in an expression system that is not related to the natural expression system, to prevent selection of binders against nontarget proteins in the protein complex that are very immunodominant. Additionally, the strategy can be adjusted in such a way that binders against the target are more likely to be obtained. This can be achieved by using elution protocols specific for the

target, such as the use of natural ligands, competitive peptides or specific domains. Alternatively, the selection can be driven towards the target by using subtractive selection techniques in which the library is preabsorbed on a (complex) sample of interest that does not contain the target protein to remove nontarget binders.

15. Refresh the washing buffer frequently to avoid contamination with phage.
16. Use only half of the eluted phage for TG1 infection and keep the remainder at 4°C as a backup when infection failed.
17. Always incubate the master plate without shaking to avoid cross contamination.
18. To reduce cross contamination, avoid formation of aerosols when transferring the clones to the induction plate and in subsequent steps when adding the helper phage and kanamycin containing medium.
19. It is always advisable to use a selection and/or screening strategy that resembles the application the binder is intended to be used for. In this case study, selections or screening could have been performed on brain sections containing Aβ deposits to select for binders that are suitable for this application. However, we hypothesized that because of the used immunization strategy most Aβ binders present in the library would be able to bind the target in IH as in IH Aβ is present in its natural context.

Acknowledgements

This work was supported by grants from the IOP Genomics Center (IGE05005), the National Institutes of Health (NIH AG021084 and AG005134) and by the Centre for Medical Systems Biology within the framework of the Netherlands Genomics Initiative (NGI)/Netherlands Organization for Scientific Research (NWO).

References

1. Marks JD, Hoogenboom HR, Bonnert TP et al (1991) By-passing immunization. Human antibodies from V-gene libraries displayed on phage. J Mol Biol 222:581–597
2. Roovers RC, van der Linden E, Zijlema H et al (2001) Evidence for a bias toward intracellular antigens in the local humoral anti-tumor immune response of a colorectal cancer patient revealed by phage display. Int J Cancer 93: 832–840
3. Sommavilla R, Lovato V, Villa A et al (2010) Design and construction of a naïve mouse antibody phage display library. J Immunol Methods 353:31–43
4. Chiliza TE, Van Wyngaardt W, Du Plessis DH (2008) Single-chain antibody fragments from a display library derived from chickens immunized with a mixture of parasite and viral antigens. Hybridoma 27:413–421
5. van Koningsbruggen S, de Haard H, de Kievit P et al (2003) Llama-derived phage display antibodies in the dissection of the human disease oculopharyngeal muscular dystrophy. J Immunol Methods 279:149–161

6. Fu Y, Shearing LN, Haynes S et al (1997) Isolation from phage display libraries of single chain variable fragment antibodies that recognize conformational epitopes in the malaria vaccine candidate, apical membrane antigen-1. J Biol Chem 272:25678–25684
7. Sahdev S, Khattar SK, Saini KS (2008) Production of active eukaryotic proteins through bacterial expression systems: a review of the existing biotechnology strategies. Mol Cell Biochem 307:249–264
8. Lang IM, Barbas CF III, Schleef RR (1996) Recombinant rabbit Fab with binding activity to type-1 plasminogen activator inhibitor derived from a phage-display library against human alpha-granules. Gene 172: 295–298
9. Roovers RC, Laeremans T, Huang L et al (2007) Efficient inhibition of EGFR signaling and of tumour growth by antagonistic anti-EFGR nanobodies. Cancer Immunol Immunother 56:303–317
10. Omidfar K, Rasaee MJ, Modjtahedi H et al (2004) Production of a novel camel single-domain antibody specific for the type III mutant EGFR. Tumour Biol 25:296–305
11. Rutgers KS, van Remoortere A, van Buchem MA et al (2011) Differential recognition of vascular and parenchymal beta amyloid deposition. Neurobiol Aging 32:1774–1783
12. Bornebroek M, Van Buchem MA, Haan J et al (1996) Hereditary cerebral hemorrhage with amyloidosis-Dutch type: better correlation of cognitive deterioration with advancing age than with number of focal lesions or white matter hyperintensities. Alzheimer Dis Assoc Disord 10:224–231
13. Sambrook J, Fritsch EF, Maniatis T (1989) Molecular cloning: a laboratory manual, vol 1–3. Cold Spring Harbor Laboratory Press, New York

Part IV

Expression of Single Domain Antibodies and Derivatives

Chapter 16

Expression of Single-Domain Antibodies in Bacterial Systems*

Toya Nath Baral and Mehdi Arbabi-Ghahroudi

Abstract

In this chapter we describe in detail the current protocols that are used to express single-domain antibodies in bacteria. Bacteria are among the most common expression systems for expressing recombinant proteins. We present different approaches for carrying out periplasmic and cytoplasmic expression, as well as small-scale and large-scale expression. In addition, we discuss the advantages and possible drawbacks of each protocol. We present data related to expression vectors, expression conditions, methods of protein extraction and purification, and yield and purity analysis of sdAbs. We also highlight important points that need to be considered before sdAbs that have been expressed in bacteria are used either in vitro or in vivo.

Key words: Single-domain antibodies, Expression, Avidity, Antibody fragment libraries, Phage display, Endotoxin

1. Introduction

Recombinant antibodies can be expressed in various formats. Such antibody fragments can be the fragments antigen binding (Fabs), single chain variable fragments (scFvs), variable light chain domains (VLs), or variable heavy chain domains (VHs) that are derived from conventional IgGs. They can also be the variable domains (VHHs) of camelid heavy chain antibodies or the variable domains (VNARs) of shark immunoglobulin new antigen receptors (IgNARs) (1). The term single-domain antibody (sdAb) is often used to describe VHs, VLs, VHHs, and VNARs (2–4). IgG antibodies or their fragments are being used increasingly in, and developed for, cancer or other disease therapies (5, 6). Antibody therapeutics that are

*This is National Research Council Canada Publication number: 50018.

Dirk Saerens and Serge Muyldermans (eds.), *Single Domain Antibodies: Methods and Protocols*,
Methods in Molecular Biology, vol. 911, DOI 10.1007/978-1-61779-968-6_16, © Springer Science+Business Media, LLC 2012

designed for treating cancer are already a multi-billion dollar a year market. A number of antibodies are already on the market and a large number are also at various stages of clinical trials. Antibody engineering techniques that are largely based on antibody expression in bacteria (7) are a driving force in the development of these bio-drugs. Genetically engineered antibody fragments that are produced in *Escherichia coli* have great potential to be used as specific targeting reagents in scientific research and in clinical trials. There is a growing interest in different engineered antibody formats, in particular because of their in vivo diagnostic and therapeutic applications. However, a major factor that can limit the applications of such antibodies is production in large amounts as soluble, stable, and functional proteins (8, 9).

Different antibody fragments, in particular scFvs, are often prone to form insoluble aggregates (also called inclusion bodies) when they are expressed at high levels in *E. coli* (8). Protein expression as inclusion bodies results in larger quantities of target proteins. However, laborious unfolding and refolding procedures need to be carried out to produce biologically functional antibody products (10). On the other hand, mammalian expression of recombinant proteins including antibodies is costly and labor-intensive (10). It takes approximately 4–6 months to produce a stable mammalian production system as compared to approximately 1 month for an *E. coli* system. While it is advantageous to use mammalian cell machinery, which makes it possible to produce glycosylated antibodies, many opportunities exist whereby antibodies can be produced effectively in *E. coli* (11). The extensive experience that researchers have with *E. coli*-based protein expression systems and the ease of genetic manipulations makes *E. coli* a highly attractive host for expressing antibodies (10). The *E. coli* machinery has also been applied in phage display technology for antibody development. By using this technology, it is possible to screen astronomical numbers of paratope repertoire sequences and isolate binding domains that are well-suited for bacterial expression, are highly specific and bind tightly to selected targets (12). Other incentives for using *E. coli* expression systems include: simple fermentation conditions, ease of scale-up, relatively short duration between transformation and protein expression, no need to worry about viral contamination that is harmful to humans, and relatively low capital costs for fermentation (10). However, *E. coli* expression has its own drawbacks. These include the possibility of bacterial endotoxins contaminating the purified products, absence of complicated folding machinery for nonsecretory eukaryotic proteins, and the lack of glycosylation if that is crucial for the function of the protein (10).

Two basic strategies can be applied to express various formats of antibody fragments in *E. coli*. The first entails directing the antibody product to the reducing environment of the cytoplasm. The second involves directing the antibody to the more oxidizing environment of the periplasmic space between the cytoplasmic and outer membranes with possible leakage into the culture medium (13). It is well established that many problems related to *in vivo* expression, correct folding, solubility, thermal stability, and conformational stability can be avoided by reducing the complexity and the size of an antibody. In this regard different antibody fragment formats have been produced by using several expression systems. Due to their simple structure, sdAbs are expressed very well in bacterial systems. This is generally not the case for several other formats. In this chapter we describe bacterial expression protocols for sdAbs which are typically VHHs of camelid heavy chain antibodies.

2. Materials

Prepare all solutions using ultrapure water (prepared by purifying deionized water to attain a sensitivity of 18 MΩ cm at 25°C) and analytical grade reagents. Prepare and store all reagents at room temperature (unless indicated otherwise). Diligently follow all waste disposal regulations when disposing waste materials.

2.1. Cloning

1. TG1 electroporation-competent cells (Stratagene, La Jolla, CA, USA).
2. pSJF2H expression vector (14).
3. pMED1 phagemid vector (15).
4. pMED2 expression vector (16).
5. Primer VHBbs1: 5′-TATGAAGACACCAGGCCGATGTGC AGCTGCAGGCG-3′.
6. Primer VHBbs2: 5′-TATGAAGACACCAGGCCCAGGCTC AGGTACAGCTGGTG-3′.
7. Primer VHBam: 5′-TATGGATCCTGAGGAGACGGTGACC TG-3′.

   Primers were purchased from Euro MWG Operon (Huntsville, AL, USA).
8. Sterile MilliQ H_2O.
9. dNTPs (New England Biolabs, Pickering, ON, Canada).
10. 10× PCR buffer (Hoffmann-La Roche Ltd., Mississauga, ON, Canada).
11. Expand high fidelity Taq DNA polymerase (Hoffmann-La Roche Ltd.).
12. LigaFast™ Rapid DNA Ligation System (Promega, Madison, WI, USA).

13. Restriction enzymes *Bbs*I, *BamH*I (New England Biolabs, Pickering, ON, Canada).
14. QIAquick PCR Purification™ kit (QIAGEN Inc., Mississauga, ON, Canada).
15. QIAquick Gel Extraction™ kit (QIAGEN Inc.).
16. Agarose gel electrophoresis equipment.
17. 1% Agarose gel.
18. Disposable electroporation cuvettes (Bio-Rad Laboratories, Mississauga, ON, Canada).
19. MicroPulser™ electroporator (Bio-Rad Laboratories) or a similar instrument.
20. SOC (per liter): 20 g Bacto tryptone, 5 g Bacto yeast extract, 0.5 g NaCl, 2.5 mM KCl, 10 mM $MgCl_2$, 20 mM glucose, and deionized H_2O. Sterilized by autoclaving.
21. Filter-sterilized ampicillin: a stock solution of 100 mg/mL in water.
22. LB/agar (per liter): 10 g Bacto tryptone, 5 g Bacto yeast extract, 10 g NaCl, 15 g bacto-agar, and deionized H_2O (17). Sterilized by autoclaving. Before pouring the plates, allow medium to cool down to 55°C. To make LB-Amp plate, add filter-sterilized ampicillin at the final concentration of 100 μg/mL.
23. Incubators for growing bacteria on plates and in liquid media.
24. Thermal Cycler (GeneAmp PCR System 9700, Applied Biosystem) or a similar instrument.

2.2. Colony PCR

1. Primer M13RP: 5′-CAGGAAACAGCTATGAC-3′.
2. Primer M13FP: 5′-GTAAAACGACGGCCAGT-3′.

   Primers were purchased from Euro MWG Operon
3. dNTPs (New England Biolabs).
4. 10× PCR buffer (Hoffmann-La Roche Ltd.).
5. Taq DNA polymerase (Hoffmann-La Roche Ltd.).
6. Agarose gel electrophoresis equipment.
7. DNA Sequencing equipment.
8. Thermal Cycler (GeneAmp PCR System 9700, Applied Biosystem) or a similar instrument.
9. QIAquick PCR Purification™ kit (QIAGEN Inc.).
10. 1% Agarose gel.
11. DNA Sequencing equipment.
12. ND-1000 spectrophotometer (NanoDrop Technologies, Wilmington, DE, USA) or a similar instrument.

2.3. Small-Scale Expression of Single-Domain Antibodies

1. B2YT medium (per liter): 16 g Bacto tryptone, 10 g Bacto yeast extract, 5 g NaCl, 4 mL glycerol, 12.32 g of K_2HPO_4, and 2.22 g KH_2PO_4.
2. Filter-sterilized ampicillin: a stock solution of 100 mg/mL in water.
3. Shaker incubator.
4. Sorvall high speed and swinging bucket bench-top (RT6000B Refrigerated) centrifuges or their equivalents.
5. Cell Density meter (Biochrome Ltd., Cambridge, UK) or equivalent.
6. Isopropyl-β-D-thio-galactopyranoside (IPTG) (Rose Scientific, Edmonton, Canada) a stock solution of 1 M in water.

2.4. Large-Scale Expression of Single-Domain Antibody

1. LB (Luria-Bertani) (per liter): 10 g Bacto tryptone, 5 g Bacto yeast extract, 10 g NaCl, and deionized H_2O. Sterilized by autoclaving.
2. LB/agar (per liter): 10 g Bacto tryptone, 5 g Bacto yeast extract, 10 g NaCl, 15 g bacto-agar, and deionized H_2O (17). Sterilized by autoclaving.
3. M9 medium (per liter): 900 mL deionized water, 100 mL 10× M9 salts sterilized by autoclaving. Add filter-sterilized 1 mL 1 M $MgCl_2$, 0.1 mL of 1 M $CaCl_2$, 5 mL of 1 mg/mL thiamine-HCl (vitamin B1), 10 mL of 20% glucose, and 20 mL of 20% casamino acids.
4. 10× M9 salts (per liter): 60 g Na_2HPO_4, 30 g K_2HPO_4, 10 g NH_4Cl, and 5 g NaCl. Sterilized by autoclaving.
5. 10× Induction medium (per 100 mL): 12 g Bacto tryptone, 24 g Bacto yeast extract, and 4 mL of glycerol. Sterilized by autoclaving.
6. Filter-sterilized ampicillin: a stock solution of 100 mg/mL in water.
7. IPTG (Rose Scientific) a stock solution of 1 M in water.
8. Wash solution: 10 mM Tris–HCl buffer, pH 8.0, and 150 mM NaCl.
9. Beckman Coulter J2-21M/E High speed centrifuge or equivalent.
10. Shaker incubator.

2.5. Periplasmic Extraction of Single-Domain Antibodies

1. Sucrose solution: 10 mM Tris–HCl buffer, pH 8.0, 1 mM EDTA, and 25% sucrose.
2. Shock solution: 10 mM Tris–HCl buffer, pH 8.0, and 0.5 mM $MgCl_2$.

3. Beckman Coulter J2-21M/E High speed centrifuge or equivalent.
4. Dialysis tubing with a cut off of 8 kDa (Biodesign Inc., Carmel, NY, USA).

2.6. Cytosolic Extraction of Single-Domain Antibodies

1. Lysis buffer: 10 mM HEPES buffer, pH 7.5, 500 mM NaCl, and 20 mM imidazole.
2. Phenylmethylsulfonyl fluoride (PMSF) (Thermo Scientific Pierce Protein Research Products, Rockford, IL, USA).
3. Dithiothreitol (DTT) (Sigma-Aldrich Canada, Ltd., Oakville ON, Canada).
4. Lysozyme (USB Corporation, Cleveland, USA).
5. DNase I (Sigma-Aldrich Canada, Ltd.).
6. Starting buffer: 10 mM HEPES (*N*-(2-hydroxyethyl) piperazine-*N*′-(2-ethanesulfonic acid)) buffer, pH 7.0, 10 mM imidazole, and 500 mM NaCl.
7. Beckman Coulter J2-21M/E High speed centrifuge or equivalent.
8. Dialysis tubing with a cut off of 8 kDa (Biodesign Inc.).
9. 0.2 μm GP Express™ Plus Membrane filtration system (MILLIPORE Corporate, Billerica, MA, USA).

2.7. Small-Scale Purification Using PureProteome™ Nickel Magnetic Beads

1. Pure Proteome™ Nickel Magnetic Beads (MILLIPORE Corporate).
2. Pure Proteome Magnetic stand (MILLIPORE Corporate).
3. Lysis buffer: 10 mM HEPES buffer, pH 7.5, 500 mM NaCl, and 20 mM imidazole.
4. Wash buffer: 10 mM Tris–HCl buffer, pH 8.0, and 150 mM NaCl.
5. Elution buffer: 10 mM HEPES buffer, pH 7.0, 500 mM imidazole, and 500 mM NaCl.

2.8. Large-Scale Purification on HiTrap™ Column

1. 5 mL HiTrap™ Chelating HP column (GE Healthcare).
2. $NiCl_2$ solution: a stock solution of at a concentration of 5 mg/mL $NiCl_2$ in water.
3. Starting buffer: 10 mM HEPES (*N*-(2-hydroxyethyl) piperazine-*N*′-(2-ethanesulfonic acid)) buffer, pH 7.0, 10 mM imidazole, and 500 mM NaCl.
4. ÄKTA FPLC purification system (GE Healthcare).
5. Dialysis tubing with a cut off of 8 kDa (Biodesign Inc.).
6. 0.2 μm GP Express™ Plus Membrane filtration system (MILLIPORE Corporate).
7. ND-1000 spectrophotometer (NanoDrop Technologies, Wilmington, DE, USA) or a similar instrument.

8. Sodium azide (Thermo Scientific Pierce).
9. Deionized H_2O.
10. Sterile phosphate-buffered saline (PBS) (17).

2.9. Gel Filtration/Size Exclusion Chromatography

1. ÄKTA FPLC purification system (GE Healthcare).
2. Superdex 75 gel filtration column (GE Healthcare) (see Chapter 21).

2.10. SDS-PAGE and Western Blotting

1. 30% polyacrylamide (Bio-Rad Laboratories).
2. 10% sodium dodecyl sulfate (SDS) in water.
3. 10% ammonium persulfate (APS) in water.
4. 1.5 M and 0.5 M Tris–HCl buffer, pH 8.8.
5. TEMED (Invitrogen, Burlington, ON, Canada).
6. Deionized H_2O.
7. 10× electrophoresis running buffer: 30.35 g Tris, 141.75 g glycine, and 10 g SDS per liter of water.
8. Isopropanol (ACP Chemicals, Inc., Montreal, QC, Canada).
9. 4× SDS loading buffer: 4 mL of glycerol, 0.4 g SDS, and 5 mL of 1.5 M Tris–HCl. Make up to 10 mL with water, and add enough bromophenol blue such that a 1× solution is dark enough to permit easy monitoring of the gel when it is being run. Just before use add 50 μL of beta-mercaptoethanol per mL of buffer.
10. SDS-PAGE (sodium dodecyl sulfate-polyacrylamide gel electrophoresis) equipment and power supply.
11. Heat block or water bath.
12. Coomassie blue dye: 50 mL of isopropylalcohol, 20 mL of acetic acid, 50 mg Coomassie blue dye, and 130 mL of water.
13. Destaining buffer: 10% acetic acid, 30% methanol, and 60% water.
14. Immobilon™ transfer membrane (MILLIPORE).
15. 10× transfer buffer; 15.1 g of Tris, 72 g of glycine, and water up to 500 mL.
16. Trans-Blot™ SD (Bio-Rad) for semidry Western blotting.
17. Sterile PBS (17). Make PBST by adding 0.1% Tween-20 (Sigma-Aldrich Canada, Ltd.) in PBS.
18. MPBS: 2% (w/v) skim milk in PBS.
19. Mouse anti-His antibody (QIAGEN Inc.).
20. Alkaline phosphatase conjugated goat anti-mouse antibody (Jackson Immunoresearch Laboratory Inc., West Grove, PA, USA).
21. AP-conjugated substrate kit (Bio-Rad Laboratories).

2.11. Affinity Measurement

BIACORE 3000 (GE Healthcare) or other surface plasmon resonance (SPR) instrument with similar capabilities (see Chapter 27).

2.12. Endotoxin Measurement

1. E-toxate kit (Sigma-Aldrich Canada, Ltd.).
2. Incubator at 37°C.
3. Parafilm®.

2.13. Endotoxin Removal

1. Deto-Gel kit (Thermo Scientific Pierce).
2. 1% deoxycholate solution in water.
3. Sterile PBS (17).

3. Methods

3.1. Cloning

All the cloning steps were performed essentially as described elsewhere (17). The VHH genes used here were identified as binders for an antigen of interest. They were isolated from a phagemid library by panning as described elsewhere (18).

1. Amplify the VHH genes from the phagemid vector (pMED1) in a total volume of 50 μL by performing colony PCR using VHBbs1 or VHBbs2 (see Note 1) and VHBam primers. *Bbs*I and *BamH*I sites are introduced at the ends of the amplified fragments by using these primers (see Note 2). Prepare each PCR reaction mix with the following ingredients:

10× PCR buffer	5.0 μL
dNTPs (2.5 mM each)	4.0 μL
VHBbs1 or VHBbs2 (10 pmol/μL)	0.5 μL
VHBam primer (10 pmol/μL)	0.5 μL
ExpandTaq DNA polymerase (5 units/μL)	0.5 μL
H_2O	41.5 μL

   Touch single colonies from the titre plates with sterile toothpicks or a P10 pipette tip and then swirl around in the PCR tubes to dislodge the bacteria into the PCR reaction solution (see Note 3). Place the reaction tubes into a thermal cycler and perform PCR by using the following program: 94°C for 5 min followed by 30 cycles of 94°C for 30 s, 55°C for 30 s, and 72°C for 30 s and as a final step of 72°C for 7 min.

2. Purify the VHH genes in a final volume of 50 μL water using a QIAquick PCR Purification™ kit.
3. Digest the purified DNA with *Bbs*I restriction endonuclease for 3 h at 37°C and then purify it in a final volume of 50 μL water by using a QIAquick PCR Purification™ kit. Re-digest with *BamH*I

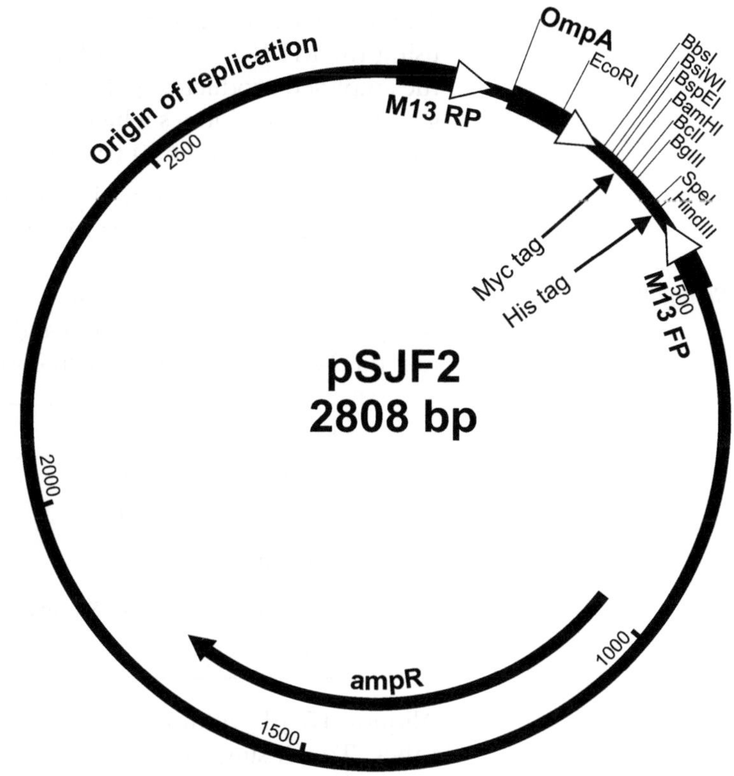


```
------------ompA--------->
CTGGCTGGTTTCGCTACCGTTGCGCAGGCCGTCTTCGTACGATCCGGACTAGCCGGATCC
                    BbsI                                 BamHI

<-----------myc-Tag----------> <------His-Tag--->
GAACAAAAACTGATCAGCGAAGAAGATCTGAACCATCACCATCACCATCACTAGTGA
                                                   stop
```

Fig. 1. Expression vector pSJF2.

restriction endonuclease for an additional 2 h at 37°C and gel-purify with a QIAquick Gel Extraction™ kit in 50 μL of water.

4. Ligate the cut fragment into *Bbs*I/*BamH*I-digested pSJF2H expression vector using LigaFast™ Rapid Ligation System (see Fig. 1) (see Note 4). This results in addition of C-terminal c-Myc and His_6 tags to the protein.
5. Prepare electrocompetent *E. coli* strain TG1 cells by following a standard protocol (17). Transform 50 μL of electrocompetent TG1 cells with 3 μL of the ligated material using a MicroPulser™ electroporator or an equivalent instrument. Transfer the electroporated cells into a tube that contains 1 mL of SOC medium and incubate it for 1 h at 37°C and at a shaking speed of 180 rpm. Alternatively, cells can be transformed by chemically prepared competent cells with a 90 s heat shock at 42°C (17).
6. Spread 100 μL of cells on to LB/Amp plates and leave the plates with their lids half open for about 5 min in a bio-hood. Cover, invert, and incubate the plates overnight at 32°C.

7. The following day, perform colony PCR (see Subheading 3.2) using the M13RP and M13FP primers. Determine the size of the amplified product by gel electrophoresis using a 1% agarose gel. The positive clones which contain the VHH genes should have a size of around 650 base pairs (see Note 5).
8. Confirm the positive clones by further sequencing their VHH genes using M13RP and/or M13FP as primers.

3.2. Colony PCR

1. Perform colony PCR in a total volume of 15 μL using the colonies that grew on the overnight plates. Prepare a master mix for 24 PCR reactions which consists of the following:

10× PCR buffer	36 μL
dNTPs (2.5 mM each)	28.8 μL
M13RP (10 pmol/μL)	7.2 μL
M13RP (10 pmol/μL)	7.2 μL
Taq DNA polymerase (5 units/μL)	3.6 μL
H_2O	277.2 μL

Aliquot 15 μL volumes from the master mix into 24 PCR tubes. Touch single colonies from the titre plates with sterile toothpicks or a P10 pipette tip and then swirl around in the PCR tubes to dislodge the bacteria into the PCR reaction solution (see Note 3). Place the reaction tubes into a thermal cycler and perform PCR by using the following program: 94°C for 5 min followed by 30 cycles of 94°C for 30 s, 55°C for 30 s, and 72°C for 30 s, and as a final step of 72°C for 7 min.

2. Apply 5 μL of the PCR mix on 1% agarose gels to identify the clones which contain a full insert of approximately 650 bp in size. Purify the remaining PCR mix for the clones which contain the full insert by using a QIAquick PCR Purification™ kit and then determine the DNA concentrations by ND-spectrophotometer. Sequence the clones using primers M13RP and/or M13FP as primers and verify the VHH sequences.

3.3. Small-Scale Expression of Single-Domain Antibodies

VHH genes are cloned in fusion with the OmpA leader sequence in pSJF2H vector. This sequence directs the expressed protein to be transported into the periplasmic space of *E. coli*. The following protein extraction protocol which is based on an osmotic shock method (19) is designed to increase the permeability of the outer membrane. It therefore enables the sdAbs to be released from the periplasm without the cells being lysed. SdAbs are partially purified by carrying out the periplasmic extraction since the periplasm contains far less endogenous protein than the cytoplasm. It is recommended to keep the fractions from various steps of the extraction at 4°C until the fractions that contain the sdAb has been verified by Western blotting.

1. Use a single clone to inoculate 2 mL of B2YT/Amp medium (100 μg/mL ampicillin) in a 15 mL Falcon tube. Incubate the cell suspension in a rotary shaker at a shaking speed of 200 rpm and at 27°C overnight.
2. Centrifuge the cells the following day for 10 min at a speed of 2,000 × *g* using bench-top centrifuge and then resuspend the pellet in 2 mL of fresh medium.
3. Add 0.5 mL of the pre-culture to 50 mL of B2YT/Amp in a 250 mL flask. Incubate the pre-culture in a rotary shaker at a shaking speed of 200 rpm and 37°C until the $OD_{600\ nm}$ reaches approximately 0.3–0.5, measured in a cell density meter.
4. Add IPTG to achieve a final concentration of 0.1 mM and then incubate the culture at 37°C and a shaking speed of 200 rpm overnight.
5. Centrifuge the cells the following day by using a bench-top centrifuge for 20 min at 4°C and a speed of 3,400 × *g*.
6. Extract the protein from the periplasm as described below (see Subheading 3.5) and purify it by using Pure Proteome™ Nickel Magnetic Beads (see Subheading 3.7).

3.4. Large-Scale Expression of Single-Domain Antibody

1. Use a single clone to inoculate 25 mL of LB/Amp. Incubate the cell suspension in a rotary shaker at a speed of 240 rpm and 37°C overnight.
2. Transfer the entire overnight culture into 1 L of M9 medium that has been supplemented with 5 μg/mL vitamin B1, 0.4% Casamino acids, and 100 μg/mL ampicillin. Incubate the culture at a speed of 180 rpm and room temperature for 30 h. Supplement the culture with 100 mL of 10× induction medium and 100 μL of 1 M IPTG and incubate for another 60 h.
3. Retain a small aliquot for SDS-PAGE and Western blotting. Centrifuge the remaining culture at 5,000 × *g* for 20 min at 4°C in a high-speed centrifuge. Keep the supernatant fraction at 4°C.
4. Re-suspend the pellet in 150 mL of wash solution. Centrifuge at 14,000 × *g* and 4°C for 10 min. Keep the supernatant fraction at 4°C. The pellet can then be subjected to periplasmic or cytosolic protein extraction.

3.5. Periplasmic Extraction of Single-Domain Antibodies

1. Re-suspend the pellet in 50 mL of sucrose solution and then incubate at room temperature for 10 min. Centrifuge at 14,000 × *g* and 4°C for 45 min (see Note 6). Keep the supernatant fraction at 4°C.
2. Re-suspend the pellet in 50 mL of ice-cold shock solution and then incubate in an ice bath for 10 min. Centrifuge at 14,000 × *g* for 25 min at 4°C. Keep the supernatant fraction at 4°C.

3. Verify whether or not the antibody has been expressed by detecting the sdAbs in the fractions that were collected during the steps that are described above. Use anti-His antibody for Western blotting (see Subheading 3.10) against the His_6 tag. Pool the fractions which contain sdAb and dialyze them against 6 L of starting buffer overnight at 4°C. Use a dialysis membrane that has 8 kDa MW cut off point.
4. Proceed with protein purification.

3.6. Cytosolic Extraction of Single-Domain Antibodies

1. Re-suspend the pellet in 100 mL of ice-cold lysis buffer comprising 10 mM HEPES, pH 7.5, 500 mM NaCl, and 20 mM imidazole. Keep everything on ice during this process and store at −20°C until further use.
2. Take out the −20°C frozen suspension and immediately add 1 mL of 100 mM PMSF to achieve a final concentration of 1 mM and 200 μL of 1 M DTT to achieve a final concentration of 2 mM. Thaw the frozen suspension at room temperature while at the same time occasionally shaking it.
3. Lyse the bacteria by adding 5 mL of freshly prepared 3 mg/mL lysozyme solution to achieve a final concentration of 100 μg/mL.
4. Incubate the mixture at room temperature for 30–50 min while occasionally shaking it until the suspension becomes viscous (see Note 7).
5. Add 200–300 μL of DNAse I (15 units/μL stock in 1 M $MgCl_2$).
6. Incubate the lysate at room temperature for an additional 20–30 min until the suspension becomes watery. Save 30 μL of the mixture for performing a Western blot.
7. Separate the soluble and insoluble fractions of the lysates by centrifuging the mixture at 4°C and 14,000 × *g* using high speed centrifuge for 20 min. Centrifuge the mixture again until the supernatant becomes clear. Save 30 μL for Western blotting.
8. Resuspend the pellet in 80 mL of ice-cold lysis buffer and keep it at −20°C. Save 30 μL of the resuspended pellet for performing a Western blot. Repeat previous steps (see Subheading 3.6, steps 2–7) if the pellet contains a lot of protein. This can be checked by Western blotting.
9. Dialyze the supernatant that was obtained by carrying out previous step (see Subheading 3.6, step 7) against starting buffer which comprises 10 mM HEPES, pH 7.5, 500 mM NaCl, 20 mM imidazole overnight, and then filter it through a 0.22 μm pore size membrane.
10. Proceed with protein purification.

3.7. Small-Scale Purification Using PureProteome™ Nickel Magnetic Beads

The C-terminal His tag in the sdAbs makes it possible to do one-step protein purification by performing immobilized metal affinity chromatography (IMAC). This can be done by using Pure Proteome™ Nickel Magnetic Beads for small-scale purification or a 5 mL HiTrap™ Chelating HP column for large-scale purification.

This protocol is for purifying 1 mL of prepared lysate. However, it can be adjusted to fit the volume of lysate accordingly.

1. Vortex the magnetic beads to resuspend them.
2. Aliquot 200 μL of the magnetic bead suspension into a 1.5 mL microcentrifuge tube. Note that 200 μL of PureProteome Nickel Magnetic Bead suspension can bind at least 200–600 μg of His-tagged protein.
3. Place the tube into the PureProteome Magnetic Stand to collect the beads. Carefully remove the storage buffer from the tube by using a pipette.
4. Resuspend the magnetic beads in 500 μL of lysis buffer and then incubate them while gently mixing them for 1 min at room temperature.
5. Place the tube back into the magnetic stand and remove the buffer.
6. Add 1 mL of the cell lysate to the magnetic beads and incubate the mixture while gently mixing it for 30 min at room temperature.
7. Place the tube back into the magnetic stand and allow the beads to migrate to the magnet. Invert the tube to remove residual beads from tube cap while the tube still seated in the magnetic stand. Alternatively, residual liquid can be removed from the cap by briefly centrifuging the tube. Capture the beads and remove the lysate.
8. Wash the magnetic beads by incubating them in 500 μL of wash buffer while gently mixing them for 1 min at room temperature.
9. Place the tube back into the magnetic stand and allow the beads to migrate to the magnet. Remove the wash buffer.
10. Repeat previous steps (see Subheading 3.7, steps 8 and 9) two more times.
11. Elute the bound protein by adding 100 μL of elution buffer. Incubate the solution while gently mixing it for 2 min at room temperature.
12. Place the tube back into the magnetic stand. Allow the beads to migrate to the magnet, and then transfer the eluted fraction into a clean collection tube.
13. Repeat previous elution steps (see Subheading 3.7, steps 11 and 12) once more. The first eluent will contain the majority

of the recombinant protein. If desired, both eluents can be combined. However, this will result in lower protein concentration overall.

3.8. Large-Scale Purification on HiTrap™ Column

1. Charge the column with Ni^{2+} by applying 30 mL of 5 mg/mL $NiCl_2$ solution. Then wash the column with 15 mL of deionized water.
2. Calibrate the column by using 15 mL of starting buffer.
3. Purify the protein using ÄKTA FPLC instrument following the instructions provided by the manufacturer. For this, load the column with the dialyzed and filtered protein extract (see Subheading 3.6) at a rate of 1 mL/min. Wash the column with the starting buffer supplemented with 10 mM of imidazole. This will remove the proteins that are nonspecifically bound to the column. Once a stable baseline is reached, elute the bound protein by using a 10–500 mM imidazole gradient. Collect the fractions of eluted proteins.
4. Examine the fractions that correspond to the elution peaks on the chromatogram to determine for the presence and purity of the VHHs by SDS-PAGE (20). Pool the sdAb fractions and dialyze them extensively against PBS. Measure the $OD_{280\ nm}$ by using Nanodrop to determine the protein concentration by using the molar extinction coefficients (21). Then add sodium azide to reach a final concentration of 0.02% and store the sdAbs at 4°C.

3.9. Gel Filtration/Size Exclusion Chromatography

Size exclusion chromatography (SEC) is also often called molecular sieve, gel permeation, or gel filtration chromatography. This analytical method is used to separate molecules based on their molecular sizes and shapes. It is based on the molecular sieve properties of a variety of porous materials. Gel filtration chromatography is a powerful and popular method for purifying and determining the molecular weights of proteins. It can be used to analyze the degree to which purified protein is pure. This method can also be used to analyze whether or not the purified protein is a monomer, dimer, or is composed of aggregates. SEC can be performed in an ÄKTA FPLC instrument using a Superdex 75 or a Superdex 200 column. The type of column that is used depends on the size of the protein to be purified. The SEC protocol is described in Chapter 21. For VHHs a single monomeric peak is typically obtained by SEC (see Fig. 2).

3.10. SDS-PAGE and Western Blotting

1. Use alcohol and Kimwipes to wipe the glass. Then set up the rest of the apparatus.
2. Prepare two 12.5% gels by adding 3.1 mL of 30% acrylamide, 3 mL of 1.5 M Tris–HCl, 1.3 mL of ddH_2O, 50 μL of 10% SDS, 36 μL of 10% APS, and 5 μL TEMED.

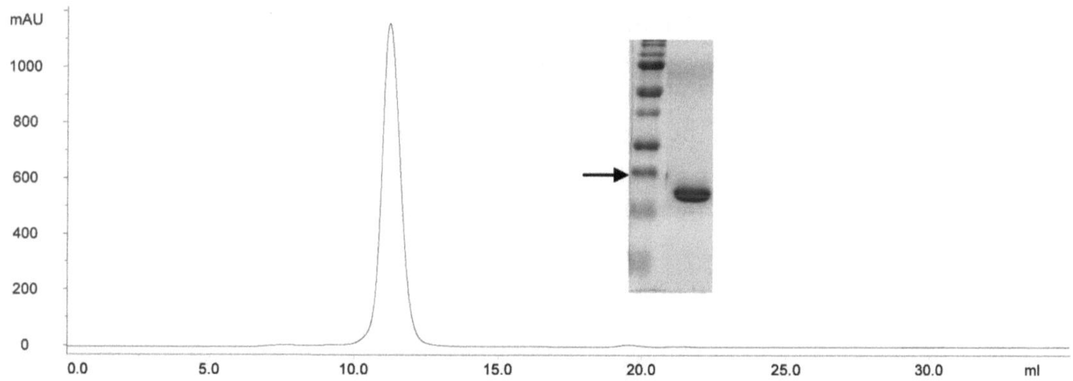

Fig. 2. A typical gel filtration/size exclusion chromatogram of a monomeric sdAb. The *inset* shows an SDS-PAGE of a typical monomeric sdAb after purification (*arrow* indicates 20 kDa).

3. Invert the tube gently after adding all of the components.
4. Pour the mixture in the gel making apparatus up to the correct level.
5. Add isopropanol on top of the acrylamide mixture and wait until the gel has polymerized.
6. Remove the isopropanol, wipe the top of the gel making apparatus using filter paper, and insert a comb into to the top of the apparatus.
7. Make staking gel by adding 1 mL of 30% acrylamide, 630 μL of 0.5 M Tris–HCl, 3.6 mL ddH_2O, 25 μL of 10% SDS, 25 μL of 10% APS, and 5 μL TEMED. Gently shake the solution. Then add the stacking gel and let it polymerise.
8. Set up the gel in the tank and make sure that the buffer is not leaking.
9. Pour in some running buffer to prevent the gel from drying out.
10. For each sample, use 4× loading dye for 1/3 of the total volume. For example, for a 30 μL sample, add 10 μL of 4× loading dye with beta-mercaptoethanol.
11. Boil each sample for 5 min and then centrifuge it before loading it on the gel.
12. Run the gel by setting the current to 20–30 mA. Check that the molecular markers separate when the current is flowing.
13. Take the gel and soak it in with the Coomassie blue dye for 1 h at room temperature.
14. Destain the gel until the protein bands can be seen clearly by using destaining solution.
15. For Western blot, immerse the gel, filter paper, and Immobilon™ membrane in the transfer solution. Place a piece of filter paper,

transfer membrane, the gel, (proteins in SDS are negatively charged), and then another piece filter paper into the transfer apparatus.

16. Set the power supply to run at 15 V and for 20 min.
17. Take the membrane and wash it four times with PBS to remove the methanol after the transfer has been completed.
18. Apply 2% MPBS (skim milk made in PBS) for 30 min to block the membrane.
19. Wash the membrane three times with PBS and add 10 mL of total primary antibody (mouse anti-His antibody) that has been diluted to the appropriate concentration in MPBS for 1 h.
20. Wash the membrane three times for 10 min with PBST.
21. Apply 1:5,000 dilution of secondary (AP-conjugated goat anti-mouse) for 30 min.
22. Wash the membrane five times with PBST for 5–10 min each time.
23. Add 100 μL each of solution A and solution B in 10 mL of AP substrate buffer to the membrane to develop it. Keep the membrane in the dark for approximately 20 min but check on it occasionally.
24. Stop the reaction by rinsing the membrane with water.

3.11. Affinity Measurements

The binding specificities of the purified sdAbs can be by using standard ELISA methods. The affinities of the sdAb-antigen interactions can also be estimated by using ELISA methods. However, SPR analyses can be performed with a BIACORE instrument if accurate binding affinities and information about the binding kinetics are desired. The affinity measurement by SPR is performed as described in Chapter 27.

3.12. Endotoxin Measurement

Endotoxin levels can be measured by using the E-toxate kit (see Note 8).

1. Make a serial dilution of endotoxin standard from 0.5 to 0.015 EU/mL in an endotoxin-free tube using endotoxin-free water.
2. Make a serial dilution of the protein samples in the same way as for the endotoxin standard.
3. Add E-toxate working solution to each tube that contains a standard or sample by inserting a pipette to just above the contents and allowing the lysate to flow down the side of the tube. This will minimize the contact and possible cross-contamination.
4. Mix the tube contents gently. Cover the mouths of each tube with parafilm and incubate it for 1 h undisturbed at 37°C.

5. Gently remove the tubes one at a time and slowly invert them by 180° while checking for evidence of gelation after 1 h of incubation. A positive test can be determined by observing the formation of a hard gel. This makes it possible to invert the tube or vial completely without disrupting the gel. All other results including soft gels, turbidity, increased viscosity, or a clear liquid are negative results.
6. The endotoxin level, EU/mL is derived by multiplying the inverse of the highest sample dilution that is positive by the lowest concentration of endotoxin standard that is positive.

3.13. Endotoxin Removal

Endotoxin is removed by using a Deto-Gel kit.

1. Regenerate 1 mL of Detoxi-Gel Resin that is pre-packed in the Detoxo-Gel column by washing with five resin-bed volumes (5 mL) of 1% sodium deoxycholate. Following this, wash it with 3–5 resin-bed volumes (15–25 mL) of PBS or water to remove the detergent.
2. Equilibrate the Detoxi-Gel Resin with 3–5 (15–25 mL) resin-bed volumes of PBS.
3. Apply the sample to the column. Add aliquots of buffer and collect the flow-through. With a gravity-flow column, the sample will begin to emerge from the column about 90% of the bed volume has been collected. For greater efficiency, stop the column flow after the sample has entered the resin bed. Then incubate the column for 1 h before collecting the samples.
4. Measure the endotoxin level as described previously (see Subheading 3.12) after removing the endotoxin.

4. Notes

1. Alternatively, primers M13RP and −96gIII can be used to amplify the VHH genes from the phagemid vector. This amplicon can be digested by *Sfi*I endonuclease and can be ligated with the *Sfi*I digested pMED2 vector, in a similar way as described for vector pSJF2H. This is particularly useful if internal *BamH*I or *Bbs*I restriction sites are present in the VHH sequences.
2. The advantage of using *Bbs*I is no extra amino acids are introduced at the N-terminal of the VHH.
3. It is important to touch the colonies very gently and therefore not to transfer too many bacterial cells into the PCR tubes. This will help to avoid "PCR smear."

4. Generally the vector is digested under the same conditions as for the insert. However, gel purification is highly recommended after the restriction enzyme digestion of the vector to avoid self-ligation. Alternatively the vector can be digested with a third enzyme such as *BspEI* or *BfaI* (see Fig. 1). A third alternative to avoid vector self-ligation is dephosphorylation the vector after digestion. A combination of any two or all three is also possible.
5. M13RP and M13FP are about 220 bp apart in an empty vector.
6. Centrifugation step is very important as the periplasmic protein contents of the bacterial cells are pushed out by the centrifugal force.
7. It is necessary to make sure that bacterial cell lysis is complete. If the lysis is complete then a clear solution can be obtained by DNAse treatment. If the lysis is not complete then sonication or further incubation with an extra amount of lysozyme might be necessary.
8. Bacterial endotoxins are lipopolysaccharides (LPSs) that are found in the cell membranes of Gram-negative bacteria. LPSs exert strong biological effects on cultured cells. Furthermore, endotoxins elicit a wide variety of pathophysiological effects in vivo by activating the host's immune system. This is particularly true in activating monocytes and macrophages, which release a range of pro-inflammatory mediators, such as tumor necrosis factor, interleukin 6, and interleukin 1. Pyrogenic reactions and shock are induced in mammals upon intravenous injection of endotoxin, even at low concentrations (22–24). Due to the high toxicity of bacterial endotoxins in vivo and in vitro, removing these molecules from the protein is crucial before it is used for cell and animal studies.

Acknowledgements

We thank Roger MacKenzie and Aaron Cowan for reviewing the manuscript. The authors declare no competing interests.

References

1. Holliger P, Hudson PJ (2005) Engineered antibody fragments and the rise of single domains. Nat Biotechnol 23(9):1126–1136
2. Muyldermans S et al (2009) Camelid immunoglobulins and nanobody technology. Vet Immunol Immunopathol 128(1–3):178–183
3. Huang L, Muyldermans S, Saerens D (2010) Nanobodies(R): proficient tools in diagnostics. Expert Rev Mol Diagn 10(6):777–785
4. De Groeve K et al (2010) Nanobodies as tools for in vivo imaging of specific immune cell types. J Nucl Med 51(5):782–789

5. Revets H, De Baetselier P, Muyldermans S (2005) Nanobodies as novel agents for cancer therapy. Expert Opin Biol Ther 5(1):111–124
6. Souriau C, Hudson PJ (2003) Recombinant antibodies for cancer diagnosis and therapy. Expert Opin Biol Ther 3(2):305–318
7. Swartz JR (2001) Advances in *Escherichia coli* production of therapeutic proteins. Curr Opin Biotechnol 12(2):195–201
8. Bothmann H, Pluckthun A (2000) The periplasmic *Escherichia coli* peptidylprolyl cis, trans-isomerase FkpA. I. Increased functional expression of antibody fragments with and without cis-prolines. J Biol Chem 275(22): 17100–17105
9. Plückthun A, Krebber A, Krebber C, Horn U, Knüpfer R, Wenderoth L, Nieba L, Proba K, Riesanberg D (1996) Antibody engineering: a practical approach. IRL Press, Oxford, pp 203–252
10. Verma R, Boleti E, George AJ (1998) Antibody engineering: comparison of bacterial, yeast, insect and mammalian expression systems. J Immunol Methods 216(1–2):165–181
11. Chan CE et al (2010) Optimized expression of full-length IgG1 antibody in a common *E. coli* strain. PLoS One 5(4):e10261
12. Kretzschmar T, von Ruden T (2002) Antibody discovery: phage display. Curr Opin Biotechnol 13(6):598–602
13. Arbabi-Ghahroudi M, Tanha J, MacKenzie R (2005) Prokaryotic expression of antibodies. Cancer Metastasis Rev 24(4):501–519
14. Tanha J, Muruganandam A, Stanimirovic D (2003) Phage display technology for identifying specific antigens on brain endothelial cells. Methods Mol Med 89:435–449
15. Doyle PJ et al (2008) Cloning, expression, and characterization of a single-domain antibody fragment with affinity for 15-acetyl-deoxynivalenol. Mol Immunol 45(14):3703–3713
16. Arbabi-Ghahroudi M, MacKenzie R, Tanha J (2009) Selection of non-aggregating VH binders from synthetic VH phage-display libraries. Methods Mol Biol 525:187–216, xiii.
17. Sambrook J, Fritsch EF, Maniatis T (1989) Molecular cloning: a laboratory manual, 2nd edn. Cold Spring Harbor Laboratory, Cold Spring Harbor, NY
18. Arbabi-Ghahroudi M, Tanha J, MacKenzie R (2009) Isolation of monoclonal antibody fragments from phage display libraries. Methods Mol Biol 502:341–364
19. Neu HC, Heppel LA (1965) The release of enzymes from *Escherichia coli* by osmotic shock and during the formation of spheroplasts. J Biol Chem 240(9):3685–3692
20. Laemmli UK (1970) Cleavage of structural proteins during the assembly of the head of bacteriophage T4. Nature 227(5259):680–685
21. Pace CN et al (1995) How to measure and predict the molar absorption coefficient of a protein. Protein Sci 4(11):2411–2423
22. Buttenschoen K, Radermacher P, Bracht H (2010) Endotoxin elimination in sepsis: physiology and therapeutic application. Langenbecks Arch Surg 395(6):597–605
23. Greisman SE, Hornick RB (1969) Comparative pyrogenic reactivity of rabbit and man to bacterial endotoxin. Proc Soc Exp Biol Med 131(4):1154–1158
24. Bentala H et al (2002) Removal of phosphate from lipid A as a strategy to detoxify lipopolysaccharide. Shock 18(6):561–566

Chapter 17

Expression of VHHs in *Saccharomyces cerevisiae*

Andrea Gorlani, Hans de Haard, and Theo Verrips

Abstract

The production of VHHs in microorganisms is relatively straightforward, however the amount of VHH produced per volume unit can vary substantially from hardly detectable to hundreds of milligrams per liter. Expression in *Escherichia coli* is more commonly used at initial research phase, since production of VHHs for large-scale application in *E. coli* is for a number of reasons not preferred. Otherwise VHH production in GRAS organisms such as *Saccharomyces cerevisiae* fits very well with industrial fermentation processes, and in fact the only commercially available VHHs are produced in *S. cerevisiae*. Immediately after the discovery of heavy chain only antibodies, which are per definition devoid of light chains, it was investigated whether many problems encountered with the production of conventional antibodies in lower eukaryotes were absent during the production of VHHs. Here we provide a protocol for the expression of VHH genes in *S. cerevisiae* in a fed-batch fermentation process. This protocol is also suitable for the production of multivalent VHHs.

Key words: *S. cerevisiae*, Fermentation, Fed-batch, Shake-flask, Heterologous protein, Downstream processing, Purification

1. Introduction

Among yeasts, *Saccharomyces cerevisiae* was reportedly used in several fermentation processes for the production of VHHs for both industrial applications and for pharmaceutical use (1–3). Despite the high variability (up to two logs) in secretion efficiency of VHHs differing only a few amino acids from each other, the highest yield so far described was achieved in *S. cerevisiae* (1) and not in *Pichia pastoris*, which is usually more favorable for the production of heterologous proteins (Verrips, unpublished data).

In this chapter, the VHH expression cassette is part of a multi-copy integration system that combines the advantage of a high copy number and a good mitotic stability (4). The selection method is based on auxotrophy complementation by the partially active

Dirk Saerens and Serge Muyldermans (eds.), *Single Domain Antibodies: Methods and Protocols*,
Methods in Molecular Biology, vol. 911, DOI 10.1007/978-1-61779-968-6_17, © Springer Science+Business Media, LLC 2012

leu2-d allele, which promotes a higher copy number of expression cassettes integrating into the rDNA locus (5). The strong GAL7 promoter used in combination with a *gal*⁻ strain does not require constant addition of galactose because this sugar cannot be metabolized (6). Especially in expensive large-scale fermentations, this has a cost reduction effect. Many signal sequences were tested for compatibility with VHH secretion in *S. cerevisiae* and the invertase leader SUC2 revealed the highest efficiency with most VHHs.

Transformation of yeast cells (*gal1* strain CEN-PK102-3A*gal1* (*gal1*:URA3, *leu2*, *ura3*) is available from EUROSCARF strains collection) is carried out following the procedure described by Gietz and Schiestl (7), which is based on the lithium acetate/single-stranded carrier DNA/PEG method. This protocol requires 4–6 days to recover the transformed colonies to be screened for secretion, and has a high transormation efficiency. Screening a large number of transformant colonies will ensure that a yeast clone with high productivity is selected for the next scaling up step.

During the initial research phase shake-flask cultivation is preferred because of low costs and possibility to screen a larger number of transformants. However, when hundreds of milligrams or more of protein are required, fermentation in a chemostat allows a higher yield of protein in a better controlled way. Fed-batch fermentation is widely used in most industrial processes (8).

Here we describe a fed-batch fermentation characterized by repeated cycles of feed-and-harvest in a small (2 L) bench-top bioreactor, with little volume increase ability. Once the batch phase is completed, the repeated feed cycles allow exploiting the benefits of high cell-density cultivation for a longer period of time than conventional fed-batch runs.

We exploited the findings of van de Laar et al. (9) and used ethanol as sole carbon source in feed. This strategy yields appreciable improvement of productivity, especially with VHHs whose secretion efficiency upon glucose cultivation is not very high.

Downstream processing, including purification, accounts for a large part of the time and costs (up to 75%) related to production of the protein. Even though the presence of COOH-terminal tags can ease the purification, most pharmaceutical and consumer goods applications do not allow presence of tags. Therefore a two-steps ion exchange strategy is described to purify tag-less VHHs from clarified fermentation medium. VHH preparations following this method are pure, stable, and withstand long-term storage in absence of stabilizers and preservatives.

Before starting the cloning work into the expression vector we recommend to check that the VHH gene codon usage is optimal for the *S. cerevisiae* system, and that no glycosylation sites are present. Even though N-glycosylation is rare in VHHs and O-glycosylation was never observed, it is worth to make sure that these typical posttranslational modifications in yeast do not affect the folding, functionality, or activity of the antibody fragment. If such glycosylation motifs are observed, the use of a yeast *pmt1* mutant strain is necessary or the N-glycosylation motif should be mutated.

2. Materials

2.1. Screening of High-Secreting Transformants

1. YNB plates: 6.7 g Yeast Nitrogen Base w/o amino acids (BD, Sparks, MD, USA), 20 g agar, 20 g glucose, distilled water. Weigh 20 g of agar in a bottle; add distilled water to 800 mL and autoclave. Prepare 6.7 g of YNB in 100 mL of distilled water and filter sterilize. Prepare 20 g of glucose in 100 mL of distilled water and autoclave separately. Melt agar in a microwave oven, add YNB and glucose solutions and pour in Petri dishes.
2. YPD Expression medium: 20 g of Peptone, 10 g of Yeast Extract, distilled water to 900 mL. Autoclave. Prepare 20 g of glucose and 5 g of galactose in 100 mL of distilled water and autoclave. Mix the two components.
3. SDS polyacrylamide gels. Standard SDS gel, with 12% polyacrylamide. SDS-PAGE running system.
4. SDS-PAGE sample buffer (4×): 80 mM Tris–HCl, pH 6.8, 33% glycerol, 6.7% SDS, 0.3 M DTT, 0.01% bromophenol blue.
5. Glycerol 60% in distilled water.
6. YNB Selective medium: prepare 6.7 g of Yeast Nitrogen Base, in 900 mL of distilled water and filter sterilize. Prepare 20 g of glucose in 100 mL of distilled water and autoclave. Mix the two components.

2.2. Fed-Batch Fermentation

If the purpose of the production is testing VHHs on cells or in animals, it is highly recommended to use LPS-free medium components since these contaminants are very difficult to eliminate quantitatively from the cultivation medium.

1. Standard bioreactor with working volume of at least 3 L. Possibility of controlling temperature, pH, dissolved oxygen tension via stirring speed. Our instrument is a Bioflow 3 (New Brunswick Scientific, NJ, USA) (see Note 1).
2. Gas analyzer for monitoring off-gas. We use a 1,440°C for O_2 and CO_2, and a Xendos 2500 for ethanol (both Servomex BV, Zoetermeer, Netherlands) (see Note 2).
3. Peristaltic pump, e.g., a Minipuls 3 (Gilson Inc., Middleton, WI, USA).

4. 2× 500 mL feed bottles and 2× 5 L containers, equipped with feed cap, air filters, and silicone tubing.
5. YNB Selective medium: prepare 6.7 g of Yeast Nitrogen Base, in 900 mL of distilled water and filter sterilize. Prepare 20 g of glucose in 100 mL of distilled water and autoclave. Mix the two components.
6. Egli trace metals: 5.5 g/L $CaCl_2 \cdot 2H_2O$, 3.75 g/L $FeSO_4 \cdot 7H_2O$, 1.4 g/L $MnSO_2 \cdot H_2O$, 2.2 g/L $ZnSO_4 \cdot 7H_2O$, 0.4 g/L $CuSO_4 \cdot 5H_2O$, 0.45 g/L $CoCl_2 \cdot 6H_2O$, 0.26 g/L $Na_2MoO_4 \cdot 2H_2O$, 0.4 g/L H_3Bo_3, 0.26 g/L KI, and 30 g/L NaEDTA. Dissolve everything in distilled water. Adjust the pH of the trace elements to 4.0 with NaOH and store at 4°C. This is a 100× solution.
7. Egli trace vitamins: 0.05 g/L biotin, 5 g/L thiamin, 47 g/L myoinositol, 1.2 g/L pyridoxin, and 23 g/L pantothenic acid. Dissolve everything in distilled water. This is a 1,000× solution.
8. Batch-phase medium: 15 g/L Yeast Extract, 2.1 g/L KH_2PO_4, 0.6 g/L $MgSO_4$, 10 mL/L Egli trace metals, 1 mL/L Egli trace vitamins, 22 g/L glucose, add distilled water to 1.5 L.
9. Feed-phase medium: it is separated in two equal volumes of nutrient feed (A) and ethanol feed (B) to avoid precipitation. (A) Nutrient feed: 50 g/L Yeast Extract, 24 g/L KH_2PO_4, 5 g/L $MgSO_4$, 40 mL/L Egli trace metals, 4 mL/L Egli trace vitamins, 10 g/L galactose add water to 2 L. (B) Ethanol feed: 670 g/L of 96% ethanol, add distilled water to 2 L.
10. Clean bottles to collect the harvested medium.

2.3. Shaker Flask Cultivation

1. YNB Selective medium: prepare 6.7 g of Yeast Nitrogen Base, in 900 mL of distilled water and filter sterilize. Prepare 20 g of glucose in 100 mL of distilled water and autoclave. Mix the two components.
2. YPD Expression medium: 20 g of Peptone, 10 g of Yeast Extract, distilled water to 900 mL. Autoclave. Prepare 20 g of glucose and 5 g of galactose in 100 mL of distilled water and autoclave. Mix the two components.
3. Erlenmeyer flask, autoclaved.

2.4. Downstream Processing: Medium Clarification and Purification

1. 0.45 μm PVDF membrane Durapore filters, 25 mm diameter (Millipore, Billerica, MA, USA) (see Note 3).
2. Filter-disc holder device, compatible with Durapore filters.
3. Sterile bottles for filtered medium.
4. Tangential-flow filtration device Vivaflow 200 (Sartorius, Goettingen, Germany).

5. Anion-exchange buffer: 25 mM sodium acetate pH 5.0.
6. 1 M Acetic acid.
7. Elution buffer: 25 mM sodium acetate pH 3.8, 500 mM NaCl.
8. PBS: For 1 L of 10× PBS dilute in distilled water 2.09 g KCl, 2.09 g KH_2PO_4, 86.0 g NaCl, 14.4 g $Na_2HPO_4{\cdot}H_2O$.
9. HiTrap Sepharose FF Q and SP 5 mL columns (GE Healthcare Europe GmbH, Munich, Germany).
10. 2 HiTrap Desalting 5 mL columns (GE Healthcare).

3. Methods

The growth time, concentration of glucose and concentration of galactose is described in Subheading 3.1. Screening of transformants, Subheading 3.2. Fed-batch fermentation and Subheading 3.3. Shaker flask cultivation is optimized for *S. cerevisiae* strain CEN-PK102-3A*gal1*. For different yeast strains these parameters might be different.

3.1. Screening for High-Secreting Transformants

1. After transformation of yeast with the method of choice (7), plate cells on a wide (20 cm) YNB plate and let grow at 30°C until colonies appear. This can take up to 4–5 days.
2. Prepare small YNB plates and when dry, pick single colonies from the transformation plate and streak onto the new plates. Each single plate can accommodate 3–4 colonies (see Note 4). Incubate in stove at 30°C for 3 days.
3. Inoculate one single colony each streak in 5 mL of YPD expression medium. Incubate in shaken incubator at 30°C at 200 rpm for 48 h.
4. Take 100 μL culture samples every 6 hours, starting at 24 h (see Note 5). Centrifuge on a table-top centrifuge for 3 min at 13,400 ×*g*. Transfer 20 μL of supernatant to a new tube and mix with SDS-PAGE sample buffer.
5. After taking the last sample (at least 48 h), run a 12% SDS-PAGE for 40 min at 200 V. Load 15 μL per time point (see Note 6).
6. Stain the gel with Coomassie Blue for 30 min and destain until protein bands appear. VHH migrate at about 15 kDa (see Note 7 and Fig. 1).
7. Reinoculate the colonies that give the best secretion of VHH in 5 mL of YPD selective medium at 30°C over night. The next day mix 1 mL of cultures with 0.5 mL of glycerol 60% and store at −80°C.

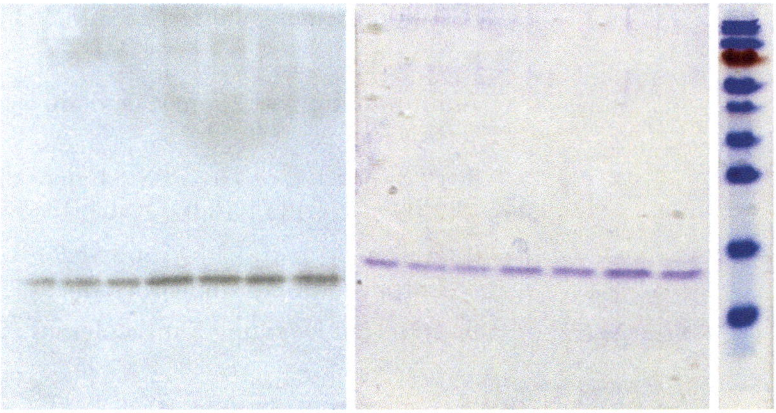

Fig. 1. Western blot (*left*) and Coomassie-stained gel of VHH D7 shake-flask production. Supernatant was sampled at 24, 30, 36, 48, 52, 56, 60 h, and 6 μL were mixed with 2 μL of sample buffer and loaded on gel.

3.2. Fed-Batch Fermentation

General knowledge on how to operate a fermenter (assembly, sterilization, monitoring run parameters) is considered part of the background of the scientist who's embarking in this production process. If fermentation equipment is not available, a simplified shake-flask protocol is also described below (see Subheading 3.3).

1. Inoculate 5 mL of selective YNB medium with the glycerol stock (see Subheading 3.1, step 7) and grow overnight at 30°C.
2. The next day inoculate 2× 50 mL of batch-phase medium with 2× 1 mL of the overnight culture and grow overnight at 30°C. This is the starter culture (see Note 8).
3. Clean and assemble the fermenter vessel but prior to closing the head plate prepare the batch-phase medium, except glucose and vitamins, and pour it into the vessel (see Note 9).

   Prepare one bottle containing glucose and connect it to a feed port of the vessel (see Note 10).

   Hand-tighten the bolts on the head plate, insert all the probes in the head plate and cover with hydrophilic cotton and aluminum foil the parts that need to be protected. Prior to autoclaving the pH probe needs to be calibrated according to the fermenter manufacturer's instructions (see Note 11).

   Autoclave the fermenter and the glucose bottle.
4. Prepare the feed-phase medium except for galactose and vitamins in a feed bottle (see Note 10). Prepare galactose in a separate bottle.

   Autoclave the feed container and the galactose separately, pour ethanol in a sterile feed bottle but do not autoclave it. Add sterile water to it.

5. Once the vessel, glucose bottle, feed container, and galactose bottle have cooled down, connect the vessel to the fermenter console according to manufacturer's instructions and air-blow the glucose in sterile conditions into the vessel. Similarly, blow the galactose in to the feed reservoir.
6. Add Egli trace vitamins (see Subheading 2.2, item 7) to the vessel and to the feed reservoir using a syringe and a filter.
7. At this point the fermenter has to be preconditioned and the dissolved oxygen (DO) probe calibrated. Growth parameters are pH 5.0, temperature 30°C, stirring should be automatically controlled by proportional–integral–derivative (PID) algorithm in order to maintain 30% minimum DO tension, 2 L/min air.
8. During preconditioning connect the feed reservoir and the ethanol reservoir to a peristaltic pump and to a feed port on the vessel via sterile silicone tubing. Set pump speed in order to obtain an initial dilution rate of 0.06 per hour with a volume of a 1.5 L.
9. When parameters in the vessel are stable (see Note 12), pour the 100 mL of full grown starter culture in the vessel in sterile conditions (see Note 13). This is the beginning of the batch phase.
10. Monitor off-gas and start feeding when ethanol concentration decreases below 300 ppm. This is the beginning of the first feed cycle (see Notes 5 and 14).
11. Feed at initial dilution rate of 0.06 per hour. If a feed-back control is connected to the pump, the concentration of ethanol in the off-gas should control the feed rate so that no accumulation of ethanol occurs in the vessel (set limit to 1,000 ppm). If no feed-back control is available, pump needs to be manually stopped when ethanol concentration increases over 1,000 ppm.
12. Feed culture with 1 L of feed-phase medium (see Subheading 2.1, item 9).
13. Pause the pump and harvest 1 L of culture in sterile conditions. Then go back to step 10 of Subheading 3.2 and repeat twice through step 12 (see Note 15).
14. End of fermentation: switch the pump off, wait for ethanol concentration in the off-gas to reach background level, switch the air flow and stirring off.
15. Harvest the whole culture in sterile conditions.
16. Switch off and disassemble the fermenter for routine cleaning and sterilization.

3.3. Shake-Flask Cultivation

1. Inoculate 2× 4 mL of YPD selective medium in a 50 mL Falcon tube with the glycerol stock and grow overnight at 30°C. This is the starter culture.
2. Prepare a 2.5 L sterile Erlenmeyer flask with 400 mL of YPD expression medium.

3. Dilute the starter culture 1:100 in YPD expression medium and grow at 30°C for 48 h shaking at 200 rpm (220 rpm if the flask is not baffled).
4. After 24 h of growth add 4 mL of 100% ethanol.
5. Harvest medium by centrifugation 15 min at 5,000 × *g*.
6. Continue further (see Subheading 3.4, step 6).

3.4. Downstream Processing: Medium Clarification and Purification

1. Centrifuge fermentation medium (see Subheading 3.3, step 7) for 15 min at 5,000 × *g*.
2. Pour supernatant in a clean container and filter it through a Durapore filter membrane (see Note 3). Collect filtered supernatant in a sterile container.
3. Prepare 2 L of anion-exchange buffer.
4. Reduce supernatant volume using a Vivaflow membrane module with 5 kDa molecular weight cut-off according to manufacturer instructions (two modules can be used in parallel to speed up tangential-flow filtration).
5. Concentrate sample to about 400 mL, then add 1 L of anion-exchange buffer and repeat by adding another liter of anion-exchange buffer when volume is 400 mL (see Note 16).
6. Make sure that pH of the sample is 5.0; if it is not, adjust pH with 1 M acetic acid.
7. Load sample on a HiTrap Sepharose FF Q 5 mL column. Many contaminating proteins remain bound whereas VHH is found in the flow-through. Collect flow-through in a sterile container.
8. Lower pH of the flow-through to 3.8 with 1 M acetic acid and load it on a HiTrap Sepharose FF SP 5 mL column. VHH will bind the cation exchange column.
9. Elute VHH with elution buffer.
10. Load eluted VHH on two HiTrap Desalting 5 mL columns connected and pre equilibrated with PBS.
11. Collect protein fraction in sterile Eppendorf tubes.

4. Notes

1. Several bioreactors are available on the market. Most of them meet the requirements listed here, so the protocol described here can be performed in most of the cases.
2. When a gas analyzer is not available, other methods have been described to measure ethanol concentration in the fermentation medium such as enzymatic assays. Nevertheless, it is very

important to be able to measure ethanol concentration "on line" as this is a fast indication of which type of metabolism yeast cells are going through.

3. Sterile filter cups, with the same pore size, are also available, but given the unavoidable turbidity of the centrifuged fermentation broth, we recommend to use disposable filter-disc, as they are cheap and easy to replace when one gets clogged.
4. We observe fluctuations in secretion efficiency of transformed *S. cerevisiae* cells. A screening of at least 15–20 transformant colonies will ensure a high-secreting one will be selected.
5. Checking secretion over time will tell how long it will take the culture to metabolize all the glucose and to uptake the galactose.
6. 15 μL of medium contain usually enough protein to be visible by Coomassie stain. If not, it's possible to perform a standard Western Blot and detect the VHH with specific antibodies. If the amount of VHH is not detectable, secretion level is too low to proceed with production.
7. Due to very few proteins secreted by yeast and usually good secretion efficiency, the VHH band stands out as the most intense on gel. Cell lysis should be avoided as the released, intracellular proteases might degrade the product.
8. Sometimes baffled flasks are used to increase aeration and growth. The effect can be appreciated when production is carried out in the flask itself, but in this case the starter culture will have enough time to consume all the glucose also in a normal Erlenmeyer flask.
9. When sugars are autoclaved with other medium components, degradation and irreversible formation of toxic (Maillard-like) compounds will cause a lower biomass yield, and in the case of galactose, it will impair induction of gene expression.
   Vitamins are heat sensitive, so they have to be added separately.
10. Make sure that the silicon tubing used to connect the bottle cap to the feed port is long enough; this will facilitate moving the fermenter in and out of the autoclave and general handling.
11. We rely on the background experience on the fermenter operator to perform these operations, as they are specific for each fermenter type.
12. It may take up to a few hours before the parameters are stable.
13. It is possible to use the bottle previously used for glucose, as that is still connected to the feed port on the vessel. Opening the bottle next to the flame and pouring the starter culture will keep the bottle sterile.

14. To our experience the culture will take 16–20 h to use all the glucose, and the ethanol produced during the glucose fermentation. Next, ethanol concentration starts decreasing. Feeding at 300 ppm of ethanol will ensure that the culture has not entered decline phase yet, so the growth rate will adjust to the dilution rate faster.
15. It is very important that, after harvesting, the monitored parameters are stable. Quite often we observed that the ethanol concentration in off-gas increased dramatically upon harvesting. Wait until ethanol has decreased before applying the next feed cycle.
16. Performing two cycles of dialysis/concentration ensures that the buffer is completely exchanged, and the sample volume —400 mL— is easily loaded on the first ion exchange column.

Acknowledgement

This work was supported by EMPRO and Bill and Melissa Foundation. Dr. T. van de Laar is kindly acknowledged for instructing A. Gorlani on fermentation procedures.

References

1. Frenken LG, van der Linden RH, Hermans PW, Bos JW, Ruuls RC, de Geus B, Verrips CT (2000) Isolation of antigen specific Llama VHH antibody fragments and their high level secretion by *Saccharomyces cerevisiae*. J Biotechnol 78:11–21
2. van der Vaart JM (2002) Expression of VHH antibody fragments in *Saccharomyces cerevisiae*. Methods Mol Biol 178:359–366
3. Thomassen YE, Verkleij AJ, Boonstra J, Verrips CT (2005) Specific production rate of VHH antibody fragments by *Saccharomyces cerevisiae* is correlated with growth rate, independent of nutrient limitation. J Biotechnol 118:270–277
4. Lopes TS, de Wijs IJ, Steenhauer SI, Verbakel J, Planta RJ (1996) Factors affecting the mitotic stability of high-copy-number integration into the ribosomal DNA of *Saccharomyces cerevisiae*. Yeast (Chichester, England) 12:467–477
5. Erhart E, Hollenberg CP (1983) The presence of a defective LEU2 gene on 2pi DNA recombinant plasmids of *Saccharomyces cerevisiae* is responsible for curing and high copy number. J Bacteriol 156:625–635
6. Johnston M (1987) A model fungal gene regulatory mechanism: the GAL genes of *Saccharomyces cerevisiae*. Microbiol Rev 51: 458–476
7. Gietz RD, Schiestl RH (2007) High-efficiency yeast transformation using the LiAc/SS carrier DNA/PEG method. Nat Protoc 2:31–34
8. Hensing MC, Rouwenhorst RJ, Heijnen JJ, van Dijken JP, Pronk JT (1995) Physiological and technological aspects of large-scale heterologous-protein production with yeasts. Antonie Van Leeuwenhoek 67:261–279
9. van de Laar T, Visser C, Holster M, Lopez CG, Kreuning D, Sierkstra L, Lindner N, Verrips T (2007) Increased heterologous protein production by *Saccharomyces cerevisiae* growing on ethanol as sole carbon source. Biotechnol Bioeng 96:483–494

Chapter 18

Stable Expression of Chimeric Heavy Chain Antibodies in CHO Cells

Vishal Agrawal, Igor Slivac, Sylvie Perret, Louis Bisson, Gilles St-Laurent, Yanal Murad, Jianbing Zhang, and Yves Durocher

Abstract

Camelid single domain antibodies fused to noncamelid Fc regions, also called chimeric heavy chain antibodies (cHCAb), offer great potential as therapeutic and diagnostic candidates due to their relatively small size (80 kDa) and intact Fc. In this chapter, we describe two approaches, limiting dilution and mini-pools, for generating nonamplified Chinese hamster ovary cell lines stably expressing cHCAb in suspension and serum-free cultures using a stringent antibiotic selection. Neither of the protocols necessitates the acquisition or implementation of expensive automated infrastructures and thus could be applied in any lab with minimal cell culture setup. The given protocol allows the isolation of stable clones capable of generating up to 100 mg/L of antibody in batch mode performed in shaker flasks.

Key words: Fc fusions, PEImax, Antibody production, Cell line development, Antibiotic selection

1. Introduction

Chimeric heavy chain antibodies (cHCAb) are generated by the fusion of camelid single domain antibody to human/mouse fragment crystallizable (Fc) (1). They represent a novel class of antibodies that were first found in Camelidae (2). Despite that these antibodies lack a light chain and are composed of a heavy chain dimer only, they are fully functional in antigen recognition (3). Due to their small size, cHCAb may offer a greater tumor penetration capability compared to the full-size antibodies and are thus viewed as a promising new class of antibodies for therapeutic, diagnostic, and imaging purposes (4). In order to develop cHCAb

Vishal Agrawal and Igor Slivac contributed equally to this chapter.

Dirk Saerens and Serge Muyldermans (eds.), *Single Domain Antibodies: Methods and Protocols*, Methods in Molecular Biology, vol. 911, DOI 10.1007/978-1-61779-968-6_18, © Springer Science+Business Media, LLC 2012

drug candidates, their continuous supply in sufficient quantity for cell-based and animal assay is required.

Mammalian cells are preferred host for the production of secreted proteins harboring posttranslational modifications that are often necessary for their optimal biological activity (5). Biomanufacturing in mammalian cells has made considerable advances in the last decades, from the early times of low-density culture of adherent cultures in presence of serum to the recent high-density cultures of suspension growing cells adapted to serum-free media. Yet, the low volumetric productivity and long development timelines in mammalian cells compared to other lower eukaryotes or microbial host systems provide a challenge to both academic and industrial researchers. Suspension-adapted Chinese hamster ovary cells (e.g., CHO-Kl, CHO-DXB11, and CHO-DG44) have been able to address these issues and are thus the predominant expression systems used to manufacture a majority of the clinically approved biologics (5, 6). A variant of the dihydrofolate reductase (dhfr)-deficient CHO-DXB11 cell line (7) has been used in this work.

A stable cell line is generated when an exogenous DNA containing a gene of interest is stably integrated into a transcriptionally active site of host genome. The integration event is random and the frequency of integration into a transcriptionally active site is extremely low. Furthermore, many integration events occur into chromosomal sites where transcription is susceptible to silencing (8). The isolation of stable cell lines expressing high level of the transgene of interest is thus a time- and labor-intensive process. Various approaches to shorten the time and lessen the labor have been developed including the use of automated colony screening and picking systems (e.g., Genetix's Clonepix™ system, http://www.genetix.com or Aviso's CellCelector™, http://www.automationpartnership.com). However, most academic labs and small biotech companies cannot afford acquiring these highly expensive systems and rather utilize the classical method of clone isolation by limiting dilution or through the use of cloning rings because of its low infrastructure costs and ease of implementation. The process of stable cell line development involves delivery of a plasmid DNA containing the gene of interest into exponentially growing host cells. Variety of biophysical methods or chemical agents can be used to that end, such as electroporation, cationic lipids, polycations, and calcium phosphate. Transfection using the polycation polyethylenimine (PEI)[1] has been shown to be a cost-effective mean to generate milligram to gram amounts of protein when performed at

[1]Use of PEI for transfection may be covered by existing intellectual property rights, including US Patent 6,013,240, European Patent 0,770,140, and foreign equivalents for which further information may be obtained by contacting licensing@polyplus-transfection.com.

Table 1
List of various eukaryotic antibiotics and their respective toxic concentration range in CHO cells

Antibiotic	Gene	Mode of action	Concentration μg/mL[a]
Blasticidin S (from *Streptomyces griseochromogenes*)	Blasticidin deaminase from *Bacillus cereus*	Inhibits protein synthesis by interfering with the peptidyl transfer reaction causing premature translation termination	1–5
Geneticin (G418)	Neomycin phosphotransferase from Tn5 or aph2	Blocks protein synthesis by interfering with protein elongation	500–1,500
Hygromycin B (from *Streptomyces hygroscopicus*)	Hygromycin phosphotransferase from *Escherichia coli*	Inhibit protein synthesis by disrupting ribosome translocation and promoting mistranslation	500–1,500
Puromycin (from *Streptomyces alboniger*)	Puromycin acetyltransferase from *Streptomyces*	Blocks protein synthesis by causing premature translation termination	5–25
Zeocin (from *Streptomyces verticillus*)	Sh ble gene from *Streptaolloteichus hindustanus*	A copper-chelated glycopeptide antibiotic that intercalates into the DNA and causes strand cleavage	10–1,000

[a]The concentration to be used should be determined as it greatly depends on the cell line, the promoter driving expression of the resistance gene, and culture medium used

large scale (9, 10). It also allowed us to generate stable transfectants expressing high yields of a secreted protein (11).

In this work, we have used PEI to efficiently generate stable CHO cell lines. An antibiotic selection cassette in the same plasmid provided the mean to kill nontransfected cells and enrich positive transfectants upon addition of the selection drug. Of all the antibiotics known for eukaryotic cells selection (see Table 1), puromycin kills nontransfected cells most quickly, in about 48–72 h. Its rapid action on the nontransfected cells makes it suitable to be used as a selective agent of choice. Selection is either performed on entire transfected population in T-flasks or on small pools (minipools) of cells distributed in 96-well plates. Consequently, for both approaches, a limiting dilution screening which basically involves seeding of approximately one cell per well of a 96-well plate is performed to identify the stable monoclonal cell lines (see Fig. 1). The top few clones are usually expanded and banked into cryovials. With this protocol, we isolated clones that could produce up to 100 mg/L of cHCAb in batch culture.

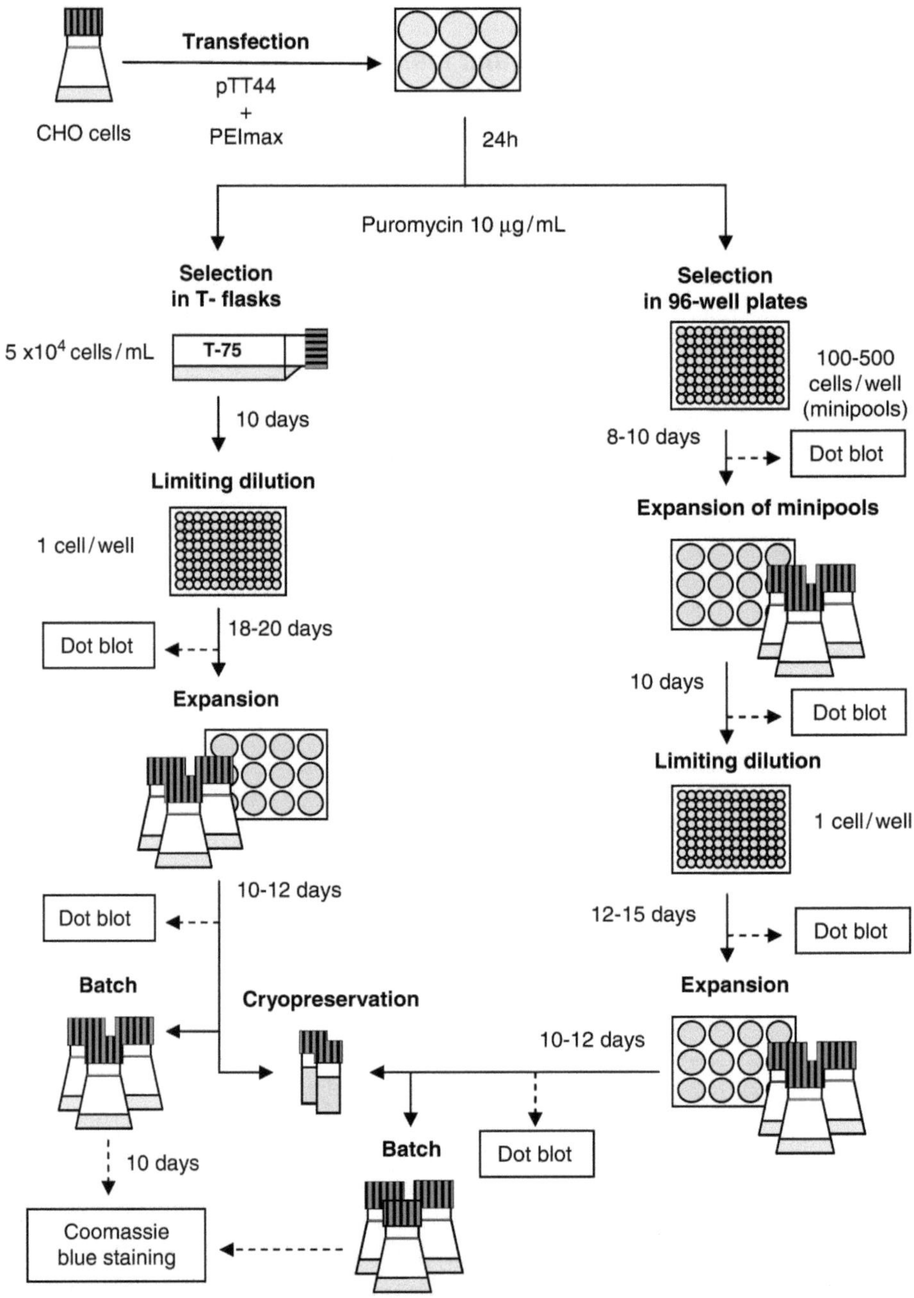

Fig. 1. Stable CHO cell line development schematic. Two strategies of stable cell line development for the production of cHCAb: limiting dilution (*left*) and minipool (*right*). Both methods require the selection of transfected cells through a stringent antibiotic marker. Whereas in limiting dilution method the clones are isolated directly from the entire selected population, minipools strategy involves the division of the transfected population into smaller pools and the clones are isolated from the highest producing minipools.

2. Materials

2.1. cHCAb Constructs

1. The cHCAb EG2-human Fc1 that recognizes the human EGF receptor was as described (12) except that the camelid sdAb portion was synthesized de novo using human-biased codons (Geneart, Regensburg, Germany).
2. The EG2-hFc1 cDNA was cloned into the pTT30 (see Fig. 2) or pTT44 vector (a modified pTT30 vector containing a S/MAR element) using EcoRI and BamHI restriction enzymes.
3. The second cHCAb (2A2-mFc2b), which recognizes the human CEACAM6 antigen, was constructed using the camelid 2A2 anti-CEACAM6 sdAb, which was selected by panning from an immune Llama library (unpublished data). The 2A2-mouse Fc2b gene was synthesized de novo by Geneart using human-biased codons and cloned into the pTT30 or pTT44 vector using EcoRI and BamHI restriction enzymes.

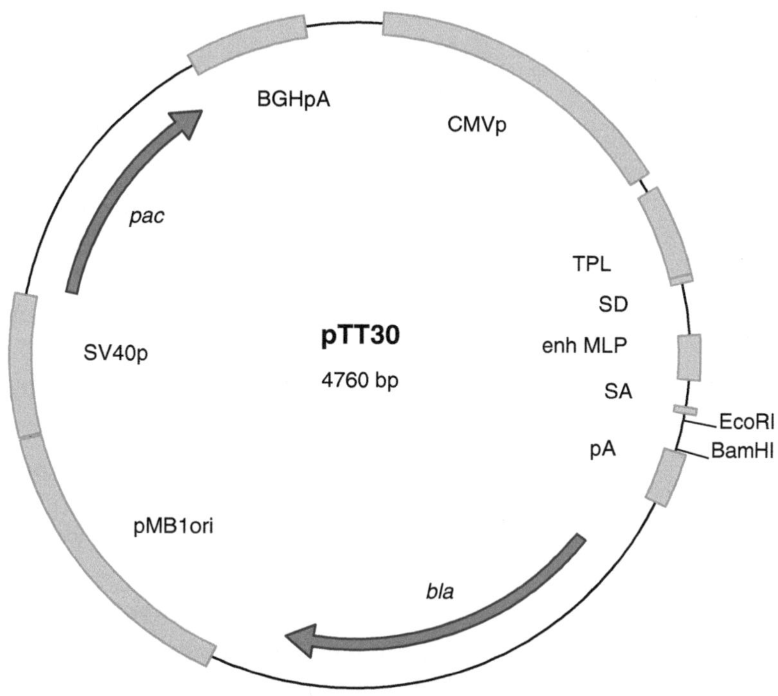

Fig. 2. pTT30 vector schematic. *CMVp* CMV promoter; *TPL* adenovirus tripartite leader; *SD* splice donor; *enh MLP* adenovirus major late promoter enhancer; *SA* splice acceptor; *pA* rabbit beta globin polyadenylation signal; *bla* beta lactamase gene; *pMB1ori* bacterial origin of replication; *SV40p* SV40 early promoter; *pac* puromycin acetyltransferase gene; *BGHpA* bovine growth hormone polyadenylation signal.

2.2. Plasmid Linearization

1. Purified supercoiled pTT30 and pTT44 plasmid preparation.
2. Pvu I restriction endonuclease (New England Biolabs, MA, USA).
3. DNA gel electrophoresis apparatus (Bio-Rad laboratories, Mississauga, ON, Canada).
4. Heating block set at 37° C.
5. Nanodrop™ (Thermo fisher scientific, Wilmington, DE, USA).
6. 3 M sodium acetate, pH 5.2.
7. 95% Ethanol.
8. 10 mM Tris–HCl, pH 7.4
9. 1 mM EDTA.

2.3. Transfection with PEI

1. CHO cells (13) adapted to suspension culture in serum-free medium.
2. CD culture medium (Invitrogen, Burlington, ON, Canada) supplemented with 8 mM glutamine and 0.18% Pluronic F68.
3. 6-well plates (Corning Inc., Lowell, MA, USA).
4. Disposable sterile plastic shaker flasks (Corning Inc., Lowell, MA, USA).
5. Humidified incubator at 37°C with 5% CO_2.
6. Orbital shaker set at 120 rpm (Analytiqs, Inc., Dorval, QC, Canada).
7. Polyethylenimine "MAX" linear, MW 25 kDa (40 kDa nominal), 3 mg/mL stock solution in water, pH 7.0 (Polysciences Inc., Warrington, PA, USA).
8. High-quality purified plasmid DNA of interest (e.g., made with Qiagen Maxi Kit or equivalent).
9. Phosphate buffered saline (PBS); 20 mM sodium phosphate, 150 mM NaCl, pH 7.2.
10. Trypan blue (0.2%w/v) or Erythrosin B (25 mg/mL) in PBS.

2.4. Selection and Screening via Limiting Dilution Strategy

1. 10 μg/mL puromycin sterile solution (Invitrogen, Burlington, ON, Canada).
2. Centrifuge (Heraeus-Thermo, Osterode, Germany).
3. Disposable sterile plastic T-75 flasks (Corning Inc., Lowell, MA, USA).
4. 6-, 12-, and 96-well plates (Corning Inc., Lowell, MA, USA).
5. Multichannel Pipette for seeding cells in 96-well plates (Rainin, Mississauga, ON, Canada).
6. Multichannel disposable solution basins (Cole-Parmer, Montreal, QC, Canada).

7. Sterile filter tips (Rainin, Mississauga, ON, Canada).
8. Humidified incubator at 37° C with 5% CO_2.
9. 15 mL: sterile falcon tubes.

2.5. Selection and Screening via Minipool Strategy

See Subheading 2.4.

2.6. Purification of cHCab

1. HiTrap MabSelect SuRe 5 mL column (GE Healthcare, Baie d'Urfe, QC, Canada).
2. HiPrep 26/10 Desalting column (GE Healthcare, Baie d'Urfe, QC, Canada).
3. 100 mM citrate buffer: 82 mM citric acid monohydrate, 18 mM trisodium citrate dihydrate, pH 3.0.
4. 1 M Tris-base pH 11 solution (should not need pH adjustment).
5. 0.45 μm bottle-top vacuum filter system (Corning Inc., Lowell, MA, USA).
6. Steritop filter unit (Millipore, Billerica, MA, USA) with a 500 mL filtrate capacity.
7. Centrifugation bottles with conical bottom (Corning Inc., Lowell, MA, USA).
8. SDS-PAGE gel electrophoresis and Western blot analysis (Bio-Rad Laboratories, Montreal, QC, Canada).
9. BM Chemiluminescence blotting substrate (POD; Roche, Laval, QC, Canada).
10. Protran nitrocellulose membrane (Whatman Inc., Piscataway, NJ, USA) for dot blot and western blot analyses.
11. Goat anti-mouse IgG (Fc specific)-peroxidase (Sigma-Aldrich, Oakville, ON, Canada).

2.7. Dot Blot Protocol

1. Protran nitrocellulose membrane (Whatman Inc., Piscataway, NJ, USA).
2. PIPETMAN® P2 (Gilson Inc, Middleton, WI, USA).
3. Shaking platform at room temperature.
4. BM Chemiluminescence blotting substrate (POD; Roche, Laval, QC, Canada).
5. Goat anti-mouse IgG (Fc specific)-peroxidase (Sigma-Aldrich, Oakville, ON, Canada).
6. Goat anti-human IgG (Fc specific)-peroxidase (Sigma-Aldrich, Oakville, ON, Canada).
7. PBST: PBS with 0.1% v/v Tween-20.
8. Kodak image station 440cf (Marketlink Scientific, Burlington, ON, Canada) or equivalent.

2.8. Cryopreservation Protocol

1. CD DG44 complete media (Invitrogen, Burlington, ON, Canada).
2. 1.8 mL cryovials (Corning Inc., Lowell, MA, USA).
3. Dimethyl sulfoxide (DMSO; Sigma-Aldrich, Oakville, ON, Canada).
4. Styrofoam boxes.
5. –80° C Freezer.
6. Liquid Nitrogen storage tank.

3. Methods

3.1. cHCAb Constructs

The gene of the cHCAb was entirely synthesized by Geneart using human-biased codons. The cHCAb constructs posses a signal peptide sequence (MEFGLSWVFLVAILKGVQC) preceded by a Kozak sequence (GCCACC). The llama 2A2 and EG2 sdAb are located between the end of the signal peptide and the hinge region of the Fc (mouse Fc2b or human Fc1, respectively). The codon-optimized constructs are flanked by EcoRI and BamHI restriction sites on the 5′ and 3′ ends, respectively, and subcloned in the pTT30 or pTT44 vector.

3.2. Plasmid Linearization

The pTT series of vectors (proprietary BRI, NRC) can be used to express high level of recombinant proteins in mammalian cells. The pTT30 and pTT44 plasmids carry two expression cassettes, one driving the expression of the cHCAb gene under the strong CMV promoter, while the other for expressing the puromycin acetyl-transferase gene under the control of the weak SV40 promoter. The pTT44 vector also bear a S/MAR sequence (unpublished) for increasing expression stability of expressing clones (14).

1. Linearize 50 μg of pTT44-EG2hFc1 plasmid at PvuI site for 3 h at 37° C (see Table 2 for details).

Table 2
Digestion reaction for the plasmid linearization

DNA (1 μg/μL)	50 μL
Buffer (10×)	10 μL
PvuI (10 U/μL)	5 μL
H_2O	35 μL
Total	100 μL

If the cHCAb gene contains a PvuI restriction site, another restriction enzyme cutting only in the prokaryotic elements (*bla* gene or ori) should be chosen

2. Ethanol precipitate the linearized plasmid by adding 0.1 volume of 3 M sodium acetate pH 5.2 and 2.5 volumes of 95% ethanol. Transfer in −20° C freezer for 2 h. Centrifuge at 10,000 × *g* for 10 min. Dissolve the plasmid pellet in 100 μL of sterile 10 mM Tris–HCl pH 7.4, 1 mM EDTA buffer.
3. Plasmid concentration is determined by absorbance at 260 nm using a Nanodrop™.
4. 50 ng of linearized plasmid is run on 0.8% agarose gel to confirm complete digestion and quality of the final product.
5. The working stock of linearized plasmid can be stored at −20° C. Long-term storage should be done at −80°C.

3.3. Transfection with PEI

1. One or two days prior to transfection, dilute the cells in a 50 mL shaker flask (10 mL working volume) to 2.5×10^5 cells/mL or 1.3×10^5 cells/mL, respectively, with CD DG44 culture medium. Transfer the flask on an orbital shaker (120 rpm) placed in the incubator (humidified 5% CO_2 and 37° C). Optimal cell density should be reached on the day of transfection (see Note 1).
2. On the day of transfection, warm the CD DG44 media to 37°C. Thaw the plasmid DNA (linearized) and PEImax.
3. Determine the cell density and viability using a hemocytometer. Cell density at transfection should range from 0.8 to 1.2×10^6 cells/mL (with a doubling time of 16–18 h) and viability should be greater than 98%.
4. Add 1.8 mL of cells to each well of a 6-well plate. Transfer the plate to the incubator on the orbital shaker (120 rpm).
5. Add 200 μL of CD DG44 media to 1.5 mL sterile eppendorf tubes.
6. Add 2 μg of DNA to each tube. Vortex gently.
7. Add 10 μg of PEImax to each tube containing DNA solution. Vortex immediately (3 times, 3 s each) after PEImax addition (see Note 2).
8. Incubate the mixture for 10 min at room temperature to allow polyplexes formation.
9. Remove the culture (see Subheading 3.3, step 4) from the incubator. Add the DNA/PEI polyplexes to the cells in a drop-wise fashion and swirl the plate gently. Return the culture to the agitator in the incubator (see Note 3).

3.4. Selection and Screening via Limiting Dilution Strategy

1. One day after transfection, determine cell density and viability on a 100 μL aliquot of transfected cells in the 6-well plate by using trypan blue (or erythrosine B) exclusion.
2. Transfected cells in the 6-well plate are diluted in 25 mL of fresh CD DG44 media at a density of 5×10^4 cells/mL in a

T-75 flask. Add puromycin at a final concentration of 10 μg/mL to initiate the selection process. Put the flask in the humidified CO_2 incubator at 37° C (see Note 4).

3. Puromycin kills the nontransfected cells (or cells expressing insufficient level of puromycin acetyltransferase) within 72 h and consequently a drop in cell viability should be observed. Media is changed by pipetting out 50% of the culture medium and adding equal volume of fresh medium with 10 μg/mL puromycin. Repeat this step every 4 days until cells reach up to 70–90% confluency.
4. Approximately 10–12 days after selection, assay for the antibody expression by performing a dot blot with the culture supernatant. At this point, viability should be greater than 90%.
5. In 15 mL sterile tubes, perform serial tenfold dilutions of the cells to obtain final cell concentrations of 0.5 or 1 cell/100 μL. For example, if the viable cell count is 1 million cells/mL. To obtain 1 cell per 100 μL, firstly dilute 15 μL of selected cells in 15 mL of medium without puromycin. Next, take 150 μL from these diluted cells and add in another tube containing 15 mL of medium without puromycin. Using a mixture of 50% fresh medium and 50% conditioned medium (without puromycin) for the limiting dilution step supports the growth of single cells as compared to the 100% fresh media (see Note 5). Make sure that the cells are not aggregated to increase clonality likelihood of emerging colonies.
6. Using a multichannel pipette, fill each well of 96-well plates with 100 μL of cell dilution (that have been transferred in sterile multichannel pipette trays). Wait for 5–10 days until the colonies start to appear. Only wells with a single colony should be taken into account for further analyses.
7. Refeed the plate by adding 100 μL of 50% fresh media and 50% conditioned media mixture. Incubate the plates for another 5 days. During that time check for the colony development every other day.
8. After another 5 days, replace 100 μL of media in marked wells with the same volume of fresh CD DG44 media. Repeat this step until the majority of the colonies grow to at least 50% confluency.
9. 18–20 days after cell plating, test for product by dot blot (see Fig. 3).
10. Based on the dot blot results and visual inspection of the colony size, pick the positive clones for expansion in 12-well plates containing 1 mL of fresh CD DG44 media without puromycin (see Note 6).
11. Incubate 12-well plates until approximately 80% confluency is reached (typically 4–5 days after plating).

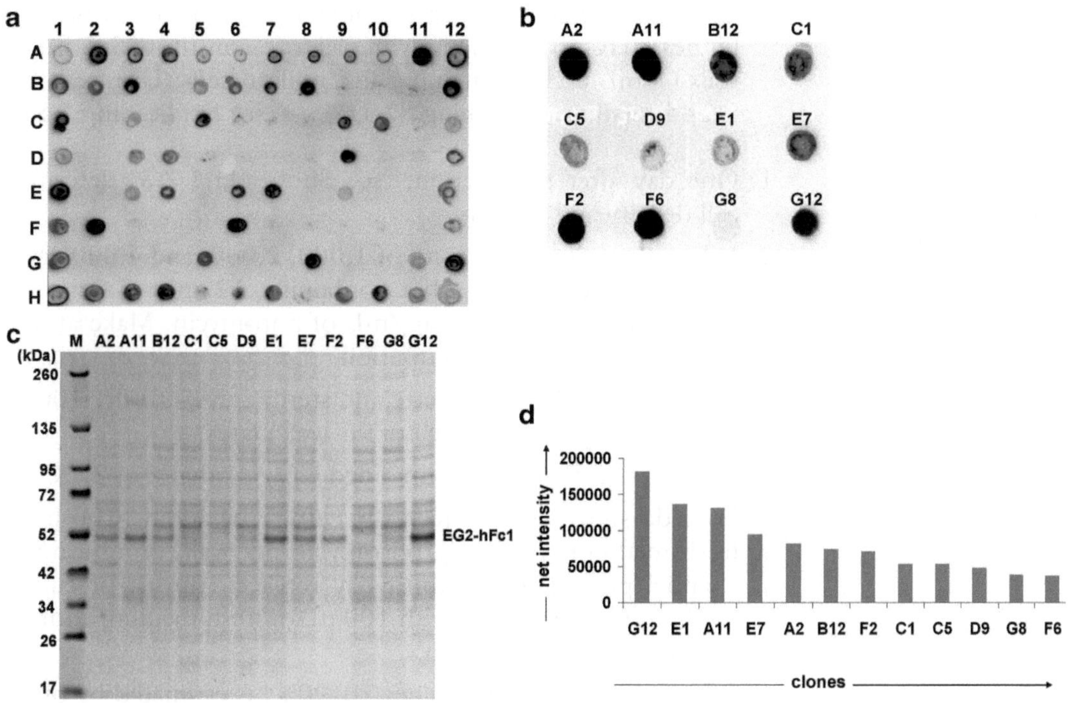

Fig. 3. Productivity analysis of isolated clones (**a**) dot blot from 96-well plate supernatants (**b**) dot blot from 12-well plate supernatants (**c**) SDS-PAGE and Coomassie staining of supernatants from 125 mL shaker flasks (**d**) clone ranking by integrating the cHCAb band intensity on Coomassie-stained SDS-PAGE.

12. Assay for the presence of antibody in media by performing a dot blot (see Fig. 3).

13. Gently detach the cells from positive wells by gently pipetting the culture medium up and down (avoid making air bubbles as this kills the cells). Transfer 75% of the resuspended cells into 125 mL shake flasks containing 10 mL of fresh CD DG44 media without puromycin. Place the flasks on an orbital shaker set at 120 rpm inside a 37°C humidified CO_2 incubator. Refill the 12-well plates with fresh media and put them back in the incubator. This is done as a precaution in case cells fail to recover after transfer.

14. When the clones in flasks reach $1–2 \times 10^6$ cells/mL, test for their productivity by cultivating them in a batch mode for 10 days. For this purpose, use new flasks and inoculate cells in 25 mL of fresh media at a density of 2.5×10^5 cells/mL. Keep the rest of the cells under regular maintenance by passing them three times a week. Check for the cell density and viability of the clones on day 10. Analyze productivity by performing a SDS-PAGE and Coomassie blue staining (see Fig. 3) to determine the best producing clones. Alternatively, antibody titers can be measured by ELISA or Protein-A/G HPLC.

15. Using cells from regular maintenances, amplify those with highest cHCAb productivity in order to constitute 3–5 frozen vials (1 mL each) containing five million cells. Use fresh CD DG44 medium containing 8% DMSO (see Subheading 3.8).

3.5. Selection and Screening via Minipool Strategy

1. One day after transfection, (see Subheading 3.3) determine cell density and viability.
2. Dilute the cells to a density of 1,000, 2,000, and 4,000 cells/mL in sterile 15 mL tubes containing 12 mL of fresh CD DG44 medium with 10 μg/mL of puromycin. Make at least 3 × 15 mL tubes for each dilution.
3. Using a multichannel pipette and sterile trays, transfer 100 μL of diluted cells to each well of 96-well plates.
4. Transfer the plates in a humidified CO_2 incubator at 37°C.
5. Four days postseeding, feed the culture by adding 100 μL of fresh medium containing puromycin per well, using a multichannel pipette. Every third day replace 100 μL of culture medium from each well with 100 μL of fresh medium containing 10 μg/mL puromycin.
6. When cell confluency reaches 70–90% (as estimated by observation using an inverted microscope), assay for the presence of antibody in supernatant by performing a dot blot.
7. Depending on the intensity of dot blot signal and relative colony size, pick chosen minipools for expansion. Transfer positive minipools from each well into a 12-well plate containing 1 mL of fresh medium/well with 10 μg/mL puromycin. 12-well plates should be kept in an incubator in static conditions (see Note 7).
8. Cells will typically reach 80–90% confluency within 4 days. Perform a dot blot for assaying the antibody in media.
9. Choose the minipools with the best producing cells and transfer 75% of the volume in 125 mL plastic shake flask containing 10 mL of fresh CD DG44 media without puromycin. Put the flasks on an orbital shaker set at 120 rpm inside an incubator. Refill the minipools in the 12-well plates with fresh medium and put them back in the incubator. This is done as precaution in case of failure to recover selected minipools.
10. After 5 days use the dot blot protocol to screen for the antibody in media from shake flasks. Check also for the cell density and viability (see Note 8).
11. At this point, the minipools with the strongest signals are chosen for subcloning by limiting dilution. Perform the limiting dilution (see Note 9; see Subheading 3.4, step 5).

3.6. Purification of cHCAb

1. Centrifuge the harvested batch culture at 3,500×*g* for 15–20 min.
2. Filter the clarified culture medium through a 0.45 μm filter unit under vacuum.
3. Load the filtered medium at 5 mL/min onto a HiTrap MabSelect SuRe Protein-A column preequilibrated with 5 column volumes (CV) of PBS. Save the flow-through for further analysis.
4. Wash the column with 5 CV of PBS at 5 mL/min. Save the wash solution for further analysis.
5. Elute the cHCAb with 5 CV of citrate buffer, pH 3.2. Collect fractions of 1 mL each and pool those containing the cHCAb.
6. The protein concentration of the purified cHCAb may be determined with a Bradford protein assay. Alternatively, concentration may be determined from the absorbance at 280 nm, using the molar extinction coefficient of the protein.
7. Load the antibody containing pool on a HiPrep desalting column equilibrated with 2 CV of PBS at 10 mL/min. Collect the fractions with cHCAb based on UV absorbance at 280 nm or Bradford assay.
8. Filter the desalted antibody using 0.22 μm cartridges. Aliquot the purified cHCAbs in sterile screw-cap 2 mL polypropylene tubes and store them at −80°C.
9. Evaluate the production and purity of cHCAbs by SDS-PAGE and Coomassie staining of collected samples including the clarified culture medium supernatant, flow-through, wash, and the eluates from the Protein-A column (see Fig. 4).

3.7. Dot Blot Protocol

1. Cut an 8×12 cm piece of nitrocellulose membrane using a clean scalpel or scissors. A grid (0.5×0.5 cm per square) may be drawn using a pencil on the membrane surface to indicate the areas where each spot will occur.
2. Using a pipette, spot 2 μL of media samples onto the nitrocellulose membrane at the center of the grid (see Note 10).
3. Dry the membrane for 30 min at room temperature. Block the membrane by immersion in 10–20 mL of blocking solution at room temperature for 30 min with gentle shaking.
4. Prepare the antibody solution by diluting a peroxidase-labeled anti-Fc (select for the appropriate species specificity) antibody in fresh blocking solution (antibody dilution is typically 1:5,000)
5. Incubate the membrane in the antibody solution for 60 min at room temperature with gentle shaking.
6. Discard the antibody solution and wash the membrane with PBST (PBS with 0.1%v/v Tween-20) three times for 5 min each.

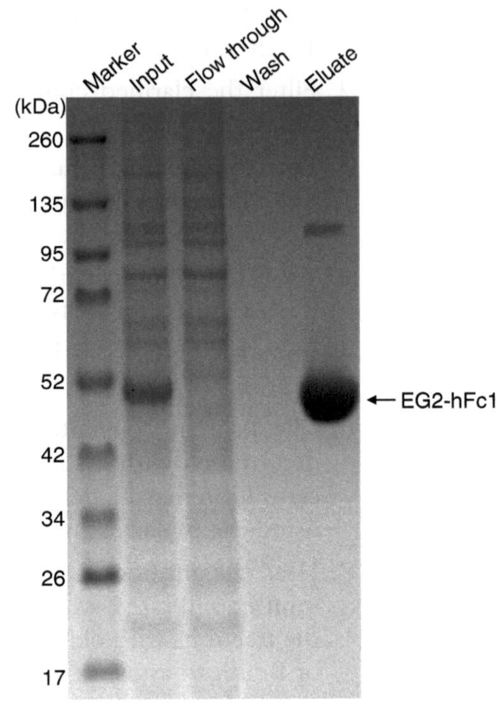

Fig. 4. Purification of cHCAb using HiTrap MAbSelect Sure™ protein A column. A 10-day batch culture was harvested and the supernatant was subjected to protein-A purification (see Subheading 3.6).

7. Incubate the membrane with chemiluminescence blotting substrate for 1 min.
8. Reveal the luminescent signal using X-ray films or other appropriate digital imaging device such as the Kodak IS440CF.

3.8. Cryopreservation Protocol

1. Prepare the freezing mixture by adding 8% (v/v) DMSO to fresh CD DG44 culture medium. Prechill this solution on ice.
2. Label the cryovials. Place in a small styrofoam box.
3. Count the cells. Determine the volume needed for cryopreservation. Cells must be in the exponential growth phase (between 8×10^5 and 1.2×10^6 cells/mL) and viability over 98%.
4. Centrifuge the cells at $200 \times g$ for 5 min. Decant the supernatant. Dissociate the cell pellet by gently tapping the tube.
5. Add the appropriate volume of freezing medium dropwise to the cells while swirling the tube to obtain the desired density (i.e., 5×10^6 to 5×10^7 cells/mL per vial).
6. Quickly aliquot the cells into the labeled vials. Immediately transfer the vials to a –80°C freezer in a styrofoam box. Do not

open the freezer door for at least 2 h. Alternatively, freeze cells at 1°C/min using a programmable cooler.

7. Transfer the vials to liquid nitrogen freezer storage (vapor phase) the following day.

4. Notes

1. CHO cells are passage three times a week and maintained in humidified incubator at 37°C with 5% CO_2. Doubling time of the cells is typically 16 h. On the day of passage, the maximum cell density should not exceed 2×10^6 cells/mL in order to prevent aggregation and reduction in viability. Emphasis on the high viability (>98%) is advised for the good transfection conditions and exponential growth of the cells. Dilution at low cell density ensures healthy cultures.
2. We use PEImax. However, different transfection reagents or methods could be used.
3. A parallel well can be transfected with GFP plasmid (e.g., pTT-GFP (10)) to estimate the transfection efficiency 24–48 h post-transfection. For this purpose, a fluorescent microscope or flow cytometer is needed.
4. If CHO cells attach poorly to the plastic surface, T-flasks with improved cell adhesion surface such as CellBind™ (Corning) can be used. This facilitates selection and elimination of dead cells and cell debris. However, this may also make the cells more difficult to detach once the selection process is finished.
5. The purpose of conditioned medium is to improve the growth of a single cell under limiting dilution conditions. Although partially depleted of some nutrients, it is enriched with cell-derived products such as growth factors. When mixed with some fresh medium, it promotes survival of cell seeded at very low densities. To prepare the conditioned medium, inoculate exponentially growing CHO cells in fresh CD DG44 medium (0.5×10^6 cells/mL) and grow them to reach at least 2×10^6 cells/mL. Collect the medium by centrifugation and filter it through a 0.2 μm sterilizing filter. Store the medium at −4°C. Warm it before use and mix it with fresh medium at a 1:1 ratio.
6. Two criteria should be considered when clones are picked using limiting dilution protocol: colony size and intensity of dot blot signal. Both of them indicate properties that are of great importance for further stable cell line establishment, i.e., growth rate and specific productivity. If the selection of clones

is performed following a minipool strategy (see Subheading 3.5), one should expect to get 5–20% of wells per 96-well plate that contain positive clones. This percentage increases the likelihood of having colonies arising from a single clone.

7. Preferable are minipools with medium-sized colonies and stronger dot blot signal. This might indicate good growth and specific productivity. Small-sized colonies with high-intensity signal could indicate high specific productivity but usually also have poor growth characteristics.
8. If the cell count is still below 1×10^6 cells/mL, media change may be required. In that case, prolong cell cultivation for 2 more days with fresh media.
9. Limiting dilution with the highest producing minipools could be initiated at 96-well plate. However, sometimes the growth and production characteristics of the minipools change substantially during expansion. So it's advisable to analyze the clones from top three minipools, if limited dilution is performed at 96- or 12-well plate stages.
10. The dot blot signal from high producing clones could be saturated and possibly result in incorrect analysis. To circumvent signal saturation, supernatants from top few clones could be diluted and reassessed.

Acknowledgment

The authors declare no competing interests. This is a NRC publication number.

References

1. Zhang J, MacKenzie R, Durocher Y (2009) Production of chimeric heavy-chain antibodies. Methods Mol Biol 525:323–336
2. Hamers-Casterman C et al (1993) Naturally occurring antibodies devoid of light chains. Nature 363:446–448
3. Hmila I et al (2008) VHH, bivalent domains and chimeric heavy chain-only antibodies with high neutralizing efficacy for scorpion toxin AahI'. Mol Immunol 45:3847–3856
4. Bell A et al (2009) Differential tumor-targeting abilities of three single-domain antibody formats. Cancer Lett 289:81–90
5. Durocher Y, Butler M (2009) Expression systems for therapeutic glycoprotein production. Curr Opin Biotechnol 20:700–707
6. Wurm FM (2004) Production of recombinant protein therapeutics in cultivated mammalian cells. Nat Biotechnol 22:1393–1398
7. Urlaub G et al (1983) Deletion of the diploid dihydrofolate reductase locus from cultured mammalian cells. Cell 33:405–412
8. Barnes LM, Bentley CM, Dickson AJ (2003) Stability of protein production from recombinant mammalian cells. Biotechnol Bioeng 81: 631–639
9. Pham PL, Kamen A, Durocher Y (2006) Large-scale transfection of mammalian cells for the fast production of recombinant protein. Mol Biotechnol 34:225–237
10. Durocher Y, Perret S, Kamen A (2002) High-level and high-throughput recombinant protein

production by transient transfection of suspension-growing human 293-EBNA1 cells. Nucleic Acids Res 30:E9

11. Loignon M et al (2008) Stable high volumetric production of glycosylated human recombinant IFNalpha2b in HEK293 cells. BMC Biotechnol 8:65
12. Zhang J et al (2009) Transient expression and purification of chimeric heavy chain antibodies. Protein Expr Purif 65:77–82
13. Urlaub G, McDowell J, Chasin LA (1985) Use of fluorescence-activated cell sorter to isolate mutant mammalian cells deficient in an internal protein, dihydrofolate reductase. Somat Cell Mol Genet 11:71–77
14. Allen GC, Spiker S, Thompson WF (2000) Use of matrix attachment regions (MARs) to minimize transgene silencing. Plant Mol Biol 43: 361–376

Chapter 19

Production of Camel-Like Antibodies in Plants

Sylvie De Buck, Vikram Virdi, Thomas De Meyer, Kirsten De Wilde, Robin Piron, Jonah Nolf, Els Van Lerberge, Annelies De Paepe, and Ann Depicker

Abstract

Transgenic plants for the production of high-value recombinant complex and/or glycosylated proteins are a promising alternative for conventional systems, such as mammalian cells and bacteria. Many groups use plants as production platform for antibodies and antibody fragments. Here, we describe how bivalent camel-like antibodies can be produced in leaves and seeds. Camel-like antibodies are fusions of the antigen-binding domain of heavy chain camel antibodies (VHH) with an Fc fragment of choice. Transient expression in *Nicotiana benthamiana* leaves allows the production of VHH-Fc antibodies within a few days after the expression plasmid has been obtained. Generation of stable *Arabidopsis thaliana* transformants allows production of scalable amounts of VHH-Fc antibodies in seeds within a year. Further, we describe how the *in planta*-produced VHH-Fc antibodies can be quantified by Western blot analysis with Fc-specific antibodies.

Key words: Molecular farming, Transient expression, Seed-specific expression, VHH-Fc antibody, *Arabidopsis thaliana*, *Nicotiana benthamiana*

1. Introduction

For some time now, plant-based systems are considered good alternatives to the conventional insect and mammalian cell lines for the production of antibodies, pharmaceuticals, industrial enzymes, and other complex heterologous proteins. Plants offer many practical, economical, and safety advantages over other systems (1). *In planta*-produced proteins are assembled correctly and harbor posttranslational modifications; the potential for production upscaling is unlimited, the production cost is lower than that of mammalian cells, and vegetative material can be grown and harvested with existing agronomical facilities. Additionally, there is no risk for contamination with mammalian viruses, human pathogens, oncogenic DNA sequences, prions, and bacterial toxins.

Dirk Saerens and Serge Muyldermans (eds.), *Single Domain Antibodies: Methods and Protocols*, Methods in Molecular Biology, vol. 911, DOI 10.1007/978-1-61779-968-6_19, © Springer Science+Business Media, LLC 2012

For the production of heterologous proteins in plants, transient and stable expression strategies have been used successfully (2–4). Transient expression in leaves has long been considered only as a pilot system to control and evaluate gene constructs, but recently, it has become an important platform for the production of heterologous proteins (5–11). Different transient expression systems have been demonstrated to be safe, fast, and yielding high amounts of heterologous proteins. A recent transient expression system is based on the pEAQ vectors that contain a deleted version of the RNA2 of the Cowpea Mosaic virus CPMV-HT (9, 10). Cloning the coding sequence of interest between the modified 5′-untranslated region and the 3′ untranslated region of the CMPV RNA2, and transferring this construct via *Agrobacterium* infiltration into *Nicotiana benthamiana* leaves, resulted in a high and rapid recombinant protein production in the leaves. Several proteins, such as the green fluorescent protein (GFP), *Discosoma* red fluorescent protein (DsRed), the hepatitis B core antigen, and the anti-HIV antibody 2G12, were produced up to more than 10 to 25% of the total soluble protein (TSP) extracted from *N. benthamiana* leaves six days after infiltration. The binary pEAQ vectors allow genes to be cloned directly by either restriction enzymes or GATEWAY recombination and allow the simultaneous high-level expression of multiple polypeptides from a single plasmid (10). To guarantee high transgene expression, the P19 suppressor of silencing was cloned onto the same T-DNA, eliminating the need for coinfiltration (10).

For the production of heterologous proteins from stable transformants, plant cell cultures as well as transgenic plants have been used (2–4), but particularly seeds of transgenic plants are considered as promising tissues because they provide a stable environment in which the recombinant proteins are protected against degradation (12). Another attractive advantage is the possibility of prolonged storage at ambient temperatures by which production can be uncoupled from extraction and purification. Moreover, the dehydrated state and the small size of most seeds allow the recombinant protein to reach a relatively high concentration that can be advantageous for extraction and downstream processing.

To obtain high seed-specific production of proteins, the potential of the regulatory sequences of the seed storage protein *arcelin-5*-encoding gene has been investigated (13). Transgenic plants transformed with *arcelin-5* gene constructs resulted in accumulation levels of 15 and 25% recombinant protein in TSP extracted from seeds of *Arabidopsis thaliana* and *Phaseolus acutifolius* (tepary bean), respectively. The transgenic plants displayed low plant-to-plant variation in *arcelin-5* expression without silencing effects in plants with complex T-DNA integration patterns (13). Based on these findings, a plant transformation vector has been developed containing a seed-specific expression cassette for the production of recombinant antibodies in dicotyledonous seeds (14). The regulatory sequences of the seed storage proteins arcelin-5I and β-phaseolin of *Phaseolus vulgaris* (common bean) were used together with an N-terminal signal peptide of the seed storage protein 2S2 for targeting the proteins to the endoplasmic reticulum. Because the highest expression levels were found upon endoplasmic reticulum retention, most gene constructs contained a C-terminal KDEL sequence (14–16). By means of this transformation vector, a variety of antibody fragments, such as a single-chain variable fragment (scFv), fused scFv-Fc proteins, and full antibodies were produced and found to accumulate reproducibly to approximately 1–5% of the *Arabidopsis* seed weight, corresponding to 5–25% recombinant protein of the extracted TSP (14–16). These *in planta*-produced antibody fragments and antibodies had the same antigen-binding activity and affinity as those produced in other production systems (14–16).

Antigen-binding domains, such as scFv and VHH proteins, have many applications, but for some purposes, bivalent antibodies perform much better. Fusion of the Fc chain to the VHH domain results in a VHH-Fc protein and by virtue of the Fc oligomerization based on the disulfide bridges in the hinge region, a stable bivalent dimeric complex is formed. This bivalency results in a strengthened antigen–antibody interaction, because avidity superimposes onto the affinity (17). Moreover, the Fc domain allows the use of secondary polyclonal antibodies in several antibody-based assays, resulting in an amplification of the signal and an increased sensitivity. ScFv and VHH proteins are produced very well in *Escherichia coli* ((17) and references therein). However, the production of complete camel antibodies or VHH-Fc fusions in *E. coli* is very inefficient. Therefore, all multimeric camel-like antibodies are produced in yeast, animal cells, baculovirus-infected insect cells, or plants. This chapter focuses on (1) the production of a camel-like antibody via transient expression in *N. benthamiana* leaves, (2) the production of a camel-like antibody in *A. thaliana* seeds, and (3) Western blot analysis with Fc-specific antibodies as a method to quantify the VHH-Fc antibody accumulation levels.

2. Materials

All buffers and solutions are made as aqueous solutions in deionized/distilled water. All reagents are prepared and stored at room temperature, unless indicated otherwise.

2.1. Infiltration of an Agrobacterium Suspension in N. benthamiana Leaves

1. A freshly grown *Agrobacterium tumefaciens* C58C1Rif^{R} (pMP90) strain (see Note 1), harboring a pEAQ-derived binary T-DNA vector (9, 10) in which the VHH-Fc-coding region is cloned in a 35S promoter driven expression cassette (see Fig. 1a). This *Agrobacterium* strain is grown on YEB medium

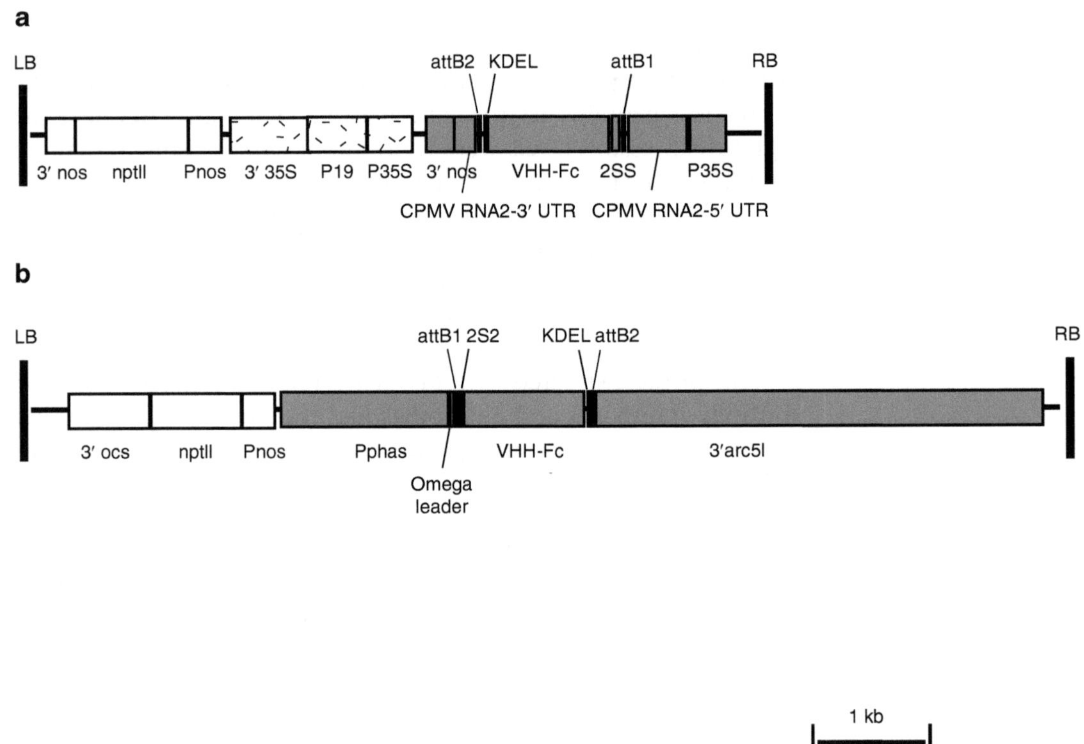

Fig. 1. Schematic outline of the different T-DNAs used. (**a**) pEAQ-derived T-DNA for transient expression of a camel-like antibody. (**b**) pPhasGW-derived T-DNA for seed-specific expression of a camel-like antibody. The different elements of each expression cassette are represented in the same filling code. *P35S* 35S promoter of the cauliflower mosaic virus promoter; *CPMV RNA-2 3′ UTR* the 3′-untranslated region of the cowpea mosaic virus RNA-2; *Pnos* nopaline synthase gene promoter; *nptII* coding sequence of the neomycin phosphotransferase gene; *3′ ocs* 3′ end of the octopine synthase gene; *Pphas* β-phaseolin gene promoter (−1 to −1470; GenBank accession no. J01263); *3′ arc5I* 3′ end of the arcelin5-I gene (3,900 bp, part of GenBank accession no. Z5020); *3′ nos* 3′ end of the nopaline synthase gene; *3′ 35S* cauliflower mosaic virus 35S terminator; *P19* P19 suppressor of the silencing gene from the tomato bushy stunt virus; *2S2* signal peptide of the *Arabidopsis* 2S2 seed storage protein gene; *Omega leader* the 5′-untranslated region of the tobacco mosaic virus (31 base pairs); *VHH-Fc* fusion protein of the VHH domain with an Fc fragment; *KDEL* endoplasmic reticulum retention signal; *LB* left border; *RB* right border; *attB1 and attB2* gateway recombination sequences.

supplemented with rifampicin (final concentration 100 mg/L), gentamycin (final concentration 40 mg/L), and kanamycin (final concentration 50 mg/L).

2. Non-transgenic *N. benthamiana* plants grown in soil for 3–4 weeks at 26°C (see Note 2).
3. Incubation shaker at 28°C (Innova 44/44R [New Brunswick Scientific, Edison, NJ] or equivalent).
4. 50-mL Falcon tubes (BD, Franklin Lakes, NJ), 12-mL ultracentrifuge tubes, and 1.5- and 2-mL microfuge tubes.
5. Spectrophotometer (DU 530 [Beckman Coulter, Brea, CA] or equivalent).
6. Disposable plastic cuvettes.

7. 1-mL syringes without needle.
8. Luria Bertani (LB) medium: 10 g of tryptone, 5 g of yeast extract, 5 g of NaCl per liter.
9. Selective antibiotic to grow the T-DNA vector containing the *A. tumefaciens* strain in liquid LB medium: kanamycin (Duchefa, Haarlem, The Netherlands) (see Note 3). The final concentration of kanamycin in the medium should be 25 mg/L.
10. 0.5 M 2-(*N*-morpholino) ethanesulfonic acid (MES).
11. 100 mM acetosyringone (Sigma-Aldrich, St. Louis, MO).
12. Infiltration solution: 10 mM $MgCl_2$, 10 mM MES, pH 5.6, 0.1 mM acetosyringone (adapted from ref. (18) and references therein).

2.2. Harvest of the Infiltrated N. benthamiana Leaves and Protein Extraction

1. Liquid nitrogen.
2. Scissors, pencils, spoon, and tongs.
3. Aluminum foil.
4. Prechilled pestle and mortar.
5. Sorvall RC5C plus Superspeed Centrifuge (Thermo Fischer Scientific, Waltham, MA).
6. Complete® protease inhibitor tablets (Roche Diagnostics, Brussels, Belgium). Dissolve one tablet of Complete® protease inhibitor in 0.5 mL of double-distilled water (ddH_2O). Stock solutions of protease inhibitors can be stored for 1–2 weeks at 2–8°C or for 12 weeks at −15 to −25°C. Just before use, add 20 μL of this protease inhibitor solution to every mL of extraction buffer to be used (see Note 4).
7. Extraction buffer (EB): 50 mM Tris(hydroxymethyl)aminomethane (Tris)–HCl, pH 8.0, 200 mM NaCl, 5 mM ethylenediaminetetraacetic acid (EDTA), 0.1% (v/v) of polyoxyethylene sorbitan monolaurate (Tween 20). Keep at 4°C until use.
8. 100% (w/v) Glycerol.

2.3. Determination of the Protein Concentration in the Leaf Extracts

1. 96-Well microtiter plates (flat bottom, untreated, polystyrene; Nunc, Roskilde, Denmark).
2. VERSAmax tunable microplate reader (Molecular Devices, Sunnyvale, CA).
3. Softmax® Pro Software 3.0 (Molecular Devices).
4. Complete® protease inhibitor and EB (see Subheading 2.2, items 6 and 7).
5. Bovine serum albumin (BSA) (Sigma-Aldrich). Make a stock solution of 100 μg/mL in water and store at −20°C in single-use aliquots.
6. Protein assay dye reagent concentrate (Bio-Rad, Hercules, CA).

2.4. A. thaliana Floral Dip Transformation

1. A freshly grown *Agrobacterium* C58C1Rif[R](pMP90) strain harboring the pPhasGW binary T-DNA vector (16) in which the VHH-Fc-coding region is cloned in a Pphas-driven expression cassette (see Fig. 1b). This *Agrobacterium* strain is grown on YEB medium supplemented with rifampicin (final concentration 100 mg/L), gentamycin (final concentration 40 mg/L), spectinomycin (final concentration 100 mg/L), and streptomycin (final concentration 300 mg/L).
2. Non-transgenic *A. thaliana* plants (L.) Heynh, ecotype Columbia 0 (see Note 5).
3. Aracon bases and sheets (Lehle Seeds, Round Rock, TX).
4. Saran wrap (Dow Chemical, Midland, MI).
5. Luria Bertani (LB) medium (see Subheading 2.1, item 8).
6. Dipping solution: 10% (w/v) of sucrose, 0.05% (v/v) of Silwet L77 (Lehle Seeds) in ddH_2O (see Note 6).

2.5. Selection of Transgenic Lines and Identification of Single-Locus Lines

1. Round Petri dishes (150 mm × 25 mm), preferably with a grid on the bottom (see Note 7), and porous tape for sealing.
2. Kl growth medium: 4.3 g/L of Murashige and Skoog (MS) salts (Gibco BRL, Gaithersburg, MD), 0.5 g/L of MES (Duchefa) supplemented with 10 g/L of sucrose. Bring this solution to pH 5.7 with 1 M KOH and complete with 8 g/L agar. Sterilize by autoclaving at 1 bar overpressure (121°C) for 20 min. Let the Kl growth medium cool down to approximately 60°C. In a flow bench, add the vitamins and the selective agents (see Subheading 2.5, items 3–6) and pour 80–100 mL of Kl growth medium in each plate when the agar is still hot. Allow the agar to set and close the plate only when the medium is at room temperature to prevent excess condensation. These sterile selective plates can be stored up to 2 months in a plastic bag at room temperature.
3. Selective agent for selection of primary transformants: kanamycin (Duchefa): final concentration 50 mg/L Kl growth medium. Make a stock solution of 100 mg kanamycin per mL water and store in single-use aliquots at −20°C (see Note 3).
4. Selective agent against fungi: nystatin (Duchefa): final concentration 50 mg/L Kl medium. Make a stock solution of 50 mg/mL in dimethylsulfoxide (DMSO) and store in single-use aliquots at −20°C (see Note 3).
5. Selective agent against *A. tumefaciens*: vancomycin. Add 800 mg vancomycin powder as such to 1 L of sterilized Kl growth medium (see Note 8).
6. Murashige & Skoog modified Vitamin Mix (Duchefa). Mix 10.4 g vitamins with 100 mL of water to obtain a 1,000× vitamin stock solution. Add 1 mL of this stock solution to 1 L of Kl medium. Store in single-use aliquots at −20°C (see Note 3).

2.6. Protein Extraction from A. thaliana Seeds

1. Grinding ball mill device MM200 (Retsch, Haan, Germany).
2. Liquid nitrogen.
3. Centrifuge 5417R (Eppendorf, Hamburg, Germany).
4. Complete® protease inhibitor and EB (see Subheading 2.2, items 6 and 7).
5. 100% (v/v) Glycerol.

2.7. Determination of the Protein Concentration in Seed Extracts

1. 96-Well microtiter plates, VERSAmax tunable microplate reader and Softmax® Pro Software 3.0 (see Subheading 2.3, items 1–3).
2. Complete® protease inhibitor and EB (see Subheading 2.2, items 6 and 7).
3. BSA (Sigma-Aldrich). Make a stock solution of 10 mg BSA in 1 mL of water and store at −20°C in single-use aliquots.
4. Lowry reagents A and B (Bio-Rad).

2.8. Western Blot Analysis to Evaluate the Accumulation Level of the VHH-Fc Antibodies

1. Mini-Protean II™ Electrophoresis Unit for protein gel electrophoresis (Bio-Rad).
2. Electro Eluter Model No 422 (Bio-Rad).
3. PowerPac HC (Bio-Rad).
4. Immobilon-P polyvinylidene fluoride (PVDF) membrane (0.45 μm pore) (Millipore, Billerica, MA).
5. Filter paper Whatman® no. 3 (GE Healthcare, Little Chalfont, UK).
6. Standard reagents for sodium dodecyl sulfate (SDS)-polyacrylamide gel electrophoresis (PAGE) (19).
7. Electrophoresis running buffer: 25 mM Tris, 192 mM glycine, 0.1% (w/v) SDS, pH 8.3 (Bio-Rad).
8. Protein sample buffer (5×): 5 mL of 0.5 M Tris–HCl, pH 6.8, 4 mL of 100% (w/v) glycerol, 0.5 g SDS, 5% (w/v) dithiothreitol (DTT), 0.01% (w/v) bromophenol blue. Add ddH_2O to a final volume of 10 mL. Store at −20°C.
9. Dual Color Precision Plus Protein standard (Bio-Rad).
10. Blotting transfer buffer: 14.41 g/L glycine, 3.024 g/L Tris, 150 mL/L methanol.
11. PBS buffer: 138 mM NaCl, 2.7 mM KCl, 10 mM Na_2HPO_4, 1.8 mM KH_2PO_4. Adjust to pH 7.2 with HCl.
12. Blocking buffer: PBS buffer supplemented with 4% (w/v) skimmed milk and 0.1% (v/v) Tween20.
13. Washing buffer: PBS buffer supplemented with 0.1% (v/v) Tween20.

14. ECL™ anti-human IgG1, horseradish peroxidase-linked whole antibody (from sheep) (NA933V) (GE Healthcare) (see Note 9).
15. Hyperfilm ECL (GE healthcare).
16. Western Lightning™ Component A and Component B (PerkinElmer, Waltham, MA).

3. Methods

3.1. Infiltration of an Agrobacterium Suspension in N. benthamiana Leaves

1. Bring 3–4 mL of LB medium, supplemented with 25 mg/L of kanamycin, in a 50-mL Falcon tube and inoculate with a colony of the *Agrobacterium* strain C58C1Rif^R (pMP90, pEAQ-VHH-Fc) from a freshly grown selective plate. Grow overnight at 28°C in a rotary shaker at 230 rpm.
2. Add 1 mL of this overnight-grown *Agrobacterium* culture to 9 mL of LB medium supplemented with 25 μg/mL of kanamycin, 200 μL 0.5 M MES (10 mM final concentration) and 2 μL of 100 mM acetosyringone (20 μM final concentration). Grow overnight at 28°C in a rotary shaker at 230 rpm.
3. Measure the optical density (OD) of the overnight-grown culture at 600 nm. As a negative control, use 1 mL of LB medium supplemented with 25 μg/mL of kanamycin, 10 mM MES, and 20 μM acetosyringone.
4. Calculate the volume of the culture needed to obtain a final concentration of $OD_{600\ nm} = 1$ and spin down at 3,000 × *g* for 10 min (see Note 10).
5. Resuspend the pellet in the calculated volume of infiltration solution and leave at room temperature for 2–3 h. Do not vortex.
6. Infiltrate the top young leaves of 3–4-week-old *N. benthamiana* plants grown at 21°C. With a 1-mL syringe without needle, infiltrate the abaxial surface of the leaves with the *Agrobacterium* suspension (see Note 11 and Fig. 2a).
7. After infiltration, dab the surface of the leaves and mark the infiltrated region with a blunt-tip permanent marker. Three to 6 days after infiltration, the infiltrated leaves can be collected for analysis.

3.2. Harvest of the Infiltrated N. benthamiana Leaves and Protein Extraction

1. Cut out the infiltrated parts of the leaf with scissors and scalpel and quickly measure the size of the infiltrated areas (see Note 12).
2. Wrap the leaf material immediately in aluminum foil and dip into liquid nitrogen (see Note 13).

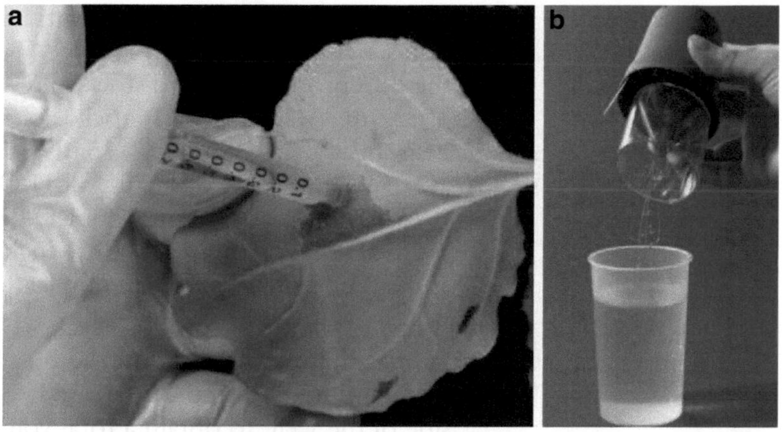

Fig. 2. Plant transformation. (**a**) *Agrobacterium* infiltration in *N. benthamiana* leaves. With a syringe, the *Agrobacterium* suspension is injected into the abaxial surface of the leaves. (**b**) Floral dip transformation of *Arabidopsis*. The flowers are dipped into the *Agrobacterium* suspension for 5–10 s.

3. Keep the prechilled pestle and mortar (see Note 14) on ice and fill the mortar with liquid nitrogen to chill it further.
4. With tweezers or gloves, pick up the foil packet from the liquid nitrogen, open it, and put the frozen leaf material into the mortar. Carefully pour some more liquid nitrogen in the mortar and grind the leaf material with the prechilled pestle. Once all the liquid nitrogen is evaporated, add some more liquid nitrogen and grind the material a second time.
5. With a chilled spoon (dipped in liquid nitrogen), transfer the powder to a chilled (nitrogen-frozen) ultracentrifuge tube. Keep on ice.
6. Add the appropriate volume of cold extraction buffer to the powder and vortex well (see Note 15).
7. Centrifuge at approximately 40,000 × *g* for 30 min at 4°C.
8. Collect the supernatant (= total protein extract) and keep on ice (see Note 16).
9. Add glycerol (100%) to a final concentration of 20% (v/v) and store at −20°C.

3.3. Determination of the Protein Concentration in the Leaf Extracts

To determine the total protein concentration in *N. benthamiana* leaf extracts, the Bradford method (20) is used.

1. Make a 1/5 dilution of the extraction buffer (=EB1/5) and a 1/5 dilution of each sample with ddH_2O (see Note 17).
2. Prepare fresh Bio-Rad dye solution, taking into account that 225 μL (=50 μL of Bio-Rad protein assay dye reagent concentrate + 175 μL of ddH_2O) will be needed per well (see Note 18).

3. To determine the protein concentration in the samples, a dilution series of BSA is used. Prepare in duplicate five dilutions of the BSA protein standard stock solution in the microtiter plate: 1 μg/mL (=2.5 μL BSA stock + 17.5 μL ddH$_2$O + 5 μL EB), 2 μg/mL (=5 μL BSA stock + 15 μL ddH$_2$O + 5 μL EB), 4 μg/mL (=10 μL BSA stock + 10 μL ddH$_2$O + 5 μL EB), 6 μg/mL (=15 μL BSA stock + 5 μL ddH$_2$O + 5 μL EB), and 8 μg/mL (=20 μL BSA stock + 5 μL EB). Include 25 μL EB1/5 in the assay as a "blank" sample in duplicate.
4. Bring 2 and 5 μL of each 1/5-diluted extract (see Subheading 3.3, step 1) on the bottom of the well (in duplicate) and add 23 and 20 μL EB1/5, respectively, to the left side of the well, to obtain a total volume of 25 μL.
5. Add to all wells (the blank, the standards and the extracts) 225 μL of Bio-Rad dye solution. Shake the plate for 10 min.
6. Read the absorbances in the VERSAmax tunable microplate spectrophotometer at 600 nm. With the Softmax Pro software, calculate the protein concentrations from the slope of the BSA standard dilution series.

3.4. A. thaliana Floral Dip Transformation

Arabidopsis transformants are obtained via *Agrobacterium*-mediated floral dip transformation (21) (see Note 5).

1. Inoculate in the morning one colony of the *Agrobacterium* strain C58C1Rif^R (pMP90, pPhasGW-VHH-Fc), from a freshly grown selective plate, in 1 mL of LB medium without antibiotic in a 50-mL tube and incubate 7–8 h at 28°C in a rotary shaker at 230 rpm.
2. Add in the evening 10 mL of LB medium and incubate overnight at 28°C in a rotary shaker at 230 rpm.
3. Measure the OD of the overnight-grown culture at 600 nm. Therefore, bring 1 mL of the culture in a cuvette. As blank, use 1 mL of LB medium. The OD should be approximately 2, corresponding to approximately 10^9 colony forming units per mL. When the value is lower, incubate the culture further at 28°C and measure the OD every 30 min.
4. Add 40 mL of freshly made dipping solution (see Note 6) to the remaining 10 mL of *Agrobacterium* suspension and mix well, but do not vortex. Use this mix immediately for the floral dip.
5. Dip the flowers of the *Arabidopsis* plants in the suspension and agitate gently for 10 s (see Fig. 2b). On average, the flowers of five plants per *Agrobacterium* suspension are dipped to obtain a sufficient number of independent transformants (see Note 19).
6. Allow the dipped plants to further grow in the greenhouse under normal growth conditions: 16 h of light/8 h of darkness,

21°C and 55% relative humidity. Cover the plants with Saran wrap for 24 h.

7. Stop watering the plants 5 weeks after the floral dip and transfer them to a room at 25°C with a 20 h light/4 h dark photoperiod and with a low humidity.
8. When the plants are dry (approximately 8 weeks after floral dip), harvest the T1 seeds and collect them in microfuge tubes (see Note 20).

3.5. Selection of Transgenic Lines and Identification of Single-Locus Lines

To select the primary transformants, harboring at least one T-DNA copy, the T1 seeds, harvested from the dipped T0 plants, are sown on selective medium. Dependent on the selective marker on the T-DNA, the appropriate antibiotic should be added to the medium. In the pPhasGW T-DNA vector, the neomycin phosphotransferase II (NPTII) resistance marker is present, so we used kanamycin as a selective antibiotic. In addition, also vancomycin and nystatin are added in the medium to avoid contamination by agrobacteria and fungi, respectively.

1. Pack 1,000 seeds (approximately 25 mg) of every dipped *Arabidopsis* plant. Keep at −70°C for 2 days. Surface-sterilize seeds and allow them to germinate on selective Kl medium (see Notes 21–23).
2. Incubate plates in a growth chamber at 21°C on a 16 h light/8 h dark cycle.
3. Identify the transformed seedlings with two pairs of green leaves on top of the cotyledons and normally expanded roots after 14–20 days of growth on the selective medium.
4. Transfer the transformed T1 plants after 3–4 weeks to soil and grow in the greenhouse (21°C, 16 h light/8 h dark cycle, 55% relative humidity).
5. Grow the plants until flowering and allow to self-fertilize. At that moment, stop watering to shorten the time that the siliques take to dry.
6. Harvest the T2 seeds.
7. As the T1 transformants are by definition hemizygous, the T-DNA locus number can be determined by the segregation ratio in the T2 generation. To identify the single-locus plants, sow 64 seeds of each T2-segregating seed stock on selective Kl medium for the T-DNA selection marker as described above (see Subheading 3.5, steps 1 and 2; Notes 7 and 24).
8. After 3–4 weeks, count the resistant (four green leaves) and sensitive (pale cotyledons and no extra leaves) seedlings. To verify the 3:1 segregation ratio, compare the ratio of the resistant to sensitive seedlings with the expected ratio from a χ^2 statistical test (22, 23).

3.6. Protein Extraction from Arabidopsis Seeds

1. Weigh 5 mg of *Arabidopsis* seeds in a 2.0-mL microfuge tube. Add two 4-mm metal balls. Chill the tubes as well as the Retsch mill holders in liquid nitrogen. Place the filled holders in the Retch MM 200 device and shake for 2 min at a mill frequency of 20 oscillations/s (see Note 25). Always use both holders to equilibrate the machine.
2. Add 900 μL of EB, mix, and vortex for 1 min (see Notes 26 and 27).
3. Centrifuge at maximal speed (approximately 20,000 × *g*) for 5 min at 4°C.
4. Collect 700 μL of the supernatant into a new microfuge tube and keep on ice.
5. Add 175 μL of 100% (v/v) glycerol (end concentration of 20%) to each protein extract and store at –20°C.

3.7. Determination of the Protein Concentration in Seed Extracts

The protein concentration in the *Arabidopsis* seed extracts is determined by the Bio-Rad dye concentrate protein assay, based on the Lowry method (13, 24) (see Note 28).

1. To determine the protein concentration in the samples, use a BSA dilution series as standard. Prepare four dilutions of the BSA protein standard stock : 1.6, 0.8, 0.4, 0.2 mg/mL of BSA in ddH_2O. Use ddH_2O as a blank sample.
2. Prepare four dilutions of each protein extract: 2.5, 5, 10, and 20×. With this dilution series of every seed extract, at least three measurements should be in the linear detection range.
3. Bring 5 μL of BSA standards, the blank, and the dilutions of the samples into a microtiter plate.
4. Add 25 μL of Component A and subsequently 200 μL of Component B into each well (see Note 29). Wrap the plate in aluminum foil and shake the plate for 15 min at room temperature.
5. Read the absorbances in a spectrophotometer at 750 nm. With the Softmax Pro software, calculate the protein concentrations from the slope of the BSA standard dilution series (see Note 30).

3.8. Western Blot Analysis to Evaluate the Accumulation Level of the VHH-Fc Antibodies

To analyze the accumulation levels of the produced VHH-Fc fragments upon transient expression in *N. benthamiana* leaves or in seeds of *A. thaliana* transformants, a Western gel blot with Fc-specific antibodies can be done. The Western blot analysis also gives information about the molecular weight and degradation products, if any, of the produced VHH-Fc antibodies (see Fig. 3).

1. Add 2 μL of protein sampling buffer to extract 1 μg of protein (see Note 31) and add ddH_2O to a final volume of 10 μL. For quantification of the recombinant protein, a number of

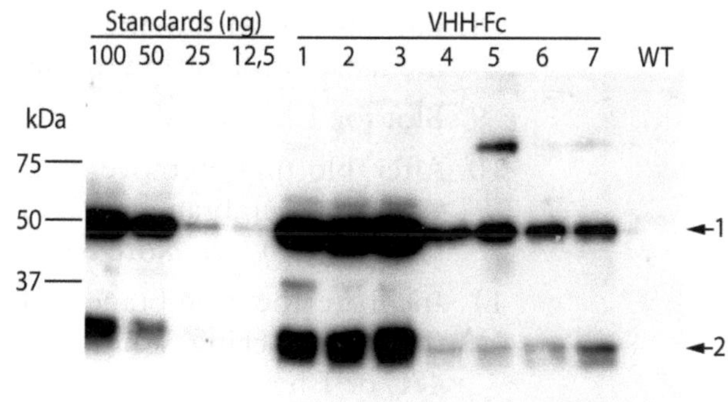

Fig. 3. Western blot analysis to evaluate the accumulation level of VHH-Fc antibody fragments in seed extracts of transgenic *Arabidopsis* plants. Two micrograms of total seed protein extract from seven different VHH-Fc transgenic lines and wild type Col-0 (WT) was loaded. To estimate the VHH-Fc accumulation levels in the different transgenic lines, protA-purified VHH-Fc from *Arabidopsis* seeds was loaded in quantified amounts as standards. The anti-human IgG, horseradish peroxidase-linked whole antibody (from sheep) was used for detection of the camel-like VHH-Fc fusions. The signal at 50 kDa (*arrow 1*) corresponds to the molecular mass of the VHH-Fc fusion, whereas that at 30 kDa (*arrow 2*) to the molecular mass of the Fc fragment and most probably results from proteolytic degradation in the linker or hinge region.

different dilutions of known amounts of the same, purified, recombinant protein can be prepared (see Fig. 3). Mix and centrifuge (approximately 20,000 × *g*) for 5 s to bring down the droplets. Boil the samples 8 min at 98°C and centrifuge again for 5 s (approximately 20,000 × *g*).

2. Make a standard gel for SDS-PAGE (19) in the Bio-Rad Mini Protean II Electrophoresis Unit™ and load the samples onto a 0.75-mm thick gel.
3. To determine the molecular weight of the produced antibody fragments in the protein extract, also load 2.5–5 μL of the Dual Color Precision Plus Protein Standard.
4. Electrophorese the sample at 180 V for 1 h (until the bromophenol blue tracking dye reaches the bottom of the gel).
5. When the dye front has reached the end of the gel, turn off the power supply. Separate the gel plates with the help of a spatula and carefully remove the stacking gel.
6. Cut two Whatman filter papers 0.5 cm larger than the gel and one PVDF membrane of the gel size (see Note 32).
7. Make a sandwich of the layers as follows: the anode, a with blotting buffer soaked sponge, a Whatman paper, the PVDF membrane, the gel, a Whatman paper, a with blotting buffer soaked sponge, and the cathode. Avoid air bubbles.

8. Put this sandwich in the Electro Eluter, add the ice box, and fill the tank with blotting transfer buffer.
9. Blot for 1 h at 50 V and 250 mA.
10. After blotting, remove the PVDF membrane carefully and wash the membrane in PBS buffer at room temperature (protein-side up) (see Note 33).
11. Incubate the membrane in blocking solution (approximately 0.2 mL blocking solution per cm^2 membrane) overnight at 4°C or 1 h at room temperature under continuous shaking.
12. Wash the membrane once for 10 min in washing buffer (at least 0.2 mL washing solution per cm^2 membrane) at room temperature under continuous shaking.
13. Add anti-human IgG, horseradish peroxidase-linked whole antibody (from sheep) to the membrane (1/5,000 dilution in blocking buffer, approximately 0.2 mL per cm^2 membrane) (see Note 34) and incubate for 1 h at room temperature under continuous shaking.
14. Wash the membrane twice for 10 min in washing buffer (at least 0.2 mL washing solution per cm^2 membrane) and once for 10 min in PBS at room temperature under continuous shaking.
15. Mix 1 mL of Component A and 1 mL of Component B and incubate the membrane for 1 min in this solution.
16. Take the membrane from the solution, place on a paper towel for a few seconds to remove excess fluid, and wrap the membrane in a plastic film.
17. Expose to a film for 1 s to 5 min (see Note 35).
18. Estimate visually the accumulation of the recombinant proteins present in the total seed extracts by comparing the signal intensity in the samples with those of the purified standards loaded on the same gel (see Subheading 3.8, step 1 and Fig. 3; Note 36).

4. Notes

1. We routinely use the *Agrobacterium* strain C58C1Rif^R, also referred to as GV3101, with the virulence plasmid pMP90 to introduce the T-DNA vectors for transient expression or stable transformation. In the original papers describing the pEAQ vectors, the *Agrobacterium* strain LBA4404 was used as carrier for the T-DNA vectors and to infiltrate the *N. benthamiana* leaves (9, 10).
2. Fifteen to 20 tobacco seeds are sown in regular soil and grown at 21°C with a photoperiod of 16 h of light/8 h of darkness

and a relative humidity of 55–60% for 1 week. Subsequently, the seedlings are transplanted per two in a pot with a diameter of 13 cm and grown under the same conditions for another 2–3 weeks. After 1 week, Peters Professional All-Purpose Fertilizer with N-P-K rating of 20-20-20 is added to the soil.

3. Prepare the selective agents as stock solutions that are more concentrated than the end concentration needed in the medium and store them after filter sterilization as aliquots in a –20°C freezer. Because the kanamycin solution is unstable, do not refreeze a defrosted aliquot.
4. The mix of extraction buffer and protease inhibitor solution should be prepared only for the samples that will be extracted at that moment, because unused mixes cannot be stored.
5. To grow *Arabidopsis* plants for floral dip transformation, Col-0 seeds are sown in regular soil and plants are grown at 22°C (day) and 18°C (night) with a photoperiod of 12 h of light/12 h of darkness and a relative humidity of 65–70%. To obtain more floral buds per dipped plant, the inflorescences are cut off when most plants have formed primary bolts. This removal will trigger the plant to produce multiple, synchronized secondary bolts. The plants are ready to dip when they have several secondary flowering stems of 10–15 cm in length and immature flowers and flower buds (approximately 2 weeks after removing the primary inflorescence).
6. The surfactant Silwet should be mixed thoroughly into the 10% sucrose solution. The mix cannot be stored and should be used immediately for the floral dip.
7. To facilitate regular spacing of seeds, plates with a grid on the bottom are convenient. For the identification of single-locus lines, two seeds are sown per square. In this manner, the plants have enough space to develop without overlap.
8. Instead of vancomycin, 300 mg/L of carbenicillin (Duchefa) can be used as antibiotic against *Agrobacterium*. Carbenicillin powder (stored at –20°C) is added as such to the sterilized K1 medium when cooled to 60°C.
9. In this experiment, the VHH domain was fused to the Fc fragment of an IgG1 human antibody. Thus, to reveal the VHH-Fc fusion, we could use an anti-human IgG, horseradish peroxidase-linked whole antibody. However, depending on which Fc (human, mouse, goat, pig, rabbit, etc.) is fused to the VHH, the respective specifically recognizing antibody should be used. The antibody dilution in the blocking buffer should be determined experimentally for each antibody.
10. For instance, given that 5 mL of *Agrobacterium* suspension is needed for the infiltration of three leaves and that the $OD_{600\ nm}$ of the culture is 3.7, the dilution of the *Agrobacterium*

suspension is calculated as follows: 5 mL/3.7 = 1.35 mL of the original 10 mL of *Agrobacterium* culture is taken and spun down. Then, the pellet can be carefully resuspended in 5 mL of infiltration solution.

11. For a perfect infiltration, hold your index finger on the adaxial side of the leaf, flip the leaf over, and put the top of the syringe (without needle) on the leaf at the position of your finger. Gently press the *Agrobacterium* suspension inside the leaf. The suspension will diffuse into the leaf, but as soon as pressure is felt, no further diffusion will happen and the infiltration can be stopped. Several infiltrations can be done with the same *Agrobacterium* suspension in one leaf.
12. To determine the volume needed of EB for the protein extraction, the infiltrated area should be measured. The easiest way is to put the infiltrated leaf area on a graph sheet and to draw a border around the leaf surface. For the protein stability, it is important that the drawing is done as quickly as possible.
13. Leaf material infiltrated with the same T-DNA construct can be frozen in the same aluminum foil package.
14. To prechill the mortar and pestle, keep both in the –20°C freezer for 10–20 min.
15. With the graph sheet (see Note 12), the surface area of the infiltrated leaf material can be calculated. By multiplying this total surface area (expressed in cm^2) by 50, the quantity (in μL) of EB to be used is obtained. If less EB is used, the supernatant will be difficult to separate from the pellet during the extraction, whereas if more is used, the protein extract might become too diluted.
16. The pellet is extremely loose, so the tubes should be transferred very carefully from the centrifuge to the working space.
17. The EB contains 0.1% (v/v) Tween20 that interferes with the Bio-Rad protein assay dye reagent concentrate; therefore, both the extraction buffer and the protein samples need to be diluted 1/5 in ddH_2O.
18. The appropriate volume of Bio-Rad dye solution should be prepared in advance in a 50-mL Falcon tube. Do not add the Bio-Rad protein assay dye reagent concentrate and the ddH_2O separately in the well, because the solution cannot be mixed well enough. As the Bio-Rad dye solution is light sensitive, cover the Falcon tube with aluminum foil when filling the plate. Also cover the plate with aluminum foil when the microtiter plate is incubated 10 min on a shaker.
19. Note that not all *A. thaliana* ecotypes can be transformed efficiently by the floral dip transformation. The transformation efficiency of Col-0 is between 0.1 and 2% of the harvested T1 seeds while that of the C24 ecotype ranges between 0.01 and

0.5%. For these ecotypes, more plants should be dipped to obtain enough transformants or an *in vitro* transformation, such as root transformation (25), should be performed.

20. The seed stocks can be stored for a long time at 4°C or at room temperature when they are kept dry. When the seeds are stored at room temperature, keep them for 1 week at 4°C before sowing because they need a vernalization period. Alternatively, the sown plates can be stored 1–4 days at 4°C.
21. In our department, the transformation efficiency of the floral dip transformation varies between 0.5 and 2%, indicating that sowing approximately 1,000 seeds results in 5–20 transformants. For optimal germination, the seeds can be kept 1 day in the dark at 4°C after sowing. The incubation step at −70°C, which can be omitted, was introduced into the protocol to reduce the egg survival of thrips within the seeds in case of an infection.
22. To efficiently spread the 1,000 seeds on the plate, collect all the seeds with a scalpel and put them on the K1 medium. Pour 5–8 mL of liquid 0.1% agarose, dissolved in water, on the K1 plate with the seeds and move the plate slowly until the agarose and the seeds are spread evenly. Leave let the plate open for 10–20 min until the agarose becomes solid.
23. Seal the plates with porous tape to allow air exchange and place them in the growth chamber under following conditions: 21°C, fluorescent (cool white) light 80 μE/m^2/s, 16 h/8 h day/night and shelves cooled at 19°C to prevent condensation against the lids of the Petri dishes.
24. In our department, more than 70% of the transformants upon floral dip transformation contain one or more T-DNAs integrated at one genetic locus (26).
25. Seed samples can also be ground manually with mortar and pestle. However, the mechanical grinding procedure is less labor-intensive and less time-consuming, with the same protein yield (27).
26. Before addition of the EB, lipids can be removed from the seeds with hexane. Add 1 mL of hexane to the seed powder, vortex, and centrifuge at maximal speed (approximately 20,000 ×*g*) for 5 min at room temperature. Discard the supernatant and repeat the hexane step. Afterwards, put the samples in the SpeedVac device at room temperature until the hexane is evaporated and the seed powder is completely dry (2–5 min).
27. When the accumulation of the recombinant protein is low, or when a more concentrated protein extract is needed, only 500 μL of EB can be added. After centrifugation, collect 400 μL of supernatant and add 100 μL of 100% (v/v) glycerol. Alternatively, 10 mg of seeds can be used to perform the extraction procedure.

28. In general, three different methods can be used to determine the total protein concentration in an *Arabidopsis* seed extract: the UV-A_{280}, the Bradford method (20), and the Lowry method (24). For *Arabidopsis* seed extracts, the measured values can differ up to 20-fold, depending on the method used. The Lowry method is the most reliable to determine the protein concentration in total *Arabidopsis* seed extracts, as demonstrated (13).
29. The final dilution factors of the samples in the plate are 115, 230, 460, and 920× (5 μL of a 2.5, 5, 10, and 20× dilution in a total volume of 230 μL).
30. In general, seed extracts prepared in this manner (see Subheading 3.6) contain 1–3 mg of protein per mL and leaf extracts 2–4 mg (see Subheading 3.2). It is good practice to bring all protein extracts to the same final protein concentration of 1 mg/mL
31. Depending on the accumulation level of the VHH-Fc antibodies and the detection sensitivity, 1–20 μg of protein can be loaded on the gel.
32. Before use, equilibrate the PVDF membrane 15 s in 100% (v/v) ethanol. Afterwards, rinse the membrane for 2 min in ddH_2O and incubate for 5 min in blotting transfer buffer.
33. Indicate the side of the membrane on which the proteins are blotted because it is especially important for the washing, blocking, and incubation steps of two membranes simultaneously. Make sure that the side of the membranes on which the proteins are blotted, are always oriented away from each other.
34. Instead of using an antibody linked to horseradish peroxidase, an antibody linked to alkaline phosphatase can be used as well. In this case, the signal is developed by addition of nitro blue tetrazolium/5-bromo-4-chloro-3-indolyl phosphate. The presence of alkaline phosphatase is visualized by formation of a blue colored precipitate on the membrane at the positions of the bands after approximately 30 min.
35. The exposure to a film should occur immediately after substrate incubation, because the light signal is only emitted for 20 up to 30 min.
36. Alternatively, you can use software tools, such as Image J, to quantify the signal strength.

Acknowledgments

The authors thank Martine De Cock for help in preparing the manuscript. This work is supported by the European Commission 6th Framework (Pharma Planta, LSHB-CT-2003-503565).

We also thank the colleagues involved in the European Cooperation in Science and Technology (COST) action "Molecular Farming: Plants as production platform for high value proteins" FA0804 for helpful discussions. V.V. and T.D.M, and K.D.W. and R.P. are indebted to the "Bijzonder Onderzoeksfonds" of the Ghent University and the "Agentschap voor Innovatie door Wetenschap en Technologie" for predoctoral fellowships, respectively.

References

1. Ma JK-C et al (2005) Plant-derived pharmaceuticals—the road forward. Trends Plant Sci 10:580–585
2. Stoger E et al (2005) Recent progress in plantibody technology. Curr Pharm Des 11: 2439–2457
3. Basaran P, Rodríguez-Cerezo E (2008) Plant molecular farming: opportunities and challenges. Crit Rev Biotechnol 28:153–172
4. De Muynck B, Navarre C, Boutry M (2010) Production of antibodies in plants: status after twenty years. Plant Biotechnol J 8:529–563
5. Gleba Y, Klimyuk V, Marillonnet S (2005) Magnifection—a new platform for expressing recombinant vaccines in plants. Vaccine 23: 2042–2048
6. Gleba Y, Klimyuk V, Marillonnet S (2007) Viral vectors for the expression of proteins in plants. Curr Opin Biotechnol 18:134–141
7. Giritch A et al (2006) Rapid high-yield expression of full-size IgG antibodies in plants coinfected with noncompeting viral vectors. Proc Natl Acad Sci USA 103:14701–14706
8. Musiychuk K et al (2007) A launch vector for the production of vaccine antigens in plants. Influenza Other Respi Viruses 1:19–25
9. Sainsbury F, Lomonossoff GP (2008) Extremely high-level and rapid transient protein production in plants without the use of viral replication. Plant Physiol 148:1212–1218
10. Sainsbury F, Thuenemann EC, Lomonossoff GP (2009) pEAQ: versatile expression vectors for easy and quick transient expression of heterologous proteins in plants. Plant Biotechnol J 7:682–693
11. Pogue GP et al (2010) Production of pharmaceutical-grade recombinant aprotinin and a monoclonal antibody product using plant-based transient expression systems. Plant Biotechnol J 8:638–654
12. Lau OS, Sun SSM (2009) Plant seeds as bioreactors for recombinant protein production. Biotechnol Adv 27:1015–1022
13. Goossens A et al (1999) The *arcelin-5* gene of *Phaseolus vulgaris* directs high seed-specific expression in transgenic *Phaseolus acutifolius* and *Arabidopsis* plants. Plant Physiol 120: 1095–1104
14. De Jaeger G et al (2002) Boosting heterologous protein production in transgenic dicotyledonous seeds using *Phaseolus vulgaris* regulatory sequences. Nat Biotechnol 20:1265–1268
15. Van Droogenbroeck B et al (2007) Aberrant localization and underglycosylation of highly accumulating single-chain Fv-Fc antibodies in transgenic *Arabidopsis* seeds. Proc Natl Acad Sci USA 104:1430–1435
16. Loos A et al (2011) Production of monoclonal antibodies with a controlled *N*-glycosylation pattern in seeds of *Arabidopsis thaliana*. Plant Biotechnol J 9:179–192
17. Harmsen MM, De Haard HJ (2007) Properties, production and applications of camelid single-domain antibody fragments. Appl Microbiol Biotechnol 77:13–22
18. Voinnet O et al (2003) An enhanced transient expression system in plants based on suppression of gene silencing by the p19 protein of tomato bushy stunt virus. Plant J 33:949–956
19. Shu L et al (1993) Secretion of a single-gene-encoded immunoglobulin from myeloma cells. Proc Natl Acad Sci USA 90:7995–7999
20. Bradford MM (1976) A rapid and sensitive method for the quantitation of microgram quantities of protein utilizing the principle of protein-dye binding. Anal Biochem 72: 248–254
21. Clough SJ, Bent AF (1998) Floral dip: a simplified method for *Agrobacterium*-mediated transformation of *Arabidopsis thaliana*. Plant J 16:735–743
22. Griffiths AJF et al (1993) An introduction to genetic analysis, 5th edn. WH Freeman, New York
23. De Neve M et al (1997) T-DNA integration patterns in co-transformed plant cells suggest

that T-DNA repeats originate from co-integration of separate T-DNAs. Plant J 11:15–29

24. Lowry OH et al (1951) Protein measurement with the Folin phenol reagent. J Biol Chem 193:265–275
25. Valvekens D, Van Montagu M, Van Lijsebettens M (1988) *Agrobacterium tumefaciens*-mediated transformation of *Arabidopsis thaliana* root explants by using kanamycin selection. Proc Natl Acad Sci USA 85:5536–5540
26. De Buck S et al (2009) The T-DNA integration pattern in *Arabidopsis* transformants is highly determined by the transformed target cell. Plant J 60:134–145
27. Van Droogenbroeck B, De Wilde K, Depicker A (2009) Production of antibody fragments in *Arabidopsis* seeds. In: Faye L, Gomord V (eds) Recombinant proteins from plants: methods and protocols, vol 483, Methods in molecular biology. Humana Press, Totowa, pp 89–101

Part V

Improvement and Applications of Single Domain Antibodies

Chapter 20

Selecting and Purifying Autonomous Human Variable Heavy (VH) Domains

Raffi Tonikian and Sachdev S. Sidhu

Abstract

Antibodies are invaluable macromolecules effectively utilized as detection reagents and therapeutics. Traditionally, researchers have relied upon the entire immunoglobulin molecule, however advances in protein engineering have ushered the use of antibody fragments as equally important biological tools such that at present, the downstream application generally dictates the antibody format employed. We provide herein robust and proven protocols for the isolation of autonomous human antibody variable heavy domains (VH). The strategy utilizes combinatorial phage-displayed libraries targeting human VH domain positions previously shown to promote autonomous behavior, and selection against a specified antigen. Subsequently, autonomous VH domains are characterized and chosen using standard biophysical methods.

Key words: Phage display, VH domain, Antibody domain, Antibody engineering, Self-folding, Light chain interface, Complementarity-determining region

1. Introduction

Antibodies are produced by the immune system to neutralize foreign agents. The most common class of antibody molecule is immunoglobulin G (IgG), a heterotetramer composed of two heavy chains and two light chains (see Fig. 1). The IgG molecule can be subdivided into two functional subunits: (1) the fragment crystallizable (Fc), which constitutes the tail of the antibody and interacts with cell surface receptors to activate an immune response, and (2) the fragment-antigen binding (Fab), which mediates antigen recognition. The Fc region comprises two pairs of constant domains (CH2 and CH3) from two paired heavy chains, whereas the Fab region consists of a variable domain followed by a constant domain from the heavy chain (VH and CH, respectively), which pair with a variable and constant domain from the light chain (VL and CL, respectively). The Fc and Fab regions are demarcated by

Dirk Saerens and Serge Muyldermans (eds.), *Single Domain Antibodies: Methods and Protocols*,
Methods in Molecular Biology, vol. 911, DOI 10.1007/978-1-61779-968-6_20, © Springer Science+Business Media, LLC 2012

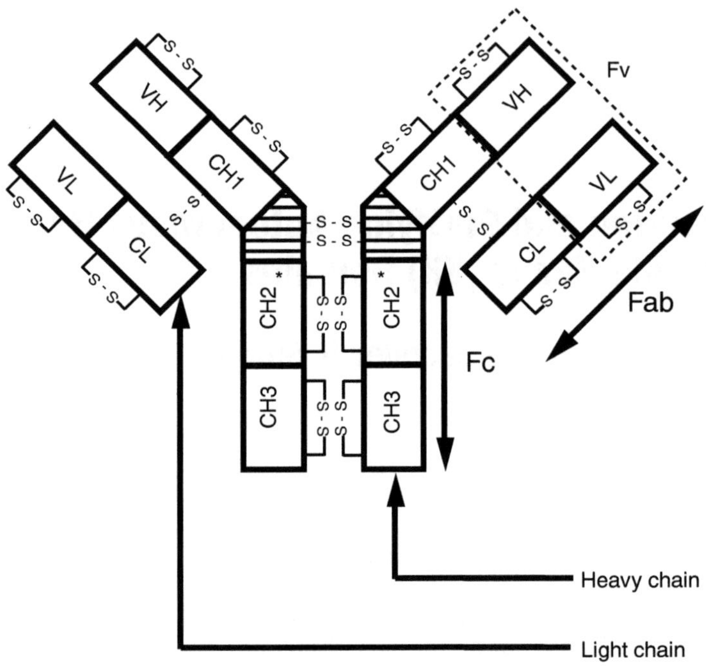

Fig. 1. The immunoglobulin G (IgG) molecule. Schematic view of an IgG heterotetramer composed of two light chains and two heavy chains. The variable and constant domains are shown in *white* and the hinge region is crosshatched. The antigen-binding fragment (Fab) and the crystallizable fragment (Fc) are labeled. Disulfide bonds (–S–S–) are shown and a glycosylation site in CH2 is denoted by an *asterisks*. The antigen-binding unit can be further reduced to the Fv consisting of the VH and VL domains (*dashed box*).

a hinge region, which contains disulfide linkages holding the two chains together (1).

As all antibodies were found to be composed of heavy and light chains, the prevailing belief was that the simplest antigen-binding unit is the variable fragment (Fv), a heterodimer of the VH and VL domains (see Fig. 1) (1). The isolation of functional single variable heavy domains (VH) from mice refuted this notion (2), and held the promise of facile production of single antibody domains in bacteria. However, the widespread use of murine and human VH domains has been hindered due to their poor solubility and propensity for aggregation.

Interest in single domain antibodies was renewed with the discovery of autonomous VH domains in camelids (camels, dromedaries, and llamas) and VH-like domains in cartilaginous fish (wobbegong and nurse sharks) (reviewed in ref. (3)). In addition to conventional antibodies, camelids also produce "heavy chain antibodies" that are devoid of light chains (4). Termed VHH (for heavy chain variable domain of a heavy chain antibody), these domains have evolved to be autonomously stable in the absence of a light chain partner. Furthermore, as VHH domains are relatively small, they exhibit increased clearance in vivo and enhanced tumor penetration, thus underscoring their potential for specialized therapeutic applications (5). As such, numerous efforts have been geared toward elucidating the structural properties underlying the autonomous behavior of camelid VHH domains and applying these to conventional VH domains, with the aim of engineering single domain antibodies with improved biophysical and therapeutic properties.

In conventional antibodies, the VH and VL domains are held in contact with one another through an interface composed mainly of hydrophobic residues. Thus, attempting to isolate the VH domain exposes these hydrophobic residues, leading to aggregation and reduced solubility. Structures of camelid VHH domains have revealed that these structural requirements can be alleviated by sequence alterations that act to collectively decrease the hydrophobicity of the former light chain interface (6–12). The most notable is the VHH tetrad, which occurs at four positions in the second framework region (13–16). In addition, the third complementarity-determining region (CDR3) makes important intramolecular contacts that sequester hydrophobic residues, thus increasing the overall solubility of the molecule. However, attempts to introduce these changes into human VH domains, a process referred to as "camelization," have brought only modest improvements in solubility and thermal stability (17).

In hindsight, it appears that camelization strategies underestimate the structural role played by the CDR3 loop in the stability and solubility of VHH domains. This places significant constraints on the design of libraries with randomized CDR3 sequences with the ultimate goal of isolating novel VH domains with desired binding properties, as it has been shown that CDR3 loop diversity is critical to the development of successful phage-displayed antibody libraries (18–20).

To gain further insight into the autonomous behavior of VH domains, we conducted a comprehensive analysis of the factors contributing to the stability and solubility of human VH domains (21). Using combinatorial phage-displayed libraries and conventional biophysical methods, the entire former light chain interface and CDR3 were analyzed in the context of the humanized monoclonal antibody 4D5, which binds to the epidermal growth factor receptor family member ErbB2 (22–24) and has been approved for cancer therapy (25, 26).

First, a phage-displayed library (referred to as library A) was created that targeted residues implicated in the stabilization of camelid VHH domains and an autonomous human VH domain. These include three of the four residues from the VHH tetrad, namely positions 37, 45, and 47 (conserved Cys residues are at positions 23 and 104 according to IMGT nomenclature) (27). In addition, position 35 was also targeted in the phage-displayed library as this position has been implicated in the stabilization of the human VH domain HEL4 (28). As VHH domains have been shown to be stabilized by interactions between the CDR3 loop and residues in the former light chain interface, the region corresponding to CDR3 was also replaced with random loops of all possible lengths ranging from 7 to 17 residues.

The library was cycled through selections for binding to protein A, isolated clones were sequenced, and the sequences were aligned and inspected for conserved motifs. Interestingly, no consensus was observed in terms of either CDR3 loop length or sequence. At positions 37 and 45, it was found that the general hydrophobic nature of the wild-type residues was conserved. At position 35, Ser/Gly was favored over the wild-type His. Position 47 was occupied by a hydrophobic residue, a charged residue, or a small residue.

A panel of selected VH domains were purified and assayed for favorable biophysical properties, which included: (1) purification in high yield in a correctly folded form, (2) existence as a monomer at high concentrations as evidenced by gel filtration and light scattering analysis, and (3) reversible folding behavior and high thermostability in temperature-induced denaturation experiments monitored by circular dichroism (CD).

The VH domain exhibiting the best behavior in these assays was used as a template for the creation of a second-generation library (referred to as library B). To delineate the residues targeted in library B, the structure of the Fv-4D5 was examined to identify all residues involved in the light chain interface, which were defined as residues that lose greater than 20 Å of solvent-accessible surface area because of contacts with the light chain. This group consisted of nine positions, including three that were randomized in library A (37, 45, 47), and six others (39, 44, 50, 91, 103, and 105). Thus, library B was designed to target these nine positions and position 35 for diversification, using a soft-randomization approach, whereby 50% of the wild-type sequence and 50% random sampling were allowed at each position.

Library B was cycled through rounds of selection for binding to protein A, and a large panel of isolated clones were sequenced and aligned to determine the distribution of amino acids at each mutagenized position. The amino acid frequencies at each position of the naïve library (prior to selection for binding to protein A) were also calculated, and these were compared to the frequencies observed among the selected clones from library B. This exercise allowed the identification of statistically significant deviations indicative of positive selective pressure for certain amino acid types at particular positions. It was found that the sequence of the parental template was mostly conserved outside of the CDR3 loop region.

As was done following selection with the initial library, the biophysical properties were tested for a panel of VH domain proteins selected from library B. Again, all selected domains showed significantly improved biophysical characteristics compared to the 4D5 VH domain.

As the CDR3 loops of camelid VH domains are involved in the stabilization of the protein fold, a shotgun alanine-scanning analysis was performed to test whether this was also the case for the VH domains selected from the phage-displayed libraries. To this end, a library was constructed allowing each CDR3 residue to vary as the wild-type or Ala with equal frequency. Following selection for binding to protein A, a number of clones were sequenced, and the WT/Ala ratio determined for each scanned position. The WT/Ala ratio correlates with the contribution of each wild-type side chain to stability, with WT/Ala ratios greater than or less than 1 indicating side chains that stabilizes or destabilizes the protein fold, respectively. The results from the shotgun alanine-scanning confirmed that the CDR3 loop is not required for the structural stability of most selected VH domains.

To conduct an in-depth analysis of all possible residues tolerated at the positions targeted in library B, a quantitative saturation scan analysis was performed. The clone exhibiting the best biophysical characteristics from library B was chosen as a template and nine positions (35, 37, 39, 44, 35, 47, 50, 91, and 105) were targeted for randomization by allowing for all possible combinations of amino acids. Again, the library was selected for binding to protein A and the percent occurrence of each amino acid at each position was calculated for a large panel of selected clones. This analysis revealed modest biases at most scanned positions, with the parental sequence among the most prevalent sequences, but no position was dominated by any single residue type. These results suggest that the stabilization of the autonomous VH domain relative to the 4D5 VH domain was achieved by cumulative effects arising from multiple mutations. In general, most of the hydrophobic residues in the former light chain interface can be replaced by smaller and/or more hydrophilic amino acids, and notably, the small hydrophilic amino acids Ser and Thr are tolerated at all positions.

Based on the saturation scanning analysis, a number of VH domains were selected and purified and their biophysical properties assayed. In almost all cases, the results from the saturation scanning analysis agreed with the biophysical tests in that mutations found to be tolerated in the combinatorial analysis yielded stabilizing effects in the biophysical tests. Taken together, these results underscore the effectiveness of the saturation scanning analysis for predicting substitutions that are well tolerated structurally by the VH domain fold.

In summary, this unbiased approach yielded numerous autonomous VH domains that do not depend on interactions between CDR3 and the former light chain interface, which is in stark contrast to camelid VHH domains. Instead, improved biophysical properties resulted from mutations that increase the hydrophilicity of the former light chain interface by replacing exposed hydrophobic residues with structurally compatible hydrophilic substitutions. It is noteworthy, that these stabilizing mutations are rarely observed in camelid VHH domains or in natural human VH domains, and could only be derived with the utilization of synthetic libraries. This work therefore outlines a general strategy that can potentially be applied to any VH domain to render it autonomous.

In the next sections, we provide detailed methods for the design and isolation of autonomous VH domains using combinatorial phage-displayed libraries. The methods rely on commonly found laboratory equipment and standard molecular biology and biophysical techniques. We provide a descriptive overview of the different technical components required to build phage-displayed VH domain libraries followed by detailed experimental protocols.

1.1. Phagemid Design

As many different vectors and formats are available, a major consideration in the generation of phage-displayed antibody domain libraries is the choice of an appropriate vector system designed to display polypeptides as fusion proteins on the surface of M13 bacteriophage (29). We prefer the use of a phagemid, which is a plasmid that contains the components required for packaging viral DNA into phage particles. A phagemid contains a double-stranded DNA (dsDNA) origin of replication, allowing replication of the phagemid as a plasmid in a bacterial host (i.e. *Escherichia coli*), and a single-stranded DNA (ssDNA) filamentous phage origin of replication (fl ori), which allows packaging into phage particles (see Fig. 2). In addition, a β-lactamase gene in the vector confers resistance to ampicillin and carbenicillin. The phagemid described here contains a P_{tac} promoter, which is inducible by isopropyl β-D-1-thiogalactopyranoside (IPTG), to drive expression of the VH domain as a fusion to the M13 bacteriophage gene-3 minor coat protein (P3). However, phagemids with other promoters may also be used. For instance, we have routinely used a phagemid with an alkaline phosphatase promoter for the display of Fabs and single-chain variable fragments (scFvs) (19, 30). The phagemid also contains a secretion signal (stII), which directs the VH-P3 fusion to the periplasm, where it is subsequently packaged into phage particles.

As mentioned above, the phagemid replicates as a double-stranded plasmid in *E. coli*. However, upon co-infection with helper phage, ssDNA replication is initiated through the fl origin of replication, which ultimately leads to the packaging of viral DNA into phage particles. While the helper phage provides all the proteins necessary for phage assembly, copies of phagemid-encoded coat protein are also incorporated into the assembling phage particles. Thus, polypeptides fused to the phagemid-encoded coat protein are displayed in linkage to their encoding viral DNA, and phage particles can be used for library screening.

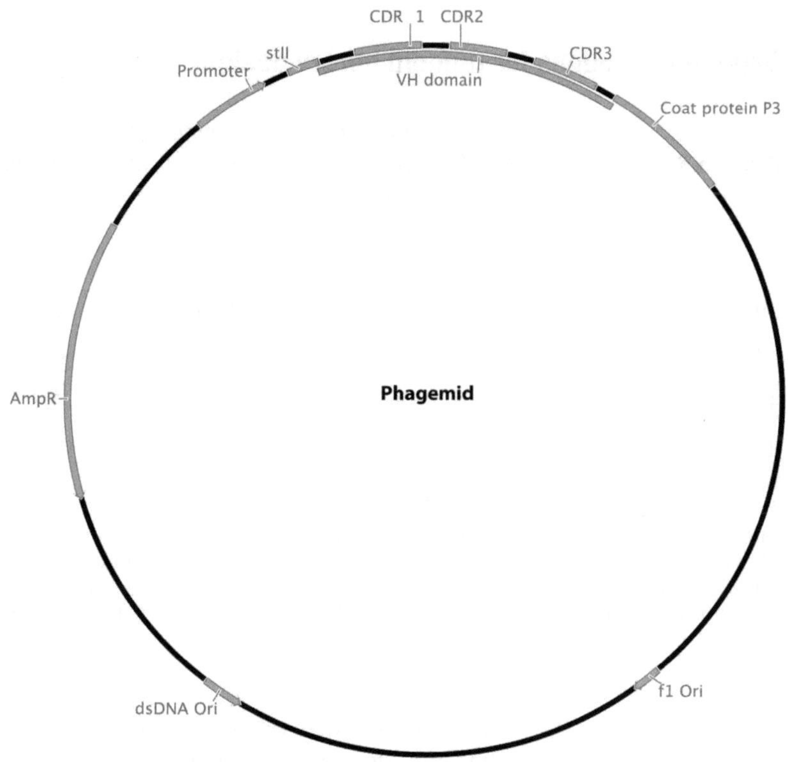

Fig. 2. A phagemid vector designed for VH domain phage display. The phagemid vectors contains origins of single-stranded (f1 ori) and double-stranded (dsDNA ori) DNA replication. A β-lactamase gene confers resistance to ampicillin and carbenicillin (AmpR). For VH domain display, the phagemid also contains a cassette consisting of a promoter that drives transcription of a VH domain fused to minor phage coat protein P3. The three complementary determining regions (CDRs) in the VH domain are also shown. A secretion signal (stII) directs the VH-P3 fusion to the periplasm, where it is incorporated into phage particles that are secreted from the *Escherichia coli* host.

1.2. Library Design

The first step in building a library of autonomous VH domains is to choose an appropriate VH domain template to clone into a suitable phagemid and target key positions for mutagenesis (21). This can be accomplished by cloning the VH domain from a Fab or scFv into the phagemid described in the previous section or one with similar vector features. In a phagemid system, antibody domain display can be achieved by inserting the VH domain of interest between the regions encoding the secretion signal and P3 (see Fig. 2).

With the VH domain cloned into the phagemid, the next important step is deciding which residues to target for mutagenesis. As described (21), a large panel of amino acid combinations at critical framework positions was tested to ascertain their effect on autonomous VH domain behavior. Although a multitude of residues were tested at several positions, the library design strategy recommended here targets framework positions that were shown to be important for the structural stability of an autonomous VH

Table 1
Degenerate codons for random library design

Position Kabat	Position IMGT	Preferred amino acids	Suggested library codon	Amino acid encoded
35	40	G, S, T	RST	A, G, S, T
37	42	Hydrophobic	NNT	A, D, G, H, I, L, N, P, R, S, T, V
39	44	Hydrophilic	RVK	A, D, E, G, H, K, N, R, S T
44	49	G, A, S, T	RST	A, G, S, T
45	50	E, H, Y	NWW	D, E, F, H, I, K, L, N, Q, V, Y
47	52	W, L, V, A, T	KSG	A, W, G, S
50	55	R	VVC	A, D, G, H, N, P, R, S, T

For each position in the 4D5 VH domain, the set of preferred amino acids as identified in Barthelemy et al. (21) is shown. The suggested library codons encode a set of amino acids that most closely resemble the preferred amino acids that were shown to promote autonomous VH domain behavior at each position. Residue numbering is provided in both the Kabat (38) and IMGT (27) nomenclature

domain. At each position, a degenerate DNA codon is inserted that encodes for particular amino acids that were found to preferentially promote VH domain solubility and stability. We recommend the use of a single mutagenic oligonucleotide that spans the entire stretch of residues targeted for mutagenesis in the VH domain framework (Table 1 and Fig. 3).

1.3. Library Construction

Very large phage-displayed VH domain libraries can be constructed by using optimized procedures that are based on the oligonucleotide-directed mutagenesis method of Kunkel et al. (31), which introduces mutations onto a single-stranded DNA (ssDNA) template (see Fig. 4). The method relies on dut$^-$/ung$^-$ bacterial strains (e.g., *E. coli* CJ236) that incorporate uracil during DNA replication. The uracil-containing ssDNA (dU-ssDNA) is used as a template onto which a mutagenic oligonucleotide is annealed. To ensure proper annealing, the mutagenic oligonucleotide must share complementarity with the template at least 15 nucleotides upstream and downstream of the sites targeted for mutagenesis. The annealed oligonucleotide primes the synthesis of a complementary DNA strand by T7 DNA polymerase. The newly synthesized DNA strand is ligated by T4 DNA ligase to form covalently closed circular double-stranded DNA (CCC-dsDNA). As the mutagenic oligonucleotide is not perfectly complementary to the template, the CCC-dsDNA contains mismatches in the region targeted for mutagenesis. Subsequently, the CCC-dsDNA is introduced into a dut$^+$/ung$^+$ *E. coli* strain host by high-efficiency electroporation. This bacterial strain resolves the CCC-dsDNA

a

```
1
GAGGTTCAGCTGGTGGAGTCTGGCGGTGGCCTGGTGCAGCCAGGGGGCTCACTCCGTTTG
 E  V  Q  L  V  E  S  G  G  G  L  V  Q  P  G  G  S  L  R  L

21                                            35    37    39
TCCTGTGCAGCTTCTGGCTTCAACATTAAAGACACCTATATCCACTGGGTGCGTCAGGCC
 S  C  A  A  S  G  F  N  I  K  D  T  Y  I  H  W  V  R  Q  A
                                   CDR1

42      44 45      47        50     52 a  53
CCGGGTAAGGGCCTGGAATGGGTTGCAAGGATTTATCCTACGAATGGTTATACTAGATAT
 P  G  K  G  L  E  W  V  A  R  I  Y  P  T  N  G  Y  T  R  Y
                                          CDR2

60
GCCGATAGCGTCAAGGGCCGTTTCACTATAAGCGCAGACACATCCAAAAACACAGCCTAC
 A  D  S  V  K  G  R  F  T  I  S  A  D  T  S  K  N  T  A  Y
    CDR2

80     82 a  b  c  83
CTACAAATGAACAGCTTAAGAGCTGAGGACACTGCCGTCTATTATTGTAGCCGCTGGGGA
 L  Q  M  N  S  L  R  A  E  D  T  A  V  Y  Y  C  S  R  W  G
                                                         CDR3

96        100 a  b  c 101
GGGGACGGCTTCTATGCTATGGACTACTGGGGTCAAGGAACCCTGGTCACCGTCTCCTCG
 G  D  G  F  Y  A  M  D  Y  W  G  Q  G  T  L  V  T  V  S  S
       CDR3
```

b

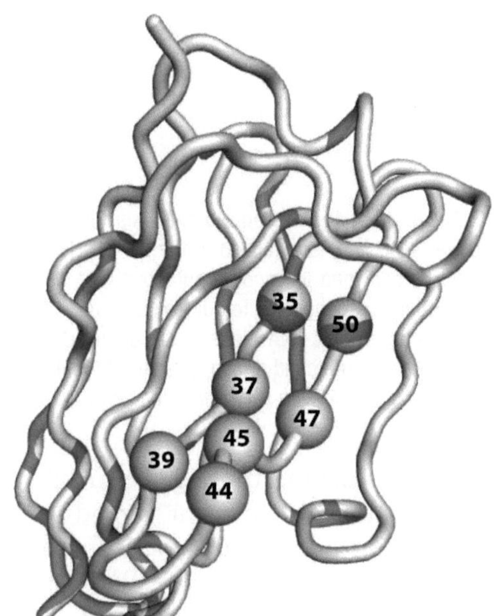

c

```
AAAGACACCTATATCRSTTGGNNTCGTRVKGCCCCGGGTAAGRSTNWWGAAKSGGTTGCAVVCATTTATCCTACGAAT
```

Fig. 3. Design of VH domain library. (**a**) Gene encoding VH-4D5. The CDRs are *underlined*. Positions targeted for randomization using oligonucleotide-directed mutagenesis include positions 35, 37, 39, 44, 45, 47, and 50. CDR definitions and residue numbering are according to the Kabat nomenclature (38). (**b**) Three-dimensional view of the VH domain library design. The VH-4D5 main chain is shown as a tube. Positions chosen for randomization are *numbered* and represented as *spheres*. The structure was visualized with the program PyMol (DeLano Scientific) using the coordinates for the crystal structure of Fv-4D5 (PDB code 1FVC). (**c**) Mutagenic oligonucleotide to create a phage-displayed VH domain library using oligonucleotide-directed mutagenesis based on the 4D5 template. The oligonucleotide is perfectly complementary to the template sequence 15 nucleotides upstream and downstream of the region targeted for randomization. Underlined degenerate codons are designed to replace the targeted positions (35, 37, 39, 44, 45, 47, 50) with amino acids found by Barthelemy et al. to be well tolerated in autonomous VH domains (21).

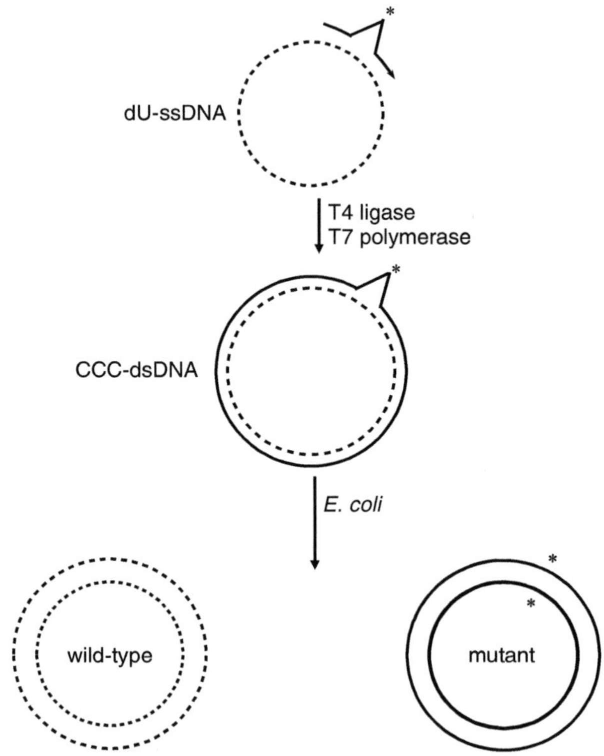

Fig. 4. Oligonucleotide-directed mutagenesis for library construction. A synthetic oligonucleotide (*solid line*) is annealed to the dU-ssDNA template (*dashed circle*). The oligonucleotide is designed to encode mutations (*asterisks*), which are flanked by perfectly complementary sequences. Heteroduplex CCC-dsDNA is enzymatically synthesized by T7 DNA polymerase and T4 DNA ligase. Heteroduplex CCC-dsDNA is introduced into an *E. coli* host where the mismatched region is repaired to either the wild-type (*circle with dashed lines*) or mutant (*circle with solid lines*) sequence.

by preferentially inactivating the uracil-containing parental strain and replicating the nascent strand containing the mutagenic oligonucleotide. The mutagenesis frequency using the procedures outlined herein is typically 50–80%.

We recommend first creating a "stop template" phagemid. This is done by using mutagenic oligonucleotides that introduce stop codons at the sites targeted for mutagenesis. The "stop template" phagemid is then used as a template for library construction, as it eliminates display of the wild-type protein on the surface of bacteriophage.

1.4. *E. coli* Electroporation and Production of Library Phage

Once the heteroduplex CCC-dsDNA has been synthesized and purified, it can be electroporated into an appropriate bacterial host to produce the phage-displayed library. The *E. coli* host must harbor the F′ episome, which allows for M13 bacteriophage infection and propagation. Once introduced into the bacterial host, the CCC-dsDNA is resolved through DNA repair and replication, and the resulting library is packaged into phage particles. The introduction of large amounts of affinity purified DNA through electroporation is an efficient way to produce highly diverse phage-displayed libraries (32). An optimized *E. coli* strain, named SS320, is ideally suited for the preparation of phage-displayed libraries, as it contains the F′ episome required for bacteriophage infection while allowing for high-efficiency transformation (32).

1.5. Selection of Autonomous VH Domains

Once the phage-displayed VH domain library has been generated, it can be used for the selection of autonomous VH domains. The procedure described herein outlines a selection strategy for binding to protein A, which is immobilized on immunosorbent plates. As described above, protein A binds to a noncontiguous, structural epitope opposite to the VH/VL interface, and therefore can serve as a screening strategy to select for structurally stable VH domains. Moreover, it has been shown that binding of a phage-displayed VH domain to this ligand is correlated with the intrinsic stability of the VH domain protein (33–35). The library of VH domains displayed on the surface of M13 bacteriophage is presented to immobilized protein A. After an incubation period, during which the displayed VH domains are allowed to bind to protein A, nonbinding phage particles are washed away with buffer containing mild detergent. The pool of structurally stable phage-displayed VH domains is eluted from the immunosorbent plate and amplified in a bacterial host (*E. coli* XL1-blue). This process is repeated over several rounds to enrich for a pool of structurally stable, autonomous VH domains.

1.6. DNA Sequencing

Following the final round of phage selection, an aliquot of the phage-infected bacteria is plated for single colonies. A single colony represents a single *E. coli* cell that has been infected with a phage displaying a unique VH domain. The DNA encapsulated by the phage clone is used as the template for a PCR to amplify the DNA fragment encoding the VH domain, which is sequenced and translated to decode the sequence of the VH domain. We recommend sequencing as many unique phage clones as possible to get a representative profile of the residues that are most prevalent at positions targeted for mutagenesis in the VH domain library. Ideally, one would select a set of representative candidates that best match the consensus profile obtained for downstream biophysical assays that test the autonomous behavior of the candidate VH domains.

1.7. Protein Purification

After a panel of VH domains has been selected for biophysical characterization, the phage display vector must be modified by the insertion of an amber stop codon between the sequence encoding the VH domain and the phage coat protein. This is done so that the VH domain is no longer produced as a fusion protein to P3 when expressed in a bacterial strain optimized for protein expression.

The amber stop codon can be introduced in the vector using the site-directed oligonucleotide mutagenesis procedure described above. For protein expression, we recommend the use of *E. coli* BL-21 cells. As our phagemid contains an IPTG-inducible P_{tac} promoter, large quantities of VH domain protein can be secreted and isolated from cells using protein A as an affinity capture reagent.

1.8. Biophysical Analysis of Autonomous VH Domains

Following purification from bacteria, the selected panel of VH domains can be analyzed using biophysical methods. The VH clone chosen for the construction of the second-generation library should ideally adhere to the following criteria: (1) purification of the correctly folded form in high yield, (2) monomeric behavior at high concentration as evidence by light scattering analysis, and (3) reversible folding behavior and high thermostability in temperature-induced denaturation experiments monitored by CD.

2. Materials

Prepare all solutions using ultrapure water (prepared by purifying deionized water to attain a sensitivity of 18 MΩ cm at 25°C) and analytical grade reagents. Prepare and store all reagents at room temperature (unless indicated otherwise). Diligently follow all waste disposal regulations when disposing waste materials.

2.1. Preparation of Helper Phage (M13KO7) Stock

1. *E. coli* XL1-Blue (Agilent Technologies, CA, USA).
2. M13KO7 (New England Biolabs, MA, USA).
3. Tetracycline stock solution: 5 mg/mL in EtOH, store at –20°C.
4. Kanamycin stock solution: 5 mg/mL in ddH_2O, filter sterilize, store at 4°C.
5. LB/tet plates: 5 g yeast extract, 10 g tryptone, 10 g NaCl. Add water to 1.0 L, adjust pH to 7.0 with NaOH, add 20 g of granulated agar. Autoclave, cool to room temperature, add 1 mL of tetracycline stock solution.
6. 2YT/kan medium: 10 g yeast extract, 16 g tryptone, 5 g NaCl. Add ddH_2O to 1.0 L, adjust pH to 7.0 with NaOH. Autoclave, cool to room temperature, add 5 mL of kanamycin stock solution.
7. 2YT/kan/tet medium: Add 1 mL of tetracycline stock solution to 1.0 L of 2YT/kan medium.
8. PEG/NaCl: 20% PEG-8000 (w/v), 2.5 M NaCl in ddH_2O. Mix and autoclave.
9. PBS: 137 mM NaCl, 3 mM KCl, 8 mM Na_2HPO_4, 1.5 mM KH_2PO_4 in ddH_2O. Adjust pH to 7.2 with HCl, autoclave.

2.2. Preparation of Electrocompetent E. coli SS320

1. 2YT/tet medium: 10 g yeast extract, 16 g tryptone, 5 g NaCl. Add ddH_2O to 1.0 L, adjust pH to 7.0 with NaOH. Autoclave, cool to 50°C, add 1 mL of tetracycline stock solution.
2. *E. coli* SS320 (Lucigen Corporation, WI, USA).
3. 2YT top agar: 16 g tryptone, 10 g yeast extract, 5 g NaCl, 7.5 g granulated agar. Add ddH_2O to 1.0 L, adjust pH to 7.0 with NaOH, heat to dissolve, autoclave.
4. LB/tet plates.
5. 2YT/kan medium.
6. 2YT/kan/tet medium.
7. Superbroth/kan/tet medium: 12 g tryptone, 24 g yeast extract, 5 mL glycerol. Add ddH_2O to 900 mL. Autoclave and cool to room temperature. Add 100 mL of autoclaved 0.17 M KH_2PO_4, 0.72 M K_2HPO_4, 1 mL of tetracycline stock solution, and 5 mL of kanamycin stock solution.
8. 1 mM Hepes, pH 7.4: Add 4.0 mL of 1.0 M Hepes, pH 7.4 (Invitrogen, CA, USA) to 4.0 L of ultrapure irrigation USP water (Braun Medical, Inc., MA, USA), filter sterilize.
9. Magnetic stir bars.
10. 10% ultrapure glycerol: Add 100 mL of ultrapure glycerol (Invitrogen, CA, USA) to 900 mL of ultrapure irrigation USP water (Braun Medical, Inc., MA, USA).
11. Liquid nitrogen.

2.3. Isolation of dU-ssDNA Template

1. *E. coli* CJ236 (New England Biolabs, MA, USA).
2. Carbenicillin: 5 mg/mL in ddH_2O, filter sterilize, store at 4°C.
3. Chloramphenicol: 10 mg/mL in ethanol, store at –20°C.
4. 2YT/carb/cmp medium: 10 g yeast extract, 16 g tryptone, 5 g NaCl. Add ddH_2O to 1.0 L, adjust pH to 7.0 with NaOH. Autoclave, cool to room temperature, add 10 mL of carbenicillin stock solution, and 1 mL of chloramphenicol stock solution.
5. Uridine: 0.25 mg/mL in ddH_2O, filter sterilize.
6. 2YT/carb/kan/uridine medium: 10 g yeast extract, 16 g tryptone, 5 g NaCl. Add ddH_2O to 1.0 L, adjust pH to 7.0 with NaOH. Autoclave, cool to room temperature. Add 10 mL of carbenicillin stock solution, 5 mL of kanamycin stock solution, and 1 mL of uridine stock solution.
7. PEG/NaCl.
8. PBS.
9. QIAprep Spin M13 Kit (Qiagen, CA, USA) which includes MP, MLB, PE, and EB buffers.

10. TAE buffer: 40 mM Tris-acetate, 1.0 mM EDTA. Adjust pH to 8.0 with HCl.
11. TAE/agarose gel: TAE buffer, 1.0% (w/v) agarose, 1:5,000 (v/v) 10% ethidium bromide.

2.4. In Vitro Synthesis of Heteroduplex CCC-dsDNA

1. 10× TM buffer: 0.5 M Tris–HCl, pH 7.5, 0.1 M $MgCl_2$.
2. 10 mM ATP (Invitrogen, CA, USA).
3. 100 mM DTT: 77 mg DTT in 10 mL of ddH_2O. Filter sterilize and store at −20°C.
4. T4 polynucleotide kinase (New England Biolabs, MA, USA).
5. 25 mM dNTP mix (Invitrogen, CA, USA).
6. T4 DNA ligase (New England Biolabs, MA, USA).
7. T7 DNA polymerase (New England Biolabs, MA, USA).
8. QIAquick PCR Purification Kit, which includes QG and PE buffers (Qiagen, CA, USA).
9. TAE/agarose gel.

2.5. E. coli Electroporation and Phage Propagation

1. 0.2 cm gap electroporation cuvette (BioRad, CA, USA).
2. BTX ECM-600 electroporation system (BTX Harvard Apparatus, MA, USA).
3. SOC medium: 5 g bacto-yeast extract, 20 g bacto-tryptone, 0.5 g NaCl, 0.2 g KCl. Add ddH_2O to 1.0 L, adjust pH to 7.0 with NaOH, autoclave. Add 5.0 mL of autoclaved 2.0 M $MgCl_2$ and 20 mL of filter sterilized 1.0 M glucose.
4. LB/carb plates: 5 g yeast extract, 10 g tryptone, 10 g NaCl. Add ddH_2O to 1.0 L, adjust pH to 7.0 with NaOH, and add 20 g of granulated agar. Autoclave, cool to room temperature, add 10 mL of carbenicillin stock solution.
5. 2YT medium: 10 g yeast extract, 16 g tryptone, 5 g NaCl. Add ddH_2O to 1.0 L, adjust pH to 7.0 with NaOH, autoclave.
6. 2YT/carb/kan medium: Add 10 mL of carbenicillin stock solution and 5 mL of kanamycin stock solution to 1.0 L of 2YT medium.
7. PEG/NaCl.
8. PBT buffer: PBS, 0.05% Tween-20, 0.5% BSA. Filter sterilize.

2.6. Affinity Selection for Binding to Immobilized Protein A

1. Maxisorp immunoplates.
2. PBS.
3. Blocking buffer: PBS, 0.5% (w/v) BSA. Filter sterilize.
4. PT buffer: PBS, 0.05% Tween20. Filter sterilize.
5. 0.1 M HCl.

6. 1.0 M Tris–HCl, pH 11.0: Dissolve 121.1 g of Tris base in 800 mL of ddH_2O, adjust to pH 11.0 with HCl, filter sterilize.
7. 2YT/tet medium.
8. *E. coli* XL1-Blue (Stratagene).
9. LB/carb plates.
10. 200 mM IPTG: dissolve 4.8 g of IPTG in ddH_2O. Filter sterilize.
11. 2YT/carb/kan/IPTG medium: Add 10 mL of carbenicillin stock solution, 5 mL of kanamycin solution, and 125 μL of IPTG stock solution to 1.0 L of 2YT medium.
12. PEG/NaCl.
13. PBT buffer.

2.7. DNA Sequencing

1. 2YT/carb/KO7 medium: Add 10 mL of carbenicillin stock solution and 10^{10} phage/mL of M13KO7 to 1.0 L of 2YT medium.
2. 96-well microtubes (VWR, USA).
3. *Taq* DNA polymerase kit (Genscript, NJ, USA).
4. PCR Mix: 19.7 μL of ddH_2O, 2.5 μL of 10× PCR Buffer (Genscript, NJ, USA), 0.25 μL of 25 mM dNTPs, 0.25 μL of each PCR primer, and 0.125 μL of *Taq* DNA polymerase.
5. TAE/agarose gel.
6. PCR clean up mix: 2 U exonuclease I and 0.2 U shrimp alkaline phosphatase (United States Biochemical, OH, USA).

2.8. VH Domain Protein Purification

1. *E. coli* BL-21 (Agilent Technologies, CA, USA).
2. LB/carb plates.
3. LB/carb medium: 5 g yeast extract, 10 g tryptone, 10 g NaCl. Add ddH_2O to 1.0 L, adjust pH to 7.0 with NaOH. Autoclave, allow to cool to room temperature and add 10 mL of carbenicillin stock solution.
4. 2YT/carb medium: To 1.0 L of 2YT medium, add 10 mL of carbenicillin stock solution.
5. 200 mM IPTG.
6. Lysis buffer: 25 mM Tris, 25 mM NaCl, 5 mM EDTA. Adjust pH to 7.1 with HCl.
7. Microfluidizer (Microfluidics, MA, USA).
8. Lysozyme.
9. 0.2 μm filtration unit (NUNC, NY, USA).
10. Protein A sepharose (GE Healthcare Life Sciences, NJ, USA).
11. Wash buffer: 10 mM Tris, 1.0 mM EDTA. Adjust to pH 8.0 using HCl.

12. 0.1 M glycine-HCl: Dissolve 11.1 g glycine-HCl in 800 mL of ddH_2O, adjust to pH 2.7 with HCl and bring volume to 1.0 L with ddH_2O.
13. 1.0 M Tris–HCl: Dissolve 121.1 g of Tris base in 800 mL of ddH_2O, adjust to pH 11.0 with HCl. Filter sterilize.

2.9. Analytical Gel Filtration and Light Scattering Analysis

1. Agilent 1100 series high pressure liquid chromatography system (Agilent Technologies, CA, USA) in line with a Wyatt MiniDawn multiangle light scattering detector (Wyatt Technology, CA, USA).
2. PBS.

2.10. Temperature-Induced Denaturation

1. J-810 spectrometer (Jasco, MD, USA).
2. PBS.

3. Methods

Prior to preparing the phage-displayed libraries, stocks of helper phage (M13KO7) and electrocompetent SS320 cells must be prepared.

3.1. Preparation of Helper Phage (M13K07) Stock

1. Inoculate 25 mL 2YT/tet media with a single colony of *E. coli* XL1-blue from a fresh LB/tet plate.
2. Incubate with shaking at 200 rpm and 37°C to mid-log phase ($OD_{550\ nm}=0.8$).
3. Make tenfold serial dilutions of M13K07 by diluting 20 μL into 180 μL of PBS (see Note 1).
4. Mix 500 μL of *E. coli* XL1-blue at exponential phase with 200 μL of each M13K07 dilution and 4 mL of 2YT top agar.
5. Pour the mixtures onto prewarmed LB/tet plates and incubate overnight at 37°C.
6. Pick a well-separated, single plaque, and inoculate 1 mL of 2YT/kan/tet media.
7. Incubate with shaking at 200 rpm and 37°C for 8 h.
8. Transfer the culture to 1.0 L of 2YT/kan media in a 4-L baffled flask (see Note 1).
9. Incubate overnight with shaking at 200 rpm and 37°C.
10. Precipitate phage particles by transferring the supernatant to a centrifuge tube containing 1/5 volume of PEG/NaCl and incubate for 5 min at room temperature.
11. Centrifuge 10 min and 4°C in a GS-3 rotor (12,000 × *g*). Decant the supernatant. Centrifuge briefly and aspirate the remaining supernatant (see Note 2).

12. Resuspend the phage in PBS to a final concentration of 10^{13} phage/mL ($OD_{268\ nm}=1.0$ for a solution containing 5×10^{12} phage/mL). The protocol yields approximately 100 mL of M13KO7 helper phage stock.
13. The stock is stable for at least 6 months at 4°C. For long-term storage, store at −80°C.

3.2. Preparation of Electrocompetent E. coli SS320

1. Inoculate 25 mL of 2YT/tet media with a single colony of *E. coli* SS320 from a fresh LB/tet plate.
2. Incubate with shaking at 200 rpm at 37°C to mid-log phase ($OD_{550\ nm}=0.8$).
3. Make tenfold serial dilutions of M13K07 by diluting 20 μL into 180 μL of PBS (see Note 3).
4. Mix 500 μL of *E. coli* SS320 at exponential phase with 200 μL of each M13K07 dilution and 4 mL of 2YT top agar.
5. Pour the mixtures onto prewarmed LB/tet plates and incubate overnight at 37°C.
6. Pick a well-separated, single plaque, and inoculate 1 mL of 2YT/kan/tet media.
7. Incubate 8 h at 37°C.
8. Transfer the culture to 250 mL of 2YT/kan media in a 2-L baffled flask.
9. Incubate with shaking at 200 rpm and 37°C overnight.
10. Inoculate six 2-L baffled flasks containing 900 mL of super-broth/kan/tet media with 5 mL of the overnight culture.
11. Incubate with shaking at 200 rpm and 37°C to mid-log phase ($OD_{550\ nm}=0.8$).
12. Chill three of the culture flasks on ice for 5 min with occasional swirling.
13. Centrifuge at 5,000 × *g* and 4°C for 10 min in a Sorvall GS-3 rotor in six 500-mL centrifuge bottles (see Note 4).
14. Decant the supernatant and add culture from the remaining flasks (these should be chilled while the first set is centrifuging) to the same tubes.
15. Repeat the centrifugation and decant the supernatant.
16. Fill the tubes with 1.0 mM Hepes, pH 7.4 and add sterile magnetic stirbars to facilitate pellet resuspension. Swirl to dislodge the pellet from the tube wall and stir at a moderate rate to resuspend the pellet completely.
17. Centrifuge at 5,000 × *g* and 4°C for 10 min in a Sorvall GS-3 rotor. Decant the supernatant, being careful to retain the stirbar. To avoid disturbing the pellet, maintain the position of the centrifuge tube when removing from the rotor.

18. Repeat previous steps (see Subheading 3.2, steps 16 and 17).
19. Resuspend each pellet in 150 mL of 10% ultrapure glycerol. Use stirbars. Do not combine the pellets.
20. Centrifuge at 5,000 × *g* and 4°C for 15 min in a Sorvall GS-3 rotor. Decant the supernatant and remove the stirbar. Remove remaining traces of supernatant with a pipette.
21. Add 3.0 mL of 10% ultrapure glycerol to one tube and resuspend the pellet by pipetting. Transfer the suspension to the next tube and repeat until all of the pellets are resuspended.
22. Transfer 350 μL aliquots into 1.5-mL microcentrifuge tubes.
23. Flash freeze with liquid nitrogen and store at −80°C (see Note 5).

3.3. Isolation of dU-ssDNA Template

Template purity dictates the success of phage-displayed library construction (see Note 6).

1. From a fresh LB/carb plate, pick a single colony of *E. coli* CJ236 harboring the appropriate phagemid into 1 mL of 2YT media supplemented with M13KO7 helper phage (10^{10} pfu/mL) and appropriate antibiotics to maintain the host F′ episome and the phagemid. For example, 2YT/carb/cmp media contains carbenicillin to select for phagemids that carry the β-lactamase gene and chloramphenicol to select for the F′ episome of *E. coli* CJ236.
2. Incubate with shaking at 200 rpm and 37°C for 2 h.
3. Add kanamycin (25 μg/mL) to select for clones that have been coinfected with M13KO7, which carries a kanamycin resistance gene.
4. Incubate with shaking at 200 rpm and 37°C for 6 h, and transfer the culture to 30 mL of 2YT/carb/kan/uridine media.
5. Incubate with shaking at 200 rpm and 37°C for 20 h.
6. Centrifuge for 10 min at and 4°C in a Sorvall SS-34 rotor (27,000 × *g*).
7. Precipitate phage particles by transferring the supernatant to a new tube containing 1/5 volume of PEG/NaCl and incubate for 5 min at room temperature.
8. Centrifuge 10 min and 4°C in an SS-34 rotor (12,000 × *g*). Decant the supernatant. Centrifuge briefly 2,000 × *g* and aspirate the remaining supernatant.
9. Resuspend the phage pellet in 0.5 mL of PBS and transfer to a 1.5-mL microcentrifuge tube.
10. Centrifuge for 5 min at 13,000 rpm in a microcentrifuge to pellet insoluble matter, and transfer the supernatant to a 1.5-mL microcentrifuge tube.

11. Add 7.0 µL of buffer MP (Qiagen) and mix. Incubate at room temperature for at least 2 min.
12. Apply the sample to a QIAprep spin column (Qiagen) in a 2-mL microcentrifuge tube. Centrifuge for 30 s at 8,000 rpm in a microcentrifuge. Discard the flow-through. The phage particles remain bound to the column matrix.
13. Add 0.7 mL of buffer MLB (Qiagen) to the column. Centrifuge for 30 s at 8,000 rpm and discard the flow-through.
14. Add 0.7 mL of buffer MLB. Incubate at room temperature for at least 1 min.
15. Centrifuge at 8,000 rpm for 30 s. Discard the flow-through. The DNA is separated from the protein coat and remains adsorbed to the matrix.
16. Add 0.7 mL of buffer PE (Qiagen). Centrifuge at 8,000 rpm for 30 s and discard the flow-through.
17. Repeat previous steps (see Subheading 3.3, steps 14–16). Residual proteins and salt are removed.
18. Centrifuge at 8,000 rpm for 30 s in a fresh 1.5-mL microcentrifuge tube to remove residual PE buffer.
19. Transfer the column to a fresh 1.5-mL microcentrifuge tube.
20. Add 100 µL of buffer EB (Qiagen; 10 mM Tris–Cl, pH 8.5) to the center of the column membrane. Incubate at room temperature for 10 min.
21. Centrifuge at 8,000 rpm for 30 s. Save the eluant, which contains the purified dU-ssDNA.
22. Analyze the DNA by electrophoresing 1.0 µL on a TAE/agarose gel.
23. Determine the DNA concentration by measuring absorbance at 260 nm ($A_{260\ nm}$ = 1.0 for 33 ng/µL of ssDNA).

3.4. In Vitro Synthesis of Heteroduplex CCC-dsDNA

1. In a 1.5-mL microcentrifuge tube, combine 0.6 µg of the mutagenic oligonucleotide, 2.0 µL of 10× TM buffer, 2.0 µL of 10 mM ATP, and 1.0 µL of 100 mM DTT. Add water to a total volume of 20 µL.
2. Add 20 U of T4 polynucleotide kinase. Incubate for 1.0 h at 37°C and use immediately for annealing (see Note 7).
3. To 20 µg of dU-ssDNA template, add 25 µL of 10× TM buffer, 0.6 µg of the phosphorylated oligonucleotide, and water to a final volume of 250 µL (see Note 8).
4. Incubate at 90°C for 3 min, 50°C for 5 min, and 20°C for 5 min.
5. To the annealed oligonucleotide/template mixture, add 10 µL of 10 mM ATP, 10 µL of 25 mM dNTP mix, 15 µL of 100 mM DTT, 30 Weiss units T4 DNA ligase, and 30 U T7 DNA polymerase.

6. Incubate overnight at 20°C.
7. Affinity purify and desalt the DNA using the Qiagen QIAquick DNA Purification Kit. Add 1.0 mL of buffer QG (Qiagen) and mix.
8. Apply the sample to two QIAquick spin columns placed in 2-mL microcentrifuge tubes. Centrifuge at 13,000 rpm for 1 min in a microcentrifuge. Discard the flow-through.
9. Add 750 μL of buffer PE (Qiagen) to each column, and centrifuge at 13,000 rpm for 1 min.
10. Transfer the column to a fresh 1.5-mL microcentrifuge tube, and centrifuge at 13,000 rpm for 1 min.
11. Transfer the column to a fresh 1.5-mL microcentrifuge tube, and add 35 μL of ultrapure irrigation USP water to the center of the membrane. Incubate at room temperature for 10 min.
12. Centrifuge at 13,000 rpm for 1 min to elute the DNA. Combine the eluants from the two columns. The DNA can be used immediately for *E. coli* electroporation, or it can be frozen for later use.
13. Electrophorese 1.0 μL of the eluted reaction product alongside the ssDNA template to monitor the reaction. Use a TAE/agarose gel with ethidium bromide for DNA visualization.

3.5. *E. coli* Electroporation and Phage Propagation

1. Chill purified CCC-dsDNA (20 μg in a minimum volume) and a 0.2-cm gap electroporation cuvette on ice.
2. Thaw a 350 μL aliquot of electrocompetent *E. coli* SS320 on ice. Add the cells to the DNA and mix by pipetting several times (avoid introducing bubbles).
3. Transfer the mixture to the cuvette and electroporate. For electroporation, follow the manufacturer's instructions using a BTX ECM-600 electroporation system with the following settings: 2.5 kV field strength, 129 Ω resistance, and 50 μF capacitance.
4. Immediately rescue the electroporated cells by adding 1 mL of SOC media and transferring to 10 mL of SOC media in a 250-mL baffled flask. Rinse the cuvette twice with 1 mL of SOC media. Add SOC media to a final volume of 25 mL.
5. Incubate with shaking at 200 rpm and 37°C for 30 min.
6. To determine the library diversity, plate serial dilutions on LB/carb plates to select for the phagemid.
7. Transfer the culture to a 2-L baffled flask containing 500 mL of 2YT/carb/kan media.
8. Incubate with shaking at 200 rpm and 37°C overnight.
9. Centrifuge the culture for 10 min at 16,000 × *g* and 4°C in a Sorvall GSA rotor.

10. Transfer the supernatant to a fresh tube and add 1/5 volume of PEG/NaCl solution to precipitate the phage. Incubate 5 min at room temperature.
11. Centrifuge for 10 min at 16,000 × *g* and 4°C in a GSA rotor. Decant the supernatant. Respin briefly and remove the remaining supernatant with a pipette.
12. Resuspend the phage pellet in 20 mL of PBT buffer.
13. Pellet insoluble matter by centrifuging for 5 min at 27,000 × *g* and 4°C in an SS-34 rotor. Transfer the supernatant to a clean tube.
14. Estimate the phage concentration spectrophotometrically ($OD_{268\ nm}$ = 1.0 for a solution of 5×10^{12} phage/mL).
15. The library can be used immediately for selection experiments (see Note 9).

3.6. Affinity Selection for Binding to Immobilized Protein A

1. Coat Maxisorp immunoplate wells with 100 μL of protein A (5 μg/mL in coating buffer) for 2 h at room temperature or overnight at 4°C (see Note 10).
2. Coat four wells with PBS alone.
3. Remove the PBS and block for 1 h with 200 μL of blocking buffer at room temperature.
4. Remove the blocking buffer and wash four times with PT buffer.
5. Add 100 μL of library phage solution in PBT buffer to each of the coated and uncoated wells. Incubate at room temperature for 2 h with gentle shaking.
6. Remove the phage solution and wash ten times with PT buffer.
7. To elute bound phage, add 100 μL of 0.1 M HCl. Incubate 5 min at room temperature. Transfer the HCl solution to a 1.5-mL microfuge tube.
8. Adjust to neutral pH by adding 1/8 volume of 1.0 M Tris–HCl, pH 11.0.
9. Add half the eluted phage solution to ten volumes of actively growing *E. coli* XL1-Blue ($OD_{550\ nm}$ < 1.0) in 2YT/tet media. Incubate with shaking at 200 rpm for 20 min at 37°C.
10. Plate serial dilutions on LB/carb plates to determine the number of phage eluted. Determine the enrichment ratio by dividing the number of phage eluted from a well coated with protein A by the number of phage eluted from the empty well.
11. Add M13KO7 helper phage to a final concentration of 10^{10} phage/mL. Incubate with shaking at 200 rpm and 37°C for 1 h.
12. Transfer the culture from the protein A-coated wells to ten volumes of 2YT/carb/kan/IPTG media and incubate overnight with shaking at 200 rpm and 37°C.

13. Isolate phage by precipitation with PEG/NaCl solution (see Subheading 3.1, steps 10–13). Resuspend in 1.0 mL of PBT buffer and estimate phage concentration spectrophotometrically ($OD_{268\ nm} = 1.0$ for a solution of 5×10^{12} phage/mL).
14. Repeat the selection cycle until the enrichment ratio has reached a maximum (see Note 11).
15. Pick individual clones for sequence analysis.

3.7. DNA Sequencing

1. Inoculate 450 μL aliquots of 2YT/carb/KO7 media in 96-well microtubes with single colonies harboring phagemids and incubate overnight with shaking at 200 rpm and 37°C.
2. Centrifuge at 4,000 rpm in microcentrifuge for 5 min and transfer 100 μL of phage supernatant to a fresh plate.
3. Sterilize the phage supernatant by incubation at 60°C for 1 h.
4. Dilute phage supernatant tenfold with with distilled water and add 2 μL to 23 μL of PCR mix. The primers should be designed to amplify the VH domain to be sequenced (see Note 12).
5. Amplify the DNA fragment using the following PCR program: 5 min at 95°C, 25 cycles of amplification (30 s at 94°C, 30 s at 55°C, 60 s at 72°C), 7 min at 72°C, and storage at 4°C.
6. Analyze representative reactions by electrophoresis on a TAE/agarose gel.
7. Dispense 2 μL of clean up mix into each well of a fresh 96-well PCR plate.
8. Transfer 5 μL of PCR product to each well and mix carefully.
9. Incubate the clean up reactions at 37°C for 15 min, at 80°C for 15 min, and store at 4°C.
10. The sample can be used directly as the template in Big-Dye terminator sequencing reactions (PE Biosystems).

3.8. VH Domain Protein Purification

1. To purify VH domains for biophysical analysis, phage display vectors must be converted to expression vectors by the insertion of an amber stop codon (TAG) between the sequence encoding the VH domain and the phage coat protein P3. This can be done using the site-directed mutagenesis technique described above.
2. Transform the VH domain expression vector into *E. coli* BL-21 cells and plate on LB/carb plates and incubate at 37°C overnight.
3. Inoculate 5 mL of LB/carb medium with a single colony and incubate overnight with shaking at 200 rpm and 37°C.
4. Use the overnight culture to inoculate 500 mL of 2YT/carb in a 2-L flask and incubate with shaking at 200 rpm and 37°C until the cells reach an $OD_{550\ nm} = 0.6–0.8$.

5. Add IPTG to a final concentration of 0.4 mM to induce VH domain expression and incubate the culture for 3 h with shaking at 200 rpm and 30°C.
6. Centrifuge the cells at 16,000 × *g* for 30 min in a Sorvall GSA rotor and decant the supernatant.
7. Freeze the cells by storing the centrifuge bottles overnight at −20°C.
8. Resuspend frozen cell pellet in 100 mL of lysis buffer. Ensure that resuspension is homogeneous with no visible cell clumps.
9. Lyse the cells with the microfluidizer.
10. If a microfluidizer is not available, the cells may be lysed with the addition of lysozyme in the resuspension buffer to a final concentration of 1 mg/mL. Incubate the cell resuspension at 4°C for 2 h with shaking on a rotator-shaker at maximal speed. Sonicate the resuspension (to shear genomic DNA) with a sonicator. We recommend short but strong pulses (e.g., 5 s ON and 5 s OFF at 40% amplitude).
11. Centrifuge the lysate in a 250 mL bottle at 30,000 × *g* for 30 min.
12. Filter the lysate by passage through a 0.2 μm filter.
13. Load onto a gravity flow protein A-Sepharose column equilibrated with five bed volumes of wash buffer.
14. Load the filtered cell lysate and allow it to flow-through.
15. Wash the column with ten bed volumes of wash buffer.
16. Elute the bound VH domain with 5 mL of 0.1 M glycine and neutralize the eluant with 1 mL of 1.0 M Tris pH 8.0.
17. The concentration of protein can be determined by the method of Bradford (36).

3.9. Analytical Gel Filtration and Light Scattering Analysis

Because many different gel filtration units are available, detailed experimental procedures may not be applicable to every laboratory. Therefore, we provide an overview of the methods used in Barthelemy et al. (21) and recommend that the procedure be followed as closely as possible with available instrumentation. In Barthelemy et al., an Agilent 1100 series high pressure liquid chromatography system (Agilent, Palo Alto, CA) in line with a Wyatt MiniDawn multiangle light scattering detector (Wyatt Technology, Santa Barbara, CA) was used.

1. Equilibrate a Superdex-75 column with PBS.
2. Inject the purified VH domain at a concentration of ~70 μM (1.0 mg/mL) in a volume of 100 μM with a flow rate of 0.5 mL/min.

3. Measure the concentration of protein using the on-line Wyatt OPTILAB DSP interferometric refractometer (Wyatt Technology), following the manufacturer's instructions.
4. Use appropriate software for light scattering data acquisition and processing.
5. Calibrate the light scattering unit and the refractometer according to the manufacturer's instructions.
6. A value of 0.185 mL/g is assumed for the d*n*/d*c* ratio of the protein.
7. Normalize the detector response by measuring the signal from monomeric bovine serum albumin.

3.10. Temperature-Induced Denaturation

As in the previous section, detailed protocols will depend on the type of instrumentation used. Therefore, we provide an overview of the thermal denaturation assays used in Barthelemy et al. (21) with a J-810 spectrometer (Jasco, Easton, MD). For a detailed overview and protocols for using circular dichroism to monitor protein secondary structure, refer to a recent article by Greenfield (37).

1. Monitor thermal denaturation of VH domains at 207 nm using a 1 cm path length CD cuvette containing protein samples at 10 μM in PBS.
2. Increase the temperature from 25 to 85°C (or higher, if necessary to achieve complete unfolding) in 2°C increments.
3. Assay the reversibility of the temperature-induced denaturation by cooling the sample to 25°C and repeating the heating program.
4. By assuming that the unfolding curves adhere to a two-state transition, calculate the fraction of folded protein using the following equation: $\alpha = (\theta_T - \theta_F)/(\theta_U - \theta_F)$, where θ_T is the observed ellipticity at any temperature; θ_F is the ellipticity of the fully folded form of the protein, and θ_U is the ellipticity of the fully unfolded form of the protein. If the raw ellipticity data of the folded and unfolded states shows no temperature dependence outside of the transition zone, θ_F is considered to be the ellipticity value observed at 25°C, and θ_U is considered to be the lowest ellipticity value observed.
5. Plot the variation of α vs. the temperature to obtain the melting curve of the VH domain under investigation. The melting temperature (T_m) is defined as the temperature at which $\alpha = 0.5$.
6. The fraction of refolded protein recovered following thermal denaturation is estimated as the α value for the sample cooled down to 25°C after heating to a temperature that induced complete unfolding.

4. Notes

1. We recommend the use of baffled culture flasks as they increase aeration and cell growth.
2. To avoid contamination, always use filtered pipette tips to manipulate phage.
3. Use a new pipette tip for each dilution.
4. In Subheading 3.2, steps 13–23 should be done in a cold room, on ice, with prechilled solutions and equipment.
5. Caution: liquid nitrogen causes burns.
6. We recommend using the Qiagen QIAprep Spin M13 Kit for dU-ssDNA purification and the following is a modified protocol that typically yields 20 μg of dU-ssDNA.
7. The phosphorylated mutagenic oligonucleotide can be stored at −20°C for a month. However, we have found that higher mutagenesis rates are achieved when the phosphorylated oligonucleotide is used immediately for the synthesis of CCC-dsDNA.
8. In cases where more than one region of the DNA is to be mutated, two or more mutagenic oligonucleotides can be added simultaneously, as long as sequences within the oligonucleotides do not overlap with each other. These DNA quantities provide an oligonucleotide:template molar ratio of 3:1, assuming that the oligonucleotide:template length ratio is 1:100.
9. Alternatively, the library can be frozen and stored at −80°C, following the addition of glycerol to a final concentration of 10%. In general, it is best to use libraries immediately, as levels of displayed proteins can be reduced over time due to denaturation or proteolysis.
10. The number of wells required depends on the diversity of the library. Ideally, the phage concentration should not exceed 10^{13} phage/mL and the total number of phage should exceed the library diversity by 1,000-fold. Thus, for a diversity of 10^{10}, 10^{13} phage should be used and, using a concentration of 10^{13} phage/mL, ten wells will be required.
11. Typically, enrichment peaks at round 4 and sorting beyond round 5 is seldom necessary. Plate serial dilutions onto LB/carb plates to isolate single colonies for DNA sequencing.
12. The mix can be made as a cocktail and dispensed into a 96-well PCR plate for high-throughput sequencing.

References

1. Padlan EA (1994) Anatomy of the antibody molecule. Mol Immunol 31:169–217
2. Ward ES, Gussow D, Griffiths AD, Jones PT, Winter G (1989) Binding activities of a repertoire of single immunoglobulin variable domains secreted from *Escherichia coli*. Nature 341:544–546
3. Saerens D, Ghassabeh GH, Muyldermans S (2008) Single-domain antibodies as building blocks for novel therapeutics. Curr Opin Pharmacol 8:600–608
4. Hamers-Casterman C, Atarhouch T, Muyldermans S, Robinson G, Hamers C et al (1993) Naturally occurring antibodies devoid of light chains. Nature 363:446–448
5. Cortez-Retamozo V, Lauwereys M, Hassanzadeh Gh G, Gobert M, Conrath K et al (2002) Efficient tumor targeting by single-domain antibody fragments of camels. Int J Cancer 98:456–462
6. Decanniere K, Desmyter A, Lauwereys M, Ghahroudi MA, Muyldermans S et al (1999) A single-domain antibody fragment in complex with RNase A: non-canonical loop structures and nanomolar affinity using two CDR loops. Structure 7:361–370
7. Desmyter A, Decanniere K, Muyldermans S, Wyns L (2001) Antigen specificity and high affinity binding provided by one single loop of a camel single-domain antibody. J Biol Chem 276:26285–26290
8. Desmyter A, Spinelli S, Payan F, Lauwereys M, Wyns L et al (2002) Three camelid VHH domains in complex with porcine pancreatic alpha-amylase. Inhibition and versatility of binding topology. J Biol Chem 277:23645–23650
9. Desmyter A, Transue TR, Ghahroudi MA, Thi MH, Poortmans F et al (1996) Crystal structure of a camel single-domain VH antibody fragment in complex with lysozyme. Nat Struct Biol 3:803–811
10. Spinelli S, Frenken L, Bourgeois D, de Ron L, Bos W et al (1996) The crystal structure of a llama heavy chain variable domain. Nat Struct Biol 3:752–757
11. Spinelli S, Frenken LG, Hermans P, Verrips T, Brown K et al (2000) Camelid heavy-chain variable domains provide efficient combining sites to haptens. Biochemistry 39:1217–1222
12. Spinelli S, Tegoni M, Frenken L, van Vliet C, Cambillau C (2001) Lateral recognition of a dye hapten by a llama VHH domain. J Mol Biol 311:123–129
13. Harmsen MM, Ruuls RC, Nijman IJ, Niewold TA, Frenken LG et al (2000) Llama heavy-chain V regions consist of at least four distinct subfamilies revealing novel sequence features. Mol Immunol 37:579–590
14. Holt LJ, Herring C, Jespers LS, Woolven BP, Tomlinson IM (2003) Domain antibodies: proteins for therapy. Trends Biotechnol 21: 484–490
15. Muyldermans S, Cambillau C, Wyns L (2001) Recognition of antigens by single-domain antibody fragments: the superfluous luxury of paired domains. Trends Biochem Sci 26:230–235
16. Nguyen VK, Hamers R, Wyns L, Muyldermans S (2000) Camel heavy-chain antibodies: diverse germline V(H)H and specific mechanisms enlarge the antigen-binding repertoire. EMBO J 19:921–930
17. Davies J, Riechmann L (1994) 'Camelising' human antibody fragments: NMR studies on VH domains. FEBS Lett 339:285–290
18. Howard GC, Kaser MR (2007) Making and using antibodies: a practical handbook. CRC Press/Taylor & Francis, Boca Raton, FL, p 394
19. Lee CV, Liang WC, Dennis MS, Eigenbrot C, Sidhu SS et al (2004) High-affinity human antibodies from phage-displayed synthetic Fab libraries with a single framework scaffold. J Mol Biol 340:1073–1093
20. Sidhu SS, Weiss GA, Wells JA (2000) High copy display of large proteins on phage for functional selections. J Mol Biol 296:487–495
21. Barthelemy PA, Raab H, Appleton BA, Bond CJ, Wu P et al (2008) Comprehensive analysis of the factors contributing to the stability and solubility of autonomous human VH domains. J Biol Chem 283:3639–3654
22. Slamon DJ, Clark GM, Wong SG, Levin WJ, Ullrich A et al (1987) Human breast cancer: correlation of relapse and survival with amplification of the HER-2/neu oncogene. Science 235:177–182
23. Slamon DJ, Godolphin W, Jones LA, Holt JA, Wong SG et al (1989) Studies of the HER-2/neu proto-oncogene in human breast and ovarian cancer. Science 244:707–712
24. Yarden Y, Sliwkowski MX (2001) Untangling the ErbB signalling network. Nat Rev Mol Cell Biol 2:127–137
25. Carter P, Presta L, Gorman CM, Ridgway JB, Henner D et al (1992) Humanization of an anti-p185HER2 antibody for human cancer therapy. Proc Natl Acad Sci U S A 89:4285–4289
26. Tokunaga E, Oki E, Nishida K, Koga T, Egashira A et al (2006) Trastuzumab and breast cancer: developments and current status. Int J Clin Oncol 11:199–208

27. Lefranc MP, Giudicelli V, Ginestoux C, Jabado-Michaloud J, Folch G et al (2009) IMGT, the international ImMunoGeneTics information system. Nucleic Acids Res 37:D1006–D1012
28. Jespers L, Schon O, James LC, Veprintsev D, Winter G (2004) Crystal structure of HEL4, a soluble, refoldable human V(H) single domain with a germ-line scaffold. J Mol Biol 337: 893–903
29. Sidhu SS (2005) Phage display in biotechnology and drug discovery. Boca Raton: Taylor & Francis, xviii, p 748
30. Fellouse FA, Wiesmann C, Sidhu SS (2004) Synthetic antibodies from a four-amino-acid code: a dominant role for tyrosine in antigen recognition. Proc Natl Acad Sci U S A 101:12467–12472
31. Kunkel TA, Roberts JD, Zakour RA (1987) Rapid and efficient site-specific mutagenesis without phenotypic selection. Methods Enzymol 154:367–382
32. Sidhu SS, Lowman HB, Cunningham BC, Wells JA (2000) Phage display for selection of novel binding peptides. Methods Enzymol 328:333–363
33. Bond CJ, Marsters JC, Sidhu SS (2003) Contributions of CDR3 to V H H domain stability and the design of monobody scaffolds for naive antibody libraries. J Mol Biol 332:643–655
34. Bond CJ, Wiesmann C, Marsters JC Jr, Sidhu SS (2005) A structure-based database of antibody variable domain diversity. J Mol Biol 348:699–709
35. de Wildt RM, Mundy CR, Gorick BD, Tomlinson IM (2000) Antibody arrays for high-throughput screening of antibody-antigen interactions. Nat Biotechnol 18:989–994
36. Bradford MM (1976) A rapid and sensitive method for the quantitation of microgram quantities of protein utilizing the principle of protein-dye binding. Anal Biochem 72:248–254
37. Greenfield NJ (2006) Using circular dichroism collected as a function of temperature to determine the thermodynamics of protein unfolding and binding interactions. Nat Protoc 1: 2527–2535
38. Kabat EA, Wu TT, Reid-Miller M, Perry H, Gottesman K (1987) Sequence of proteins of immunological interest. National Institutes of Health Research, Bethesda, p 2387

Chapter 21

Solubility and Stability Engineering of Human VH Domains*

Dae Young Kim, Wen Ding, and Jamshid Tanha

Abstract

Solubility and stability are amongst the factors contributing to the therapeutic efficacy of biologics. Human antibody heavy chain variable domains, VHs, are one class of biologics; improving VH biophysical properties is the focus of significant protein engineering efforts. Here, we describe an efficacy engineering approach which involves the introduction of a disulfide linkage in the VH core and which improves both VH solubility and stability. More specifically, we describe protocols for generation of disulfide engineered human VHs and their characterization in terms of disulfide linkage formation, non-aggregation, and stability. Our solubility/stability engineering approach may be applied to other VHs.

Key words: Human VH, Single-domain antibody, Disulfide linkage, Solubility, Stability, Melting temperature

1. Introduction

Like many other recombinant antibody fragments, human VH fragments are a promising class of therapeutics (1, 2). However, the generation of VH therapeutics requires extra efforts and care due to the general tendency of VHs to aggregate. Thus, a number of approaches have been developed for obtaining non-aggregating VHs (3–13). Some of the same approaches have additionally improved VHs stability.

Disulfide linkages involving pairs of Cys residues are a significant stabilizing force in proteins including antibodies (14–16). An example is the highly conserved disulfide linkage between Cys22 and Cys92 (Kabat numbering system[1]) (17) in VH domains. This disulfide linkage, buried in the core of the VH, pins together the

*This is National Research Council Canada Publication 50016.

[1] Kabat amino acid positions 22, 92, 49 and 69 correspond to amino acid positions 23, 104, 54 and 78, respectively, in IMGT numbering system (http://www.imgt.org/).

Dirk Saerens and Serge Muyldermans (eds.), *Single Domain Antibodies: Methods and Protocols*, Methods in Molecular Biology, vol. 911, DOI 10.1007/978-1-61779-968-6_21, © Springer Science+Business Media, LLC 2012

two β-sheets which make up the overall fold of the protein. Recently, in a number of studies it was shown that the engineering of an additional disulfide linkage in camelid heavy chain antibody variable domains (termed VHHs) drastically increased VHH stability (18–21). Similar to the Cys22/Cys92 disulfide linkage, the engineered disulfide linkage is also in the interior of the VHH and ties the two β-sheets together. It was not obvious however, if the introduction of a homologous disulfide linkage in human VHs would reduce VH aggregation tendencies as well as increase their stability. In this chapter we demonstrate that this indeed is the case. We use HVHAm302 which is an aggregating human VH (10) as an example to demonstrate that the engineering of the aforementioned extra disulfide linkage in the core of human VH domains significantly

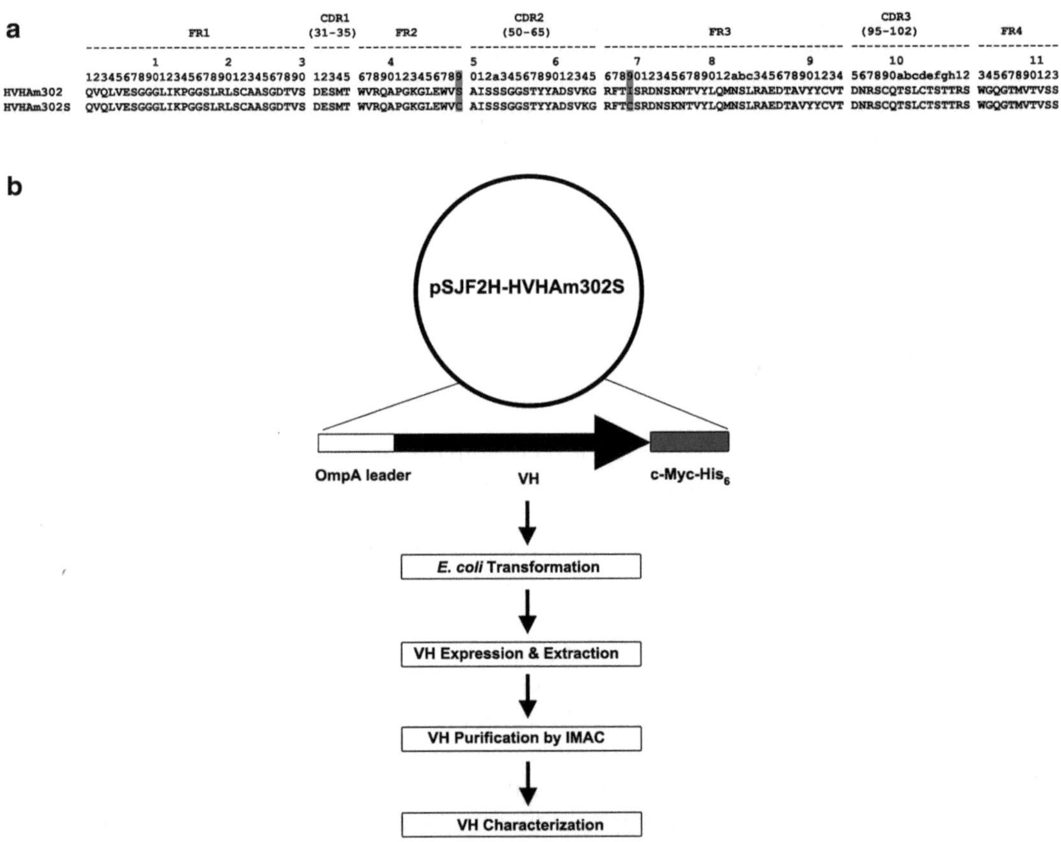

Fig. 1. An overall scheme showing the generation and characterization of HVHAm302S, a human VH with an engineered disulfide linkage. (**a**) An amino acid comparison between HVHAm302S and the wild type VH, HVHAm302. The mutational difference between the two VHs is highlighted in *gray*. The engineered cysteine residues in the mutant VH do form an extra disulfide linkage compared to the wild type VH (see text). The residues are numbered according to the Kabat numbering system (17). *CDR* complementarity-determining region; *FR* framework region. (**b**) Schematic work flow chart. HVHAm302S VH gene (*black*) was cloned in the expression vector pSJF2H in fusion with the OmpA leader sequence (*white*) and the c-Myc-His$_6$ tag (*gray*). *Arrow* denotes the expression direction of VH. The OmpA (outer membrane protein A) leader peptide directs the expressed VH to the *Escherichia coli* periplasm for proper folding. *IMAC* immobilized-metal affinity chromatography.

improves not only their stability but also reduces aggregation. The mutant version of HVHAm302 VH, termed HVHAm302S (see Fig. 1), has two Cys mutations compared to HVHAm302 VH (Ser49Cys and Ile69Cys)[1] and thus is expected to have one more disulfide linkage than HVHAm302 VH. Here, we present protocols on the cloning, expression, and purification of disulfide linkage engineered VHs and characterization of the engineered VHs. With respect to characterization, protocols include mass spectrometry (MS) analysis, size exclusion chromatography, and thermostability analysis by circular dichroism (CD) spectroscopy. The overall protocol scheme is depicted in Fig. 1.

2. Materials

All solutions and media were prepared with distilled and deionized water (ddH_2O). Autoclaving of solutions was performed on liquid cycle at 121°C, 15 lb/in. and 20 min. Filter-sterilized solutions were prepared using 0.2 µm filter units (see Note 1).

2.1. Cloning and Expression of Mutant VHs

1. pSJF2H-HVHAm302S plasmid[2] (contains the gene for the mutant VH HVHAm302S) (see Note 2).
2. M13RP: 5′-TCACACAGGAAACAGCTATGAC-3′ (10 pmol/µL) (see Note 3).
3. M13FP: 5′-CGCCAGGGTTTTCCCAGTCACGAC-3′ (10 pmol/µL).
4. *Escherichia coli* TG1 electroporation-competent cells (Stratagene, La Jolla, CA; see Note 4).
5. SOC medium: Dissolve 20 g tryptone, 5 g yeast extract, 0.5 g NaCl in 950 mL ddH_2O, add 10 mL of 0.25 M KCl. Adjust the pH to 7.0 with 5 M NaOH, add ddH_2O to 1 L, sterilize by autoclaving. Add 5 mL of autoclave-sterilized 2 M $MgCl_2$ and 20 mL of filter-sterilized 1 M glucose.
6. Autoclave-sterilized 50% (v/v) glycerol. Store at room temperature.
7. LB medium: Dissolve 10 g tryptone, 5 g yeast extract, and 10 g NaCl in 900 mL ddH_2O, add ddH_2O to 1 L, sterilize by autoclaving.
8. Filter-sterilized ampicillin (100 mg/mL). Store in 1 mL aliquots at −20°C.
9. LB/ampicillin agar plates (see Note 5).

[2] All plasmid constructs are available to researchers free of charge.

10. Disposable 0.22 μm filter units.
11. Disposable inoculation loops.
12. Miniprep plasmid purification kit.
13. Electroporation cuvettes.
14. Electroporator.

2.2. Extraction and Purification of Mutant VHs

1. Cell lysis buffer (CLB): 50 mM Tris–HCl, 25 mM NaCl, 2 mM EDTA, pH 8.0. Autoclave and store at 4°C.
2. PMSF (phenylmethyl sulfonyl fluoride, 100 mM): Dissolve 174 mg PMSF in 10 mL of isopropanol, store in 1 mL aliquots at −20°C.
3. Hen egg white lysozyme: Prepare at 3 mg/mL in CLB, store at −20°C.
4. DNase I: Prepare fresh at 15 units/mL in 1 M $MgCl_2$.
5. 6× His tag® antibody [HIS-1] (alkaline phosphatase) conjugate (abcam, Cambridge, MA; see Note 6).
6. Alkaline phosphatase substrate solutions for Western blotting.
7. Filter-sterilized $NiCl_2 \cdot 6H_2O$ (5 mg/mL).
8. 5 mL HisTrap™ FF immobilized-metal affinity chromatography (IMAC) column (GE Healthcare, Baie d'Urfé, QC, Canada; see Note 7).
9. Buffer A: 10 mM HEPES buffer, 0.5 M NaCl, pH 7.0. Dissolve 29.22 g NaCl in 900 mL of ddH_2O. Add 10 mL of 1 M HEPES buffer, pH 7.0, and ddH_2O to 1 L. Sterilize by autoclaving, store at room temperature.
10. Buffer B: 10 mM HEPES buffer, 0.5 M NaCl, 0.5 M imidazole, pH 7.0. Dissolve 29.22 g NaCl and 34.04 g imidazole in 900 mL of ddH_2O. Add 10 mL of 1 M HEPES buffer, pH 7.0. Adjust the pH to 7.0 with 10 M HCl and add ddH_2O to 1 L. Sterilize by autoclaving, store at room temperature.
11. Phosphate-buffered saline (PBS): Dissolve 8 g NaCl, 0.2 g KCl, 1.44 g Na_2HPO_4, and 0.24 g KH_2PO_4 in 1 L of ddH_2O, pH 7.4. Sterilize by autoclaving, store at room temperature.
12. Sodium azide.
13. Filter-sterilized 0.5 M EDTA, pH 8.0.
14. Dialysis membranes (≤10 kDa MWCO).
15. SDS-PAGE (sodium dodecyl sulfate-polyacrylamide gel electrophoresis) and Western blotting reagents and equipments.
16. ÄKTA FPLC purification system (GE Healthcare).
17. ND-1000 spectrophotometer (Thermo Scientific, Wilmington, DE) or a similar instrument (see Note 8).

2.3. Disulfide Linkage Mapping of Mutant VHs by MS

1. Sequencing-grade trypsin (Roche Diagnostics Canada, Laval, QC, Canada): Prepare at 100 μg/mL in 1 mM HCl, store at 4°C (see Note 9).
2. Trypsin digestion buffer (TDB): 0.1 M Tris–HCl, pH 8.5. Filter-sterilize, store at room temperature.
3. HPLC-grade acetonitrile and water (Sigma, Mississauga, ON, Canada).
4. ACS-grade formic acid (EMD, Gibbstown, NJ).
5. Ultrafree®-0.5 centrifugal filter device with Biomax®-5 ultrafiltration membrane (5 kDa MWCO) (Millipore, Billerica, MA).
6. 180 μm I.D. × 20 mm 5 μm symmetry® C18 trap and 100 μm I.D. × 10 cm 1.7 μm BEH130C18 column (Waters, Milford, MA).
7. SDS-PAGE reagents and equipment.
8. NanoAcquity UPLC system coupled to a Q-TOF Ultima™ hybrid quadrupole/time of flight (TOF) mass spectrometer (Waters).
9. Q-TOF 2™ hybrid quadrupole/TOF mass spectrometer (Waters).
10. Masslynx™ 4.0 software (Waters).
11. Max Ent 1 and Max Ent 3 programs under the Masslynx™ 4.0 software (Waters).
12. Mascot™ database searching system (Matrix Science, London, UK).

2.4. Assessment of Aggregation State of Mutant VHs by Analytical Size Exclusion Chromatography

1. Filtered and degassed ddH_2O. Degas the filtered water with a conventional water aspirator.
2. Filtered and degassed PBS (see Subheading 2.2, item 11). Degas the filtered PBS with a conventional water aspirator.
3. Superdex™ 75 10/300 GL size exclusion column (bed volume: 24 mL; bed dimensions: 10 mm × 300 mm) (GE Healthcare; see Note 10).

2.5. Thermal Stability Assessment of Mutant VHs by CD Spectroscopy

1. N_2 gas supply.
2. Stock HCl.
3. Ethanol.
4. 6 M guanidine hydrochloride.
5. 0.1 M sodium phosphate buffer: 77.4 mL of 1 M Na_2HPO_4, 22.6 mL of 1 M NaH_2PO_4 in 900 mL of ddH_2O, pH 7.4. Sterilize by autoclaving, store at room temperature.
6. Hellmanex™ II cuvette cleaning solution (Hellma, Plainview, NY). Dilute 2 mL of Hellmanex™ II in 98 mL of ddH_2O, store at room temperature.

7. Ultrafree®-0.5 centrifugal filter device with Biomax®-5 ultrafiltration membrane (5 kDa MWCO) (Millipore).
8. 1-mm cuvette (Hellma).
9. Spectrophotometer (see Subheading 2.2, item 17).
10. J-815 CD spectropolarimeter (Jasco, Easton, MD).
11. Peltier PTC-423 heat control unit (Jasco).
12. Software and data analysis: Jasco J-815 software and GraphPad Prism graphing software (version 4.02 for Windows; GraphPad Software, San Diego, CA; www.graphpad.com).

3. Methods

3.1. Cloning and Expression of Mutant VHs

In this step, pSJF2H-HVHAm302S plasmid containing the gene for HVHAm302S VH is used to transform *E. coli* cells. Next, the transformed bacterial cells are first grown in a minimal medium then in a rich induction medium containing IPTG to induce VH expression. The expression protocol is designed to be performed under low temperature (25–30°C) and IPTG concentration, and although 5 days in duration, it consistently yields milligram quantities of purified protein per liter of bacterial culture.

1. Mix 1 μL (a few nanograms) of pSJF2H-HVHAm302S (see Note 11) with 25 μL of *E. coli* TG1 electroporation-competent cells in an ice-cold electroporation cuvette. Transform cells using an electroporator and settings suggested by the manufacturer (22) (see Notes 12 and 13).
2. Immediately following electroporation, transfer the cells to a 15-mL sterilized Falcon tube containing 1 mL of SOC medium. Incubate in a shaker incubator for 30 min at 37°C and 230 rpm.
3. Spread 50 μL of the transformation solution on an LB/ampicillin agar Petri dish. Keep the remaining transformation solution overnight at 4°C (see Note 14). Incubate the plate in an incubator overnight at 32°C (see Note 15).
4. In the morning, touch individual colonies on the plate (5–10 colonies) with disposable inoculation loops and inoculate 2-mL LB/ampicillin media in 15-mL Falcon tubes by swirling the loops in the media. Use the same loop to make a reference plate of the individual colonies (see Note 16). Grow the cell cultures at 37°C and 230 rpm for 20 h.
5. In the morning, purify plasmid DNA from the cell cultures using a miniprep plasmid purification kit according to the supplier's instructions (see Note 17).

6. Confirm the sequence of the construct using M13RP or M13FP as primer (see Note 18).
7. Refer to your reference plate (see Subheading 3.1, step 4) and make a permanent stock of the positive clone (see Note 19).
8. Proceed with periplasmic expression of the positive clone as described in Chapter 16.

3.2. Extraction and Purification of Mutant VHs

Following the VH expression, the cells are lysed by a lysozyme-mediated cell lysis method and the soluble fraction containing the VH is recovered. The success of expression is assessed by performing Western blot on the soluble fraction using an antibody which detects VH by binding to its C-terminal His_6 tag. The His_6 tag is also used to purify the VH in one step and under mild conditions by IMAC.

1. Following expression, pellet the cells by centrifugation at 5,000 × *g* and 4°C for 10 min. Repeat the centrifugation step if the supernatant is turbid.
2. Resuspend the cell pellet in 100 mL of ice-cold CLB (see Notes 20 and 21) and immediately add 1 mL of 100 mM PMSF.
3. Initiate the cell lysis by adding 5 mL of freshly-thawed 3 mg/mL lysozyme to the cell suspension. Incubate the mixture at room temperature for 1 h with occasional shaking until the suspension becomes viscous.
4. Add 250 μL of freshly-prepared DNase I solution to the cell lysate. Incubate the lysate at room temperature for 1 h until the solution becomes watery. Save 30 μL as "total" for Western blotting.
5. Centrifuge the lysate at 14,000 × *g* and 4°C for 20 min to separate the soluble and insoluble fractions. Transfer the supernatant to new centrifuge bottle and repeat the centrifugation. Decant the soluble fraction and remove/save 30 μL as "soluble" for Western blotting. Resuspend the insoluble fraction in CLB to be used as "insoluble" for Western blotting. Keep both fractions at 4°C or −20°C.
6. Perform Western blotting on "total," "soluble", and "insoluble" samples using 6x His tag® antibody [HIS-1] (alkaline phosphatase) as the detecting agent (23). Include a His_6-tagged protein, e.g., VH, as a positive control. Proceed with the dialysis of the soluble fraction (see Subheading 3.2, step 5), if the presence of protein in the "soluble" sample is confirmed by Western blotting.
7. Dialyze the soluble fraction against 6 L of Buffer A at 4°C for 4–6 h using dialysis tubing with ≤10 kDa MWCO. Repeat the dialysis once more. Filter the dialyzed solution using 0.22 μm filter units and add Buffer B to a final concentration of 10 mM imidazole. Keep at 4°C while preparing for the IMAC purification of the VH.

8. To purify the VH, charge a 5-mL HisTrap™ FF IMAC column with 25 mL of 5 mg/mL $NiCl_2 \cdot 6H_2O$. Subsequently wash the column with 25 mL of ddH_2O.
9. Perform IMAC protein purification on an ÄKTA FPLC purification instrument according to the instructions provided by the manufacturer using Buffer A/2% Buffer B as the equilibration buffer and a gradient of 10–500 mM imidazole for elution of column-bound VH.
10. Following purification, confirm the presence and purity of the VH in the eluted peak fractions by SDS-PAGE (23) (see Note 22). Pool the VH-containing fractions and dialyze extensively against PBS (see Note 23).
11. Recover the dialyzed material and measure $A_{280\ nm}$ for determination of VH concentration (24) (see Note 24). Add EDTA and sodium azide to the VH prep to a final concentration of 0.5 mM and 0.02%, respectively. Store the purified VH at 4°C (see Note 25).

3.3. Disulfide Linkage Mapping of Mutant VHs by MS

In this section, MS is used to verify if the cysteine residues at positions 49 and 69 of HVHAm302S mutant form a disulfide linkage. To this end, the molecular weights of the VHs and the tryptic fragments thereof are determined by MS. The obtained information is then used to verify the presence of disulfide linkage between Cys49 and Cys69. The wild type VH, HVHAm302, is also included in the analysis for comparison.

In steps (1–6), the VHs are buffer-exchanged into a buffer feasible for the subsequent trypsin digestion experiment followed by the trypsin treatment of the VHs to produce a pool of peptides for subsequent MS analysis. Here we employ spin columns to exchange buffers, however, buffer exchange can also be achieved by dialysis (see Note 26).

1. Wash an Ultrafree®-0.5 (5 kDa MWCO) spin column attached to a collecting microtube by adding 500 μL of ddH_2O into the column and centrifuging with a microfuge at 12,000 rpm and 4°C for 10 min.
2. Add the VH solution (~300 μg, already centrifuged to remove particulates) to the spin column. Centrifuge the column at 12,000 rpm and 4°C in a microfuge until ~50 μL of the solution remains in the column (this may take ~15 min). Discard the flow-through.
3. Add 500 μL of TDB to the column and centrifuge (see Subheading 3.3, step 2). Repeat this step once more. Transfer the remained 50 μL of VH solution to a new microtube and determine the concentration of the VH (see Subheading 3.2, step 11). Adjust the protein concentration to 0.5 mg/mL with TDB.

4. Add 25 μL of 100 μg/mL trypsin solution to 100 μL of the protein sample. Vortex gently, then centrifuge briefly to consolidate the content of the tube. Incubate the reaction mixture in a 37°C water bath for 2 h. Incubate a protease negative control mixture (25 μL of TDB plus 100 μL of protein sample) under the same conditions.
5. Mix 10 μL of the trypsin digested protein solution as well as the negative control solution with 10 μL of 2× SDS-PAGE sample loading buffer. Treat the solutions at 95°C for 5 min, then centrifuge briefly to consolidate the contents of the tube. Use 10 μL in reducing SDS-PAGE analysis and verify the success of the digestion using the control sample gel profile as the reference.
6. Proceed with the MS analysis of the tryptic peptides (see Subheading 3.3, steps 7–17). Figure 2 shows the overall scheme for the preparation of VH tryptic peptides for subsequent MS analysis. It can be seen from the reducing SDS-PAGE profile that both HVHAm302S and HVHAm302 (control) have been successfully digested by trypsin into small peptides (compare "Trypsin(−)" lanes with "Trypsin(+)" lanes).

   In steps (7–17), the molecular weights of VHs are first measured by infusion electrospray ionization (ESI)-MS. Subsequently, the molecular masses of the tryptic peptides of VHs are determined and the peptide fragment ion information is obtained using nano-flow reversed-phase liquid chromatography tandem MS (MS^2) with data dependent analysis (DDA) to verify the presence of disulfide linkage between Cys49 and Cys69 (25).
7. Resuspend an aliquot of the VH protein stock solution in 50%/50% acetonitrile/ddH$_2$O to a concentration of ~5 pmol/μL and infuse the protein solution at a flow rate of 1 μL/min into the ESI source of a Q-TOF 2™ mass spectrometer (see Note 27).
8. Deconvolute the mass spectra of VHs using the Max Ent 1 program under Masslynx™ software to determine the molecular weights of the VHs.
9. Perform the DDA of the trypsin-treated VHs (a collection of peptides) (see Subheading 3.3, step 6) in 0.1% formic acid using nano-flow reversed-phase liquid chromatography MS (see Note 28).
10. Load the tryptic peptides onto a 180 μm I.D. × 20 mm 5 μm symmetry® C18 trap.
11. Elute the peptides from a 100 μm I.D. × 10 cm 1.7 μm BEH130C18 column using a linear gradient of 0–36% solvent B (acetonitrile + 0.1% formic acid) for 36 min, 36–90% solvent B for 2 min at a flow rate of ~0.3 μL/min. Solvent A is ddH$_2$O + 0.1% formic acid.

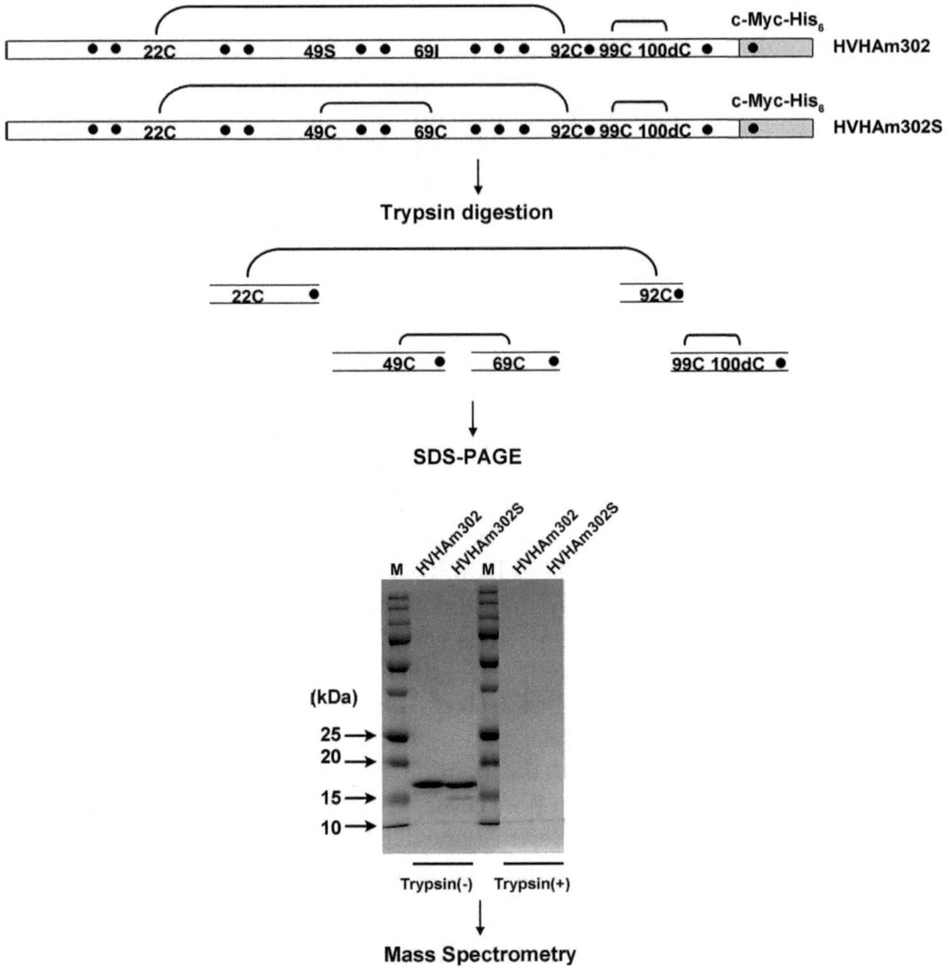

Fig. 2. VH tryptic fragment preparation for subsequent disulfide linkage mapping of VHs by MS. Putative disulfide linkages between Cys pairs (denoted as C's) are shown by *curved lines*. *Closed circles* represent potential trypsin cleavage sites. Upon trypsin digestion, HVHAm302S is expected to yield one more set of disulfide-linked doublet peptide than HVHAm302. Tryptic fragments are too small to be detected on the SDS-PAGE gel [lane "Trypsin(+)"]. M denotes the lane with standard proteins.

12. Search the peptide MS^2 spectra against the VH sequences for VH identification using the Mascot™ database searching algorithm (see Note 29).
13. Extract the theoretical disulfide-linked peptide masses from the LC-MS chromatograms of VHs (see Table 1) (see Notes 30 and 31).
14. Deconvolute the MS^2 spectra of the disulfide-linked peptides using the MaxEnt 3 program for de novo sequencing.
15. De novo sequence the disulfide-linked peptides with one peptide treated as a modification via a disulfide bond which remains intact under collision induced dissociation (CID) (25).

Table 1
Disulfide linkage determination of VHs by MS

VH	Tryptic peptides[a]	MW_{for} (Da)	MW_{exp} (Da)	ΔMW (MW_{for} – MW_{exp}) (Da)
HVHAm302	SCQTSLCTSTTR	1284.54	1284.55	-0.01
	LSCAASGDTVSDESMTWV R AEDTAVYYCVTDNR	3630.55	3630.52	0.03
HVHAm302S	SCQTSLCTSTTR	1284.54	1284.56	-0.02
	GLEWVCAISSSGGSTYYAD SVK FTCSR	2889.28	2889.30	-0.02
	LSCAASGDTVSDESMTWV R AEDTAVYYCVTDNR	3630.55	3630.52	0.03

[a]Major tryptic peptides with disulfide linkages between "bold" cysteine residues are shown. The spaces in between the two disulfide connected fragments in the longer peptides represent sequences in the VH which are lost by trypsinization. MW_{for}: formula (expected) molecular weight; MW_{exp}: molecular weight determined experimentally by MS.

16. Determine the disulfide linkage positions by the presence of y fragment ion series containing the disulfide linkage of the expected disulfide-linked peptides from each VH (see Note 32). A typical MS^2 spectrum of a disulfide-linked peptide demonstrating the exact disulfide linkage positions is shown in Chapter 25.
17. The determined disulfide-linked peptides from the VHs are recorded in Table 1. It can be seen that HVHAm302S mutant, in addition to the two disulfide linkages which is also present in HVHAm302, has a third one between Cys49 and Cys69.

3.4. Assessment of Aggregation State of Mutant VHs by Analytical Size Exclusion Chromatography

In this step, size exclusion chromatography employing Superdex™ 75 is used to assess the aggregation state of VH domains. Non-aggregating VHs should give chromatograms with a single, symmetrical peak with elution volumes expected for a monomeric VH (see Note 33). In contrast, the chromatogram profiles of aggregating VHs, in addition to the monomeric peaks, consist of additional peaks which elute earlier (see Note 34). Percent monomer can be calculated by area integration of the peaks and used as a quantitative measure of VH aggregation tendency (the higher the % monomer of a VH, the lower its aggregation tendency).

1. Wash a Superdex™ 75 size exclusion column with 50 mL of filtered and degassed ddH_2O and subsequently equilibrate with 50 mL of filtered and degassed PBS at a pump speed of 0.5 mL/min (see Note 23).
2. Inject and elute 200 μL of purified VH and obtain the chromatogram (see Notes 35–37).
3. Integrate monomeric and aggregate peaks to obtain % monomer.

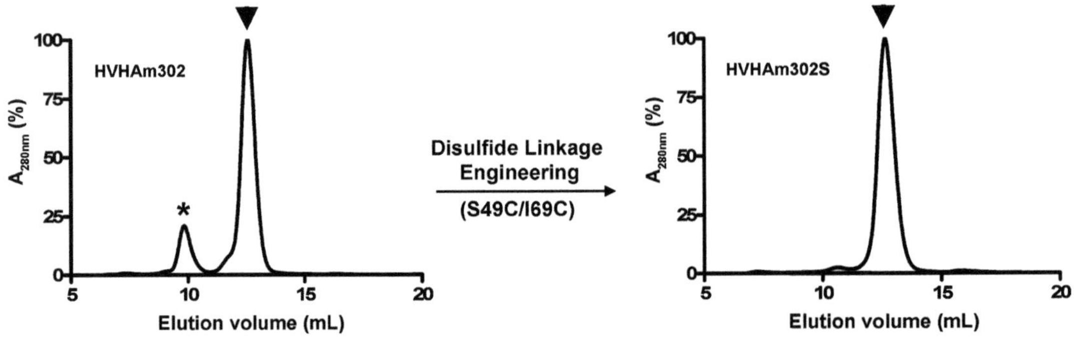

Fig. 3. Comparison of size exclusion chromatogram of HVHAm302S VH with that of HVHAm302. For each chromatogram, background absorbance was subtracted and all peaks were normalized with respect to the monomeric peak (marked by *arrowheads*) which was set to 100%. HVHAm302S is homogeneously monomer while HVHAm302 forms a considerable amount of aggregates (possibly dimeric aggregates) represented by the peak marked by the *asterisk*.

4. Figure 3 shows that the disulfide linkage engineering involving Ser49Cys/Ile69Cys mutations significantly improves HVHAm302 solubility. In contrast to HVHAm302, which forms non-monomeric species (% monomer = 82%), HVHAm302S is essentially devoid of such forms and exist primarily as monomers.

3.5. Thermal Stability Assessment of Mutant VHs by CD Spectroscopy

The thermal stability of the VH is assessed in terms melting temperature (T_m) by CD spectroscopy measurements.

1. Turn on the Jasco-815 CD spectropolarimeter, N_2 gas supply and prewarm the lamp for at least 30 min. Ensure the water level is at capacity in the Peltier heat control unit.
2. Buffer exchange the purified HVHAm302S VH into 0.1 M sodium phosphate buffer using a Millipore Ultrafree®-0.5 (5 kDa MWCO) spin column attached to a collecting microtube as described by the manufacturer.
3. Measure $A_{280\ nm}$ for determination of the protein concentration using a spectrophotometer (see Note 24) and prepare 0.5 mL of HVHAm302S at 50 μg/mL in 0.1 M sodium phosphate buffer.
4. Set the following CD spectropolarimeter parameters:

Data collection range	180–260 nm
Scan speed	50 nm/min
Data pitch	1 nm
Bandwidth	1 mm
Temperature range	30–96°C
Temperature ramp	1°C/min
Data collection	Every 2°C
Accumulations	4

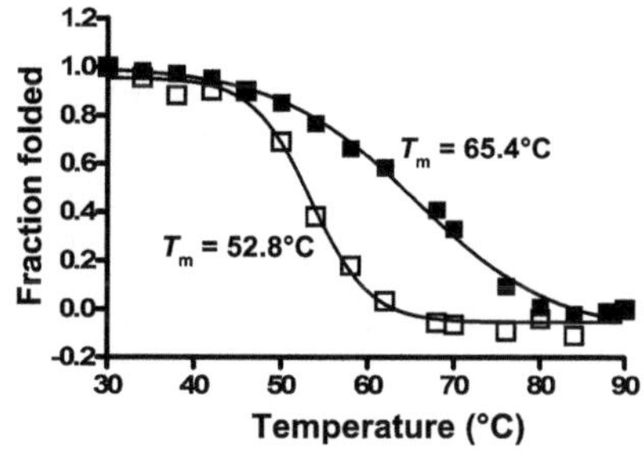

Fig. 4. Stability comparison between HVHAm302S (*closed square*) and HVHAm302 (*open square*) VHs in terms of T_m. Heat-induced protein unfolding curves were constructed from ellipticity values obtained at 205 nm.

5. Wash a 1-mm cuvette thoroughly (see Notes 38 and 39). Add 150 μL of 0.1 M sodium phosphate buffer (see Note 40). Perform a "buffer blank" scan at 30°C from 180 to 260 nm to confirm the cuvette is clean. Save the data.
6. Remove the 0.1 M sodium phosphate buffer from the cuvette and replace it with 150 μL of the mutant VH at 50 μg/mL (see Note 41). Perform the temperature induced unfolding experiment using the parameters described (see Subheading 3.5, step 4).
7. Smooth the spectra of the sample and the buffer blank using the Jasco software. Subtract the buffer blank response from the sample response. The VH exhibits a large change in ellipticity at 205 nm (see Note 42). Convert the raw ellipticity data (in millidegrees) at 205 nm at each temperature to molar ellipticity and then to the fraction of protein folded (see Note 43).
8. Export the converted data from Excel into GraphPad Prism, plot the fraction of protein folded vs. temperature and perform nonlinear regression analysis (see Fig. 4). The temperature at which 50% of the mutant VH is unfolded represents the melting temperature (T_m).
9. Repeat the procedure for the wild type VH control.
10. Figure 4 clearly demonstrates that the presence of an extra disulfide linkage between amino acid positions 49 and 69 drastically increases HVHAm302 stability. While HVHAm302 has a T_m of 52.8°C, HVHAm302S with the extra disulfide linkage has a T_m of 65.4°C, higher by over 12°C.

4. Notes

1. We typically use Millipore's 0.2 μm MILLEx®-GV filter units for sterilizing small volumes and 0.2 μm GP Express™ Plus Membrane filtration system for sterilizing large volumes.

2. The expression plasmid in the construct is pSJF2H (11).
3. Prepare the primer solutions in autoclaved ddH_2O and always store at −20°C to prevent their degradation. We typically prepare a 100× (100 pmol/μL) stock solution and 10× working solutions in 100 μL aliquots.
4. A more cost-effective approach is to prepare electrocompetent cells in house (22).
5. Mix 15 g agar, 10 g tryptone, 5 g yeast extract, and 10 g NaCl in a total volume of 1 L of ddH_2O. Sterilize the solution by autoclaving. Allow the solution to cool to about 60°C and then add 1 mL of 100 mg/mL filter-sterilized ampicillin. Mix the solution by shaking and pour in 20 mL volumes in Petri dishes. Partly cover the plates with lids and leave the plates for 10 min at room temperature for the media to solidify. Leave the plates overnight at room temperature in order to ensure they are not contaminated and then store them away at 4°C. Stored plates are usable up to around 1 month.
6. Other vendors offer similar products. We prefer to use conjugated anti-His tag antibodies for Western blotting, since they avoid the additional step of including the secondary antibody conjugate.
7. We routinely use 5-mL HisTrap™ FF IMAC columns. However, comparable columns are available from other vendors, e.g., Bio-Rad. When protein expression is low we recommend using 1-mL columns to reduce background binding of bacterial proteins.
8. In contrast to conventional spectrophotometers, the ND-1000 spectrophotometer or instruments with similar technology measures absorbance at very low volumes (1 μL) and without the use of cuvettes.
9. We highly recommend using sequencing-grade trypsin. Nonsequencing grade trypsin may have other enzyme contaminants, e.g., chymotrypsin, which may result in unwanted protease cleavages, thus making the interpretation of MS data difficult.
10. We routinely use Superdex™ 75 columns for assessing the aggregation status of single-domain antibodies and purification of monomeric species from IMAC-purified antibody preps. However, GE Healthcare's Superdex™ 200 columns (10/300 GL size exclusion columns) can also be used for these purposes.
11. pSJF2H-HVHAm302S was constructed synthetically at Geneart Inc. (Toronto, ON, Canada). This approach, although convenient, is not cost-effective when the number of constructs is too many. Alternatively, the construction and cloning of mutants can be achieved using a previously described method (12).

12. Newer electroporators have pre-programmed settings for electroporation of *E. coli*.
13. Avoid introducing air bubbles or too much salt in your cuvettes to avoid arcing during electroporation and transformation failure as a result. To rid electroporation mixtures of air bubbles flick gently the side and bottom of the cuvette.
14. If in the morning no colonies are obtained, plate the entire remaining transformation solution which has been kept at 4°C.
15. With *E. coli* TG1, we incubate plates at 32°C as opposed to 37°C to avoid the formation of satellite colonies. As a result of the lower incubation temperature, a longer incubation time may be necessary for the appearance of visible colonies on the plate.
16. To make a reference plate of colonies, touch the surface of an LB/ampicillin agar plate with the colony-inoculated loops to form spots. Label the spots for each clone, and incubate the plate overnight at 32°C. In the morning, seal the plate air-tight with parafilm and store at 4°C for later reference (see Subheading 3.1, step 7).
17. We routinely use the QIAprep Spin MiniPrep™ kit from QIAGEN Inc. (Mississauga, ON, Canada) which has a purification capacity of up to 20 μg of molecular biology grade plasmid DNA.
18. One primer gives enough sequencing read coverage and thus it is not necessary to use both M13RP and M13FP for DNA sequencing.
19. To prepare a permanent stock of a clone, touch the respective colony on the reference plate with a disposable inoculation loop and swirl the loop in a 2-mL LB/ampicillin medium in a 15-mL sterile Falcon tube. Incubate the culture at 37°C and 230 rpm for 20 h. Add 0.7 mL of the bacterial culture and 0.3 mL of sterile 50% glycerol to a sterile cryogenic vial. Vortex briefly to mix and store at -80°C.
20. To re-suspend the cells, put a magnetic bar inside the container then vortex the cell solution.
21. If there are time constraints, the unsuspended bacterial pellet in CLB can be stored at –20°C and processed at a later time. To continue with the cell lysis, add PMSF first then thaw/resuspend the cells. This can be carried out by incubation at 37°C and occasional shaking.
22. Our chromatograms typically consist of an early peak which corresponds to nontarget proteins, e.g., bacterial proteins, and a late one which corresponds to the eluted VH. If the VH aggregates extensively, a peak corresponding to the aggregating species is also observed and elutes after than that for non-aggregating species.

23. We observe that our single-domain antibodies are more soluble in 10 mM HEPES, 150 mM NaCl, 3 mM EDTA, pH 7.4 than in PBS.
24. Calculate protein concentration using the following formula: $[\text{protein}]_{\text{mg/mL}} = (A_{280\ \text{nm}} \times \text{molecular weight}) \div \text{extinction coefficient}$. Commercial protein analysis softwares, e.g., Laser gene v6.0, DNASTAR, Inc., or online freeware, e.g., ExPASy ProtParam tool at http://us.expasy.org/tools/protparam.html, can be used for calculation of molar extinction coefficient and molecular weight.
25. We frequently observe that the C-terminal c-Myc-His tag of our single-domain antibodies is removed within a few months of storage at 4°C, the VH domain itself, however, remains intact for much longer periods. It might be feasible to store single-domain antibodies at −20°C for complete integrity.
26. For dialysis of small volumes (few hundred microliters range) we typically use Slide-A-Lyzer® dialysis cassettes from Pierce (Rockford, IL).
27. The Q-TOF 2™ hybrid quadrupole/TOF mass spectrometer was calibrated by infusing a 5 pmol/μL myoglobin solution for determination of VH molecular weights. All the molecular weights of VHs were determined to be within 40 ppm mass accuracy using infusion ESI-MS.
28. Set the DDA parameters as follows: ion intensity threshold = 50 counts; survey scan time = 1 s; number of components = 3. Peptides were fragmented using CID.
29. The identification coverage of each protein from the analysis of their proteolytic digests using nanoRPLC-MS^2 with DDA was more than 30%. The cut off ion score of 30 above which ion scores indicate identity was used for accepting individual MS^2 spectra for protein identification.
30. The theoretical molecular weights of disulfide-linked peptides were calculated using the Protein/peptide editor under the Masslynx™ software.
31. The theoretical disulfide-linked peptide ions appeared prominent in the survey scan of the DDA experiment.
32. The theoretical disulfide-linked peptide fragment ions were dominant in the MS^2 spectra of the expected disulfide-linked peptides. The annotated MS^2 spectra of disulfide-linked peptides are not shown.
33. There are typically some variations in the elution volumes of monomeric fractions (5, 10).
34. Unlike the monomeric peaks for the non-aggregating VHs, those for aggregating VHs may not be symmetrical but display tailing which could be due to nonspecific interaction of the VH with the column material.

35. As little as 50 μL of protein preparation may be sufficient to give a reliable signal (a mAU peak value of around 50 or higher). When the peak mAU values are too low, particularly when lower than 10, a reliable statement with regards to the VH aggregation states cannot be made.

36. Use the same concentration when comparing different VHs as protein concentration is a factor in aggregation formation.

37. We routinely export the chromatographic data as Excel files and subsequently feed the data into the graphing software GraphPad Prism for flexible data manipulation and multiple chromatogram presentations on the same graph.

38. The choice of cuvette path length depends on the working VH concentration. Cuvettes with longer path lengths (larger volumes) may need to be used with lower concentrations in order to obtain a significant CD signal.

39. Wash all cuvettes thoroughly before use and between samples. Rinse the cuvette with ddH_2O followed by 2–3 washes with a commercial cleaning solution from suppliers such as Hellma, with a combination of 30% HCl and 70% ethanol, or with 6 M guanidine hydrochloride followed by ddH_2O and ethanol. After washing allow the cuvette to air dry. Ideally, soak the cuvettes overnight when possible. In all cases, perform a CD scan on the empty cuvette to ensure there is no residual protein remaining.

40. Avoid using buffers with high absorbance in the wavelength range used (e.g., buffers with high salt concentration) as they would increase the noise. This is particularly important for VHs as they are essentially β-strand proteins and as a result give only a modest CD signal change upon denaturation.

41. It is critical to use the same concentration and buffer when comparing different VHs as protein concentration is a factor in aggregation formation and T_ms are a function of buffer composition.

42. We consistently find the biggest difference in signal (ellipticity) between native and denatured VHs at wavelengths of 205–220 nm. In our thermal unfolding experiments, we calculated T_ms for VHs using the ellipticity at 205 nm since it gave the highest goodness of fit (R^2).

43. Ellipticity (θ) from the CD spectropolarimeter is given in millidegrees (mdeg). Export the raw mdeg data to a program such as Excel. To convert from mdeg to molar ellipticity ($[\theta]$) in deg cm^2/dmol, use the following formula: $[\theta] = (\text{mdeg} \times \text{mean residue weight})/(\text{pathlength in mm} \times \text{antibody concentration in mg/mL})$ (26). The mean residue weight, MRW = (molecular weight of the antibody/number of backbone amino acids). To convert from molar ellipticity to the fraction of protein folded (FF) (27), use the following formula: $\text{FF} = ([\theta] - [\theta_U])/([\theta_F] - [\theta_U])$ where $[\theta]$ is the molar ellipticity at each temperature

point (calculated above in this Note), $[\theta_U]$ is the molar ellipticity of the fully unfolded protein (in this case the $[\theta_{205\,nm}]$ at 96°C), and $[\theta_F]$ is the molar ellipticity of the fully folded protein (in this case the $[\theta_{205\,nm}]$ at 30°C).

References

1. Holliger P, Hudson PJ (2005) Engineered antibody fragments and the rise of single domains. Nat Biotechnol 23:1126–1136
2. Holt LJ et al (2003) Domain antibodies: proteins for therapy. Trends Biotechnol 21:484–490
3. Davies J, Riechmann L (1995) Antibody VH domains as small recognition units. Biotechnology (N Y) 13:475–479
4. Tanha J et al (2001) Optimal design features of camelized human single-domain antibody libraries. J Biol Chem 276:24774–24780
5. Jespers L et al (2004) Aggregation-resistant domain antibodies selected on phage by heat denaturation. Nat Biotechnol 22:1161–1165
6. To R et al (2005) Isolation of monomeric human V_Hs by a phage selection. J Biol Chem 280:41395–41403
7. Tanha J et al (2006) Improving solubility and refolding efficiency of human V_Hs by a novel mutational approach. Protein Eng Des Sel 19:503–509
8. Christ D, Famm K, Winter G (2007) Repertoires of aggregation-resistant human antibody domains. Protein Eng Des Sel 20:413–416
9. Famm K et al (2008) Thermodynamically stable aggregation-resistant antibody domains through directed evolution. J Mol Biol 376:926–931
10. Arbabi-Ghahroudi M et al (2009) Aggregation-resistant V_Hs selected by in vitro evolution tend to have disulfide-bonded loops and acidic isoelectric points. Protein Eng Des Sel 22:59–66
11. Arbabi-Ghahroudi M, MacKenzie R, Tanha J (2009) Selection of non-aggregating V_H binders from synthetic V_H phage-display libraries. Methods Mol Biol 525:187–216
12. Arbabi-Ghahroudi M, MacKenzie R, Tanha J (2010) Site-directed mutagenesis for improving biophysical properties of V_H domains. Methods Mol Biol 634:309–330
13. Kim DY, Tanha J (2010) Sodium dodecyl sulfate-polyacrylamide gel electrophoresis for screening nonaggregating human antibody heavy chain variable domains. Anal Biochem 403:117–119
14. Glockshuber R, Schmidt T, Plückthun A (1992) The disulfide bonds in antibody variable domains: effects on stability, folding in vitro, and functional expression in *Escherichia coli*. Biochemistry 31:1270–1279
15. Betz SF (1993) Disulfide bonds and the stability of globular proteins. Protein Sci 2:1551–1558
16. Proba K, Honegger A, Plückthun A (1997) A natural antibody missing a cysteine in V_H: consequences for thermodynamic stability and folding. J Mol Biol 265:161–172
17. Kabat EA et al (eds) (1991) Sequences of proteins of immunological interest. US Department of Health and Human Services, US Public Health Service, Bethesda, MD
18. Hagihara Y, Mine S, Uegaki K (2007) Stabilization of an immunoglobulin fold domain by an engineered disulfide bond at the buried hydrophobic region. J Biol Chem 282: 36489–36495
19. Chan PH et al (2008) Engineering a camelid antibody fragment that binds to the active site of human lysozyme and inhibits its conversion into amyloid fibrils. Biochemistry 47: 11041–11054
20. Saerens D et al (2008) Disulfide bond introduction for general stabilization of immunoglobulin heavy-chain variable domains. J Mol Biol 377:478–488
21. Hussack G et al (2011) Engineered single-domain antibodies with high protease resistance and thermal stability. PLoS ONE 6:e28218
22. Tung WL, Chow KC (1995) A modified medium for efficient electrotransformation of *E. coli*. Trends Genet 11:128–129
23. Sambrook J, Fritsch EF, Maniatis T (eds) (1989) Molecular cloning: a laboratory manual. Cold Spring Harbor Laboratory, Cold Spring Harbor, NY
24. Pace CN et al (1995) How to measure and predict the molar absorption coefficient of a protein. Protein Sci 4:2411–2423
25. Wu SL et al (2009) Mass spectrometric determination of disulfide linkages in recombinant therapeutic proteins using online LC-MS with electron-transfer dissociation. Anal Chem 81:112–122
26. Greenfield NJ (2006) Using circular dichroism spectra to estimate protein secondary structure. Nat Protoc 1:2876–2890
27. Greenfield NJ (2006) Analysis of the kinetics of folding of proteins and peptides using circular dichroism. Nat Protoc 1:2891–2899

Chapter 22

Improvement of Proteolytic Stability Through In Silico Engineering

Lucy Rutten, Hans de Haard, and Theo Verrips

Abstract

VHHs usually display high physical and proteolytic stability, but in some cases stability needs to be increased further for their intended applications. The high thermal stability is due to the stable 3D structure of VHHs, which consists of a sandwich of nine beta-strands with a high number of intramolecular interactions, resulting in a very compact structure. Because of this compact structure, relatively low numbers of (basic) amino acids are accessible for proteases, explaining their usually high proteolytic stability. The high stability of VHHs is required when used as therapeutics given orally and nasally or when used as microbicides given, e.g., intra-vaginally. When given orally, VHHs should be stable at the low pH in the stomach and be resistant against all proteases in the intestines. Here a method is described to predict the proteolytic susceptibility of VHHs and to subsequently increase the proteolytic stability through genetic engineering.

Key words: VHHs, Proteolytic stability, Engineering, Bioinformatics, 3D structure

1. Introduction

Protein stability refers on the one hand to physical stability, i.e., thermodynamic stability. The net stability of a protein is defined as the difference in free energy between the native and denatured state. On the other hand protein stability can also refer to chemical stability or proteolytic stability. For the use of proteins as drugs or as additives to food or personal care products, proteins should remain stable under and after all conditions they are expected to encounter. In this case the protein stability mainly refers to functional stability, which should be fully retained. To use VHHs as nasal or oral drugs, they should be chemically stable, in particular at the very low pH in the stomach and in the presence of proteases such as pepsin and trypsin present in the stomach and intestinal tract, respectively, and the proteases produced by intestinal flora. To use VHHs as vaginal microbicides, they should be resistant to

Dirk Saerens and Serge Muyldermans (eds.), *Single Domain Antibodies: Methods and Protocols*,
Methods in Molecular Biology, vol. 911, DOI 10.1007/978-1-61779-968-6_22, © Springer Science+Business Media, LLC 2012

proteases secreted by e.g., *lactobacilli* and should not only remain stable at the low pH of the vagina but also even retain its affinity against its target at that pH.

VHHs, as well as conventional antibodies, have been shown to remain stable when injected intravenously (1–4). This is not so surprising because upon active immunization of camelids these antibodies are selected "in vivo" for serum stability. In contrast, proteins selected from synthetic libraries do not always display high stability in the serum. VHHs have been shown to have superior stability compared to conventional antibodies (5–7). The lower stability of conventional antibodies may mainly be caused by the structure of conventional antibodies, which consist of multiple chains that usually dissociate at lower temperatures than at which the domains unfold. VHHs have been shown to remain intact and functional even up to 90°C (8). Furthermore, due to their larger structure as compared to VHHs, conventional antibodies generally have more protease cleavage sites. Some VHHs have been shown to be fully functional under extreme conditions such as in the presence of detergents (9) or to be able to refold to their native state after temperature denaturation with or without the ligand present (10, 11). Inherent to the multi-domain nature of conventional antibodies, their refolding after denaturation is very problematic.

Physical stability of VHHs can be studied basically with all methods that can distinguish between a folded and unfolded state. These methods include circular dichroism (CD) spectroscopy, differential scanning calorimetry (DSC), urea gradient gel electrophoresis, tryptophan fluorescence, nuclear magnetic resonance (NMR), and electrospray ionization mass spectrometry (ESI-MS) (11). The melting temperature of a protein is the best descriptor of thermo stability and can be measured best via either CD spectroscopy or DSC in which the temperature is changed gradually or stepwise to a higher temperature, possibly followed by a change to a lower temperature. Methods for studying VHH functionality under certain conditions or after being exposed to certain conditions or proteases are functional assays like ELISA, isothermal titration calorimetry (ITC), and surface plasmon resonance (SPR) measurements. Proteolytic degradation after exposure to proteases, however, can be studied easily by using sodium dodecyl sulfate-polyacrylamide gel electrophoresis (SDS-PAGE) or Western blotting.

When VHHs do not meet the desired stability for use in intended applications, they can be engineered randomly or rationally on DNA level. Random engineering can be performed by making use of the VHH DNA sequence to generate a secondary library with DNA shuffling to select proteolytically stable VHHs with retained binding affinities (12). Rational engineering of VHHs, and proteins in general, to increase thermal stability, can be performed for example by changing glycines into alanines and alanines into prolines to rigidify the main chain. Moreover additional disulfide bridges can be introduced to stabilize the folded structure (reviewed by ref. (13)). These methods, however, are not yet straightforward. The rational removal of protease cleavage sites using site-directed mutagenesis may be more straightforward. VHHs susceptible to certain proteases often contain many putative cleavage sites. Most such sites cannot be accessed by proteases due to their positions in the structure. Therefore bioinformatics and crystal structures or structural models are most valuable to predict the most probable cleavage sites. In general, only the putative cleavage sites (1) that have certain surrounding amino acids allowing optimal binding in the protease active site, (2) that show flexibility (e.g., high B-factors in crystal structures) and (3) that are exposed well to the outside of the protein, are the sites that are indeed susceptible to protease cleavage.

Here a method is described to predict the position of protease cleavage sites in VHHs, by applying bioinformatics. As an example we describe the prediction of the accessible trypsin cleavage site present in an anti-rotavirus-VHH (14), which contains 11 arginines and lysines after which trypsin may cleave the protein. The power of this prediction method is confirmed by removing the most likely cleavage site by genetic engineering, which resulted in a VHH that is resistant to trypsin cleavage.

2. Materials

The method described here is based on bioinformatics, for which a computer is needed with an Internet connection. This method can easily be used with standard programs such as a web browser and a spreadsheet program.

3. Methods

3.1. Sequence-Based Prediction of Putative Proteolytic Cleavage Sites

1. Predict the putative proteolytic cleavage sites with the OPAL program. The online program OPAL (http://www.oppf.ox.ac.uk/opal/OPAL.php) predicts trypsin cleavage sites and their probability of cleavage, subdivided into four classes (see Note 1). To predict other protease cleavage sites, another online tool, i.e., Peptide Cutter is available (see Note 2).
2. Enter the protein amino acid sequence (see Note 3).
3. Select "Trypsin Cleavage" and "all classes" and click on "Send."
4. Collect list of putative proteolytic cleavage sites in a table. The program provides a list with the putative trypsin cleavage sites. An example of a list, shown here, is obtained by using the

Table 1
List of classes of putative trypsin cleavage sites in VHH1 obtained by the program OPAL

Class of trypsin cleavage site	At position P1[a]	P3–P2–P1–P1′
Class 1	27	SGRT
Class 1	38	WFRQ
Class 1	66	KGRF
Class 1	71	IARV
Class 1	84	MNRL
Class 3	43	PGKE
Class 3	64	AGKG
Class 3	75	NAKN
Class 4	17	GDRL
Class 4	45	KERE

[a]The positively charged amino acids R or K are at the P1 position, so at the first line the R is at position 27

sequence of an anti-rotaviral VHH, which has been shown to undergo cleavage by trypsin at one site in the protein (Table 1) (see Note 4).

3.2. 3D Structure Generation/Modeling

1. Download protein coordinates, when available, from the Protein Data Bank (see Note 5). When a high resolution 3D structure of the VHH of interest is available, it can be used to determine the surface accessibility of the amino acids predicted to be involved in putative proteolytic cleavage sites.
2. Generate a tentative 3D model, if no high resolution 3D structure is available. To date quite a number of VHH structures have been deposited at the Protein Data Bank. These structures can form the basis for modeling a VHH with an unknown 3D structure. Using the SWISS-MODEL SERVER (http://swissmodel.expasy.org) a model can be generated automatically, by just providing the amino acid sequence of the VHH.
3. Choose the "Modelling" "Automated Mode." Fill in your e-mail address and project title and enter the VHH sequence, after which the "Submit Modelling Request" should be selected. Figure 1 shows the model that was obtained for the anti-rotaviral VHH.

3.3. Determining the Accessible Surface

1. Determine the accessible surface and buried surface with the WHAT IF Web Interface (http://swift.cmbi.ru.nl/servers/html/index.html) (15).

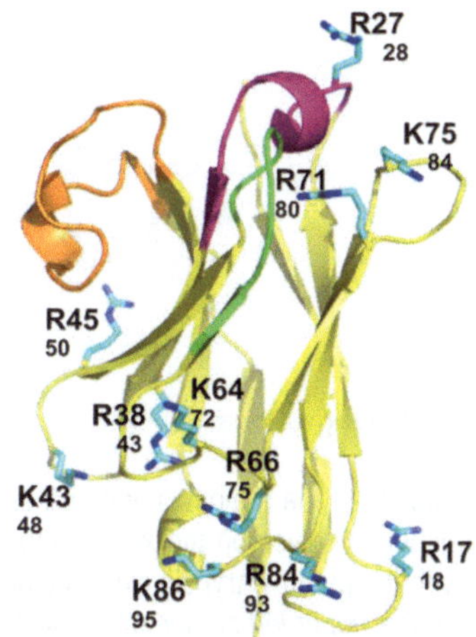

Fig. 1. Structural model of VHH1 against rotavirus. The backbone is schematically represented by a ribbon diagram. CDR1 is colored *magenta*, CDR2 *green*, CDR3 *orange*, and the framework is colored *yellow*. Site chains of all positively charged amino acids, i.e., arginines (R) and lysines (K), in the structure are depicted in all atom model and are labeled with one-letter amino acid codes with the number of the position of the residue in the sequence. The nitrogen atoms are colored *blue* and the carbon atoms are in *cyan*. The IMGT numbering is shown in *small characters* below the sequential numbering.

2. Choose "Accessibility" from the list of Classes. Then choose "Buried surface. Calculate the surface buried relative to the residue in vacuum."
3. Upload the PDB file (see Subheading 3.2, step 3).
4. Copy and paste the results in a spreadsheet. The WHAT IF program provides the accessible surface for each atom in each amino acid in the last column (see Note 6). Copy the total residue accessibility percentages of the basic amino acids and the accessibility percentages for the C-atom of the basic amino acid (P1) and the N-atom of the following amino acid (see Note 7) and paste it into a spreadsheet.

3.4. Generating the Trypsin Susceptibility Plot

1. Use a spreadsheet to generate a plot by setting out the class of the potential cleavage site against the accessible surface percentage of the lysine or arginine in the site (see Note 8) (see Fig. 2a).
2. Omit the sites with an accessibility of "0" for the main chain C- or N-atom, because they are very unlikely targets for trypsin. Only the potential cleavage sites with an accessible scissile bond can be cleaved by trypsin (see Note 9) (see Fig. 2b). Arginine 27 is in both Fig. 2a, b the most likely target for trypsin cleavage (class 1 with a surface accessibility of the arginine of 75.7%) at the left upper corner of the charts.
3. Mutate the most likely residue that is targeted by trypsin digestion. We mutated Arg27 to an alanine and observed that proteolytic degradation by trypsin was abrogated (see Fig. 3). Binding affinity against the target was not affected at all and

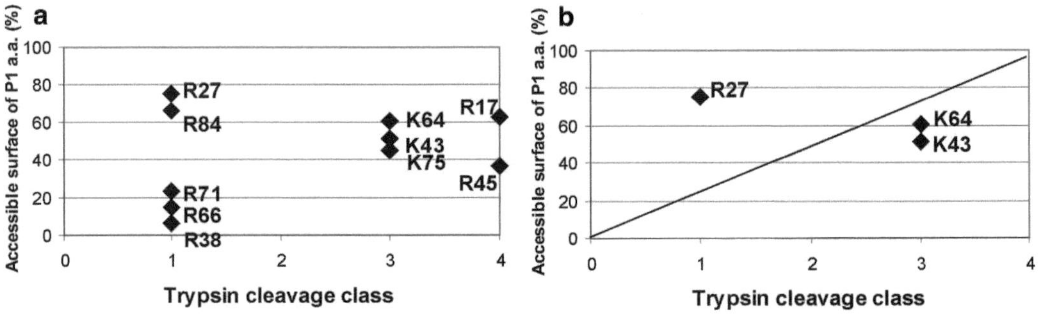

Fig. 2. Trypsin cleavage probability of the arginines and lysines in VHH1. (**a**) All putative trypsin cleavage sites are given. The class of trypsin cleavage sites is given on the *x*-axis, and the surface accessibility of the P1 residue is given on the *y*-axis. (**b**) The same as (**a**) with the putative trypsin cleavage sites removed that have a non-accessible scissile bond. The trypsin cleavage site that is in the *upper left corner* is the most probable trypsin cleavage site.

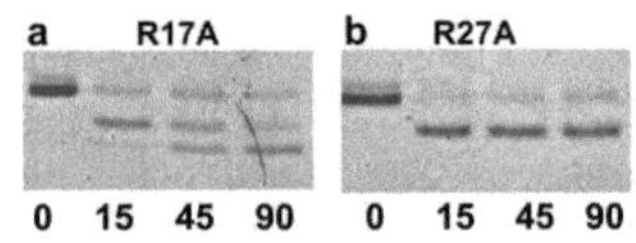

Fig. 3. Digestion of R17A and R27A by trypsin on a Coomassie stained SDS-PAGE gel. (**a**) Tryptic digest of R17A VHH1 before (=0), and 15, 45, and 90 min digestion by trypsin. Wild-type VHH1 as well as the mutants K64A, K86A, and R45A show the same digestion pattern. (**b**) As (**a**), but R27A. This mutant is cleaved once between the protein-tag and the VHH, but the intrinsic trypsin cleavage site has been removed.

neither was the expression level. In this example the arginine that has the best accessibility in the plot indeed is the one that is target for the actual trypsin digestion.

4. In conclusion, when observing cleavage of a VHH by, e.g., trypsin, using trypsin digestion followed by SDS-PAGE analysis, out of many potential cleavage sites, the actual cleavage site can be predicted by making use of bioinformatics. By using the method described above to predict the most probable cleavage site, a lot of experimental mutagenesis can be avoided (see Note 10). The lysine or arginine in the most probable cleavage site can be specifically mutated or even the residue at the P1′ site can be mutated into, e.g., a proline to abrogate trypsin digestion.

4. Notes

1. Class 1 cleavage sites have arginine in position P1 and have the highest cleavage rates. Class 2 cleavage sites have lysine in position P1 and have the second highest cleavage rates. Class 3 cleavage sites have some inhibition of cleavage by residues in positions P3–P1′. Class 4 cleavage sites have considerable

inhibition by residues in positions P3–P1′ and have the lowest cleavage. The cleavage site sequences displayed have the pattern P3–P2–P1–P1′, where subsite P1 is the numbered position stated. The protein is cleaved between P1 and P1′.

2. With the PeptideCutter tool in the program Expasy (http://ca.expasy.org/tools/peptidecutter/) a great number of putative proteolytic cleavage sites, e.g., for caspases, pepsin, proteinase K, thrombin, enterokinase, and many more, can be predicted. By choosing all proteases the program will provide a huge number of putative proteolytic cleavage sites, of which a number of interesting ones can be chosen. For example, if the focus is on obtaining a VHH that is stable in the gut, it should not be cleaved by e.g., pepsin and trypsin.
3. In the OPAL program, the sequence should be introduced in FASTA format. The first line in a FASTA format starts with a ">" (greater-than) symbol directly followed by a title of choice, followed by an "Enter" and the sequence represented using single-letter codes (in capitals).
4. Not all sequences with an arginine or lysine can be cleaved by trypsin. In our example, for instance, at one of the 11 basic amino acids, i.e., K86, the VHH cannot be cleaved by trypsin at all, because it is followed by a proline, so this one does not appear in the list (Table 1). The numbering of the amino acids is in the actual order as they appear in the sequence. As a consequence the numbering differs from the IMGT and Kabat numbering, which are usually used for VHH sequences.
5. At the Protein Data Bank (PDB) (http://www.rcsb.org/pdb/home/home.do) structures of VHHs can be searched for. If the structure of interest is found it can be downloaded as a file in PDB format. Choose the "download file" option "PDB File (text)."
6. In the WHAT-IF output the percentage is given in the last column, the surface accessibility of the atom in the structure relative to what it would be in vacuum.
7. First of all, the side chain of a key residue for proteolytic cleavage should be accessible. The NZ of lysines and the NH1 and NH2 of arginines should be accessible. Although, these are often exposed to the outside of the VHH, they can still be involved in a salt-bridge formation, which makes it more unlikely that it is recognized by the protease. For a protease to be able to cleave a protein, the scissile bond (the bond to be cleaved) should also be accessible to the protease. The scissile bond consists of the main chain C-atom of the P1 residue (a basic residue in the case of trypsin) and main chain N-atom of the P1′ residue.
8. By looking at the percentage of accessible surface of arginines and lysines and not at the actual accessible surface area, arginines

which have a larger molecular surface than lysines will not provide larger numbers and thus they will not, solely based on their surface area, be favored above lysines in the plot.

9. In our example three of the potential cleavage sites have scissile bonds that are non-buried in the model. Two of these sites belong to the class 3 trypsin cleavage sites, which display some inhibition of cleavage by residues in positions P3–P1′ and are therefore not very likely to be cleaved by trypsin. One putative cleavage site involving arginine 27 that has a non-buried scissile bond belongs to a class 1 trypsin cleavage site.
10. We do not want to claim that the method described here works perfect for all VHHs, because the structural modeling may not be fully correct and even a crystal structure, which is a kind of snapshot, does not represent the VHH structure in solution. This method, which consumes little time and effort, can certainly aid to pinpoint the residues that are most likely prone to protease cleavage and the ones that are certainly not, resulting in saving a lot of time normally needed for generating and testing many different mutants.

References

1. Els Conrath K, Lauwereys M, Wyns L, Muyldermans S (2001) Camel single-domain antibodies as modular building units in bispecific and bivalent antibody constructs. J Biol Chem 276:7346–7350
2. Cortez-Retamozo V, Backmann N, Senter PD, Wernery U, De Baetselier P, Muyldermans S, Revets H (2004) Efficient cancer therapy with a nanobody-based conjugate. Cancer Res 64:2853–2857
3. Harmsen MM, Van Solt CB, Fijten HP, Van Setten MC (2005) Prolonged in vivo residence times of llama single-domain antibody fragments in pigs by binding to porcine immunoglobulins. Vaccine 23:4926–4934
4. Coppieters K, Dreier T, Silence K, de Haard H, Lauwereys M, Casteels P, Beirnaert E, Jonckheere H, Van de Wiele C, Staelens L, Hostens J, Revets H, Remaut E, Elewaut D, Rottiers P (2006) Formatted anti-tumor necrosis factor alpha VHH proteins derived from camelids show superior potency and targeting to inflamed joints in a murine model of collagen-induced arthritis. Arthritis Rheum 54:1856–1866
5. Dumoulin M, Conrath K, Van Meirhaeghe A, Meersman F, Heremans K, Frenken LG, Muyldermans S, Wyns L, Matagne A (2002) Single-domain antibody fragments with high conformational stability. Protein Sci 11:500–515
6. Arbabi Ghahroudi M, Desmyter A, Wyns L, Hamers R, Muyldermans S (1997) Selection and identification of single domain antibody fragments from camel heavy-chain antibodies. FEBS Lett 414:521–526
7. Frenken LG, van der Linden RH, Hermans PW, Bos JW, Ruuls RC, de Geus B, Verrips CT (2000) Isolation of antigen specific llama VHH antibody fragments and their high level secretion by *Saccharomyces cerevisiae*. J Biotechnol 78:11–21
8. van der Linden RH, Frenken LG, de Geus B, Harmsen MM, Ruuls RC, Stok W, de Ron L, Wilson S, Davis P, Verrips CT (1999) Comparison of physical chemical properties of llama VHH antibody fragments and mouse monoclonal antibodies. Biochim Biophys Acta 1431:37–46
9. Dolk E, van der Vaart M, Lutje Hulsik D, Vriend G, de Haard H, Spinelli S, Cambillau C, Frenken L, Verrips T (2005) Isolation of llama antibody fragments for prevention of dandruff by phage display in shampoo. Appl Environ Microbiol 71:442–450
10. Dolk E, van Vliet C, Perez JM, Vriend G, Darbon H, Ferrat G, Cambillau C, Frenken LG, Verrips T (2005) Induced refolding of a temperature denatured llama heavy-chain antibody fragment by its antigen. Proteins 59: 555–564

11. Perez JM, Renisio JG, Prompers JJ, van Platerink CJ, Cambillau C, Darbon H, Frenken LG (2001) Thermal unfolding of a llama antibody fragment: a two-state reversible process. Biochemistry 40:74–83
12. Harmsen MM, van Solt CB, van Zijderveld-van Bemmel AM, Niewold TA, van Zijderveld FG (2006) Selection and optimization of proteolytically stable llama single-domain antibody fragments for oral immunotherapy. Appl Microbiol Biotechnol 72:544–551
13. Eijsink VG, Bjork A, Gaseidnes S, Sirevag R, Synstad B, van den Burg B, Vriend G (2004) Rational engineering of enzyme stability. J Biotechnol 113:105–120
14. van der Vaart JM, Pant N, Wolvers D, Bezemer S, Hermans PW, Bellamy K, Sarker SA, van der Logt CP, Svensson L, Verrips CT, Hammarstrom L, van Klinken BJ (2006) Reduction in morbidity of rotavirus induced diarrhoea in mice by yeast produced monovalent llama-derived antibody fragments. Vaccine 24:4130–4137
15. Hekkelman ML, Te Beek TA, Pettifer SR, Thorne D, Attwood TK, Vriend G (2010) WIWS: a protein structure bioinformatics Web service collection. Nucleic Acids Res 38:W719–W723

Chapter 23

Selection of Human VH Single Domains with Improved Biophysical Properties by Phage Display

Kip Dudgeon, Romain Rouet, Kristoffer Famm, and Daniel Christ

Abstract

Human antibody variable heavy (VH) domains tend to display poor biophysical properties when expressed in isolation. Consequently, the domains are often characterized by low expression levels, high levels of aggregation, and increased "stickiness." Here, we describe methods that allow the engineering of human VH domains with improved biophysical properties by phage display. The engineered domains withstand challenging conditions, such as high temperature and acidic pH. Engineered human single domains are a promising new class of antibody fragments and represent robust research tools and building blocks for the generation of antibody therapeutics.

Key words: Human VH domains, Aggregation, Phage display

1. Introduction

Human heavy chain variable (VH) domains tend to have poor biophysical properties when expressed in the absence of light chain partners (1–3). This includes low expression in bacteria and they readily aggregate upon concentration. They also generally do not unfold reversibly upon heating and have an unfortunate tendency to "stick" to gel-filtration matrices. These features are in marked contrast to single domains from camels and llamas (4) and initially prevented the wider use of human domains as research tools and therapeutics.

More recently, we have described phage display methods for the selection of aggregation-resistant human VH domains. These fully human domains display favorable properties in the absence of any "camelising" mutations. For this purpose, we have utilized geneIII display on filamentous bacteriophage using a multivalent system (2, 5, 6). A key aspect of the method is based on the fact that the phage particle is surprisingly resistant to physical and

Dirk Saerens and Serge Muyldermans (eds.), *Single Domain Antibodies: Methods and Protocols*,
Methods in Molecular Biology, vol. 911, DOI 10.1007/978-1-61779-968-6_23, © Springer Science+Business Media, LLC 2012

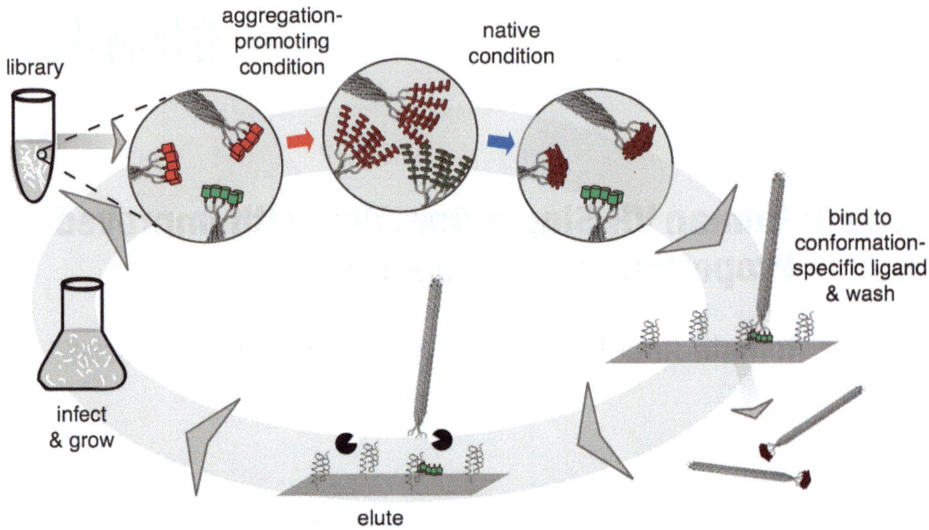

Fig. 1. Selection of VH domains with improved biophysical properties by phage display. Human VH domains are displayed on filamentous bacteriophage in a multivalent format. The domains are first exposed to aggregation-promoting conditions (heat or acid), followed by return to native conditions (room temperature, neutral pH). Human VH domains on phage that resist aggregation are then captured using a conformation-specific ligand (antigen or superantigen). After wash and elution steps, phages are amplified by infection of *E. coli* bacteria.

chemical challenges (such as temperatures exceeding 80°C and low pH) (7, 8). This allows the exposure of the displayed proteins to highly aggregation-promoting conditions, without affecting viability of the phage particle. A second feature of the method relates to the use of conformation-specific superantigens, such as protein A from *Staphylococcus aureus*. Protein A can be used as a probe for folded domains, as it selectively binds to a conformational epitope on folded VH, but does not bind to unfolded or aggregated domains (9). Alternatively, antigen binding can also be used as a selective pressure (2), particularly for VH domains that do not bind to protein A (e.g., domains other than VH3).

The selection process is outlined in Fig. 1 and essentially follows the established phage display selection cycle (10). For selection, a library of human VH domains is displayed on phage in a multivalent phage format. This format (rather than phagemid) is essential to achieve high local concentration of the VH domains on the tip of the bacteriophage. This can be achieved by cloning of VH genes from phagemid libraries into a multivalent phage vector. As the generation of libraries in phage vectors requires high quality DNA preparations, we provide a protocol for the in vitro amplification of phage DNA using Phi29 polymerase (11).

As a source of the domains, single framework synthetic human antibody libraries can be utilized (such as Tomlinson I/J or ETH-2) (12, 13). From these libraries, VH genes can be amplified either from the naïve repertoires or from antigen selections. Alternatively, additional diversity can be introduced through PCR or oligonucleotide-based mutagenesis methods. Once a repertoire of VH domains on phage has been generated, the displayed domains are exposed to aggregation-promoting conditions. Such conditions include temperatures significantly above the T_m of the domains (such as 80°C), or alternatively acidic conditions (such as pH 3) (14). Human VH domains that resist aggregation are next captured by binding to a conformation-specific ligand (such as antigen or superantigen). Finally, the selected domains are produced in a periplasmic expression vector and their aggregation propensity analyzed by size exclusion chromatography.

2. Materials

2.1. Amplification of VH genes by PCR

1. FdMyc phage vector (derived from FdTet (15), with a *c-Myc* tag introduced between the *Not*I site and geneIII).
2. Thermocycler (BioRad, Foster City, CA, USA).
3. Thermostable DNA polymerase and reaction buffers (e.g., Expand High Fidelity PCR System (Roche Applied Science, Mannheim, Germany)).
4. dNTPs: deoxynucleoside triphosphates (New England Biolabs, Ipswich MA, USA).
5. 2% Agarose gel: dissolve agarose in TBE buffer (2 g per 100 mL), melt agarose in microwave, and add SYBRSafe (Invitrogen, Carlsbad, CA, USA) or Ethidium Bromide to appropriate working concentration.
6. QIAprep Spin miniprep kit (Qiagen, Hilden, Germany).
7. QIAquick PCR purification kit (Qiagen, Hilden, Germany).
8. Primers used in cloning of VH genes into FdMyc phage vector (restriction sites are shown in italic). These will amplify VH3 domains such as present in the Tomlinson I/J or ETH-2 libraries; the use of other VH domains may require changes to the sequences shown in bold:
   (a) ApaLI_VHFwd: 5′-ACGC *GTGCAC* **AGGTGCA GCTGTTGG**-3′ (anneals in the 5′- region of VH genes and introduces *ApaLI* site).
   (b) VHNotI_Rev: 5′-CTGTTA *GCGGCCGC* **GCTCGAG ACGGTGACCAG**-3′ (anneals in the 3′-region of VH genes and introduces *Not*I restriction site).
9. Restriction enzymes *ApaLI*, *Not*I, and restriction enzyme buffers (New England Biolabs, Ipswich MA, USA).
10. Agarose for gel electrophoresis (Lonza, Basel, Switzerland).
11. TBE buffer: 10.6 g/L Tris base, 5.5 g/L boric acid, 4 mL/L of 0.5 M EDTA, pH 8.0.

12. 100 bp ladder DNA length marker (New England Biolabs, Ipswich MA, USA).
13. PCR purification kit, Plasmid miniprep kit (Qiagen, Hilden, Germany).
14. GoTaq polymerase (Promega, Fitchburg, WI, USA).
15. Water: use sterile, highly pure water such as autoclaved MilliQ (Millipore, Billerica, MA, USA).

2.2. Cloning of VH Genes into FdMyc Phage Display Vector

1. *Phi*29 DNA polymerase and 10× *Phi*29 Buffer (New England Biolabs, Ipswich, MA, USA).
2. Random hexamers (50 μM stock) (Applied Biosystems, Carlsbad, CA, USA).
3. BSA (100×) (New England Biolabs, Ipswich MA, USA).
4. 2× TY medium: 16 g/L bacto-tryptone, 10 g/L yeast extract, 5 g/L NaCl.
5. Amicon Ultra filter unit (10 kDa MWCO) (Millipore, Billerica, MA, USA).
6. Restriction enzymes *ApaLI*, *Not*I, and *Dpn*I and restriction enzyme buffers (New England Biolabs, Ipswich, MA, USA).
7. Sephacryl S-1000 resin (GE Healthcare, Little Chalfont, UK).
8. FLPC system, e.g., AKTA purifier (GE Healthcare, Little Chalfont, UK).
9. T4 DNA ligase and buffer (New England Biolabs, Ipswich, MA, USA).
10. *Escherichia coli* TG1 (Agilent, Santa Clara, CA, USA).
11. Colony PCR buffer: 2% of formamide, 1× *Taq* buffer, 200 μM dNTPs, 400 nM μL of each forward (FdMycFwd4) and reverse (G3Seq6) primers, 1.25 units of GoTaq polymerase.
12. FdMyc sequencing primers:
    (a) FdMycFwd4: 5′-AAATTCACCTCGAAAGCAAGC-3′.
    (b) G3seq6: 5′-CCCTCATAGTTAGCGTAACGA-3′.
13. Agarose for gel electrophoresis (Lonza, Basel, Switzerland).
14. TBE buffer: 10.6 g/L Tris base, 5.5 g/L boric acid, 4 mL/L of 0.5 M EDTA, pH 8.0.
15. 100 bp ladder DNA mass markers (New England Biolabs, Ipswich MA, USA).
16. PCR purification kit, Plasmid miniprep kit (Qiagen, Hilden, Germany).
17. GoTaq polymerase (Promega, Fitchburg, WI, USA).
18. 10 mM Tris–HCl, pH 8.5: 1.21 g/L Tris base, pH 8.5 using 5 M HCl.

2.3. Phage Production and Purification

1. *E. coli* TG1 (Agilent, Santa Clara, CA, USA).
2. TYE/tet agar (15 g/L agarose, 8 g/L NaCl, 10 g/L Bacto-tryptone, 5 g/L Yeast extract (Oxoid, Hampshire, UK) MilliQ water up to 1 L, autoclave), supplemented with 15 μg/mL tetracycline.
3. 2× TY/tet medium: 2× TY medium supplemented with 15 μg/mL tetracycline.
4. 0.45 μm vacuum filter unit (Corning, Midland, MI, USA).
5. 20% polyethylene glycol (PEG 6.000), 2.5 M NaCl.
6. PBS buffer: 8 g/L NaCl, 0.2 g/L KCl, 1.44 g/L Na_2HPO_4, 0.24 KH_2PO_4, pH 7.4.

2.4. Selection of Heat-Refoldable VH Domains on Phage

1. 96-well MaxiSorp Immunoplate (Nunc, Roskilde, Denmark).
2. Recombinant protein A (Sigma, St Louis, MO, USA).
3. Carbonate buffer: 100 mM $NaHCO_3$, 30 mm Na_2CO_3, pH 9.6.
4. PBST: 0.1% Tween-20 diluted in PBS.
5. 4% MPBS: 4 g/L skim-milk powder diluted in PBS.
6. 2% MPBS: 2 g/L skim-milk powder diluted in PBS.
7. Trypsin (Sigma, St Louis, MO, USA).
8. 2× TY medium.
9. TYE/tet agar: TYE agar supplemented with 15 μg/mL tetracycline.
10. *E. coli* TG1 (Agilent, Santa Clara, CA, USA).

2.5. Selection of Acid-Resistant VH Domains on Phage

1. 96-well MaxiSorp Immunoplate (Nunc, Roskilde, Denmark).
2. Recombinant protein A (Sigma, St Louis, MO, USA).
3. Carbonate buffer: 100 mM $NaHCO_3$, 30 mm Na_2CO_3, pH 9.6.
4. PBST: 0.1% (v/v) Tween-20 diluted in PBS.
5. 4% MPBS.
6. 2% MPBS.
7. HN7: 10 mM *N*-2-Hydroxyethylpiperazine-*N'*-2-ethanesulfonic acid [HEPES], 10 mM NaCl, pH 7.0.
8. 200 mM Citrate, pH 3.0.
9. 1 M Tris, pH 7.4.
10. Trypsin (Sigma, St Louis, MO, USA).
11. 2× TY medium.
12. TYE/tet agar.
13. *E. coli* TG1 (Agilent, Santa Clara, CA, USA).

2.6. Analysis of Aggregation-Resistance by Phage ELISA

1. Shaking incubator at 30°C.
2. 1.5 mL tubes (Eppendorf, Hamburg, Germany).
3. 2× TY medium.
4. 2× TY/tet medium.
5. 96-well MaxiSorp Immunoplate (Nunc, Roskilde, Denmark).
6. NHS-PEO_4-biotin (Pierce, Rockford, IL, USA).
7. PBS buffer.
8. PBST.
9. 4% MPBS.
10. 1 M Tris–HCl, pH 7.5.
11. 3 M Tris, pH 7.5.
12. 2 M Glycine-HCl, pH 2.5.
13. 2% BSA in PBS: 2 g/L bovine serum albumin (BSA)(Sigma, St Louis, MO, USA) dissolved in PBS buffer.
14. Thermocycler (BioRad, Foster City, CA, USA).
15. PCR strip tubes with strip caps (Axygen, Union City CA, USA).
16. Extravidin-HRP (Sigma, St Louis, MO, USA).
17. TMB substrate solution (BD Biosciences, San Diego CA, USA).
18. 1 M H_2SO_4.
19. ELISA plate washer and plate reader.
20. Platform shaker.

2.7. Cloning of VH Genes into Periplasmic Expression Vector

1. Primers used in cloning of VH genes into pET12a expression vector (restriction sites in italic). These will amplify VH3 domains such as present in the Tomlinson I/J or ETH-2 libraries; the use of other VH domains may require changes to the sequences shown in bold:
   (a) VH_SalIFwd: 5′-ACGC *GTCGAC* **AGTCGACGCA GGTGCAGCTGTTGG**-3′ (anneals in the 5′-region of VH gene and introduces *Sal*I restriction site).
   (b) VH_BamHIRev: 5′-CTGTTA *GGATCC* **GCTCGAGA CGGTGACCAG**-3′ (anneals in the 3′-region of VH gene and introduces *Bam*HI restriction site).
2. Colony PCR buffer: 2% of formamide, 1× *Taq* buffer, 200 μM dNTPs, 400 nM μl of each forward (T7Pro) and reverse (T7Term) primers, 1.25 units of GoTaq polymerase.
3. pET12a sequencing primers:
   (a) T7 Pro: 5′- TAATACGACTCACTATAGG-3′ (anneals approximately 150 bp upstream of insert in pET12a).
   (b) T7 Term: 5′- GCTAGTTATTGCTCAGCGG-3′ (anneals approximately 150 bp downstream of insert in pET12a).

4. Expand High Fidelity PCR kit (Roche Applied Science, Mannheim, Germany).
5. dNTPs (New England Biolabs, Ipswich, MA, USA).
6. pET12a expression vector (Novagen, Gibbstown, NJ, USA).
7. Restriction enzymes *Sal*I, *Bam*HI, and buffers; T4 ligase and buffer (New England Biolabs, Ipswich MA, USA).
8. TYE agar.
9. TYE/amp/tet/glu agar: TYE agar containing 100 μg/mL ampicillin, 15 μg/mL tetracycline, and 4% glucose.
10. *E. coli* BL21Gold (Agilent, Santa Clara, CA, USA).
11. Agarose for gel electrophoresis (Lonza, Basel, Switzerland).
12. TBE buffer.
13. 100 bp ladder DNA length marker (New England Biolabs, Ipswich, MA, USA).
14. PCR purification kit, Plasmid miniprep kit (Qiagen, Hilden, Germany).
15. GoTaq polymerase (Promega, Fitchburg, WI, USA).

2.8. Expression and Purification of Soluble VH Domains

1. *E. coli* BL21Gold (Agilent).
2. TYE/amp/tet/glu agar: TYE agar supplemented with 100 μg/mL ampicillin, 15 μg/mL tetracycline, 4% (v/v) glucose.
3. 2× TY/amp/tet/glu medium: 2× TY medium supplemented with 100 μg/mL ampicillin, 15 μg/mL tetracycline, 4% (v/v) glucose.
4. Sorvall centrifuge and centrifuge bottles (500 mM).
5. IPTG: Isopropyl β-D-1-thiogalactopyranoside (Gold Biotechnology, St. Louis MO, USA).
6. Disposable cuvettes (Eppendorf, Hamburg, Germany).
7. Spectrophotometer (Eppendorf, Hamburg, Germany).
8. 2.5 L baffled flasks.
9. rProtein A sepharose fast flow (GE Healthcare, Little Chalfont, UK).
10. Gravity flow column (BioRad, Foster City, CA, USA).
11. 0.1 M Glycine-HCl, pH 3.0.
12. Amicon Ultra centrifugal filter unit (10 kDa MWCO) (Millipore).
13. PBS buffer.
14. 0.45 μM vacuum filter unit (Corning, Lowell, MA, USA).
15. Periplasmic preparation buffer 1: 100 mM Tris–HCl, pH 8.0, 1 mM EDTA, 20% (w/v) sucrose.
16. Periplasmic preparation buffer 2: 5 mM $MgSO_4$.

17. Complete Mini EDTA free protease inhibitor (Roche Applied Science, Mannheim, Germany).
18. SnakeSkin dialysis tubing (Pierce, Rockford, IL, USA).

2.9. Characterization of Aggregation-Resistant VH Domains by Size Exclusion Chromatography

1. FLPC system, e.g., AKTA purifier (GE Healthcare, Little Chalfont, UK).
2. Superdex 75,10/300 GL gel filtration column (GE Healthcare, Little Chalfont, UK).
3. SpinX centrifuge tube filters 0.22 μm (Corning, Midland, MI, USA).
4. Thermocycler (BioRad, Foster City, CA, USA).

3. Methods

3.1. Amplification of VH Genes by PCR

1. Prepare the template DNA of VH (in phagemid vector or other) using a suitable DNA purification method such as a QIAprep Spin Miniprep kit and as specified by manufacturer.
2. Amplify DNA encoding the VH domains of interest, introducing *ApaL*I and Not*I* restriction enzyme sites for cloning into FdMyc vector. This can be achieved by PCR using the primers ApaLI_VHFwd and VHNotI_Rev. For this purpose, set up a PCR reaction using a suitable system such as the Expand High Fidelity PCR kit (Roche). Following the manufacturer's instructions, PCR reactions are performed in a total volume of 100 μL containing 1× buffer 2 (includes 1.5 mM $MgCl_2$), 200 μM dNTPs, 400 nM of each primer, 200 ng of template DNA, and 5 units of polymerase (Roche kit).
3. Heat reaction mix to 94°C for 5 min. Proceed with 25 cycles at 94°C (1 min), 55°C (1 min), and 72°C (1 min). Incubate at 65°C for 10 min for final elongation.
4. Analyze PCR products on a 2% agarose gel in TBE buffer to confirm correct size of PCR product (approximately 500 bp).
5. Purify amplified DNA fragments using a QIAquick PCR purification kit, eluting purified DNA in 30 μL of EB buffer.
6. Digest the PCR fragments overnight with *ApaL*I and *Not*I restriction enzymes, using restriction enzyme buffer NEB2 supplemented with BSA, overnight at 37°C.
7. Purify the digested fragments using a QIAquick PCR purification kit, eluting in 30 μL of EB buffer.

3.2. Cloning of VH Genes into FdMyc Phage Display Vector

1. Set up a *Phi*29 DNA amplification reaction containing 100 μL of 10× *Phi*29 buffer, 500 μM dNTPs, 50 μM random hexamers, and 1 μg of FdMyc template DNA (see Note 1), adjust volume

to 1 mL with sterile MilliQ water. Divide this reaction mixture into 5 × 200 μL aliquots in thin-walled PCR tubes and heat to 72°C for 5 min, before cooling to 30°C. Combine the samples into one tube.

2. Add 10 μL of BSA (100×) and 2.5 μL of *Phi*29 DNA polymerase. Incubate at 30°C for 6 h. Heat-inactivate polymerase by heating to 70°C for 20 min, cool to 4°C (the sample should be highly viscous at this stage).
3. Digest the amplified DNA by adding 300 μL of NEB2 buffer (10×), 30 μL of BSA (100×), 200 units of *ApaL*I and 400 units *Not*I restriction enzymes, and 30 units of *Dpn*I restriction enzyme. Adjust volume to 3 mL with sterile MilliQ water. Incubate overnight at 37°C, shaking at 250 rpm.
4. Concentrate the digested DNA to a final volume of 500 μL using an Amicon Ultra centrifugal filter unit (10 kDa MWCO), while rinsing the unit with 500 μL of 10 mM Tris–HCl, pH 8.5 on several occasions throughout the process.
5. Purify digested DNA using Sephacryl S-1000 column and a FLPC machine (e.g., AKTA purifier) in using running buffer (10 mM Tris, 100 mM NaCl, pH 7.4). Combine the main peak fractions and concentrate to approximately 50 ng/μL using an Amicon Ultra centrifugal filter unit (10 kDa MWCO).
6. Clone digested PCR products (see Subheading 3.1, step 7) into *ApaL*I/*Not*I digested FdMyc phage vector. Use a molar ratio of insert to vector of approximately 3:1 in a 10 μL reaction, using 400 units of T4 DNA ligase and 1× T4 DNA ligase buffer. Incubate at 23°C for 1 h and purify using a QIAquick PCR purification kit, eluting with 20 μL of 20% EB buffer diluted in sterile MilliQ water. Transform DNA into *E. coli* TG1 and grow single colonies overnight on a TYE/tet agar plate.
7. Screen for positive clones by PCR. For this, set up a 50 μL PCR reaction containing 48 μL of colony PCR buffer containing 400 nM each of FdMycFwd4 and G3Seq6 primers and 2 μL of bacterial overnight culture.
8. Heat reaction mixes to 94°C for 10 min. Proceed with 35 cycles of 94°C (30 s), 50°C (30 s), and 72°C (1 min). Incubate at 65°C for 10 min for final elongation.
9. Analyze PCR products on a 2% agarose gel in TBE buffer to confirm correct size of PCR product. Positive clones yield a PCR product of around 650 bp.
10. Confirm correct sequence of clones by DNA sequencing.

3.3. Phage Production and Purification

1. Inoculate 5 mL of 2× TY/tet medium with transformed TG1 bacteria and grow at 37°C, shaking at 250 rpm, until $OD_{600\ nm}$ reaches >1.

2. Inoculate 100 mL of 2× TY/tet medium in a conical flask with overnight culture to an $OD_{600\ nm}$ 0.1. Incubate overnight at 30°C (16–20 h), shaking at 250 rpm.
3. Centrifuge at 3,220 × *g* for 30 min at 4°C.
4. Filter the supernatant by passing through a 0.45 μm filter unit (do not use a 0.22 μm filter at this step).
5. Add 1/5 volume of 20% (w/v) polyethylene glycol (PEG), 2.5 M NaCl to supernatant. Incubate for at least 1 h on ice.
6. Centrifuge at 3,220 × *g* for 30 min at 4°C (phage in pellet). Resuspend each pellet in 4 mL of PBS.
7. Repeat PEG precipitation by adding 1 mL of 20% PEG, 2.5 M NaCl to phage solution. Incubate for 15 min on ice.
8. Centrifuge 3,220 × *g*, 30 min (phage in pellet).
9. Resuspend phage pellet in 1 mL of PBS or a smaller volume if appropriate.
10. Measure $OD_{260\ nm}$ (dilute 1/100) to estimate the number of phage using the following formula:

$$\text{Phage/mL} = OD_{260\ nm} \times 100 \times 22.14 \times 10^{10}.$$

11. Store phage at 4°C until further use.

3.4. Selection of Heat-Refoldable VH Domains on Phage

1. Coat an Immunotube or 96-well MaxiSorp Immunoplate plate with 50 μL/well of protein A at a concentration of 10 μg/mL, diluted in carbonate buffer pH 9.6. Incubate overnight (approximately16 h) at room temperature (23°C). Wash plate once with PBST and block the plate with 4% MPBS for more than 2 h. Wash the plate three times with PBST before use.
2. Dilute 10^{10} phages into 10 μL of PBS (1×10^{12} TU/mL). Heat phage to 80°C for 10 min then cool to 4°C for 10 min. Dilute phage to 800 μL in 2% MPBS and capture heat-refoldable domains on the protein A-coated plate (50 μL/well) by incubating at room temperature for 2 h, shaking gently.
3. Wash wells ten times with PBS and elute protein A-bound phage in 1 mg/mL trypsin in PBS for 10 min at room temperature.
4. Use the eluted phage to infect exponentially growing *E. coli* TG1 by incubation at 37°C for 30 min. Pellet bacteria by centrifugation at 3,220 × *g* for 20 min at 4°C. Resuspend cells in 1 mL of 2× TY medium and plate onto TYE/tet agar. Grow cells overnight at 37°C.
5. Select individual colonies, grow phage, and perform the heat-refoldable phage ELISA screen as described in Subheading 3.6 to determine the heat-refoldability of the clone.

3.5. Selection of Acid-Resistant VH Domains on Phage

1. Coat an Immunotube or 96-well MaxiSorp Immunoplate plate with 50 μL/well of protein A at a concentration of 10 μg/mL, diluted in carbonate buffer pH 9.6. Incubate overnight

(approximately16 h) at room temperature (23°C). Wash plate once with PBST and block the plate with 4% MPBS for more than 2 h. Wash the plate three times with PBST before use.

2. Dilute approximately 1×10^{10} phages in 5 μL of HN7 (2×10^{12} TU/mL) and add equal volumes of 200 mM citrate, pH 3.0 (final pH is 3.2). Incubate phage at 37°C for 2 h and neutralize reaction by adding equal volumes of 1 M Tris–HCl, pH 7.4. Dilute phage to 800 μL in 2% MPBS and capture acid-resistant domains on the protein A-coated plate (50 μL/well) by incubating at room temperature for 2 h, shaking gently.
3. Proceed as described earlier (see Subheading 3.4, steps 3–5) above, following the protocol for the acid-resistant phage ELISA screen as described below (see Subheading 3.6).

3.6. Analysis of Aggregation-Resistance by Phage ELISA

1. Coat a 96-well MaxiSorp Immunoplate plate with 50 μL/well of protein A or antigen at a concentration of 5–10 μg/mL diluted in carbonate buffer, pH 9.6. Incubate overnight (approximately16 h) at room temperature (23°C). Wash plate once with PBST and block the plate with 4% MPBS for more than 2 h. Wash the plate three times with PBST before use.
2. Inoculate 3 mL of 2× TY/tet medium in a 15 mL round bottom tube with VH-FdMyc clone (transformed in *E. coli* TG1) and incubate overnight at 30°C, shaking at 260 rpm (see Note 2).
3. The following day, transfer 1 mL of bacterial culture to a 1.5 mL tube and centrifuge at 16,000 × *g* for 10 min at 4°C.
4. Transfer supernatant, containing phages, into a fresh 1.5 mL tube and add NHS-PEO_4-biotin to a final concentration of 50 μM and incubate for 2 h at room temperature (see Note 3). Quench biotinylation reaction by adding 1 M Tris–HCl, pH 7.5 to a final concentration of 100 mM for 1 h at room temperature. Incubate for 1 h at room temperature.
5. Subject the VH domains to the desired denaturing conditions, as follows:
   (a) *Heat-refoldability*: Transfer half of the biotinylated phages into PCR strip tubes (100 μL per tube) and incubate tubes in a PCR machine preheated at 80°C for 10 min. Remove tubes and incubate them at 4°C for 10 min. Allow samples to equilibrate to room temperature for 15 min before adding to antigen/protein A-coated plate.
   (b) *Acid-resistance*: Add 250 μL of biotinylated phage samples to tubes containing 50 μL of 2 M Glycine-HCl, pH 2.5. This will result in a final pH of approximately 3.0. Incubate for 3 h at 37°C and neutralize by adding 200 μL of 3 M Tris, pH 7.5.
6. Add treated and untreated biotinylated phages to protein A/antigen-coated plates at 50 μL/well. Incubate for 1 h at room temperature on platform shaker.

7. Wash ELISA plate three times with PBST and incubate with 50 μL/well of extravidin-HRP (diluted 1:2000 in 2% BSA in PBST). Incubate for 30 min at room temperature on platform shaker.
8. Wash ELISA plate three times with PBST and develop with 50 μL/well TMB substrate. Incubate at room temperature for 30 min or until sufficient color has developed.
9. Stop reaction by adding 50 μL/well of 1 M H_2SO_4.
10. Read ELISA plate at 450 nm (reference at 630 nm).
11. Determine the retained protein A binding after treatment by expressing the absorbance of the treated sample as a percentage of the untreated sample.

3.7. Cloning of VH Genes into Periplasmic Expression Vector

1. Prepare the template DNA of VH in FdMyc using a suitable DNA purification method such as a QIAprep Spin Miniprep kit.
2. PCR-amplify the DNA encoding the VH genes of interest, introducing *Sal*I and *BamH*I restriction enzyme sites for cloning into the pET12a vector. This can be achieved by PCR using the primers VH_*Sal*IFwd and VH_*Bam*HIRev. For this purpose, set up a PCR reaction using a suitable system such as the Expand High Fidelity PCR kit (Roche). Following the manufacturer's instructions, PCR reactions are performed in a total volume of 100 μL containing 1× buffer 2 (includes 1.5 mM $MgCl_2$), 200 μM dNTPs, 400 nM primers each, 200 ng of template DNA, and 5 units of polymerase (Roche kit).
3. Heat reaction mix to 94°C for 5 min. Proceed with 25 cycles at 94°C (1 min), 55°C (1 min), and 72°C (1 min). Incubate at 65°C for 10 min for final elongation.
4. Analyze PCR products on a 2% agarose gel in TBE buffer to confirm correct size of PCR product (approximately 500 bp).
5. Purify amplified DNA fragments using a QIAquick PCR purification kit, eluting purified DNA in 30 μL of EB buffer.
6. Digest the PCR fragments overnight with *Sal*I and *BamH*I restriction enzymes, using restriction enzyme buffer NEB3 supplemented with BSA, overnight at 37°C.
7. Purify the digested fragments using a QIAquick PCR purification kit, eluting in 30 μL of EB buffer.
8. Clone digested PCR products into *Sal*I/*BamH*I-digested pET12a vector. Use a molar ratio of insert to vector of approximately 3:1 in a 10 μL reaction, using 400 units of T4 DNA ligase and 1× T4 DNA ligase buffer. Incubate at 23°C for 1 h and purify using a QIAquick PCR purification kit, eluting with 20 μL of water. Transform DNA into *E. coli* BL21Gold and grow single colonies overnight on a TYE/amp/tet/glu agar plate.
9. Screen for positive clones by PCR. For this, set up a 50 μL PCR reaction containing 48 μL of colony PCR buffer containing

400 nM each of T7Pro and T7Term primers and 2 μL of bacterial overnight culture.

10. Heat reaction mixes to 94°C for 10 min. Proceed with 35 cycles of 94°C (30 s), 50°C (30 s), and 72°C (1 min). Incubate at 65°C for 10 min for final elongation.
11. Analyze PCR products on a 2% agarose gel in TBE buffer to confirm correct size of PCR product. Positive clones yield a PCR product of around 650 bp.
12. Confirm sequence of clones by DNA sequencing.

3.8. Expression and Purification of Soluble VH Domains

1. Freshly transform DNA preparation of VH in pET12a into *E. coli* BL21Gold, plate on TYE/amp/tet/glu agar, and incubate overnight at 37°C.
2. Inoculate 5 mL of 2× TY/amp/tet/glu medium with a single colony and incubate overnight at 37°C, shaking at 260 rpm.
3. Inoculate 1 L 2× TY/amp/tet/glu medium in a 2.5 L baffled flask with overnight culture to an $OD_{600\ nm}$ 0.1 and incubate at 37°C, 260 rpm until $OD_{600\ nm}$ 0.5–0.7.
4. Transfer culture to 2×500 mL centrifuge bottles and spin down at 3,220×*g* for 20 min at 4°C.
5. Discard supernatant and resuspend bacterial pellet in 1 L 2× TY/amp/tet (no glucose) medium containing 1 mM IPTG.
6. Incubate at 30°C for 24–42 h. If expressing for 42 h, re-induce after 24 h by adding IPTG (1 mM final) and ampicillin (100 μg/mL final) after 24 h of growth.
7. Spin down bacteria at 6,400×*g* for 15 min at 4°C.
8. Filter supernatant through a 0.45 μm vacuum filter (see Note 4).
9. Add PBS-washed rProtein A sepharose to the filtered supernatant (5 mL of sepharose per liter of culture) and incubate overnight at 4°C on a roller.
10. Transfer beads to a gravity flow column then run the supernatant by gravity.
11. Wash beads twice with 10 mL of PBS.
12. Elute the antibody by adding 15–20 mL of 0.1 M Glycine – HCl, pH 3.0 and collecting 1 mL fractions. Neutralize by adding 250 μL of 1 M Tris–HCl, pH 8.0 to each fraction.
13. Measure $OD_{280\ nm}$ of eluted fractions and combine those containing protein.
14. Concentrate antibody and change buffer to PBS using an Amicon Ultra centrifugal filter unit (10 kDa MWCO).
15. Measure final concentration of purified protein by measuring $OD_{280\ nm}$.
16. Store purified VH protein at 4°C if used within days to weeks, otherwise snap freeze in liquid nitrogen and store at −20°C.

3.9. Characterization of Aggregation-Resistance VH Domains by Size Exclusion Chromatography

1. Prepare 1 mL of purified VH protein at 10 μM (see Note 5) (diluted into PBS).
2. Aliquot 5 × 100 μL into PCR tubes and heat at 80°C for 10 min, 4°C for 10 min. Combine the aliquots and transfer to a 1.5 mL tube. Centrifuge both the heated and unheated samples at 16,000 × *g* for 10 min at 4°C.
3. Remove the supernatant, transfer to a 0.22 μm SpinX filter unit and briefly centrifuge at 16,000 × *g* for 2 min at 4°C.
4. Run 500 μL of the unheated and heated sample sequentially on a Superdex-G75 gel filtration column, equilibrated with PBS, at a flow rate of 0.5 mL/min.
5. Calculate the recovery of the VH by measuring the area under the curve of the heated sample, expressed as a percentage of the unheated sample.

4. Notes

1. Best results are obtained using FdMyc ssDNA as a template for Phi29 amplification. Grow TG1 cells transformed with FdMyc overnight (approximately 16 h) at 30°C in 2× TY medium supplemented with 15 μg/mL tetracycline. Remove cells by centrifugation and PEG precipitate phage as described previously (see Subheading 3.3, steps 4–7). Once purified phages are obtained, isolate ssDNA using QIAprep Spin M13 Kit according to the manufacturer's instructions.
2. Leaving a sterile tip in the 15 mL tube after inoculation improves aeration.
3. Biotinylate 2× TY medium as a negative control.
4. Optional step—Periplasmic extraction of VH protein:
   (a) Resuspend bacterial pellet in 50 mL of periplasmic preparation buffer 1, add complete Mini EDTA free protease inhibitor tablet and incubate on ice for 1 h.
   (b) Centrifuge at 17,000 × *g* for 15 min at 4°C and transfer supernatant into 50 mL tube.
   (c) Resuspend pellet in 50 mL of periplasmic preparation buffer 2 and incubated on ice for 30 min.
   (d) Centrifuge at 17,000 × *g* for 15 min at 4°C and transfer supernatant into 50 mL tube.
   (e) Dialyse extractions 1 and 2 against PBS in SnakeSkin dialysis tubing overnight at 4°C, using a magnetic stirrer (change dialysis buffer multiple times).

(f) Combine dialysed extractions 1 and 2 and filter through 0.45 μm filter unit.

(g) Purify VH protein as described in Subheading 3.8, steps 9–16.

5. Guideline only. Protein concentration may have to be adapted depending on VH domain.

Acknowledgements

Protocols are based on methods originally developed by D. Christ and others in Greg Winter's group at the MRC Laboratory of Molecular Biology and were modified in our laboratory at the Garvan Institute. This work was funded by the Garvan Institute of Medical Research, the Australian National Health and Medical Council, the Cancer Institute NSW, and the United Kingdom Medical Research Council.

References

1. Ewert S, Huber T, Honegger A, Pluckthun A (2003) Biophysical properties of human antibody variable domains. J Mol Biol 325: 531–553
2. Jespers L, Schon O, Famm K, Winter G (2004) Aggregation-resistant domain antibodies selected on phage by heat denaturation. Nat Biotechnol 22:1161–1165
3. Tomlinson IM, Walter G, Marks JD, Llewelyn MB, Winter G (1992) The repertoire of human germline V_H sequences reveals about fifty groups of V_H segments with different hypervariable loops. J Mol Biol 227:776–798
4. Ewert S, Cambillau C, Conrath K, Pluckthun A (2002) Biophysical properties of camelid V_{HH} domains compared to those of human V_H3 domains. Biochemistry 41:3628–3636
5. Christ D, Famm K, Winter G (2007) Repertoires of aggregation-resistant human antibody domains. Protein Eng Des Sel 20:413–416
6. Dudgeon K, Famm K, Christ D (2009) Sequence determinants of protein aggregation in human V_H domains. Protein Eng Des Sel 22:217–220
7. Holliger P, Riechmann L, Williams RL (1999) Crystal structure of the two N-terminal domains of g3p from filamentous phage fd at 1.9 A: Evidence for conformational lability. J Mol Biol 288:649–657
8. Kristensen P, Winter G (1998) Proteolytic selection for protein folding using filamentous bacteriophages. Fold Des 3:321–328
9. Jansson B, Uhlen M, Nygren PA (1998) All individual domains of staphylococcal protein A show Fab binding. FEMS Immunol Med Microbiol 20:69–78
10. Lee CM, Iorno N, Sierro F, Christ D (2007) Selection of human antibody fragments by phage display. Nat Protoc 2:3001–3008
11. Christ D, Famm K, Winter G (2006) Tapping diversity lost in transformations-*in vitro* amplification of ligation reactions. Nucleic Acids Res 34:e108
12. Ascione A, Flego M, Zamboni S, De Cinti E, Dupuis ML, Cianfriglia M (2005) Application of a synthetic phage antibody library (ETH-2) for the isolation of single chain fragment variable (scFv) human antibodies to the pathogenic isoform of the hamster prion protein (HaPrPsc). Hybridoma (Larchmt) 24: 127–132
13. de Wildt RM, Mundy CR, Gorick BD, Tomlinson IM (2000) Antibody arrays for high-throughput screening of antibody-antigen interactions. Nat Biotechnol 18: 989–994
14. Famm K, Hansen L, Christ D, Winter G (2008) Thermodynamically stable aggregation-resistant antibody domains through directed evolution. J Mol Biol 376:926–931
15. Zacher AN 3rd, Stock CA, Golden JW 2nd, Smith GP (1980) A new filamentous phage cloning vector: Fd-tet. Gene 9:127–140

Chapter 24

Improvement of Single Domain Antibody Stability by Disulfide Bond Introduction

Yoshihisa Hagihara and Dirk Saerens

Abstract

The successful medical application of single domain antibodies largely depends on their functionality. This feature is partly determined by the intrinsic stability of the single domain. Therefore a lot of research has gone into the elucidation of rules to uniformly increase stability of antibodies. Recently, a novel intra-domain disulfide bond was independently discovered by two research groups, after either rational design or careful investigation of the naturally occurring camelid antibody repertoire. By introducing this particular disulfide bond within a single domain antibody, the conformational stability can be increased in general. In this chapter it is described how to introduce this extra intra-domain disulfide bond and how to estimate the biophysical and biochemical impact of this cystine on the domain.

Key words: Disulfide bond, Thermal stability, Chemical stability, Circular dichroism, Fluorescence, Surface plasmon resonance

1. Introduction

Antibodies and antibody-derived fragments constitute excellent building blocks for therapeutic and diagnostic tools. However problems with insufficient stability hampered immediate widespread application of antibodies and antibody-derived fragments. Even single domain antibodies do not generally posses the necessary intrinsic stability upon isolation. Many techniques have been proposed to tackle this problem either before (1), during (2, 3), or after (4) their isolation. The stability of a protein in vitro is defined by two concepts, the resistance against harsh conditions and the thermodynamic stability. The resistance of the protein against environmental stress is generally probed by incubation of the protein in an extreme, nonphysiological condition followed by measuring the residual activity at physiological conditions. Conversely, the thermodynamic stability is measured by following

Dirk Saerens and Serge Muyldermans (eds.), *Single Domain Antibodies: Methods and Protocols*,
Methods in Molecular Biology, vol. 911, DOI 10.1007/978-1-61779-968-6_24, © Springer Science+Business Media, LLC 2012

the conformational change upon variance of temperature, denaturant concentration, or pH.

The variable domains of camelid heavy-chain antibodies (VHH or Nanobody—Nb) are known to be remarkably stable (5). For example, they are highly resistant to heat as compared to conventional antibodies. After incubating at 90°C and cooling down to room temperature, most VHHs are still able to bind their antigen in contrast to mouse monoclonal antibodies (6, 7). This reveals the highly efficient refolding process of the VHHs after heat treatment (8, 9). This remarkable reversibility of (un-)folding is also observed upon acid treatment. This property is used to make affinity beads with immobilized VHH against human IgG, commercialized as a substitution of protein A or G column for IgG purification (IgSelect: GE Healthcare, Buckinghamshire, UK). Additionally, the thermodynamic stability of these camelid single domain antibodies is comparable to that of domains of conventional antibodies (5, 8–10).

Several examples exist and nicely illustrate the application of VHHs in extreme environments. Van der Vaart et al. examined the possibility of oral administration of VHHs to treat diarrhea caused by rotavirus (11). Although the VHHs neutralized rotavirus effectively in vitro, complete inhibition of the infection could not be obtained. For effective rotavirus inhibition, VHHs should resist the acidic pH of the gut. In another example, Ladenson et al. suggested that an anti-caffeine VHH can be used for measurement of caffeine in hot coffee by dipstick format (7). In this case, the single domain antibody needs to be folded correctly and be able to bind to the antigen at elevated temperature. To accomplish that goal, not only folding reversibility but also increased thermodynamic stability is required. Since not every single domain antibody is endowed with the necessary intrinsic stability for optimal performance in the foreseen application, additional antibody engineering needs to be performed.

An elegant solution to increase the stability of single domain antibodies was discovered from the study of the variable domains of heavy-chain antibodies from *Camelidae*. It is based on two amino acid substitutions within the framework to form an additional intra-domain disulfide bond while having minimal effects on antigen affinity. Such extra disulfide bond can be inserted between amino acid positions 49 and 69 (Kabat numbering; the positions are 54 and 78 in IMGT numbering, [http://www.imgt.org/]), and significantly increased the thermodynamic stability (12, 13) (see Figs. 1 and 2). Strikingly these mutations were found independently either by prediction based on the crystal structure of llama VHH (12), or in a naturally occurring camelid VHH (13). So far, the significant stabilizing effect of this disulfide bond was observed in several different VHHs, suggesting that the extra disulfide bond between those amino acid positions universally increases the thermodynamic stability of single domain antibodies. To our knowledge,

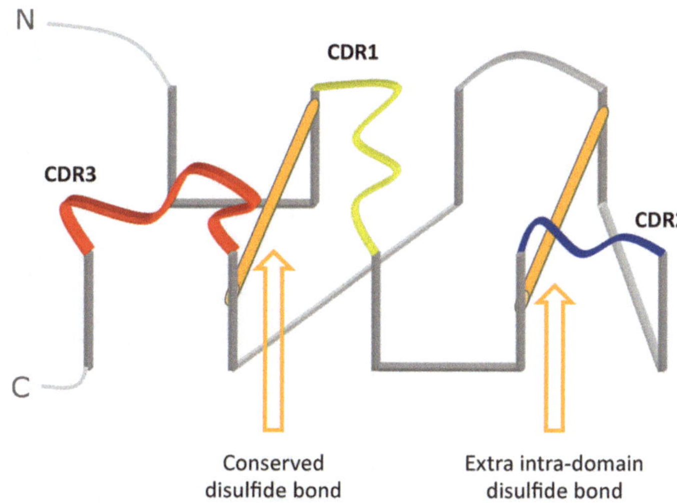

Fig. 1. Structural representation of a VHH containing the extra intra-domain disulfide bond. The framework is represented in *gray*. The CDR1, CDR2, and CDR3 are labeled and colored in *yellow*, *blue*, and *red*, respectively. Both the conserved and extra intra-domain disulfide bonds are labeled and shown in *orange* tubes.

equivalent antibody engineering of VH and VL would most likely result in similar stability increase due to the conserved nature of the hydrophobic core around those amino acid residues within VH, VL, and VHH. In this chapter, the methods to introduce this disulfide bond and to estimate the impact of the extra intra-domain disulfide bond on the domain are described.

2. Materials

Materials which are not described step-by-step should be prepared either by following the instructions from manufacturers/suppliers of the kits, reagents, etc. or according to Sambrook and Russell (14). In addition, prepare all solutions using ultrapure water (prepared by purifying deionized water to attain a sensitivity of 18 MΩ cm at 25°C) and analytical grade reagents. Prepare and store all reagents at room temperature (unless indicated otherwise). Diligently follow all waste disposal regulations when disposing waste materials.

2.1. PCR-Based Mutagenesis Using PCR Product as a Megaprimer

1. PCR primers: Design the forward and reverse primers for your single domain antibody. These primers should ideally be about 30 bp long and have t_m-values of more than 55°C. The primers are designed having a TGT or TGC codon in the middle of the primers (see Note 1). The primer with the mutation at position 49 and 69 is the forward and reverse primer, respectively.

```
              1        10        20         30          40        50         60         70        80        90        100        110            120          Tm(°C)  Cm (M)  Ref.
IMGT          |********|*********|****** ***|******** *|*********|***** ****|***** ****|*********|*********|*********|**** *****|*12*123***** **|********
              1         10        20         30             40        50         60         70        80        90         100            110
KABAT         |********.|*********|***** ****|*****a. bc****|*********| **abc***** **|****.*****|*********|**abc*******|** *******|abcdefgh** *******|***
              <--------framework-1-----> <----CDR-H1---><-framework-2><-------CDR-H2-------><--------- framework-3 ---------><-----CDR-H3----><framework4>

cAbhCG        QVQLQESGG GLVQAGGSLRLSCAAS GRTGSTYDMG     WFRQAPGKERESVAA INW   DSART YYASSVR GRFTISRDNAKKTVYLQMNSLKPEDTAVYTC GAGEGGTW        DS WGQGTQVTVSS   64             12
cABhCG 2SSVHH QVQLQESGG GLVQAGGSLRLSCAAS GRTGSTYDMG     WFRQAPGKERESVCA INW   DSART YYASSVR GRFTCSRDNAKKTVYLQMNSLKPEDTAVYTC GAGEGGTW        DS WGQGTQVTVSS   74             12

cAbPSA-N8     DVQLQESGG.GLVQPGGSLRLSCAAS GFLFSDTY.... MTWARQAPGKGLEWLGG ISKDGSGT.. LYEDSVE.GRFTISRDNAKNTLYLQMNSLKSEDTALYYC STGALLP..T...RP... QGQGTQVTVSS   52     1.24    13
cAbPSA-C12    DVQLQESGG.GLVRPGGSLRLSCAAS GFLFSGTY.... MTWARQAPGKGLEWLCG INKDGSGT.. LYADSVE.GRFTCSRDNAKNTLYLQMNSLKSEDTALYYC STGALLP..T...RP... QGQGTQVTVSS   62     1.87    13

cAbBCII10_1-0-0 QVQLVESGG.GSVQAGGSLRLSCTAS GGSEYSYSTFS. LGWFRQAPGQEREAVAA IASMGGLT.. YYADSVK.GRFTISRDNAKNTVTLQMNNLKPEDTAIYYC AAVRGYFMRLPSSHNFRY WGQGTQVTVSS   78     3.28    13
cAbBCII10_1-0-1 QVQLVESGG.GSVQAGGSLRLSCTAS GGSEYSYSTFS. LGWFRQAPGQEREAVCA IASMGGLT.. YYADSVK.GRFTCSRDNAKNTVTLQMNNLKPEDTAIYYC AAVRGYFMRLPSSHNFRY WGQGTQVTVSS   87     3.77    13

cAbAn33_1-0-0 DVQLVESGG.GSVQAGGSLRLSCAVS GSTYSPCT.... TGWYRQAPGKEREWVSS ISSPGTI... YYQDSVK.GRFTISRDNAKNTVYLQMNSLQREDTGMYYC QIQCGVR..S...IREY. WGQGTQVTVSS   71     2.12    13
cAbAn33_1-0-1 DVQLVESGG.GSVQAGGSLRLSCAVS GSTYSPCT.... TGWYRQAPGKEREWVCS ISSPGTI... YYQDSVK.GRFTCSRDNAKNTVYLQMNSLQREDTGMYYC QIQCGVR..S...IREY. WGQGTQVTVSS  >90     3.62    13

cAbGFP4_1-0-0 QVQLVESGG.ALVQPGGSLRLSCAAS GFPVNRYS.... MRWYRQAPGKEREWVAG MSSAGDRS.. SYEDSVK.GRFTISRDDARNTVYLQMNSLKPEDTAVYYC NVNVGFE..Y........ WGQGTQVTVSS   70     2.14    13
cAbGFP4_1-0-1 QVQLVESGG.ALVQPGGSLRLSCAAS GFPVNRYS.... MRWYRQAPGKEREWVCG MSSAGDRS.. SYEDSVK.GRFTCSRDDARNTVYLQMNSLKPEDTAVYYC NVNVGFE..Y........ WGQGTQVTVSS   76     2.43    13
```

Fig. 2. Amino acid sequences of wild-type VHHs and mutants with extra disulfide bonds (12, 13). Both IMGT (http://www.imgt.org/) and Kabat numbering (26) are shown. The cysteines are indicated in *bold* and those for extra disulfide bonds are *underlined*. The mid-point temperature of thermal unfolding (t_m-value) and the mid-point of chemical denaturation (C_m-value) at neutral pH are shown for each protein.

2. PCR reagents. High fidelity DNA polymerase without terminal transferase activity, such as *Pfu* turbo (Agilent Technologies, Santa Clara CA, USA). When dNTP is not supplied with enzyme, usually 2 mM dNTPs Mixture (TOYOBO, Osaka, Japan) should suffice.
3. *Dpn*I (TOYOBO, Osaka, Japan).
4. Thermocycler and agarose gel electrophoresis equipment.
5. QIAquick Gel Extraction Kit (Qiagen, Hilden, Germany).

2.2. Examination of Disulfide Bond Formation by Ellman's Assay

1. UV-2500PC (Shimadzu, Kyoto, Japan) or equivalent measurement instrument.
2. Micro cuvette (Shimadzu, Kyoto, Japan). The micro cuvette requires 100 μL of sample solution. The volume of reagents may differ depending on the number of samples and which measurement instrument used.
3. 1 M Na-phosphate (pH 6.5). Filter through a 0.22 μm membrane and store at room temperature.
4. Assay solution for protein concentration determination: 7.5 M GdmCl, 25 mM Na-phosphate, pH 6.5. Prepare as follows: add 2.5 mL of 1 M Na-phosphate (pH 6.5) to 71.64 g of GdmCl, gradually add H_2O till solid GdmCl is completely dissolved, adjust the volume to 100 mL with H_2O, filter through a 0.22 μm membrane and store at room temperature.
5. 1 M Tris–HCl (pH 8.5). Filter through a 0.22 μm membrane and store at room temperature.
6. 8 M GdmCl in 0.2 M Tris–HCl (pH 8.5). Prepare as follows: add 10 mL of 1 M Tris–HCl (pH 8.5) to 38.2 g of GdmCl, gradually add H_2O till solid GdmCl is completely dissolved, adjust the volume to 50 mL with H_2O, store at room temperature.
7. 10 mM 5,5′-dithiobis(2-nitrobenzoic acid) (DTNB) in 0.2 M Tris buffer (pH 8.5). Prepare as follows: take 2 mg of solid DTNB in a 1.5 mL microtube, dissolve DTNB to a concentration of 10 mM by adding 505 μL of 0.2 M Tris–HCl (pH 8.5). Prepare just before use (see Note 2).
8. Ellman's assay solution. Prepare as follows: dilute the DTNB solution (10 mM) with nine volumes of 8 M GdmCl in 0.2 M Tris–HCl (pH 8.5). The final concentration of DTNB is 1 mM. Prepare just before use.

2.3. Thermal Unfolding Monitored by Circular Dichroism

1. Spectropolarimeter J-820 with PTC-423L Peltier device type temperature controller (Jasco, Tokyo, Japan) or equivalent measurement instrument.
2. Synthetic quartz cell (GL Science, Tokyo, Japan): 621021006 with light path 10 mm width and height 450 mm.

3. Purified protein (>95% pure as determined on Coomassie stained SDS-PAGE).
4. 1 M K-phosphate (pH 6.3). Filter through a 0.22 μm membrane and store at room temperature.
5. 5 M NaCl. Filter through a 0.22 μm membrane and store at room temperature.
6. 10× measurements buffer: 200 mM K-phosphate, 1.5 M NaCl, pH 6.3. Prepare as follows: mix 400 μL of 1 M K-phosphate (pH 6.3) with 600 μL of 5 M NaCl and 1 mL of H_2O (see Note 3).

2.4. Denaturant-Induced Unfolding Monitored by Fluorescence

1. Amino-Bowman series-2 luminescence spectrometer (Thermo Fisher Scientific, Waltham MA, USA) or equivalent measurement instrument.
2. Precision Cells made of Quartz Suprasil (Hellma, Müllheim, Germany). A 101-QS with light path 10 mm with maximum volume of 2 mL.
3. Purified protein (>95% pure as determined on Coomassie stained SDS-PAGE) at a concentration of 3 mg/mL.
4. 50 mM Na-phosphate buffer (pH 7.0). Filter through a 0.22 μm membrane and store at room temperature.
5. 200 mM Na-phosphate buffer (pH 7.0). Filter through a 0.22 μm membrane and store at room temperature.
6. 7 M GdmCl stock solution: 66.87 g of GdmCl, 100 mL of 200 mM Na-phosphate (pH 7.0). Prepare as follows: add H_2O to completely dissolve the GdmCl, adjust the pH to 7.0 with NaOH, and add H_2O to a final volume of 100 mL.

2.5. Measurement of Affinity by Surface Plasmon Resonance

1. Biacore machine such as 2000, 3000, or T100.
2. Biacore consumables such as CM5 chips (GE Healthcare, Buckinghamshire, UK).
3. Purified protein (>95% pure as determined on Coomassie stained SDS-PAGE).
4. HBS-EP Biacore buffer: 0.01 M HEPES, 0.15 M NaCl, 3.4 mM EDTA, 0.005% surfactant Tween-20, pH 7.4 (GE Healthcare, Buckinghamshire, UK).

3. Methods

Methods which are not described step-by-step should be carried out either by following the instructions from manufacturers/suppliers of the kits, reagents, etc. or according to Sambrook and Russell (14).

3.1. PCR-Based Mutagenesis to Introduce the Novel Intra-Domain Disulfide Bond

In the original paper (12), both Cys mutations were introduced one at a time. In a recent preparation of the mutated gene with two new cysteines, a PCR product was used as megaprimer for "QuickChange" mutagenesis (Agilent Technologies, Santa Clara CA, USA) (15–17).

1. Prepare the megaprimer. Each primer is diluted to 10 μM in H_2O. About 10 ng of template plasmid with the wild-type sequence are mixed with both primers (1 μL, 10 pmole) and PCR reaction reagents in a final reaction volume of 100 μL. The PCR reaction can be carried out following the standard protocol described in the manual of the polymerase using a thermocycler. Confirm the proper amplification of the PCR product by agarose gel electrophoresis (see Note 4).
2. Purify the reaction mixture using QIAquick Gel Extraction Kit (Qiagen, Hilden, Germany) with addition of isopropanol and absorption of DNA in the spin column, as described in the protocol for the purification of enzymatic reaction shown in manual provided by the manufacturer. Elute the PCR product, i.e., the megaprimer, with 30 μL of H_2O (see Note 5).
3. Mutate the plasmid containing the wild-type single domain antibody gene using megaprimer from the previous step. Mix 50 ng template plasmid, 10 μL of megaprimer (see Subheading 3.1, step 2), and PCR reaction reagents. Adjust the reaction volume to 25 μL with H_2O. Set the PCR cycles to 20 and extension time to 2 min/kb of template plasmid (see Note 6). This PCR process of annealing template and megaprimer is generally carried out at 51°C and extension process is carried out at 68°C.
4. Add 1 μL of *Dpn*I to the PCR reaction and incubate at 37°C for 1 h. Clean up the reaction mixture by QIAquick Gel Extraction Kit and elute with 30 μL of H_2O.
5. Transform the cleaned reaction mixture using electrocompetent *Escherichia coli* XL-1 Blue provided by the kit manufacturer (Agilent, Santa Clara CA, USA) (see Note 7).
6. Pick several colonies to verify the sequence of plasmids for the introduction of desired mutation and the absence of unintended mutations at other positions within the single domain antibody coding region (see Note 8).
7. Expression of wild-type and mutant single domain antibodies is performed as described in other chapters of this volume.

3.2. Examination of Disulfide Bond Formation by Ellman's Assay

1. Determine the protein concentration using UV absorption of Trp, Tyr, and Cys. Based on the amino acid composition, calculate the molar extinction coefficient using the published parameters, in which molar extinction coefficients of Trp, Tyr, and half-cystine at 280 nm were 5,690, 1,280, and 120 M cm

in 6 M GdmCl and 20 mM phosphate (pH 6.5), respectively (18) (see Note 9). Dilute the stock protein solution (about 1 mg/mL) with four volumes of assay solution for protein concentration determination (7.5 M GdmCl and 25 mM Na-phosphate (pH 6.5)). Measure the UV-spectra of buffer (6 M GdmCl and 20 mM phosphate prepared by mixing one volume of water and four volume of assay solution for protein concentration determination) for baseline and protein sample. The protein concentration is estimated by absorption at 280 nm using the calculated extinction coefficient.

2. Prepare the protein solution adjusting the single domain antibody concentration between 20 and 50 μM, which corresponds to about 0.3–0.6 mg/mL.
3. Mix the same volume of assay buffer and protein solution, and prepare the reference solution including the same volume of water and assay solution. Promptly add the solutions to the sample and reference cuvettes.
4. Monitor the absorption at 412 nm at room temperature until there is no further increase of absorption.
5. Read the endpoint absorption at 412 nm is used for estimation of molar concentration of free thiol. The molar extinction coefficient of reduced 2-nitro-5-thiobenzoic acid (TNB) is originally estimated to be 13,600 and this value has been widely used including our lab (19) (see Note 10). The single domain antibody with the extra intra-domain disulfide encompasses either four or six cysteines, depending on the absence or presence of an interloop disulfide bond (see Note 11).

3.3. Thermal Unfolding Monitored by Circular Dichroism

Mid-point temperature of thermal unfolding (t_m) is the good index for thermal stability of protein. Measurement of the t_m-value using circular dichroism (CD) requires only a small amount of sample and is easy to perform.

1. Start the spectropolarimeter at least 30 min earlier than measurements.
2. Dilute the protein to a concentration of about 0.05 mg/mL using 10× measurement buffer and water in 10 mm cuvette by mixing with stirrer (see Note 12). The required sample volume is usually 2 mL and thermocouple should be dipped into the solution.
3. Measure the CD spectrum at far-UV region from 255 to 200 nm at 25 and 95°C to define the wavelength at which to monitor the conformational change induced by heat. Determine the wavelength whereby the difference between folded and unfolded spectra is the largest. As for VHHs, the spectra of native and unfolded states with extra disulfide bonds showed relatively large difference at 235 nm (see Fig. 3a) (see Note 13).

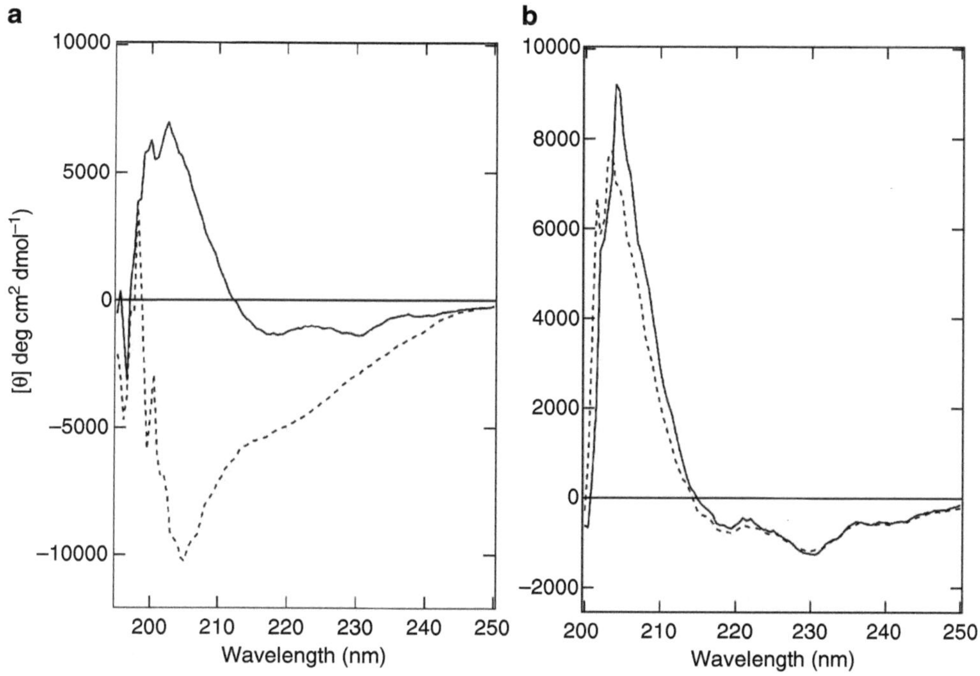

Fig. 3. CD spectra of the VHH cAbhCG with extra disulfide bond at different conditions in 20 mM K-phosphate (pH 6.3) and 150 mM NaCl. (**a**) CD spectra of the VHH with extra disulfide bond (20 μM) were measured at 15°C (*solid line*) and 92°C (*broken line*). To obtain the good spectra for reader's clarity, a 1 mm cuvette was used. (**b**) The reversibility of thermal unfolding was checked by measuring CD spectra of sample (4 μM) before (*solid line*) and after (*broken line*) thermal unfolding using 10 mm cuvette at 15°C. The spectra were similar between before and after unfolding, suggesting that thermal unfolding is reversible at the experimental condition.

4. Discard the sample and prepare new sample as described above (see Subheading 3.3, step 2).
5. Adjust the temperature of the cell holder to the start temperature. Set the cuvette with new sample in cell holder and start mixing with the stirrer. To draw the correct baseline, it is best to set the start temperature at least 20°C lower than the expected t_m-value (see Note 14). The end point temperature can be about 20°C higher than t_m-value of the wild-type single domain antibody. For example, the VHH with extra disulfide bond is very stable and the end point temperature can be more than 90°C.
6. Measure the CD spectrum at far-UV region from 255 to 200 nm at the starting temperature (see Fig. 3b).
7. Gradually increase the temperature at the rate of 1°C/min and collect the data every 0.1 or 0.2°C (see Fig. 4a).
8. After completing the measurements, immediately start cooling the sample by setting the temperature of cell holder to initial value. After temperature of sample is reached to the initial temperature, measure the CD spectrum. Comparison of the

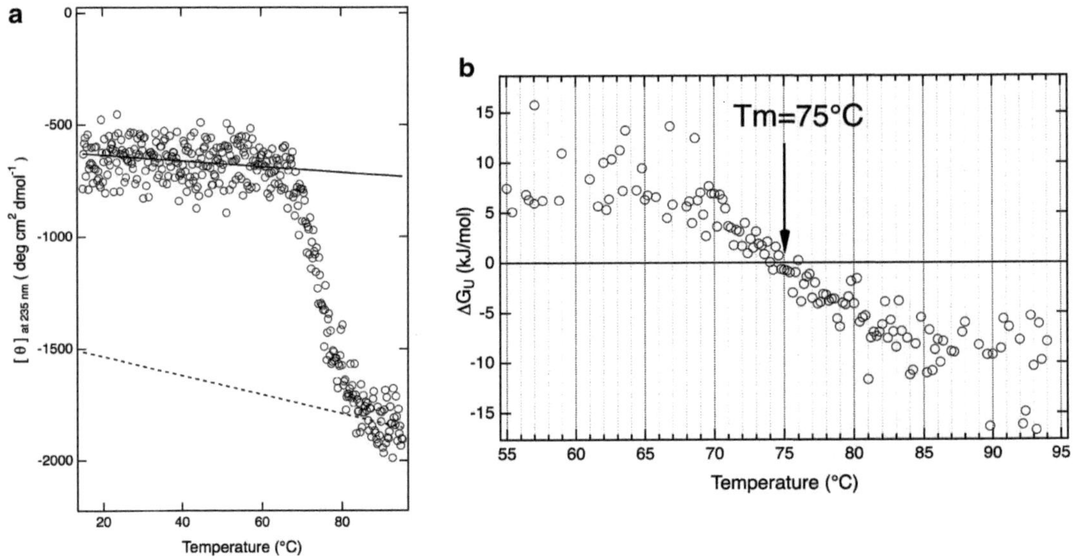

Fig. 4. Unfolding curves monitored at 235 nm (**a**) and temperature dependence of ΔG_U (**b**) of VHH (cAbhCG) with extra disulfide bond. (**a**) The unfolding curve was measured in 20 mM K-phosphate (pH 6.3) and 150 mM NaCl at the protein concentration of 4 μM in 10 mm cuvette. *Solid* and *broken lines* show baselines for the native and unfolded states, respectively. (**b**) Temperature dependence of ΔG_U was calculated by Eqs. 2, 3, 4, 5, and 6. The cross point of ΔG_U and *zero line* indicates that t_m-value at this condition was 75°C.

spectra recorded before and after thermal unfolding gives the information of reversibility of the reaction (see Fig. 3b).

9. Record the spectra and ellipticity at measured wavelength of buffer solution as blank.

10. Store the data as a text file. Usually analysis of the CD data is performed using Igor Pro (WaveMetrics, Inc., Lake Oswego, OR, USA), but other software can be used. First, subtract the blank and convert the observed ellipticity θ_{obs} to mean residue ellipticity (θ) using following equation:

$$[\theta] = \theta_{obs} 100 / (cln) \quad (1)$$

where *c*, *l*, and *n* are molar concentration of protein, path length (cm), and number of amino acid of the protein, respectively. Subsequently, draw the base lines of the native BL_N and unfolded states BL_U. The baselines and fraction of unfolding protein, $Fra_U(t)$, can be described as:

$$BL_N(t) = BL_N(0) - tBL_{N,slope} \quad (2)$$

$$BL_U(t) = BL_U(0) - tBL_{U,slope} \quad (3)$$

$$Fra_U(t) = (BL_N(t) - Unf_{obs}(t)) / (BL_N(t) - BL_U(t)) \quad (4)$$

where t and $\mathrm{Unf}_{\mathrm{exp}}(t)$ is the temperature (°C) and observed unfolding curve, respectively. The equilibrium constant of unfolding reaction is:

$$\mathrm{K_U}(t) = \mathrm{Fra_U}(t) / (1 - \mathrm{Fra_U}(t)) \quad (5)$$

Gibbs free energy of unfolding can be calculated using following equation:

$$\Delta \mathrm{G_U}(t) = -R(t + 273.15)\ln K_{\mathrm{U}}(t) \quad (6)$$

where R is gas constant (8.314 J/mol/K).

The plot of $\Delta G_{\mathrm{U}}(t)$ against t is shown in Fig. 4b. The t_{m}-value is defined as the temperature where the $\Delta G_{\mathrm{U}} = 0$, the temperature at the cross point of ΔG_{U} and zero line gives the t_{m}-value.

3.4. Denaturant-Induced Unfolding Monitored by Fluorescence

Mid-point concentration of denaturant-induced unfolding (C_{m}) is the concentration of denaturating agent where half of all the protein in a sample is denatured. This C_{m}-value is the good index for conformational stability of protein and can be used to compare stabilities among different single domain antibodies. Measurement of the C_{m}-value using fluorescence requires much larger amounts of protein as compared to CD measurements.

1. Prepare the intrinsic fluorescence measurement instrument. Set the measurement temperature at 25°C. The excitation wavelength is set at 280 nm. The emission scan is usually performed from wavelengths 300–420 nm at a scan rate of 1 nm/s.
2. Dissolve the protein in 50 mM Na-phosphate buffer (pH 7.0) to a concentration of about 1 mg/mL.
3. Prepare various GdmCl concentrations. Calculate for a total volume of 2 mL, the volume required from the 7 M GdmCl stock and 50 mM Na-phosphate buffer (pH 7.0) for preparation of different GdmCl concentration between 0 and 6 M GdmCl in a volume of 1.950 mL (see Note 15). Prepare the different concentrations as calculated.
4. Add 50 μL of the protein solution (see Subheading 3.4, step 2) in each tube containing different GdmCl concentrations in order to have a final volume of 2 mL (see Note 16).
5. Prepare reference samples of the concentration series without protein, i.e., the protein volume as specified previously (see Subheading 3.4, step 4) is replaced by 50 μL of 50 mM Na-phosphate buffer (pH 7.0).
6. Gently shake the samples and incubate them overnight at room temperature.
7. Record the intrinsic fluorescence spectrum from 300 to 420 nm for each GdmCl concentration in ascending order. Spectra obtained from cAbPSA-N8 (see Fig. 5a) and cAbPSA-C12 (see Fig. 5b) at 0 and 5 M GdmCl are provided as examples.

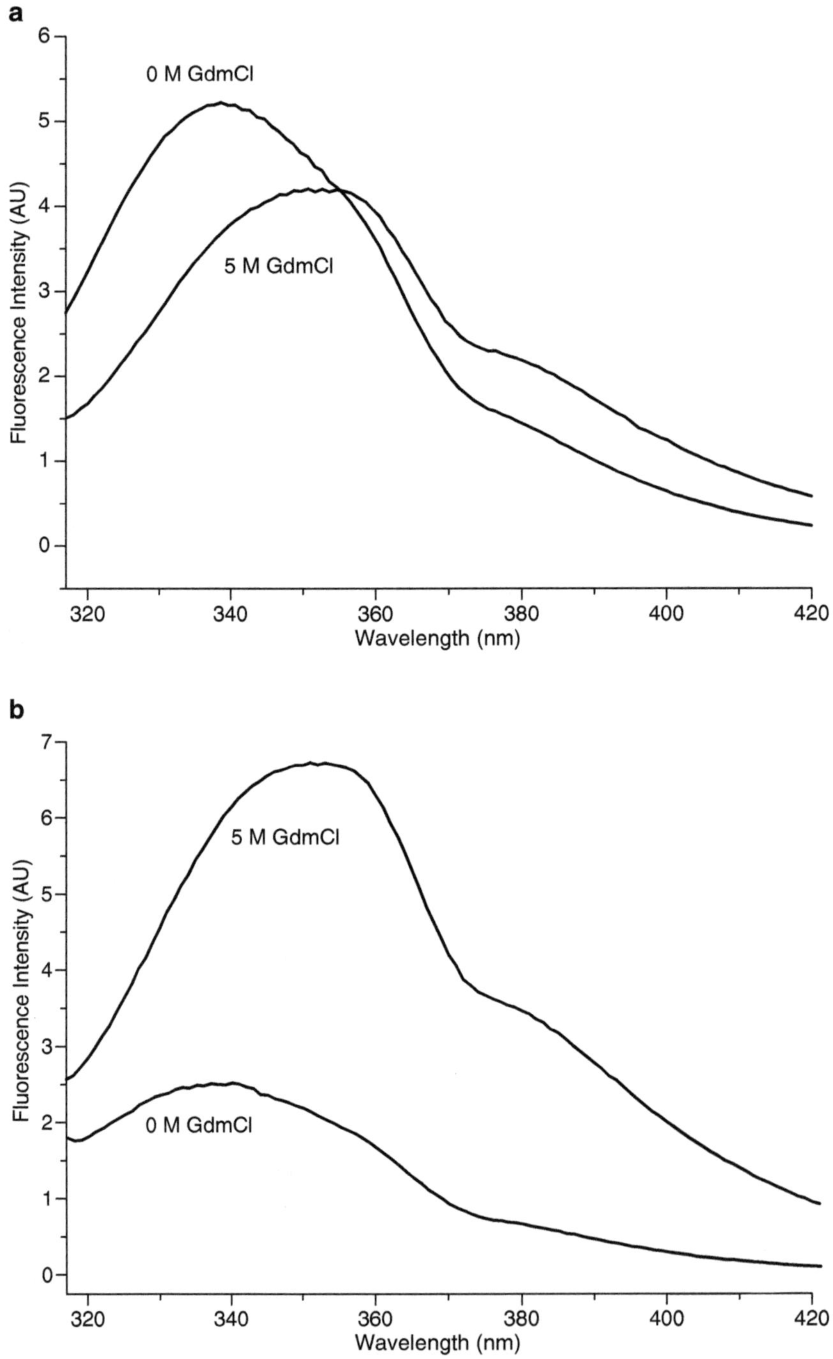

Fig. 5. Tryptophan fluorescence spectra of cAbPSA-N8 (**a**) and cAbPSA-C12 (**b**) at 0 and 5 M GdmCl concentrations. The spectra were recorded at 25°C and the excitation wavelength was 280 nm.

8. Correct the recorded signal for the background of the solution for all measured samples.
9. Store the data as a text file. Usually analysis of the intrinsic fluorescence data is performed using Origin (OriginLab, USA),

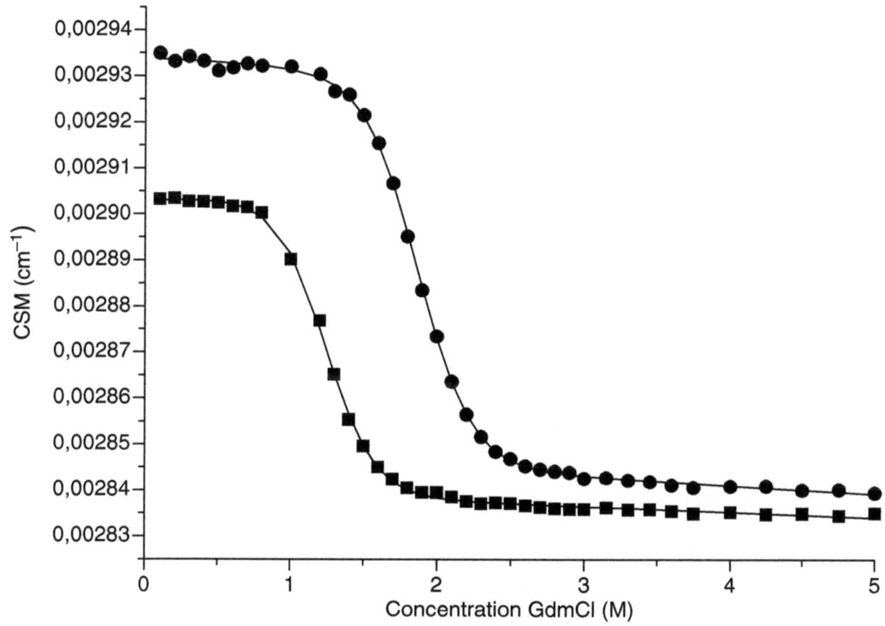

Fig. 6. GdmCl-induced denaturation of cAbPSA-N8 (*filled square*) and cAbPSA-C12 (*filled circle*) as shown by the changes in the mass center of the tryptophan fluorescence spectrum (CSM). The data were analyzed on the basis of a two-state model, and the *lines* represent the best fit to Eq. 8.

but other software programs can be used. Plot the unfolding data as detailed below (see Fig. 6). The fluorescence spectra are usually described as a function of concentration of GdmCl by the center of spectral mass (CSM), which is the weighted mean of the fluorescence:

$$\mathrm{CSM} = \frac{\sum(\upsilon_i F_i)}{\sum F_i} \quad \text{and} \quad \upsilon_i = \frac{1}{\lambda_i} \tag{7}$$

where υ_i is the wavenumber, λ_i the wavelength, and F_i the fluorescence intensity at υ_i. Alternatively, $F_{340\ \mathrm{nm}}/F_{360\ \mathrm{nm}}$ as a function of GdmCl concentration represents the shift in fluorescence, since the signal is most sensitive to GdmCl at those wavelengths. Fitting of unfolding data is determined by fitting CSM and/or $F_{340\ \mathrm{nm}}/F_{360\ \mathrm{nm}}$ into the following model (5):

$$y_{\mathrm{obs}} = \frac{[(y_{\mathrm{N}} + px) + (y_{\mathrm{U}} + qx)e^{(M(x-C_{\mathrm{m}})/a)}]}{1 + e^{(M(x-C_{\mathrm{m}})/a)}} \tag{8}$$

where x is the GdmCl concentration, M a measure for the dependence of $\Delta G°$ to GdmCl concentration, y_{obs} the measured fluorescence at denaturant concentration x, and y_{N} and y_{U} the signal for the native and unfolded state, respectively.

This model is based on the assumption of (un-)folding via a simple two-state mechanism ($\mathrm{N} \rightleftarrows \mathrm{U}$), which is exact for most VHHs (5).

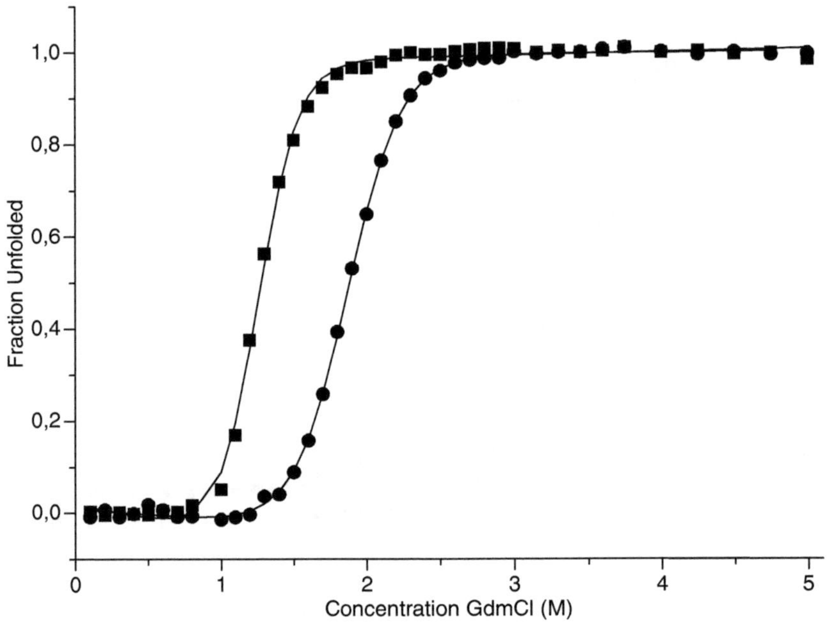

Fig. 7. Fraction of cAbPSA-N8 (*filled square*) and cAbPSA-C12 (*filled square*) unfolded as a function of GdmCl concentration. The values were calculated from the data from Fig. 6 and according to the Eqs. 2, 3, 4, and 5.

Fitting of the unfolding data into Eq. 8, and plotting the fraction unfolded against the concentration of GdmCl (see Fig. 7), yields C_m-values. The fraction of unfolded can be calculated according to the Eqs. 2, 3, 4, and 5, with changing the temperature (°C) to the concentration (*M*). Since conformational stability was determined from equilibrium chemical unfolding experiments, the free energy of folding ΔG° could be determined by:

$$C_m = \frac{\Delta G^\circ}{M} \qquad (9)$$

10. In order to validate the ΔG° values, reversibility experiments need to be carried out. Two samples of each protein are prepared: one sample contains 50 μg of protein and 0.5 M GdmCl into 50 mM Na-phosphate buffer (pH 7.0) in a total volume of 2 mL. This sample represents the native state of the protein. The second sample contains 50 μg of protein and 5 M GdmCl into 50 mM Na-phosphate buffer (pH 7.0) in a total volume of 200 μL, which reflects the unfolded state of the protein. Samples are incubated at room temperature overnight. The next day, the second sample is diluted with 1.8 mL 50 mM Na-phosphate buffer (pH 7.0), creating an identical environmental condition for the protein as the first sample. Fluorescence of both samples is subsequently measured as described above in Subheading 3.4, steps 7 and 8. Both spectra should be identical in order to prove that chemical unfolding by GdmCl is completely reversible (see Note 17).

3.5. Measurement of Affinity by Surface Plasmon Resonance

1. Prepare the Biacore system (GE Healthcare, Buckinghamshire, UK) for surface plasmon resonance (SPR) analysis (see Note 18). Set the measurement temperature at 25°C. Perform the necessary maintenance before starting the measurements, e.g., Desorb and Prime according to the manufacturer recommendations. Insert a CM5 chip, dock, and perform the necessary startup procedures such as Prime and Normalize according to the manufacturer recommendations.
2. The following is the example of experiment of which the antigen is human chorionic gonadotropin (hCG). Dissolve hCG (Sigma-Aldrich Co., MO, USA) in H_2O to a final concentration of 5 mg/mL.
3. Subsequently mix the 5 μL of hCG stock solution and 495 μL of 10 mM Na-Acetate pH 6.0 (see Note 19) at 20°C. This hCG solution is used for immobilization to sensor chip (CM5 sensor chip from GE Healthcare, Buckinghamshire, UK) by amine coupling (see Note 20).
4. According to the manual of your SPR system, set the target resonance unit to 1,000 and immobilize the antigen (see Note 21).
5. Prepare the serial dilution of the single domain antibody. In the case of the cAbhCG, of which K_D is about 20 nM, we used 15.6, 31.3, 62.5, 125, 250, and 500 nM dilution samples. Insert the concentration samples into the Biacore and measure the binding curves at 25°C using kinetic mode. The regeneration buffer is 20 mM HCl (pH 1.8) (see Note 22).
6. Analyze the kinetic data using the software with the equipment, such as BIAevaluation (GE Healthcare, Buckinghamshire, UK).

4. Notes

1. Usage of both Cys codons (TGT and TGC) are more than 30% in *E. coli*, *Saccharomyces cerevisiae*, and human.
2. The solution containing DTNB should be kept in the dark.
3. Avoid the use of Tris-based buffers, since the pH of Tris-based buffer significantly changes dependent on the temperature (20). The temperature dependencies of other buffers are described by Fukada and Takahashi (21).
4. If the template plasmid is different from that used in the second PCR reaction, add 1 μL of *Dpn*I to the reaction mixture and incubate at 37°C for 1 h. Ensure that the plasmid DNA template is isolated from a dam+ *E. coli* strain. The majority of the common used *E. coli* strains are dam+. Plasmid DNA isolated from dam− strains, e.g., JM110 and SCS110, is not suitable.

5. Other methods for PCR product purification can be used. As the PCR product of this experiment is a short double-strand DNA, the methods should be applicable to the small fragment less than 100 bp.
6. The speed of extension depends on the enzyme. In the case of *Pfu* turbo, 2 min/kb of template is required.
7. The eluted DNA (3 μL) gives thousands of colonies.
8. The amount of template plasmid, PCR cycles, and annealing temperature can be changed if the experiment is failed, as in the case of no mutants obtained.
9. Slightly different molar extinction coefficients of these amino acids are also reported (22). When these parameters are used, molar extinction coefficient can be calculated via Expasy Protparam tool (http://expasy.org/tools/protparam.html).
10. There are a number of reports that extinction coefficient of DTNB is sensitive to the environments, such as temperature and ionic strength (23–25). Nevertheless, the deviation between experimental conditions is less than 5% at most.
11. In our preparation of VHH (cAbhCG) with extra disulfide bond using *Pichia pastoris*, about 8% of total cysteines is reduced. There can be two incompletely oxidized species: VHH with no disulfide bond and VHH with one disulfide bond. If the latter is the most of the case, about 16% of total cAbhCG mutant has only one disulfide bond. The heat treatment at 65°C for 2 h and subsequent purification using gel filtration decreased the number of reduced cysteines to less than 5% of total cysteines.
12. This protein concentration (0.05 mg/mL) is higher than that for proteins including helical structure, since the difference of CD spectrum between the native and thermal unfolded states is not large (see Fig. 3a).
13. At the shorter wavelength, such as at 210 nm, the difference is larger than at 235 nm; however, the signal to noise ratio decreases. Thus, the wavelength of 235 nm is preferably selected for thermal stability in the case of VHH with extra disulfide bond.
14. If the t_m-value of a sample is unknown, start around 10°C. If condensation is a problem at low temperatures, increase the flow of N_2-gas or increase the initial temperature slightly, for example, to 15°C.
15. Since 50 μg (50 μL) of VHH is required per single measurement and around 50 measurement points are required for good data analysis, about 3 mg of purified VHH is required for the complete measurement of chemical unfolding.

16. This is a very delicate step during the preparation of the samples, since any minor change of the total volume will introduce measurement errors in the unfolding curve. It is advised to take time to prepare these samples.
17. The intrinsic fluorescence spectra should be imposable before further thermodynamic analysis is performed. If these are not imposable, then the unfolding is not a two-state process and the thermodynamic parameters calculated (see Subheading 3.4, step 9) do not have a physical meaning.
18. Other machinery to measure kinetics based on SPR of QCM can be applied.
19. pH is the critical factor for immobilization. It is important to confirm the pH of buffer before immobilization. It is recommended to perform a rigorous analysis on the most optimal immobilization pH before performing the actual immobilization. It is recommended to check Biacore manual for further instructions.
20. In addition to antigen immobilization, VHH with histidine tag also can be immobilized by Ni-NTA sensor chip. In our experience, coupling the antigen on the CM5 chip and injecting different VHH concentrations to determine the K_D-value gives better results than using the Ni-NTA sensor chip.
21. According to the molecular weight of the antigen to be coupled onto the CM5 chip, determine the most optimal amount to be coupled according to the Biacore manual.
22. In most cases for protein–protein interactions, 10 mM glycine-HCl (pH 2.0–2.5) is an excellent regeneration buffer. It is, however, recommended to do a rigorous regeneration analysis to determine the most optimal regeneration condition according to the Biacore manual.

Acknowledgements

No financial interest is declared by the authors. We would like to thank Ms. Kaede Lilian-Komaba, Ir. Jochen Govaert, and Dr. Ir. Cécile Vincke for critically reading the manuscript.

References

1. Vincke C, Loris R, Saerens D, Martinez-Rodriguez S, Muyldermans S, Conrath K (2009) General strategy to humanize a camelid single-domain antibody and identification of a universal humanized nanobody scaffold. J Biol Chem 284:3273–3284
2. Jespers L, Schon O, Famm K, Winter G (2004) Aggregation-resistant domain antibodies selected on phage by heat denaturation. Nat Biotechnol 22:1161–1165
3. Famm K, Hansen L, Christ D, Winter G (2008) Thermodynamically stable aggregation-resistant

antibody domains through directed evolution. J Mol Biol 376:926–931
4. Saerens D, Pellis M, Loris R, Pardon E, Dumoulin M, Matagne A, Wyns L, Muyldermans S, Conrath K (2005) Identification of a universal VHH framework to graft non-canonical antigen-binding loops of camel single-domain antibodies. J Mol Biol 352:597–607
5. Dumoulin M, Conrath K, Van Meirhaeghe A, Meersman F, Heremans K, Frenken LG, Muyldermans S, Wyns L, Matagne A (2002) Single-domain antibody fragments with high conformational stability. Protein Sci 11:500–515
6. van der Linden RH, Frenken LG, de Geus B, Harmsen MM, Ruuls RC, Stok W, de Ron L, Wilson S, Davis P, Verrips CT (1999) Comparison of physical chemical properties of llama VHH antibody fragments and mouse monoclonal antibodies. Biochim Biophys Acta 1431:37–46
7. Ladenson RC, Crimmins DL, Landt Y, Ladenson JH (2006) Isolation and characterization of a thermally stable recombinant anti-caffeine heavy-chain antibody fragment. Anal Chem 78:4501–4508
8. Ewert S, Cambillau C, Conrath K, Pluckthun A (2002) Biophysical properties of camelid V(HH) domains compared to those of human V(H)3 domains. Biochemistry 41:3628–3636
9. Perez JM, Renisio JG, Prompers JJ, van Platerink CJ, Cambillau C, Darbon H, Frenken LG (2001) Thermal unfolding of a llama antibody fragment: a two-state reversible process. Biochemistry 40:74–83
10. Hagihara Y, Matsuda T, Yumoto N (2005) Cellular quality control screening to identify amino acid pairs for substituting the disulfide bonds in immunoglobulin fold domains. J Biol Chem 280:24752–24758
11. van der Vaart JM, Pant N, Wolvers D, Bezemer S, Hermans PW, Bellamy K, Sarker SA, van der Logt CP, Svensson L, Verrips CT, Hammarstrom L, van Klinken BJ (2006) Reduction in morbidity of rotavirus induced diarrhoea in mice by yeast produced monovalent llama-derived antibody fragments. Vaccine 24:4130–4137
12. Hagihara Y, Mine S, Uegaki K (2007) Stabilization of an immunoglobulin fold domain by an engineered disulfide bond at the buried hydrophobic region. J Biol Chem 282: 36489–36495
13. Saerens D, Conrath K, Govaert J, Muyldermans S (2008) Disulfide bond introduction for general stabilization of immunoglobulin heavy-chain variable domains. J Mol Biol 377:478–488
14. Sambrook J, Russell DW (2001) Molecular cloning: a laboratory manual, 3rd edn. Cold Spring Harbor Lab Press, Plainview
15. Weiner MP, Costa GL, Schoettlin W, Cline J, Mathur E, Bauer JC (1994) Site-directed mutagenesis of double-stranded DNA by the polymerase chain reaction. Gene 151:119–123
16. Barik S (1997) Mutagenesis and gene fusion by megaprimer PCR. Methods Mol Biol 67: 173–182
17. Miyazaki K, Takenouchi M (2002) Creating random mutagenesis libraries using megaprimer PCR of whole plasmid. Biotechniques 33: 1033–1038
18. Edelhoch H (1967) Spectroscopic determination of tryptophan and tyrosine in proteins. Biochemistry 6:1948–1954
19. Ellman GL (1958) A colorimetric method for determining low concentrations of mercaptans. Arch Biochem Biophys 74:443–450
20. Bates RG, Robinson RA (1973) Tris (hydroxymethyl) aminomethane. Useful secondary pH standard. Anal Chem 45:420
21. Fukada H, Takahashi K (1998) Enthalpy and heat capacity changes for the proton dissociation of various buffer components in 0.1 M potassium chloride. Proteins 33:159–166
22. Pace CN, Vajdos F, Fee L, Grimsley G, Gray T (1995) How to measure and predict the molar absorption coefficient of a protein. Protein Sci 4:2411–2423
23. Eyer P, Worek F, Kiderlen D, Sinko G, Stuglin A, Simeon-Rudolf V, Reiner E (2003) Molar absorption coefficients for the reduced Ellman reagent: reassessment. Anal Biochem 312: 224–227
24. Riddles PW, Blakeley RL, Zerner B (1983) Reassessment of Ellman's reagent. Methods Enzymol 91:49–60
25. Riddles PW, Blakeley RL, Zerner B (1979) Ellman's reagent: 5,5′-dithiobis(2-nitrobenzoic acid)–a reexamination. Anal Biochem 94:75–81
26. Kabat EA, Wu TT, Perry HM, Gottsman KS, Foeller C (1991) Sequences of proteins of immunologic interest, 5th edn. Public Health Service, National Institutes of Health, US Department of Health and Human Services, Bethesda

Chapter 25

Characterization of Single-Domain Antibodies with an Engineered Disulfide Bond*

Greg Hussack, C. Roger MacKenzie, and Jamshid Tanha

Abstract

Camelidae single-domain antibodies (VHHs) represent a unique class of emerging therapeutics. Similar to other recombinant antibody fragments (e.g., Fabs, scFvs), VHHs are amenable to library screening and selection, but benefit from superior intrinsic biophysical properties such as high refolding efficiency, high solubility, no tendency for aggregation, resistance to proteases and chemical denaturants, and high expression, making them ideal agents for antibody-based drug design. Despite these favorable biophysical characteristics, further improvements to VHH stability are desirable when considering applications in adverse environments like high heat, low humidity, pH extremes, and the acidic, protease-rich gastrointestinal tract. Recently, the introduction of a disulfide bond into the hydrophobic core of camelid VHHs increased antibody thermal and conformational stability. Here, we present additional protocols for characterizing the effects of the introduced disulfide bond on a panel of llama VHHs. Specifically, we employ mass spectrometry fingerprinting analysis of VHH peptides to confirm the presence of the introduced disulfide bond, size exclusion chromatography, and surface plasmon resonance to examine the effects on aggregation state and target affinity, and circular dichroism spectroscopy and protease digestion assays to assess the effects on thermal and proteolytic stability. The disulfide bond stabilization strategy can be incorporated into antibody library design and should lead to hyperstabilized single-domain antibodies (VHHs, VHs), and possibly Fabs and scFvs, if selection pressures such as denaturants or proteases are introduced during antibody selection.

Key words: Single-domain antibody, Antibody engineering, Disulfide bond, Stability, Melting temperature, Protease resistance

1. Introduction

In recent years, recombinant antibody fragments (e.g., scFvs, Fabs, VHHs, VNARs, VHs, VLs) have been explored as alternatives to monoclonal antibodies, a highly successful class of biological therapeutics. A drawback to some recombinant antibody formats is their poor stability, which is one of the key determinants of antibody

*This is National Research Council Canada Publication 50015.

Dirk Saerens and Serge Muyldermans (eds.), *Single Domain Antibodies: Methods and Protocols*, Methods in Molecular Biology, vol. 911, DOI 10.1007/978-1-61779-968-6_25, © Springer Science+Business Media, LLC 2012

efficacy. A number of strategies have been explored to enhance antibody stability in the context of increased thermal stability, pH stability, protease resistance, serum half-life, and reduced aggregation tendency. For example, some strategies include: selection of antibodies from display libraries panned in the presence of proteases (1), heat (2, 3), acidic pH (4), or other selection pressures (5), introduction of disulfide bonds (6) and other stabilizing mutations (7, 8), random mutagenesis (9, 10), and PEGylation (11).

Of all the recombinant antibody formats, VHHs are considered one of the most stable with high solubility, high thermal, chemical, and conformational stability, inherent protease resistance, and lack of tendency to aggregate (12–14). However, further stability enhancements of these domains are desirable for applications in harsh environments such as the gastrointestinal tract which compromises protein integrity due to high acidity (stomach) and protease contents (e.g., pepsin, trypsin, chymotrypsin). Recently, it was shown that introducing artificial disulfide bonds into the hydrophobic core of *Camelidae* VHHs resulted in increased thermal and conformational stability with only minor reductions in antigen binding affinity (15–17).

In this chapter we provide additional protocols on the functional characterization of VHHs with introduced disulfide bonds (see Chapter 24). Specifically, we describe protocols for the characterization of *Clostridium difficile* toxin A-specific llama VHHs with an introduced disulfide bond in the hydrophobic core at positions 54 and 78 (IMGT numbering system; http://www.imgt.org/). These disulfide bond mutant VHHs are referred to as "DSB-2 VHHs" throughout this chapter. Using mass spectrometry (MS), we confirm the presence of the engineered disulfide bond through VHH mass analysis and *de novo* sequencing of VHH proteolytic peptides harboring the introduced disulfide bond. Using size exclusion chromatography and surface plasmon resonance (SPR) analyses, we examine the effects of the mutations on VHH aggregation profiles and toxin-binding affinity, respectively. Circular dichroism (CD) spectroscopy is used for comparing VHH midpoint thermal unfolding temperatures (T_ms) among wild-type (WT) and DSB-2 VHHs. Finally, protocols for determining VHH resistance to the major gastrointestinal proteases, pepsin, trypsin, and chymotrypsin, are provided. The following protocols describe a basic strategy to characterize introduced disulfide bonds in llama VHHs, but should be extendable to all VHHs and possibly to other single-domain antibodies (e.g., VHs).

2. Materials

All solutions were prepared with distilled and deionized water (ddH_2O). Filter-sterilized solutions were prepared using 0.2 μm filter units (see Note 1).

2.1. Disulfide Linkage Mapping of DSB-2 VHHs by MS

1. CNBr. Prepare a 10 mg/mL stock in 0.1 M HCl, protect from light and store at 4° C.
2. Sequencing-grade trypsin (Roche Diagnostics Canada, Laval, QC, Canada) (see Note 2).
3. 10× PBS, pH 7.3 (18).
4. 1 M HCl.
5. 1 M Tris–HCl buffer: 121.4 g Tris-base, in 1 L of ddH_2O. Adjust to pH 8.6 with 3 M HCl, filter-sterilize, store at 4° C.
6. SDS-PAGE (sodium dodecyl sulfate-polyacrylamide gel electrophoresis) reagents and equipment.
7. ND-1000 spectrophotometer (Thermo Scientific, Wilmington, DE) or similar instrument (see Note 3).
8. HPLC-grade acetonitrile and water (Sigma, Mississauga, ON, Canada).
9. ACS-grade formic acid (EMD, Gibbstown, NJ).
10. Ultrafree®-0.5 centrifugal filter device with Biomax®-5 ultrafiltration membrane (5 kDa MWCO) (Millipore, Billerica, MA).
11. 180 μm I.D. × 20 mm 5 μm symmetry®C18 trap and 100 μm I.D. × 10 cm 1.7 μm BEH130C18 column (Waters, Milford, MA).
12. NanoAcquity UPLC system coupled to a Q-TOF Ultima™ hybrid quadrupole/time of flight (TOF) mass spectrometer (Waters).
13. Q-TOF 2™ hybrid quadrupole/TOF mass spectrometer (Waters).
14. Masslynx™ 4.0 software (Waters).
15. MaxEnt 1 and MaxEnt 3 programs under the Masslynx™ 4.0 software (Waters).
16. Mascot™ database searching system (Matrix Science, London, UK).

2.2. Assessing Non-aggregation State and Toxin A Binding Affinity of DSB-2 VHHs by Size Exclusion Chromatography and SPR Analyses

1. Superdex™ 75 10/300 GL size exclusion column (bed volume: 24 mL; bed dimensions: 10 mm × 300 mm) (GE Healthcare, Baie-d'Urfé, QC, Canada).
2. Filtered and degassed ddH_2O. Degas the filtered water with a conventional water aspirator.
3. Filtered and degassed PBS (18). Degas the filtered PBS with a conventional water aspirator.
4. Purified *C. difficile* toxin A (TcdA).
5. Appropriate control (reference) protein for Biacore.
6. HBS-E buffer: 10 mM HEPES, 150 mM NaCl, 3 mM EDTA, pH 7.4. This buffer can be purchased from GE Healthcare.

If not purchased from GE Healthcare, it should be thoroughly degassed before use.

7. Surfactant P20 (GE Healthcare).
8. Amine coupling kit containing *N*-hydroxysccinimide (NHS), *N*-ethyl-N′-(3-dimethylaminopropyl) carbodiimide hydrochloride (EDC), and ethanolamine (GE Healthcare).
9. 10 mM acetate buffer, pH 4.0.
10. 1 M ethanolamine, pH 8.5.
11. CM5 sensor chips (GE Healthcare).
12. BIACORE 3000 (GE Healthcare) or other SPR instrument with similar capabilities.

2.3. Measuring DSB-2 VHH Thermal Stability by CD Spectroscopy

1. Buffer P: 1.4 g Na_2HPO_4, 0.24 g KH_2PO_4, pH 7.3, in 1 L of ddH_2O. Filter-sterilize, store at room temperature.
2. Ultrafree®-0.5 centrifugal filter device with Biomax®-5 ultrafiltration membrane (5 kDa MWCO) (Millipore).
3. Spectrophotometer (see Subheading 2.1, item 7).
4. 5-mm cuvette (Hellma, Plainview, NY).
5. J-815 CD spectropolarimeter (Jasco, Easton, MD).
6. Peltier PTC-423 heat control unit (Jasco).
7. N_2 gas supply.
8. Software and data analysis: Jasco J-815 software and GraphPad Prism graphing software (version 4.02 for Windows; GraphPad Software, San Diego, CA; "www.graphpad.com").
9. Hellmanex™ II cuvette cleaning solution (Hellma). Dilute 2 mL of Hellmanex™ II in 98 mL of ddH_2O, store at room temperature.
10. Stock HCl.
11. Ethanol.
12. 6 M guanidine hydrochloride.

2.4. Measuring DSB-2 VHH Protease Resistance

1. 1 M HCl.
2. 10× PBS, pH 7.3 (18).
3. 1 M NaOH.
4. Protease inhibitor cocktail (Sigma).
5. $CaCl_2$. Prepare 100 mM stock, store at 4° C.
6. Porcine stomach pepsin (460 units/mg; Sigma).
7. Sequencing-grade chymotrypsin (Roche Diagnostics Canada).
8. Sequencing-grade trypsin (see Subheading 2.1, item 2).
9. SDS-PAGE reagents and equipment.
10. Coomassie Blue stain.

11. AlphaImager3400™ camera (Alpha Innotech Corp., San Leandro, CA).
12. AlphaEaseFc™ software package (version 7.0.1; Alpha Innotech Corp.).

3. Methods

For illustrative purposes, we provide details on the partial characterization of two VHH DSB-2 mutants, namely A4.2m and A5.1m, which are llama single-domain antibodies with specificity for *C. difficile* toxin A. In characterizing the DSB-2 mutants, the WT VHHs without mutations (A4.2 and A5.1) serve as controls.

Construct the DSB-2 VHHs by introducing two cysteine residues into the WT VHHs at positions 54 and 78 (IMGT numbering system) using a PCR-based mutagenesis method (see Chapter 24). Transform TG1 *Escherichia coli* cells with the mutant VHH construct (see Chapter 14) and express and purify the VHHs by immobilized metal-affinity chromatography (IMAC) (see Chapter 16).

3.1. Disulfide Linkage Mapping of DSB-2 VHHs by MS

To determine if the introduced cysteine residues are creating a disulfide bond, two methods may be used. The first method is an Ellman's assay (see Chapter 24). The second method, used here, employs electrospray ionization MS mass determination of the VHHs and MS^2 peptide mass fingerprinting to accurately determine proteolytic VHH peptides harboring the introduced disulfide bond. Both methods are complementary; however, the Ellman's assay uses significantly more protein and in contrast to the MS approach presented here does not identify the Cys pairs which form the disulfide bond. Detailed protocols for all MS experiments (mass determination and peptide mass fingerprinting) are described in Chapter 21.

1. Measure the concentration ($A_{280\ nm}$) of the purified DSB-2 VHHs using a spectrophotometer (18) (see Note 4).
2. Before MS^2 analysis, create proteolytic peptides of DSB-2 VHHs by digestion with CNBr and trypsin. Digest with CNBr first, by preparing the following reaction:

Purified DSB-2 VHH (see Note 5)	50 μg
10× PBS	10 μL
1 M HCl	10 μL
CNBr	40 μL
ddH_2O	add to 100 μL

Incubate the digestion for 14–16 h at room temperature, in the dark.

3. Perform the trypsin digestion next day by adding the following components directly to the overnight CNBr digest:

1 M Tris–HCl, pH 8.6	100 μL
Trypsin (100 μg/mL)	60 μL

Incubate the digestion reaction for 2 h at 37°C. Remove and analyze 2–3 μg by SDS-PAGE under nonreducing conditions to confirm complete digestion. Run the same quantity of undigested DSB-2 VHH as a control.

4. Continue on with the MS^2 analysis of peptides to determine disulfide bond formation between Cys54 and Cys78 as described in Chapter 21.

Figure 1 shows the annotated MS^2 fragment ion series of the A4.2m disulfide-linked peptide indicating the exact position of the introduced disulfide bond.

a

QVKLEESGGGLVQAGGSLRLSCAASGRTFNTLSMGWF
RQAPGKEREFVCAVSRSGGSTYYADSVKGRFTCSRDN
AKNTVYLQMNSLKPEDTAVYYCAAAATKSNTTAYRLS
FDYWGQGTQVTVSS*GSEQKLISEEDLNHHHHHH*

b

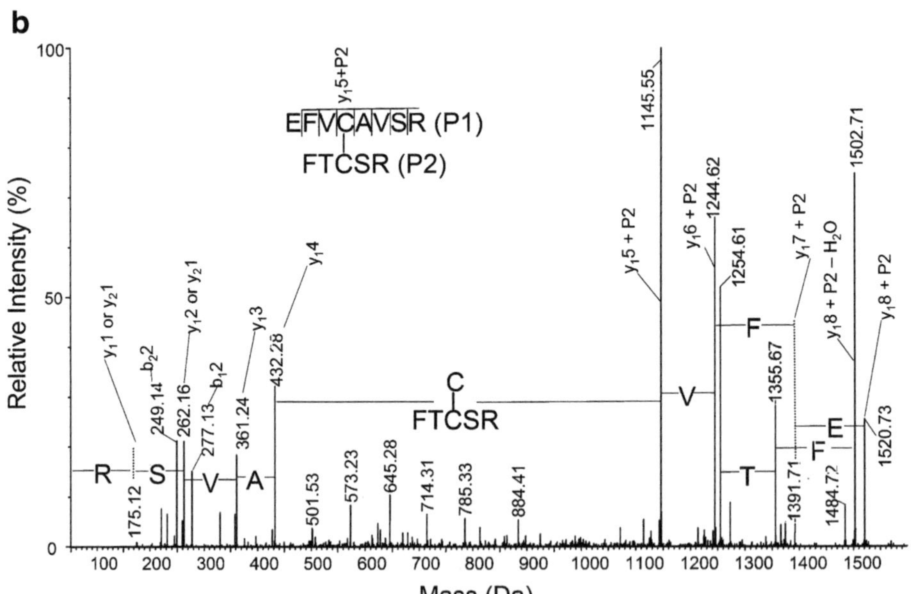

Fig. 1. MS confirms the formation of Cys54–Cys78 disulfide bond in DSB-2 VHHs. (**a**) Amino acid sequence of DSB-2 VHH A4.2m with the extra C-terminal c-Myc and His_6 sequences shown in italics. The cysteine residues introduced at positions 54 and 78 (*bolded*) and the resulting disulfide bond (*dashed line*) are shown. Two peptides (*underlined*) linked by the introduced disulfide bond were generated by digestion of A4.2m with CNBr and trypsin. These tryptic peptides were positively identified by MS^2 analysis in (**b**). (**b**) MaxEnt 3 deconvoluted MS^2 spectrum of the A4.2m disulfide-linked peptide.

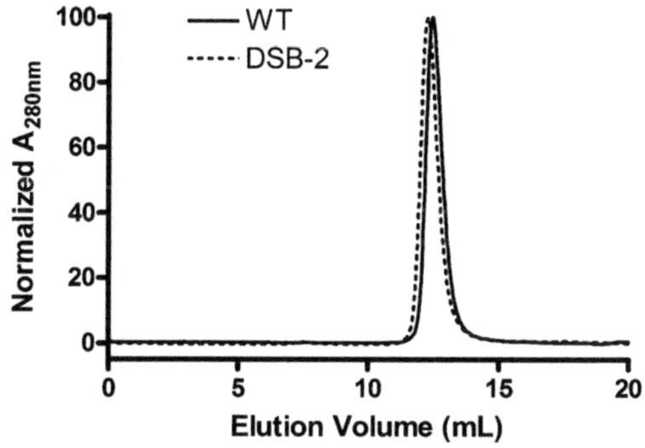

Fig. 2. Representative size exclusion chromatography profiles of WT and DSB-2 VHHs. For illustrative purposes, the profiles of A4.2 (WT and DSB-2 VHHs) are shown. The chromatograms were generated by comparing the two VHHs on a Superdex 75™ size exclusion chromatography column. The profiles indicate that the DSB-2 mutant, like the WT, is a non-aggregating monomer with an essentially superimposable elution volume.

3.2. Assessing Non-aggregation State and Toxin A Binding Affinity of DSB-2 VHHs by Size Exclusion Chromatography and SPR Analyses

1. Determine the aggregation state of DSB-2 VHHs by size exclusion chromatography as described in Chapter 21. As an example, the size exclusion chromatography profiles for A4.2 WT and DSB-2 mutant are shown in Fig. 2. Similar to the WT, the DSB-2 mutant has the chromatogram profile which is characteristic of non-aggregating single-domain antibodies demonstrating that the engineered disulfide linkage does not promote VHH aggregation or interdomain disulfide bond formation.
2. Determine the toxin A binding affinity of DSB-2 VHHs by SPR as described in Chapter 14. Equilibrium dissociation constants, K_Ds, for binding of DSB-2 VHHs A4.2m and A5.1m to toxin A were similar or higher than those for WT VHHs. For example, the K_Ds of WT and DSB-2 A4.2 were 24 and 20 nM, respectively, while the K_Ds of WT and DSB-2 A5.1 were 3 and 17 nM, respectively. This demonstrates that the engineered disulfide linkage has a modest effect on VHH affinity.

3.3. Measuring DSB-2 VHH Thermal Stability by CD Spectroscopy

The thermal stability of the DSB-2 VHHs is assessed in terms of midpoint thermal unfolding temperature (T_m) by CD spectroscopy measurements. The WT VHHs are also included in the analysis for comparison.

1. Turn on the Jasco-815 CD spectropolarimeter, N_2 gas supply, and prewarm the lamp for at least 30 min. Ensure the water level is at capacity in the Peltier heat control unit.
2. Buffer exchange the purified DSB-2 VHH into buffer P using a Millipore Ultrafree®-0.5 (5 kDa MWCO) spin column attached to a collecting microtube as described by the manufacturer.

3. Measure $A_{280\ nm}$ for determination of the protein concentration using a spectrophotometer (see Note 4) and prepare 1.5 mL of DSB-2 VHH at 50 μg/mL in buffer P.
4. Set the following CD spectropolarimeter parameters:

Data collection range	190–250 nm
Scan speed	20 nm/min
Data pitch	0.5 nm
Bandwidth	1 mm
Temperature range	30–96° C
Temperature ramp	1° C/min
Data collection	every 2° C
Accumulations	4

5. Wash a 5-mm cuvette thoroughly (see Notes 6 and 7). Add 1.5 mL of buffer P (see Note 8). Perform a "buffer blank" scan at 30° C from 190–250 nm to confirm the cuvette is clean. Save the data.
6. Remove the buffer P from the cuvette and replace it with 1.5 mL of DSB-2 VHH at 50 μg/mL (see Note 9). Perform the temperature-induced unfolding experiment using the parameters described (see Subheading 3.3, step 4).
7. Smooth the spectra of the sample and the buffer blank using the Jasco software. Subtract the buffer blank response from the sample response. The DSB-2 VHHs exhibit the largest change in ellipticity at 215 nm (see Note 10). Convert the raw ellipticity data (in millidegrees) at 215 nm at each temperature to molar ellipticity and then to the fraction of protein folded (see Note 11).
8. Export the converted data from Excel into GraphPad Prism, plot the fraction of protein folded vs. temperature, and perform nonlinear regression analysis (see Fig. 3). The temperature at which 50% of the DSB-2 VHH is unfolded represents the melting temperature (T_m).
9. Repeat the procedure for the other DSB-2 VHH and WT controls.

Figure 3 depicts typical thermal unfolding curves of WT and DSB-2 VHHs. A5.1 (WT VHH) and A5.1m (DSB-2 VHH) temperature-induced unfolding profiles are shown as examples. The midpoint unfolding temperatures, T_ms, of A5.1 and A5.1m are 73.1°C and

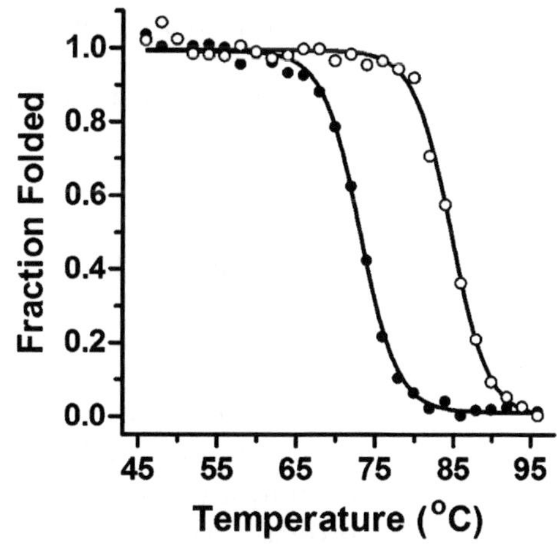

Fig. 3. Typical thermal unfolding curves of WT and DSB-2 VHHs. A5.1 (WT VHH) and A5.1m (DSB-2 VHH) temperature-induced unfolding is shown as *filled* and *open circles*, respectively. The midpoint unfolding temperatures, T_ms, of A5.1 and A5.1m are 73.1° C and 84.7° C, respectively.

84.7° C, respectively, demonstrating the drastically stabilizing effect of the extra disulfide linkage between Cys54 and Cys78.

3.4. Measuring DSB-2 VHH Protease Resistance

DSB-2 VHH resistance profiles to the major gastrointestinal proteases, pepsin, trypsin, and chymotrypsin, are determined by digestion assays. The WT VHHs are also included in the analysis as controls. To measure the sensitivity of WT and DSB-2 VHHs to pepsin, trypsin, and chymotrypsin, purified VHHs are incubated at 37° C for 1 h in the presence or absence of protease and analyzed by SDS-PAGE. To begin, a range of protease concentrations is explored (0.1 μg/mL, 1 μg/mL, 10 μg/mL, 100 μg/mL) to find the optimal sensitivity range (see Note 12).

1. Protease solutions are to be prepared fresh each day. Prepare a working solution of pepsin, trypsin, and chymotrypsin (1 mg/mL stock each) diluted in 1 mM HCl.
2. Perform pepsin digestion at pH 2.0 and trypsin and chymotrypsin digestions at pH 7.3 as follows:

   (a) Pepsin

Purified DSB-2 VHH	4.8 μg
10× PBS	2 μL
1 M HCl	1 μL
Pepsin (1 mg/mL)	2 μL
ddH$_2$O	add to 20 μL

(b) Trypsin and chymotrypsin

Purified DSB-2 VHH	4.8 μg
10× PBS	2 μL
10× $CaCl_2$	2 μL
Trypsin or chymotrypsin (1 mg/mL)	2 μL
ddH_2O	add to 20 μL

These digestion reactions contain a final protease concentration of 100 μg/mL. For lower final protease concentrations (e.g., 10 μg/mL and 1 μg/mL), dilute the stock protease to 100 μg/mL and 10 μg/mL, respectively. In all cases, include a control reaction mixture where protease is replaced with water. Incubate the digestion reactions at 37° C for 1 h. Immediately neutralize the digestion and control reactions by adding 1 μL of 1 M NaOH (pepsin) or protease inhibitor cocktail (trypsin and chymotrypsin).

3. Analyze the digested and control VHHs by running equivalent volumes on SDS-PAGE gels (under reducing conditions) (see Note 13). Stain the gel with Coomassie Blue, destain, photograph using AlphaImager™ or similar camera, and determine the band intensity of the digested VHH relative to no-protease control using AlphaImager software or similar imaging software. Each digestion experiment should be repeated three times and analyzed on unique SDS-PAGE gels.
4. Repeat the procedure for the other DSB-2 VHH and WT controls.

Head-to-head comparisons of A4.2 and A4.2m VHHs digested with various concentrations of pepsin are shown as an example (see Note 14 and Fig. 4). It is clear that VHHs with the engineered

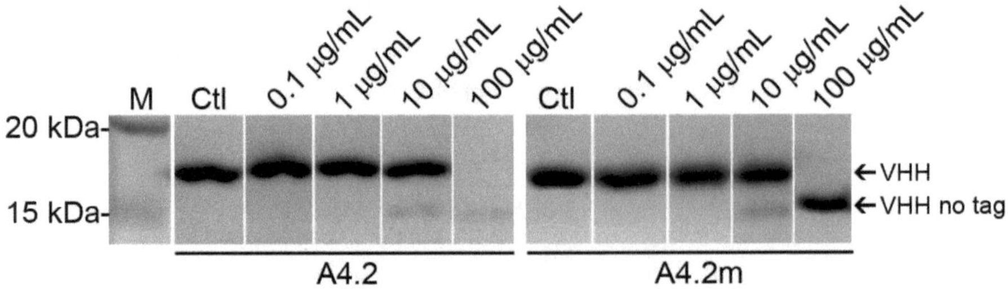

Fig. 4. Sensitivity of WT and DSB-2 VHHs to various concentrations of pepsin. A4.2 and A4.2m VHHs were incubated with various concentrations of pepsin (0.1–100 μg/mL) for 1 h at 37° C, neutralized and analyzed by sodium dodecyl sulfate-polyacrylamide gel electrophoresis (SDS-PAGE) under reducing conditions. The DSB-2 mutant A4.2m was considerably more resistant than A4.2 at the highest pepsin concentration (100 μg/mL). The band ~2 kDa below the expected VHH size represents the VHH variant ("VHH no tag") with cleaved C-terminal c-Myc and His_6 tags. This can be confirmed by MS analysis (21). M: protein molecular weight standards; *Ctl* control VHH incubated at 37° C for 1 h without protease.

disulfide bond are more resistant to pepsin degradation relative to their WT VHH counterparts. This stability gain is not at the expense of trypsin and chymotrypsin stability as the WT and DSB-2 VHHs had comparable resistance to trypsin and chymotrypsin (data not shown).

4. Notes

1. We typically use Millipore's 0.2 μm MILLEx®-GV filter units for sterilizing small volumes and the 0.2 μm GP Express™ Plus Membrane filtration system for sterilizing large volumes.
2. Werecommendusingsequencing-gradetrypsin.Nonsequencing grade trypsin may have other enzyme contaminants.
3. In contrast to a conventional spectrophotometer, the ND-1000 spectrophotometer (or instruments with similar technology) measures absorbance at very low volumes (1 μL) and without the use of cuvettes.
4. Calculate protein concentration using the following formula: $[\text{protein}]_{\text{mg/mL}} = (A_{280\ \text{nm}}$ x molecular weight) ÷ extinction coefficient. Commercial protein analysis software, e.g., Laser gene v6.0, DNASTAR, Inc. (Madison, WI), or online freeware, e.g., ExPASy ProtParam tool at http://us.expasy.org/tools/protparam.html, can be used for calculation of molar extinction coefficient and molecular weight.
5. We perform VHH digestions in PBS, pH 7.3, but other buffers may also be compatible with the digestion reaction.
6. The choice of cuvette pathlength depends on the working VHH concentration. Cuvettes with longer pathlengths (larger volumes) may need to be used with lower concentrations in order to obtain a significant CD signal.
7. Wash all cuvettes thoroughly before use and between samples. Rinse the cuvette with ddH_2O followed by 2–3 washes with a commercial cleaning solution from suppliers such as Hellma, with a combination of 30% HCl and 70% ethanol, or with 6 M guanidine hydrochloride followed by ddH_2O and ethanol. After washing allow the cuvette to air dry. Ideally, soak the cuvettes overnight when possible. In all cases, perform a CD scan on the empty cuvette to ensure there is no residual protein remaining.
8. Avoid using buffers with high absorbance in the wavelength range used (e.g., buffers with high salt concentration) as they would increase the noise. This is particularly important for VHHs as they are essentially β-strand proteins and as a result give only a modest CD signal change upon denaturation.

9. It is critical to use the same concentration and buffer when comparing different VHHs as protein concentration is a factor in aggregation formation and T_ms are a function of buffer composition.
10. We consistently find the biggest difference in signal (ellipticity) between native and denatured VHHs at wavelengths of 210–220 nm. In our thermal unfolding experiments, we calculated T_ms for all VHHs using the ellipticity at 215 nm since it was a local minimum. For other users, this local minimum may differ.
11. Ellipticity (θ) from the CD spectropolarimeter is given in millidegrees (mdeg). Export the raw mdeg data to a program such as Excel. To convert from mdeg to molar ellipticity ($[\theta]$) in deg cm^2/dmol, use the following formula: $[\theta]$ = (mdeg x mean residue weight)/(pathlength in mm x antibody concentration in mg/mL) (19). The mean residue weight is the molecular weight of the VHH (in Da)/the number of backbone amino acids. To convert from molar ellipticity to the fraction of protein folded (FF) (20), use the following formula: $FF = ([\theta]-[\theta_U])/([\theta_F]-[\theta_U])$ where $[\theta]$ is the molar ellipticity at each temperature point (calculated above in this note), $[\theta_U]$ is the molar ellipticity of the fully unfolded protein (in this case the $[\theta_{215\ nm}]$ at 96° C), and $[\theta_F]$ is the molar ellipticity of the fully folded protein (in this case the $[\theta_{215\ nm}]$ at 30° C).
12. Final protease concentrations of 0.1–100 μg/mL were initially tested. Proteases (pepsin, trypsin, and chymotrypsin) are all dissolved in 1 mM HCl. Make sure to prepare fresh 1 mM HCl each time when diluting the proteases. From a 1 mg/mL working stock solution, all protease concentrations can be made by making 1:10 dilutions in 1 mM HCl.
13. Always perform reducing SDS-PAGE on the digested VHHs to detect protease nicks which occur at sites between disulfide linkage(s). Such nicks may go undetected on a nonreducing SDS-PAGE gel since the disulfide linkage(s) would hold the digested fragments together.
14. VHHs digested with higher concentrations of proteases are preferentially cleaved within their C-terminal c-Myc epitope tag. As shown in Fig. 4, the result is a band approximately 2 kDa lower than that observed for undigested VHHs. We have confirmed this band to be structurally intact VHH by MS analysis, as shown for human VHs (21).

References

1. Sieber V, Plückthun A, Schmid FX (1998) Selecting proteins with improved stability by a phage-based method. Nat Biotechnol 16: 955–960
2. Jespers L et al (2004) Aggregation-resistant domain antibodies selected on phage by heat denaturation. Nat Biotechnol 22:1161–1165
3. Arbabi-Ghahroudi M et al (2009) Aggregation-resistant V_Hs selected by *in vitro* evolution tend to have disulfide-bonded loops and acidic isoelectric points. Protein Eng Des Sel 22: 59–66
4. Famm K et al (2008) Thermodynamically stable aggregation-resistant antibody domains through directed evolution. J Mol Biol 376:926–931
5. Jermutus L et al (2001) Tailoring in vitro evolution for protein affinity or stability. Proc Natl Acad Sci U S A 98:75–80
6. Young NM et al (1995) Thermal stabilization of a single-chain Fv antibody fragment by introduction of a disulphide bond. FEBS Lett 377:135–139
7. Wörn A, Plückthun A (1998) Mutual stabilization of V_L and V_H in single-chain antibody fragments, investigated with mutants engineered for stability. Biochemistry 37: 13120–13127
8. Arbabi-Ghahroudi M, MacKenzie R, Tanha J (2010) Site-directed mutagenesis for improving biophysical properties of V_H domains. Methods Mol Biol 634:309–330
9. Chao G et al (2006) Isolating and engineering human antibodies using yeast surface display. Nat Protoc 1:755–768
10. Harmsen MM et al (2006) Selection and optimization of proteolytically stable llama single-domain antibody fragments for oral immunotherapy. Appl Microbiol Biotechnol 72:544–551
11. Kubetzko S et al (2006) PEGylation and multimerization of the anti-p185HER-2 single chain Fv fragments 4D5: effects on tumor targeting. J Biol Chem 281:35186–35201
12. Holliger P, Hudson PJ (2005) Engineered antibody fragments and the rise of single domains. Nat Biotechnol 23:1126–1136
13. Arbabi-Ghahroudi M, Tanha J, MacKenzie R (2005) Prokaryotic expression of antibodies. Cancer Metastasis Rev 24:501–519
14. Hussack G, Tanha J (2010) Toxin-specific antibodies for the treatment of *Clostridium difficile*: current status and future perspectives. Toxins 2:998–1018
15. Hagihara Y, Mine S, Uegaki K (2007) Stabilization of an immunoglobulin fold domain by an engineered disulfide bond at the buried hydrophobic region. J Biol Chem 282:36489–36495
16. Saerens D et al (2008) Disulfide bond introduction for general stabilization of immunoglobulin heavy-chain variable domains. J Mol Biol 377:478–488
17. Chan PH et al (2008) Engineering a camelid antibody fragment that binds to the active site of human lysozyme and inhibits its conversion to amyloid fibrils. Biochemistry 47:11041–11054
18. Sambrook J, Fritsch EF, Maniatis T (eds) (1989) Molecular cloning: a laboratory manual. Cold Spring Harbor Laboratory, Cold Spring Harbor, NY
19. Greenfield NJ (2006) Using circular dichroism spectra to estimate protein secondary structure. Nat Protoc 1:2876–2890
20. Greenfield NJ (2006) Analysis of the kinetics of folding of proteins and peptides using circular dichroism. Nat Protoc 1:2891–2899
21. To R et al (2005) Isolation of monomeric human V_Hs by a phage selection. J Biol Chem 280:41395–41403

Chapter 26

Affinity Maturation of Single-Domain Antibodies by Yeast Surface Display

Akiko Koide and Shohei Koide

Abstract

Although single-domain antibodies derived from libraries prepared either after animal immunization or naïve animals generally exhibit reasonable affinity, it is often desirable to further improve their affinity. This chapter describes protocols for improving the affinity of single-domain antibodies using quantitative library sorting by yeast surface display. An example is included where we also exploit a complementary strength of phage display in generating larger sequence diversity prior to library sorting with yeast surface display.

Key words: Antibody engineering, Molecular recognition, Combinatorial libraries, Phage display

1. Introduction

Single-domain antibodies are increasingly utilized within diverse applications. Affinity is a critical parameter for the performance of antibodies. High affinity is essential for sensitive detection, efficient antigen capture, and effective inhibition of the function of an antigen. Single-domain antibodies derived from immunized animals generally show good affinity, with a typical equilibrium dissociation constant (K_D) value in the nM range (1, 2). However, it is often desirable to increase the affinity of such initial antibody leads. This chapter describes a systematic method for affinity maturation of single-domain antibodies.

Affinity maturation is a direct evolution technique which has great similarities with the somatic hypermutation within the immune system. Amino acid diversity is introduced into the initially identified antibody to construct a large collection of mutants ("library") from which variants with increased affinity are identified. Therefore, two key considerations should be made before the affinity maturation is initiated: (1) how amino acid diversity will be

Dirk Saerens and Serge Muyldermans (eds.), *Single Domain Antibodies: Methods and Protocols*,
Methods in Molecular Biology, vol. 911, DOI 10.1007/978-1-61779-968-6_26, © Springer Science+Business Media, LLC 2012

generated and (2) in which way the improved variants will be identified.

Strategies for generating amino acid diversity can be categorized in two fundamentally different manners in terms of locations of introduced diversity: random and targeted approaches. Random mutagenesis using techniques such as error-prone PCR is straightforward, and it does not require detailed knowledge of the structure–function relationship of the wild type antibody. However, random mutagenesis does not concentrate mutations in regions that are important for antigen binding or bias amino acid compositions toward those expected to be beneficial for increasing affinity. As such, the probability of obtaining variants with improved affinity from a library constructed using random mutagenesis is generally low.

Targeted introduction of amino acid diversity requires prior knowledge of how an antibody recognizes its antigen. Detailed studies on the sequence diversity and on the structural basis for antigen recognition have established a considerable body of knowledge on how single-domain antibodies function in general (2–5). As in the conventional immunoglobulins, the overall fold of single-domain antibodies is essentially constant among different variants, and the antigen-binding site is primarily constituted of residues in the complementarity determining regions (CDRs). Therefore, although there is a certain level of idiosyncrasy for each antibody, one can safely assume that portions of the CDRs, three surface loops in the case of camelid VHHs, are intimately involved in antigen binding. Therefore, altering these CDR residues would affect antigen-binding properties. Thus, approaches that generate amino acid diversity into CDRs and their immediate vicinity are particularly suited for antibodies. Targeted diversification can be further refined by the knowledge of the importance of individual residues. One may not wish to diversify residues that are highly critically important for binding, because any substitution of such a position is likely to lead to a large loss of binding. Based on these considerations, custom combinatorial libraries are generated.

Phage display and yeast surface display are the most commonly used techniques for directed evolution of antibodies (6–8). They have complementary strengths and weaknesses. One can generate larger libraries in the order of 10^{10} clones in phage display, while yeast surface display libraries are typically in the order of 10^7 clones due to lower efficiency of transforming yeast than *E. coli*. Therefore, it is more convenient to generate a library in the phage-display format. Because VHHs are almost always identified from a phage-display library, it is particularly straightforward to introduce amino acid diversity into a VHH already in a phage-display vector.

Affinity maturation requires the ability to discriminate variants with improved affinity from the starting clone. This requirement is distinct from that for de novo discovery of rare functional clones from a large library in which the predominant majority is nonfunctional. Screening of a yeast surface display library using fluorescence-activated cell sorting (FACS) is particularly powerful in terms of quantitative discrimination of closely related clones (see Fig. 1) (9). FACS interogates individual yeast cells for binding, and accordingly there is no direct competition for antigen between different variants of antibodies. Furthermore, it is straightforward to perform selection based on the dissociation rate constant in the yeast surface display format (8). Although yeast surface display requires access to a flow cytometer, a flow cytometry "core facility" is increasingly common at major research institutions. In contrast, it is difficult to discriminate clones with similar affinity using phage display. Phage display selection recovers a population of variants that bind to an antigen with a particular threshold from a large mixture, and selection relies on different levels of recovery of clones from such a mixture. As such, variants with similar levels of affinity (less than tenfold difference in K_D) often are recovered with equal efficiency. In the example shown below, we combined the two molecular-display methods so that we could take advantage of the strengths of both. Large libraries were first constructed in the phage display format, and the best clones were identified using yeast surface display. We were able to increase the affinity of a VHH by >100 fold to a sub-nM K_D (10).

2. Materials

2.1. Yeast Display of the Starting VHH Clone

1. *YPD medium*: 20 g Bacto-peptone, 10 g yeast extract, 20 g glucose per liter water. For plates, add 20 g/L Bacto-agar.
2. *SD-CAA medium*: For 1 L, mix 1.5 g of "Yeast Nitrogen Base w/o amino acids w/o ammonium sulfate" (BD Difco; http://www.bd.com), 5 g $(NH_4)_2SO_4$, 10.25 g $Na_2HPO_4{\cdot}7H_2O$, 8.56 g $NaH_2PO_4{\cdot}H_2O$, 5 g Casamino acids, and 960 mL of water and autoclave the solution. Add 40 mL of sterile 50% glucose and mix well. For plates, add 20 g/L Bacto-agar.
3. *SG-CAA medium*: For 1 L, mix 1.5 g of "Yeast Nitrogen Base w/o amino acids w/o ammonium sulfate" (BD Difco), 5 g $(NH_4)_2SO_4$, 10.25 g $Na_2HPO_4{\cdot}7H_2O$, 8.56 g $NaH_2PO_4{\cdot}H_2O$, 5 g Casamino acids, and 900 mL of water and autoclave. Add 100 mL of sterile 20% galactose and mix well.
4. *TBS*: 50 mM Tris–HCl, 100 mM NaCl, pH 8.0.
5. *BSS*: TBS and 1 mg/mL BSA.
6. *BSST*: BBS and 0.5% (v/v) Tween20.
7. EBY100 (Invitrogen; http://www.invitrogen.com).
8. pYD1 (Invitrogen).

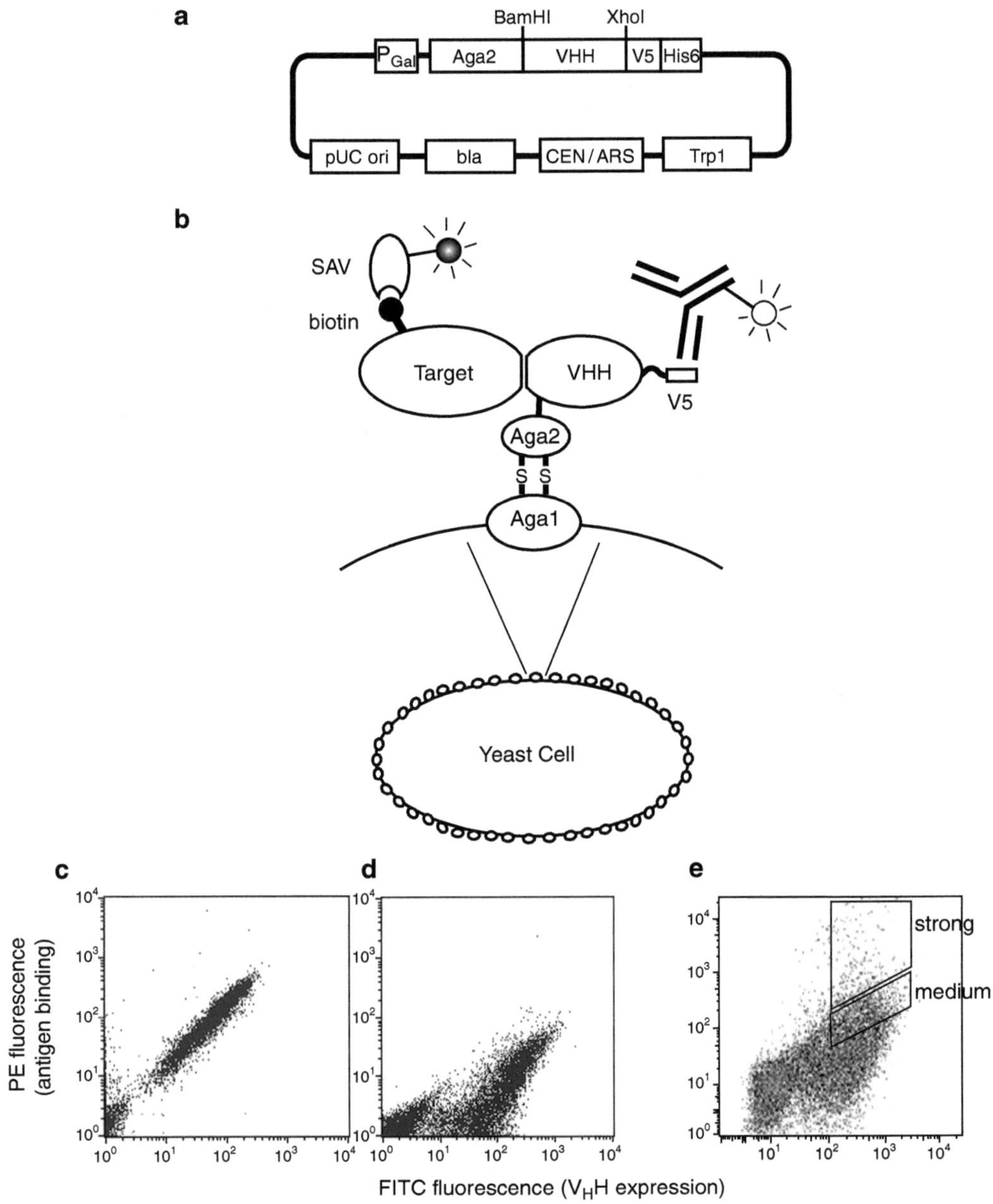

Fig. 1. The concept of yeast display and flow cytometry analysis. (**a**) Schematic drawing of a vector used for yeast display of VHH. The *E. coli*–yeast shuttle vector expresses the Aga2-VHH fusion protein under the control of the P_{gal} promotor. (**b**) A labeling scheme of VHH displayed on the surface of yeast cells. Approximately 50,000 copies of an Aga2 fusion protein are typically displayed on the surface of a single cell, with considerable variation among cells (8). The level of surface display is determined by detecting the V5 tag with an antibody and subsequently with a secondary antibody labeled with a fluorescence dye (not shown for simplicity), while binding of a biotinylated target is detected with streptavidin (SAV) labeled with another dye. (**c**, **d**) Flow cytometry analysis of yeast cells displaying a VHH. The *horizontal axis* shows the intensity of FITC fluorescence emission that indicates the level of surface display. The *vertical axis* shows the intensity of PE fluorescence emission that indicates the degree of antigen binding. Each *dot* represents data for a single yeast cell. (**c**) Shows a typical profile for a clone exhibiting strong binding, which gives a high binding to display ratio. (**d**) Is for a clone with weak binding. (**e**) A flow cytometry profile of a combinatorial library of a VHH. Regions containing variants with strong and medium levels of binding are designated.

2.2. Labeling Yeast Cells for Flow Cytometry Analysis

1. Rabbit anti-V5 antibody and anti-rabbit IgG-FITC conjugate (Sigma-Aldrich; http://www.sigmaaldrich.com/).
2. Anti-rabbit IgG-AlexaFluor647 conjugate, Streptavidin (SAV)-R-Phycoerythrin (PE) (SAV-PE) conjugate and Neutravidin (NAV)-PE conjugate were from Invitrogen (http://www.invitrogen.com).
3. Biotinylation reagent EZ-Link NHS-LC-Biotin was purchased from Pierce (http://www.piercenet.com/).
4. Yeast DNA preparation kit was purchased from Zymo Research (http://www.zymoresearch.com).

2.3. Affinity Measurement by Ligand Titration Using Yeast Surface Display

1. MultiScreenHTS-HV Plate with Durapore membrane (catalog number MSHVN4510, Millipore; http://www.millipore.com).

2.4. Scanning Mutagenesis

1. See refs. (11, 12).

2.5. Design, Construction, and selection of Phage-Display Affinity Maturation Library

1. See refs. (7, 10, 13, 14).

2.6. Construction of a Yeast Display Library

1. See Subheading 2.1.

2.7. FACS Screening of Improved Clones Based on Equilibrium Binding

1. See Subheadings 2.1 and 2.2.

2.8. FACS Screening of Improved Clones Based on Dissociation Kinetics

1. See Subheadings 2.1 and 2.2.

3. Methods

An affinity maturation project involves several major steps as follows. (1) Determination of the affinity of the starting antibody clone. We used yeast surface display for this purpose (see Note 1 and Subheading 3.1). (2) Identification of residues that are important for antigen recognition. (3) Library construction. (4) Library sorting. (5) Characterization of new clones.

3.1. Yeast Display of the Wild Type VHH Clone

1. The gene for the starting VHH clone is subcloned in the pYD1 vector using appropriate restriction sites (see Note 2). The resulting plasmid, termed pGalAgaVHH, encodes the fusion protein, Aga2-VHH-V5 tag-His tag, under the P_{Gal} promoter (see Fig. 1).
2. Transform yeast strain EBY100 (15) with the pGalAgaVHH plasmid (16) and select trp^{+} transformants on a SD-CAA agar plate at 30°C.
3. Inoculate a 3-day-old colony in 2 mL of SD-CAA media and incubate with shaking at 30°C for 24 h. The SD-CAA media is used for growing yeast cells without inducing the Aga2-VHH fusion.
4. Measure $OD_{600\ nm}$ of the culture and determine the volume of the culture that makes 1.5 mL at $OD_{600\ nm} = 0.4$. Transfer this volume of the culture to a 1.5 mL microtube. For example, if the $OD_{600\ nm}$ of the preculture is 3, 0.2 mL of the preculture is used.
5. Centrifuge the preculture at 8,000 rpm in a microfuge for 10 s, remove the supernatant using a 200 μL pipetter. Suspend the cells in 30 μL of sterile water and transfer into 1.5 mL of SG-CAA in sterile test tube with 16 mm diameter. The SG-CAA media is used to induce the expression of the Aga2-VHH fusion.
6. Incubate with shaking at 30°C for 20–34 h.
7. Measure $OD_{600\ nm}$ of the culture and transfer the culture in a microtube, centrifuge at 8,000 rpm in a microfuge for 10 s, and remove the supernatant by decantation.
8. Add 1 mL of ice-cold BSS and suspend the cells by vortexing, then centrifuge the tube at 8,000 rpm in a microfuge for 20 s, and remove the supernatant by decantation.
9. Add an appropriate volume of BSS so that the cell density is 10^8/mL after suspension. For EBY100, $OD_{600\ nm}$ of 1 corresponds to 10^7 cells/mL. Thus, for example if the $OD_{600\ nm}$ is 2, suspend cells from 1.5 mL culture in 300 μL of BSS.
10. Store the induced cells at 4°C. Cells can be kept at 4°C for up to a week.

3.2. Labeling Yeast Cells for Flow Cytometry Analysis

1. Take 10^6 induced cells (10 μL of the cell suspension, see Subheading 3.1, step 10).
2. Dilute the primary antibody for surface display (i.e., rabbit anti-V5 antibody) to a final concentration of 5 ng/μL in BSS. About 5 μL of diluted primary antibody is needed for each sample.
3. Dilute a biotinylated target in BSS (see Note 3). One sample requires 5 μL of the diluted target. Take into account that the target will be further diluted by fourfold after mixed with yeast cell suspension. If the K_D value for the system is unknown, try the final antigen concentration of 0.1 and 1.0 μM.

4. Mix 10 μL of yeast cells, 5 μL of the diluted primary antibody, and 5 μL of the diluted biotinylated target. Prepare another sample with no target as a control.
5. Incubate the samples on a rotator at 4°C for 40 min.
6. Centrifuge at 8,000 rpm in a microfuge for 20 s, withdraw, and discard supernatant completely using a 200 μL pipetter (see Note 4).
7. Suspend cells in 100 μL of BSST by vortex.
8. Repeat previous two steps (see Subheading 3.2, but using BSS, and then step 6 again.
9. Prepare secondary detection solutions in appropriate quantities. For each sample, 20 μL each of the following solutions are needed. FITC-conjugated anti-rabbit antibody diluted 100 fold in BSS, and SAV-PE diluted 100 fold in BSS (see Note 5).
10. Incubate on a rotator at 4°C for 40 min.
11. Centrifuge for 20 s at 8,000 rpm in a microfuge and remove as much supernatant as possible with a 200 μL pipetter.
12. Suspend the cells in 100 μL of BSST by vortexing.
13. Centrifuge for 20 s and remove as much supernatant as possible with a 200 μL pipetter.
14. Suspend the cells in 100 μL of BSS by vortexing.
15. Centrifuge for 20 s and remove as much supernatant as possible with a 200 μL pipetter.
16. Suspend the cells in 300 μL BSS and analyze cells using a flow cytometer (see Note 6).

3.3. Affinity Measurement by Ligand Titration Using Yeast Surface Display

1. Prepare serial dilutions of the biotinylated antigen in BSS. The concentration range should cover 1/5 to 40 times of the expected K_D value (the final concentrations during actual binding reaction will be 1/4 of these concentrations).
2. For each diluted target, mix 10 μL of the target solution and 10 μL of the cell suspension above (see Subheading 3.1, step 9) contains 10^6 induced cells (see Notes 6 and 7 for preparing samples for low target concentrations).
3. Incubate the samples on rotator in 4°C for 40 min.
4. Because a titration often involves many samples, cell washing is performed in a 96-well format using vacuum filtration. Wash the wells of a 96-well filter plate with Durapore membrane by adding 100 μL BSS to a sufficient number of wells and apply vacuum to pass the solution through the filter membrane. Break vacuum.
5. Transfer the cell suspensions with target in the washed wells.
6. Apply vacuum to remove the solution. Discontinue vacuum.

7. Add 200 μL of BSST to each well and apply vacuum to remove BSST. Discontinue vacuum.
8. Repeat previous step except using BSS instead of BSST.
9. Prepare an appropriate quantity of diluted SAV-PE solution (100-fold dilution) in BSS. Each sample needs 20 μL of the solution. Add 20 μL of the solution to each well.
10. Place the filter plate on ice in a small container and place the container on a shaker. Shake it for 40 min.
11. Place the filter plate on the vacuum manifold and apply vacuum to remove reaction solution.
12. Wash each well with 200 μL BSST (see Subheading 3.3, step 7).
13. Wash each well with 200 μL BSS.
14. Suspend cells in 300 μL BSS and measure fluorescence intensity using a flow cytometer.
15. Determine the mean fluorescence of the PE signal as a function of ligand concentration and determine the K_D value by nonlinear least-squares fitting (see Fig. 1; Note 8).
16. Repeat the titration if the determined K_D value is outside the ligand concentration range used.

3.4. Scanning Mutagenesis

The goal is to gain the knowledge of critical and noncritical residues, which will guide library design. Scanning mutagenesis can be performed individually, where each residue in CDR is mutated to alanine or serine and the change in affinity is measured using the method described above (11). Alternatively, so-called shotgun scanning mutagenesis can be performed (12).

3.5. Design, Construction, and Selection of Phage-Display Affinity Maturation Library

Several factors need to be considered in designing combinatorial libraries for affinity maturation. The scanning mutagenesis experiments above will identify residues with different levels of contribution to binding energetics. Residues that are highly important for binding, operatively those that Ala-substitution reduces affinity more than ten times (i.e., K_D increases by >10), would be unchanged. Other residues are diversified. The theoretical size of a library should be kept smaller or similar to the physical size limit of phage-display libraries (approximately 10^{10}). Thus, we often generate multiple libraries in which a subset of residues, e.g., residues within one CDR, are diversified and also a subset of codons ("reduced genetic code") are used (10, 13) in such a way that the total number of encode sequences is less than 10^9 (see Fig. 2).

1. Design libraries and construct phage display libraries. A library can be constructed using any of established mutagenesis methods (7, 14). It is important to avoid the situation that the library contains a large fraction of the starting clone. Because the starting clone binds to the antigen with significant affinity, if it is present at a high concentration, it can overwhelm higher

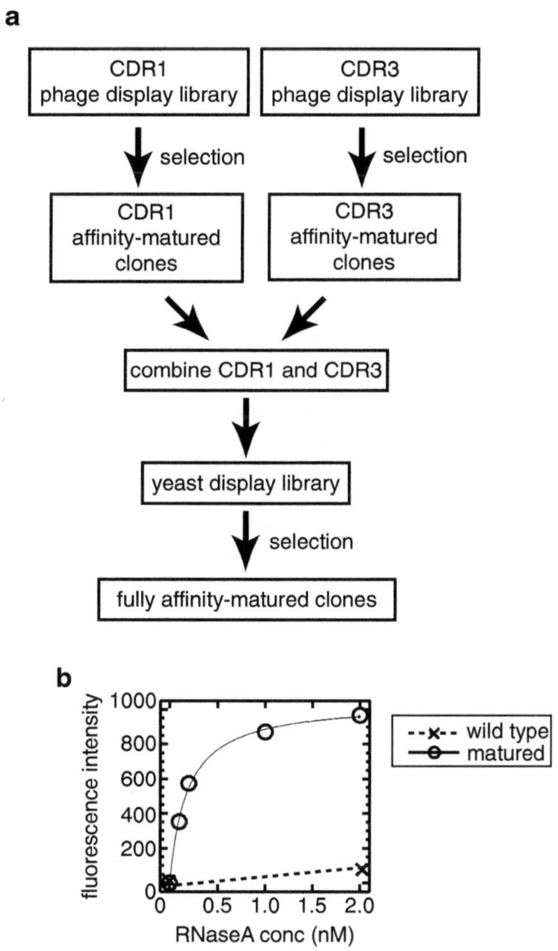

Fig. 2. Affinity maturation strategy. (**a**) Outline of a strategy used for maturation of an anti-RNaseA VHH. In this case, CDR1 and CDR3 were diversified, because the available crystal structure indicated CDR2 were not involved in antigen binding. (**b**) Antigen titration curves of the starting and matured clones, as measured using yeast surface display. Reproduced with permission from ref. (10).

affinity variants that are present at much lower concentrations. The starting clone can be easily eliminated from a library by making a library using a template that has a stop codon in a region to be diversified (see Note 9).

2. Perform two or three rounds of phage display selection. Detailed protocols for phage-display library selection have been described in another volume of this series (14). The goal here is to enrich functional sequences and eliminate the vast number of nonfunctional sequences.

3.6. Construction of a Yeast Display Library

Construct a yeast display library for affinity maturation by transferring enriched VHH sequences from phage display selection. It is convenient to use homologous recombination in yeast where a PCR product is mixed with a vector that has been digested with restriction enzymes (17). No in vitro ligation is required. The CDR sequences can be easily "shuffled" in the process of yeast library construction as described below.

1. Using standard procedures, PCR-amplify DNA fragments that contain segments of the VHH gene from the enriched phage libraries (see Note 10).
2. Assemble the PCR fragments into one large fragment that encodes the entire VHH gene by PCR. Mix 0.1 μg each of purified initial PCR products and perform three PCR cycles without primers in total of 20 μL. Dilute the product to 50 times and perform PCR in total of 50 μL, with primers that respectively anneal to the 5′- and 3′-extremes of the VHH gene and also contain a 60-base overlap with the yeast display vector (see Note 11).
3. Transform EBY100 with the PCR fragment and the yeast display vector digested with restriction enzymes that remove existing VHH fragment (e.g., BamHI and XhoI in Fig. 1a). Mix 30 μg of the digested vector and 15 μg of the assembled PCR fragment and use them for EBY100 competent cells prepared from 300 mL culture in YPD media in 30 of 1.5 mL microtubes. Follow the high efficiency LiAc method carry out yeast transformation (15).
4. Pool transformants and grow them in 600 mL of the SD-CAA medium for 2 days at 30°C with shaking. Take a small portion and titer on a SD-CAA plate and determine the total number of the transformants, i.e., the total size of the library.
5. Transfer sufficient number of cells as determined by $OD_{600\ nm}$ (50 times over the total size of the library) to 200 mL of the SG-CAA medium to induce surface display.
6. Harvest the induced cells, wash the cells with BSS, and suspend the cells in BSS.

3.7. FACS Screening of Improved Clones Based on Equilibrium Binding

When affinity-matured clones are expected to have K_D values greater than 10 nM range, one can readily discriminate those from lower-affinity clones based on equilibrium binding. A good starting ligand concentration is 1/10 of the K_D of the starting clone. Comprehensive analysis and discussion on the conditions for library sorting are found in Boder and Wittrup (18). Binding profiles of the starting clone and of the library are compared using FACS, and cells exhibiting higher levels of binding are recovered. After two cycles of such sorting, individual clones are analyzed quantitatively (see Subheading 3.3; Note 12).

3.8. FACS Screening of Improved Clones Based on Dissociation Kinetics

When the K_D is lower than 10 nM, it is difficult to discriminate clones based on the level of target binding under equilibrium (18). In such a situation, library sorting based on dissociation kinetics should be employed. According to the relationship, $K_D = k_{off}/k_{on}$, for a simple binding reaction, variants exhibiting slower dissociation rate usually have smaller K_D, i.e., tighter binding. Library sorting based on the dissociation rate involves two steps. First the dissociation kinetics of the starting clone is determined, and then a library is sorted under conditions in which most of the starting clone is eliminated.

1. Grow and induce yeast cells harboring the display vector for the starting clone.
2. Incubate the induced cells with 1 nM biotinylated target in BSS for 30 min.
3. Wash the cells and then incubate them in BSS containing 1 μM nonbiotinylated target and incubate at 4°C.
4. Take samples at intervals (e.g., 1, 15 min, 1.5, 5, and 16 h after previous step), and stain the cells with SAV-PE immediately after sampling.
5. Measure the PE intensities of the cells using FACS. Plot the PE intensity as a function of time and determine the half life of the decay.
6. Incubate the induced cells for a library with 1 nM biotinylated target in BSS for 30 min.
7. Wash the cells and incubate them with buffer containing 1 μM nonbiotinylated target for a period equal to 8–10 times the half-life determined in step e (i.e., time required to eliminate >99% of the binding of the starting clone).
8. Label cells with SAV-PE and antibodies for FACS analysis (see Subheading 3.2).
9. Recover cells exhibiting high expression and binding using a sorter (see Note 6).
10. Grow and induce recovered clones individually (see Subheading 3.2) and measure binding affinity (see Subheading 3.3).
11. Isolate the plasmid from yeast cells exhibiting desired binding property using the yeast DNA preparation kit and use the DNA for sequencing and cloning.

4. Notes

1. It is important to construct a yeast display vector for the starting clone, because it serves as a reference in setting conditions for library sorting (18). It is also important to characterize selected clones side by side with the starting clone (10).
2. We have eliminated the Express tag from the vector, because the tag cross-react with the commonly used anti-FLAG antibodies.

Such cross-reactivity is undesirable because we often use an antigen that contains the FLAG tag.

3. Follow the manufacturer's instructions for preparing a biotinylated antigen. However, it is important to keep the number of biotin modifications per antigen molecule low. This is because "overbiotinylation" can significantly reduce the solubility and also potentially mask the epitope for the antibody of interest.
4. Centrifuged yeast cells are loosely packed. Remove the supernatant as soon as possible after centrifugation.
5. For a FACS analyzer with a 488 nm laser, a dye combination of FITC and PE can be used with proper compensation between the FITC and PE channels. For a FACS analyzer with multiple lasers, it is desirable to select a dye combination that requires no compensation, such as APC and PE.
6. We advise that one performs flow cytometer analysis and cell sorting with an experience user of a specific instrument to be used.
7. When the target concentration is 1–10 nM, final volume of target binding solution was increased to 200 μL. For 0.1–1 nM, final volume of 2 mL was used. In these cases, the number of yeast cells was kept unchanged (10^6 cells/sample).
8. Fitting can be performed using a common data analysis program, such as Origin (Origin Lab), Kaleidagraph (Synergy Software) and Igor Pro (Wavemetrics).
9. Before constructing a library, substitute the codon for the first residue of CDRs to the ochre stop codon (TAA). In this way, this "stop mutant" does not display a VHH molecule on the surface of phage and consequently it is not efficiently recovered during library sorting. Only those library members in which the stop codon is replaced with a nonstop codon are displayed. For library construction see another volume of this series (14).
10. For example, the 5′-half of the VHH gene, containing CDR1 and CDR2, and the 3′-half of the VHH gene, containing CDR3, can be amplified separately. For efficient recombination, there should be 20–30 bases of overlap between PCR products.
11. Although yeast cells can be transformed with multiple overlapping PCR fragments, the use of a single, preassembled fragment gives a greater number of transformants than multiple fragments in our experience.
12. To avoid selecting false positive clones that bind to SAV, SAV-PE and NAV-PE should be used alternately in successive rounds of library sorting.

Acknowledgments

This work was supported by the National Institutes of Health grants R01 GM090324 and RC1 DA028779 to SK.

References

1. Muyldermans S (2001) Single domain camel antibodies: current status. J Biotechnol 74:277–302
2. Muyldermans S, Cambillau C, Wyns L (2001) Recognition of antigens by single-domain antibody fragments: the superfluous luxury of paired domains. Trends Biochem Sci 26:230–235
3. De Genst E, Silence K, Decanniere K, Conrath K, Loris R, Kinne J, Muyldermans S, Wyns L (2006) Molecular basis for the preferential cleft recognition by dromedary heavy-chain antibodies. Proc Natl Acad Sci U S A 103:4586–4591
4. Decanniere K, Desmyter A, Lauwereys M, Ghahroudi MA, Muyldermans S, Wyns L (1999) A single-domain antibody fragment in complex with RNase A: non-canonical loop structures and nanomolar affinity using two CDR loops. Structure 7:361–370
5. Desmyter A, Transue TR, Ghahroudi MA, Thi MH, Poortmans F, Hamers R, Muyldermans S, Wyns L (1996) Crystal structure of a camel single-domain VH antibody fragment in complex with lysozyme. Nat Struct Biol 3:803–811
6. Sidhu SS, Koide S (2007) Phage display for engineering and analyzing protein interaction interfaces. Curr Opin Struct Biol 17:481–487
7. Sidhu SS, Lowman HB, Cunningham BC, Wells JA (2000) Phage display for selection of novel binding peptides. Methods Enzymol 328:333–363
8. Boder ET, Wittrup KD (2000) Yeast surface display for directed evolution of protein expression, affinity, and stability. Methods Enzymol 328:430–444
9. VanAntwerp JJ, Wittrup KD (2000) Fine affinity discrimination by yeast surface display and flow cytometry. Biotechnol Prog 16:31–37
10. Koide A, Tereshko V, Uysal S, Margalef K, Kossiakoff AA, Koide S (2007) Exploring the capacity of minimalist protein interfaces: interface energetics and affinity maturation to picomolar KD of a single-domain antibody with a flat paratope. J Mol Biol 373:941–953
11. Clackson T, Wells JA (1995) A hot spot of binding energy in a hormone-receptor interface. Science 267:383–386
12. Weiss GA, Watanabe CK, Zhong A, Goddard A, Sidhu SS (2000) Rapid mapping of protein functional epitopes by combinatorial alanine scanning. Proc Natl Acad Sci U S A 97: 8950–8954
13. Fellouse FA, Wiesmann C, Sidhu SS (2004) Synthetic antibodies from a four-amino-acid code: a dominant role for tyrosine in antigen recognition. Proc Natl Acad Sci U S A 101: 12467–12472
14. Koide A, Koide S (2007) Monobodies: antibody mimics based on the scaffold of the fibronectin type III domain. Methods Mol Biol 352:95–109
15. Gietz RD, Schiestl RH (2007) High-efficiency yeast transformation using the LiAc/SS carrier DNA/PEG method. Nat Protoc 2:31–34
16. Gietz RD, Woods RA (2002) Transformation of yeast by lithium acetate/single-stranded carrier DNA/polyethylene glycol method. Methods Enzymol 350:87–96
17. Ma H, Kunes S, Schatz PJ, Botstein D (1987) Plasmid construction by homologous recombination in yeast. Gene 58:201–216
18. Boder ET, Wittrup KD (1998) Optimal screening of surface-displayed polypeptide libraries. Biotechnol Prog 14:55–62

Chapter 27

Multivalent Display of Single-Domain Antibodies

Jianbing Zhang and C. Roger MacKenzie

Abstract

Antigen-binding fragments, such as single-domain antibodies (sdAbs), can now be readily isolated by in vitro technologies. Antibody fragment libraries derived from immune or nonimmune sources are presented in a molecular display format, typically phage display, and binders to individual antigens are selected from the libraries by a so-called panning process. Nonimmune libraries can serve as sources of binders to a wide range of targets but yield antigen-binding fragments that generally have much lower affinities than those obtained from immune sources. Here we describe a strategy for constructing pentameric sdAbs termed pentabodies. Pentamerization introduces avidity which can greatly enhance the binding of low affinity sdAbs to antigens presented on surfaces.

Key words: Single-domain antibodies, Pentabodies, Multivalency, Avidity, Antibody Fragment libraries, Phage display

1. Introduction

With the refinement of in vitro antibody generation technologies over the past 2 decades, it is now possible to routinely isolate antibody fragments that bind to essentially any member of the human proteome (1). Compared to hybridoma technology, in vitro antibody isolation approaches offer several advantages such as no requirement for animal care, reduced time and cost for antibody selection, and the capability of isolating antibodies against targets that do not elicit an immune response in animals (1). The antibody fragments can be the fragments antigen binding (Fabs), single chain variable fragments (scFvs), variable light chain domains (VLs), or variable heavy chain domains (VHs) from conventional IgGs; they can also be the variable domains (VHHs) of camelid heavy chain antibodies or the variable domains (VNARs) of shark immunoglobulin new antigen receptors (IgNARs) (2). The term

Dirk Saerens and Serge Muyldermans (eds.), *Single Domain Antibodies: Methods and Protocols*,
Methods in Molecular Biology, vol. 911, DOI 10.1007/978-1-61779-968-6_27, © Springer Science+Business Media, LLC 2012

single-domain antibody is often used to describe VHs, VLs, VHHs, and VNARs (3). Phage display libraries of antigen binding fragments from nonimmune sources can serve as single pot sources of binders to a wide variety of antigens but the affinities of binders from such sources are typically significantly lower than the affinities of binders from immune sources. Introduction of avidity can dramatically improve functional affinity for antigen when the target is available for multivalent binding such as on a Western blot, a cell surface, or a tissue section. Fusion of sdAbs to the pentamerization domain of verotoxin, also known as shiga-like toxin, has been shown to be a highly effective means of enhancing binding to immobilized antigen; these pentavalent sdAbs have been termed pentabodies (4). Single-domain antibodies are ideal antigen binding fragments for construction of such multivalent reagents because of high expressions levels and stability. Moreover, naturally occurring sdAbs such as VHHs do not aggregate, as often happens with scFvs, the most logical candidates for constructing equivalent molecules based on conventional antibodies. However, methods have been described for the selection of nonaggregating sdAbs from human VH libraries (5, 6). Here we describe the construction, expression, purification, and partial characterization of a pentabody, ES1, for which the sdAb building block is AFAI, a VHH isolated by panning a nonimmune llama VHH library against the A549 non-small lung carcinoma cell line (7).

2. Materials

Prepare all solutions using distilled and deionized water (ddH$_2$O) with a sensitivity of 18 MΩ cm at 25 °C) and analytical grade reagents. Prepare and store all reagents at room temperature (unless indicated otherwise). As required, sterilize water and solutions using 0.2 μM filter units. Diligently follow all disposal regulations for hazardous waste materials.

2.1. Assembly of ES1 Gene

1. The gene encoding sdAb AFAI (see Fig. 1), accession number AJ617283 (see Note 1).
2. Pentamerization vector pVT2 (see Fig 1), accession number AJ619719 (see Note 2).
3. Primer AFAI-F: 5′-GAAGAAGAAGACAACAGGCCGATG TGCAGCTGCAGGCGTC-3′.
4. Primer AFAI-R: 5′-GAAGAAGGGCCCTGAGGAGACGGT GACCTGGG-3′.
5. dNTPs (New England BioLabs Ltd. Mississauga, ON, Canada).
6. 10× PCR buffer (Hoffmann-La Roche Ltd., Mississauga, ON, Canada).

a

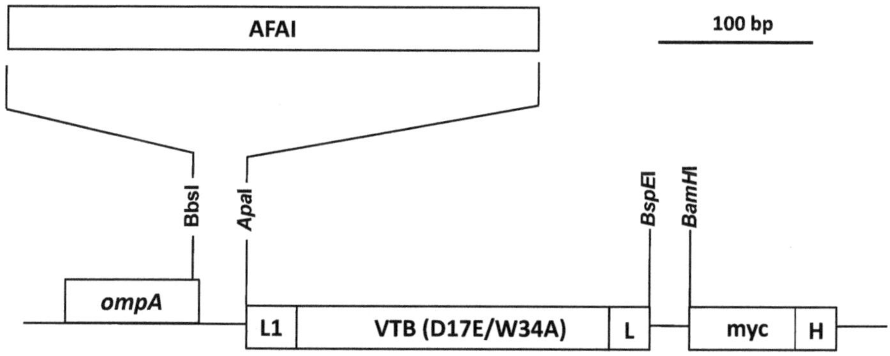

AFAI	sdAb AFAI
ompA	*ompA* leader sequence MKKTAIAIAVALAGFATVAQA
L1	Linker sequence GGGSGGGGS
VTB	D17E/W34A mutant of VTB
L	Linker sequence GGGGS
Myc	c-Myc detection tag EQKLISEEDLN
H	5× histidine purification tag HHHHH

b

DVQLQASGGGVVQPGGSLRLSCAAHDPIFDKNLMGWGRQ
APGKQREYVATISGSGGTNYASSVEGRFTISRDNAKKTV
YLQMNDLKPEDTAVYYCNSAFAIWGQGTQVTVSS

c

TPDCVTGKVEYTKYNDEDTFTVKVGDKELFTNRANLQSL
LLSAQITGMTVTIKTNACHNGGGFSEVIFR

Fig. 1. Construction of the pentabody ES1. (**a**) Schematic drawing of the cloning strategy. (**b**) Amino acid sequence of AFAI. (**a**) Amino acid of VTB (D17E/W34A). The OmpA leader sequence is removed during secretion of the protein into the periplasm.

7. Expand high fidelity Taq DNA polymerase (Hoffmann-La Roche Ltd.).
8. QIAquick Gel Extraction™ kit (QIAGEN, Mississauga, ON, Canada).
9. QIAquick PCR purification™ kit (QIAGEN).
10. Restriction Endonucleases *Bbs*I, *Apa*I and NE buffer 4 (New England BioLabs).
11. LigaFast™ Rapid DNA Ligation System, including T4 DNA ligase buffer and T4 DNA ligase (Promega, Madison, WI, USA).
12. TG1 electroporation-competent cells (Stratagene, La Jolla, CA, USA).
13. LB agar (8).
14. Sterile ampicillin.
15. Sterile 70% glycerol.
16. Sterile ddH_2O.

17. 0.2 μm MILLEX®-GV filter units (Millipore, Toronto, ON, Canada). Use these units for small volumes, e.g., antibiotic solutions.
18. Disposable electroporation cuvettes.
19. Agarose gel electrophoresis equipment.
20. Thermocycler for performing polymerase chain reactions (PCR).
21. ND-1000 spectrophotometer (NanoDrop Technologies, Wilmington, DE, USA) or a similar instrument.
22. MicroPulser™ electroporator (Bio-Rad Laboratories, Mississauga, ON, Canada) or a similar instrument.
23. Cell densitometer (Fisher Scientific, Nepean, ON) or any standard spectrophotometer.
24. Sterile toothpicks.
25. 15, 25, and 37° C water baths.

2.2. Expression and Purification of ES1

1. M9/Amp: M9 medium (8) supplemented with 5 μg/mL vitamin B1, 0.4% casamino acids and 100 μg/mL ampicillin.
2. Filter-sterilized IPTG (isopropyl-β-D-thio-galactopyranoside).
3. 10× induction medium: 12% tryptone, 24% yeast extract, and 4% (v/v) glycerol.
4. Wash solution: 10 mM Tris–HCl, pH 8.0, 150 mM NaCl.
5. Sucrose solution: 10 mM Tris–HCl, pH 8.0, 1 mM EDTA, 25% sucrose.
6. Shock solution: 10 mM Tris–HCl, pH 8.0, 0.5 mM $MgCl_2$ (keep on ice).
7. Anti-c-Myc tag monoclonal antibody (Jackson ImmunoResearch Inc., Cambridgeshire, UK).
8. Starting buffer: 10 mM HEPES (*N*-[2-hydroxyethyl]piperazine-*N′*-[2-ethanesulfonic acid]), 10 mM imidazole, 500 mM NaCl, pH 7.0.
9. Dialysis membrane (10 kDa MW cut-off).
10. SDS-PAGE (sodium dodecyl sulfate-polyacrylamide gel electrophoresis) and Western blotting equipment.
11. $NiCl_2{\cdot}6H_2O$ (5 mg/mL).
12. Elution buffer: 10 mM HEPES, 1 M imidazole, 500 mM NaCl, pH 7.0.
13. Sodium phosphate buffer: 6.7 mM Na_2HPO_4, 3.3 mM NaH_2PO_4, 150 mM NaCl, 0.5 mM EDTA, pH 7.0.
14. Sodium azide.
15. 5-mL HiTrap™ Chelating HP column (GE Healthcare, Baie-d-Urfé, QC, Canada).
16. ÄKTA FPLC purification system (GE Healthcare) or similar instrument.

2.3. Analysis of AFAI and ES1 Binding to CEACAM6-A

1. Recombinant CEACAM6-A, the N-terminal domain of CEACAM6 (gift from Helix BioPharma Corp., Aurora, ON, Canada).
2. AFAIKL2, AFAI with a C-terminal lysine (gift from Helix BioPharma Corp.).
3. ES1, a pentameric version of AFAI (7).
4. Superdex™ 75 10/300 GL and Superdex™ 200 10/300 GL gel filtration columns (GE Healthcare).
5. HBS-E buffer: 10 mM HEPES, pH 7.4, 150 mM NaCl, 3 mM EDTA. This buffer can be purchased from GE Healthcare. If not purchased from GE Healthcare, it should be thoroughly degassed before use.
6. Surfactant P20 (GE Healthcare).
7. Amine coupling kit containing *N*-hydroxysuccinimide (NHS), *N*-ethyl-*N′*-(3-dimethylaminopropyl)carbodiimide hydrochloride (EDC), and ethanolamine (GE Healthcare).
8. Immobilization buffer: 10 mM acetate buffer, pH 4.0 (see Note 3).
9. Blocking solution: 1 M ethanolamine, pH 8.5.
10. CM5 sensor chips (GE Healthcare).
11. BIACORE 3000 (GE Healthcare) or other surface plasmon resonance (SPR) instrument with similar capabilities.

3. Methods

3.1. Assembly of ES1 Gene

1. Amplify the AFAI gene by PCR using a plasmid containing the AFAI gene as template and AFAI-F and AFAI-R as primers. This reaction amplifies the intact AFAI gene and adds the *Bbs*I and *Apa*I to the 5′- and 3′-ends of the gene, respectively.

   dNTPs (2.5 mM each): 4 μL

   10× PCR buffer: 5 μL

   Primers AFAI-F and AFAI-R (10 μM): 0.5 μL each

   Plasmid template (1 ng/μL): 1 μL

   Expand high fidelity Taq DNA polymerase (3.5 U/μL): 0.5 μL

   Sterile ddH_2O: 39 μL

   Place the reaction tubes in a thermocycler and synthesize the DNA fragment with a program consisting of a preheating step at 94 °C for 5 min and 30 cycles of 94 °C for 30 s, 55 °C for 30 s, and 72 °C for 1 min. Clean the PCR product, designated PCR1, with a QIAquick PCR purification Kit™.
2. Digest pVT2 with *Bbs*I and *Apa*I.

pVT2 (500 ng/μL): 6 μL

NE Buffer 4: 2 μL

*Apa*I (50 U/μL): 1 μL

Sterile ddH_2O: 11 μL

Place the reaction in a 25 °C water bath and incubate for 2 h. After the *Apa*I digestion, add 1 μL of *Bbs*I (20 U/μL), place the reaction in a 37 °C water bath and continue the reaction overnight (see Note 4).

3. Digest the PCR product with *Bbs*I and *Apa*I.

   PCR1 (500 ng/μL): 6 μL

   NE Buffer 4: 2 μL

   *Apa*I (50 U/μL): 1 μL

   sddH_2O: 11 μL

   Place the reaction in a 25 °C water bath and incubate for 2 h. Add 1 μL of *Bbs*I (20 U/μL) after the reaction, place the mixture in a 37 °C water bath and continue the reaction for overnight (see Note 3).

4. Purify from gel the *Bbs*I and *Apa*I digested pVT2 and the PCR product using a QIAquick Gel Extraction™ kit. Determine the concentration of both DNA products based on $OD_{260\ nm}$ measurements on a ND-1000 spectrophotometer.
5. Ligate the PCR product into pVT2.

   *Bbs*I and *Apa*I digested pVT2 (~100 ng/μL): 4 μL

   *Bbs*I and *Apa*I digested PCR product (~50 ng/μL): 4 μL

   T4 DNA ligase buffer: 1 μL

   T4 DNA ligase (3 U/μL): 1 μL

   Place the reaction tube in a 15 °C water bath and incubate for 4 h.

6. Purify digested vector with a QIAquick PCR purification kit and water elution.
7. To transform *Escherichia coli* TG1, add 0.5 μL of ligation mixture to 40 μL of TG1 competent cells for electroporation and transform the TG1 cells using a MicroPulser™ or an equivalent instrument. Transfer the transformed cells to 1 mL of LB medium and incubate at 37 °C and 180 rpm for 1 h. Plate 2, 10, and 100 μL of the culture on an LB plate supplemented with 100 μg/mL ampicillin plates. Sediment the remaining cells by centrifugation at 4,400 × *g* for 15 min, remove most of the medium, resuspend the cells in the remaining medium (~100 μL) and plate them on a fourth plate.

8. Perform colony PCR (see Subheading 3.1, step 1) except using bacterial cells grown on the plates as template. After mixing all reagents except the template and aliquoting the mixture into PCR tubes (12 μL each), use a sterile toothpick to touch a colony and then dip it into a PCR tube. Repeat this step for a total of 20 colonies and perform PCR (see Subheading 3.1, step 1). Perform agarose gel electrophoresis to determine the size of the PCR products.
9. Isolate plasmids from clones with PCR products of ~400 bp, and confirm the integrity of the clones by sequencing the plasmids using AFAI-F and AFAI-R as primers.

3.2. Expression and Purification of ES1

Monomeric and pentameric sdAbs are cloned in fusion with the OmpA leader sequence to direct expressed protein to the periplasm. The osmotic shock method described below (9) is designed to increase the permeability of the outer membrane and release monomers and pentamers from the periplasm, without lysing the cells. Since the protein content of the periplasm is much less than that of the cytoplasm, the periplasmic extraction step results in partial purification of the expressed recombinant protein. The presence of c-Myc and His_5 tags at the C-terminus of monomers and pentamers allows for expression verification by Western blotting using commercially available anti-c-Myc or anti-His tag antibodies. The presence of the C-terminal His_5 tag in VHHs allows for one-step protein purification by immobilized metal affinity chromatography (IMAC) using a HiTrap™ Chelating HP column (see Note 5). The protocols described below are largely identical to those outlined for large-scale expression and purification of (see Chapter 16).

1. Use a single positive clone to inoculate 100 mL of M9/Amp. Incubate in a rotary shaker at 200 rpm for 24 h at 25 °C.
2. Transfer 30 mL of the above preculture to 1 L of M9/Amp. Incubate the culture at 200 rpm for 24 h at 25 °C followed by supplementation with 100 mL of 10× induction medium and 100 μL of 1 M IPTG. Incubate for another 48 h at 25 °C.
3. Reserve a small aliquot for Western blotting (see Subheading 3.2, step 7) and centrifuge the remaining culture at 5,000 × *g* for 20 min at 4 °C. Keep the supernatant fraction at 4 °C.
4. Resuspend the pellet in 150 mL of wash solution. Centrifuge at 14,000 × *g* for 10 min at 4 °C. Keep the supernatant fraction at 4 °C.
5. Resuspend the pellet in 50 mL of sucrose solution and incubate at room temperature for 10 min. Centrifuge at 14,000 × *g* for 45 min at 4 °C. Keep the supernatant fraction at 4 °C.
6. Resuspend the pellet in 50 mL of ice-cold shock solution and incubate in an ice bath for 10 min. Centrifuge at 14,000 × *g* for 25 min at 4 °C. Keep the supernatant fraction at 4 °C.

7. Verify expression by detecting the presence of monomers and pentamers in fractions (see Subheading 3.2, steps 3–6) by Western blotting against the c-Myc tag (10) using anti-c-Myc antibody (see Note 6). Pool the fractions which contain monomers and pentamers and dialyze against 6 L of starting buffer overnight at 4 °C using a dialysis membrane with a 10 kDa MW cutoff.
8. Proceed with protein purification.
9. Charge the column with Ni^{2+} with 30 mL of a 5 mg/mL $NiCl_2{\cdot}6H_2O$ solution and subsequently wash the column with 2–5 column volumes of deionized water.
10. Perform purification on an ÄKTA FPLC purification instrument according to the instructions provided by the manufacturer. After loading the extract on the column in starting buffer, elute bound protein using the elution buffer with a 10 mM–1 M imidazole gradient.
11. Analyze the fractions corresponding to the eluted peaks on the chromatogram for the presence and purity of the monomeric and pentameric sdAbs by SDS-PAGE (11). Pool the fractions containing pure monomer or pentamer product and dialyze extensively against sodium phosphate buffer. Dissolve any precipitate by the addition of EDTA to give a final concentration of up to 3 mM. Measure $OD_{280\ nm}$ for determination of protein concentration from molar extinction coefficients (12), add sodium azide at a final concentration of 0.02%, and store the monomeric and pentameric sdAbs at 4 °C.

3.3. Analysis of AFAI and ES1 Binding to CEACAM6-A

Standard ELISA methods can be employed to determine the binding specificities of, and approximate affinities of the sdAb–antigen interactions. However, accurate binding affinities and information on the kinetics of binding can be determined by SPR analyses.

1. Isolate nonaggregated monomeric and pentameric sdAbs prior to SPR analysis by Superdex 75 and Superdex 200 size exclusion column chromatography, respectively (column volumes = 25 mL). Equilibrate the columns with 2–5 column volumes of HBS-E buffer containing 0.005% surfactant P20 at a pump speed of 0.5 mL/min, inject 200 μL of IMAC-purified protein and collect the monomer or pentamer peak fractions. Determine the protein concentrations.
2. Carry out SPR experiments at 25 °C using a BIACORE 3000 instrument with HBS-E containing 0.005% surfactant P20 as the running buffer.
3. Activate the CM-dextran surface on a CM5 sensor chip with a 7 min injection of a mixture of 50 mM NHS and 200 mM EDC at a flow rate of 5 μL/min. Inject 50 μg/mL antigen diluted in 10 mM acetate buffer, pH 4.0, for 3 min and block

the surface with a 7 min injection of 1 M ethanolamine, pH 8.5 (see Note 7).

4. Analyze monomer and pentamer interaction with antigen using an appropriate reference surface. Inject 10 or 20 μL of six or more different concentrations of monomer over both the active and reference surfaces at a flow rate of 50 μL/min to collect a data set for K_D determination.
5. Analyze the data using BIA evaluation software 4.1 (GE Healthcare). Calculate the K_Ds for monomer binding to antigen by steady state affinity fitting and/or from rate constants. Determine the approximate dissociation rate constants for monomer and pentabody binding to antigen by analyzing one or more portions of the dissociation phase (see Notes 8–10).

4. Notes

1. AFAI, which recognizes carcinoembryonic antigen-related cell adhesion molecule 6 (CEACAM6), has been described previously (7).
2. This vector was constructed previously (13) and serves to fuse an sdAb to either the N-, C- or both termini of a D17E/W34A mutant of the B-subunit of verotoxin 1. Use of this mutant, which has a ~10^6-fold reduction in binding affinity to its receptor CD77 (14), will prevent the constructed pentabodies from binding to kidney epithelial cells or other human cells expressing CD77.
3. The immobilization pH may differ for other antigens and is dictated by the isoelectric point of the antigen. At the immobilization pH the antigen should have a positive charge to attract it to the negatively charged CM5 sensor chip surface. However, the immobilization pH should not be lower than pH 3.5.
4. For digestion of DNA with two restriction enzymes, efficient digestion of the DNA by either enzyme should be examined by single digestion and subsequent agarose gel electrophoresis. For digestion of PCR products, where efficient digestion is often undetectable on agarose gel, examination of the digestion of a plasmid bearing the restriction site(s) can be used as a control.
5. The pentabodies actually have five His_5 tags. Accordingly, they bind more tightly to IMAC columns than monomers which have only one His_5 tag, eluting at a higher imidazole concentration. Due to their stronger retention on metal ion columns, pentabodies can often be purified from cell lysates (see Chapter 16) by IMAC, whereas this is generally not feasible with monomers.

6. Commercially available anti-His-tag antibodies can also be used for detection. The monomers and pentamers are generally found in both the "sucrose" and "shock" fractions.
7. The surface density should be high enough to achieve maximum binding valency.
8. The valency of binding of a pentabody to an antigen surface depends on numerous factors and in almost all instances is likely to be heterogeneous, i.e., a mixture of binding valencies. To ensure maximum binding valencies high antigen density surfaces should be used and pentabody concentrations should be kept relatively low, since at high pentabody concentrations competition for available antigen leads to lower binding valencies. The lower binding valencies at higher pentabody concentrations are manifested in faster dissociation rate constants (see Fig. 2).
9. The heterogeneity of pentabody binding to antigen makes it impossible to accurately calculate functional affinities for these interactions and consequently to derive accurate numbers for the increase in functional affinity conferred by the introduction of avidity. The heterogeneity of binding valency is manifested in faster dissociation rate constants at the beginning of SPR sensorgram dissociation phases, relative to later stages in the dissociation (see Fig. 2). A reasonable estimate of the avidity gain can be made by comparing the dissociation rate constant of the monomer with that of the pentamer at various stages in the dissociation phase. In the example provided here the monomer off-rate was 7×10^{-1}/s, whereas that of the pentamer was as slow as 5.3×10^{-4}/s, indicating an avidity gain of over 1,000-fold.
10. The pentabodies described here, with a nine amino acid linker between the sdAb and VTB, are probably not able to bind to larger antigens with high valency (with a molecular weight of 13 kDa, the CEACAM6-A fragment used in the studies described here is relatively small). To increase binding valency with larger antigens longer linkers should be considered—e.g., $(GGGGS)_4$.

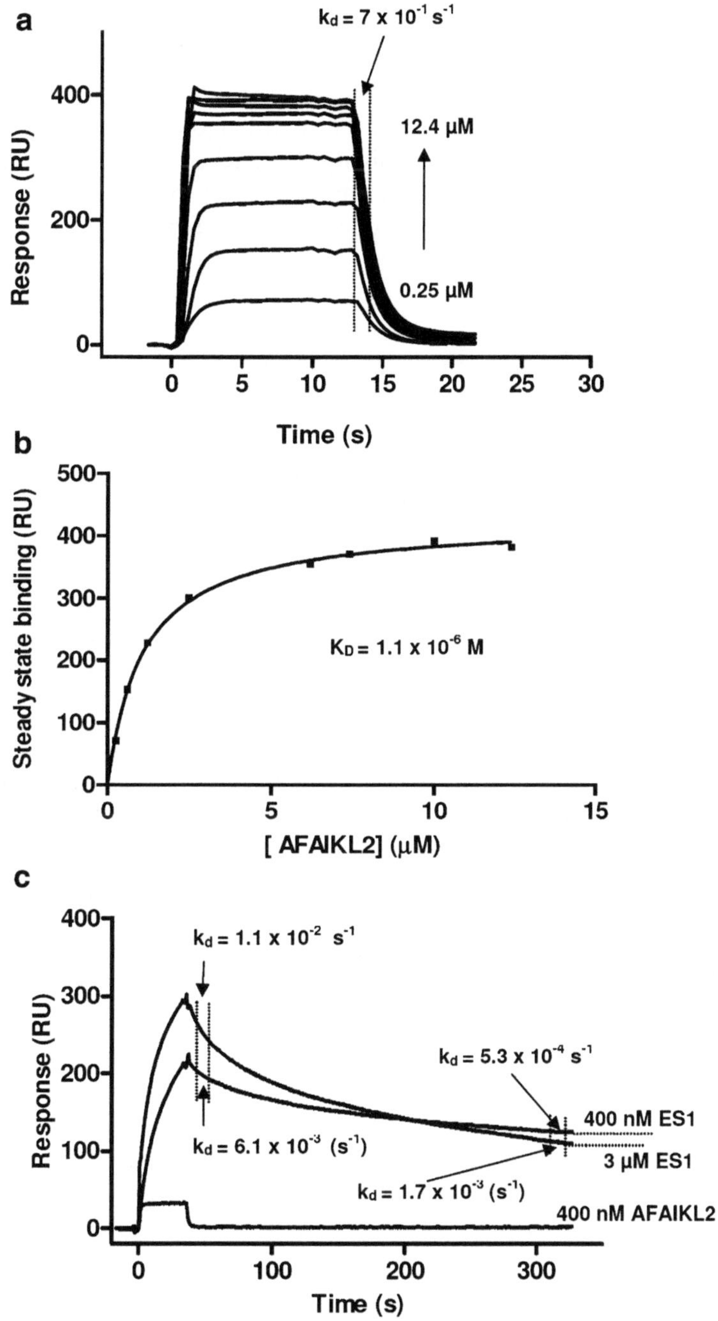

Fig. 2. SPR analysis of AFAIKL2 and ES1 binding to immobilized CEACAM6-A. (**a**) Injection of AFAIKL2 at concentrations of 0.25–12.4 μM over a 1,750 resonance unit (RU) surface. (**b**) Fitting of the equilibrium data in A to a steady-state affinity model. (**c**) Injection of 400 nM AFAIKL2, 400 nM ES1 and 3 μM ES1 over a 1,050 RU surface. For ES1, the dissociation rate constants at early and late stages in the dissociation phase are indicated.

Acknowledgement

We thank Heman Chao and colleagues at Helix BioPharma Corp. for supplying AFAIKL2 and the CEACAM6-A antigen. We thank Thanh-Dung Nguyen for performing the SPR analyses. The authors declare no financial conflict of interest.

References

1. Dübel S et al (2010) Generating recombinant antibodies to the complete human proteome. Trends Biotechnol 28:333–339
2. Holliger P, Hudson PJ (2005) Engineered antibody fragments and the rise of single domains. Nat Biotechnol 23:1126–1136
3. Muyldermans S et al (2010) Camelid immunoglobulins and nanobody technology. Vet Immunol Immunopathol 128:178–183
4. Zhang J et al (2004) Pentamerization of single-domain antibodies from phage libraries: a novel strategy for generation of high-avidity antibody reagents. J Mol Biol 335:49–56
5. Jespers L et al (2004) Aggregation-resistant domain antibodies selected on phage by heat denaturation. Nat Biotechnol 22:1161–1165
6. Arbabi-Ghahroudi M et al (2008) Aggregation-resistant V_Hs selected by in vitro evolution tend to have disulfide-bonded loops and acidic isoelectric points. Protein Eng Des Sel 22:59–66
7. Zhang J et al (2004) A pentavalent single-domain antibody approach to tumor antigen discovery and the development of novel proteomics reagents. J Mol Biol 341:161–169
8. Sambrook J, Fritsch EF, Maniatis T (eds) (1989) Molecular cloning: a laboratory manual. Cold Spring Harbor Laboratory, Cold Spring Harbor
9. Anand NN et al (1991) Synthesis and expression in *Escherichia coli* of cistronic DMA encoding an antibody fragment specific for a *Salmonella* serotype B O-antigen. Gene 100:39–44
10. MacKenzie CR et al (1884) Effect of C_λ-C_κ domain switching on Fab activity and yield in *Escherichia coli*: synthesis and expression of two anti-carbohydrate Fabs. Biotechnology (N Y) 12:390–395
11. Laemmli UK (1970) Cleavage of structural proteins during the assembly of the head of bacteriophage T4. Nature 227:680–685
12. Pace CN et al (1995) How to measure and predict the molar absorption coefficient of a protein. Protein Sci 4:2411–2423
13. Stone E et al (2007) The assembly of single domain antibodies into bispecific decavalent molecules. J Immunol Methods 318: 88–94
14. Soltyk AM et al (2002) A mutational analysis of the globotriaosylceramide-binding sites of verotoxin VT1. J Biol Chem 277: 5351–5359

Chapter 28

Methods for Determining the PK Parameters of AlbudAbs™ and of Long Serum Half-Life Drugs Made Using the AlbudAb™ Technology

Daniel Rycroft and Lucy J. Holt

Abstract

Increasing serum residence time of drugs by means of fusing them to albumin-binding domain antibodies (AlbudAbs™) has previously been documented. AlbudAbs™ provide a valuable method for increasing the efficacy of drugs by extending the time for which therapeutic levels of drug are present in the body and also for increasing the convenience to the patient by reducing the need for frequent dosing. Here, we describe methods that could be used preclinically to determine the suitability of drug-AlbudAbs™ for development. Particular focus is given to suggested *in vivo* study design which could enable the fitting of accurate PK parameters, assay methods for concentration determination of AlbudAbs™ in blood samples, and to the protocols used to fit PK parameters to AlbudAb™ concentration data. Whilst the examples cited here are focussed on the AlbudAb™ technology, similar methods could be used for assessing the success of other half-life extension technologies (drug Fc fusions, PEGylated drugs).

Key words: AlbudAb™, Domain Antibody, dAb™, Antibody fragment, Therapeutic, PK, Half-life

1. Introduction

Drugs with extended serum half-life can be dosed less frequently (e.g., weekly) than their first-generation counterparts that must be dosed frequently (e.g., daily or twice a day) whilst achieving similar or better efficacy. Biopharm drugs with extended serum half-lives either promise to make or have already made a significant impact on dosing regimens for patients in a variety of diseases, e.g., Albiglutide for type II diabetes (1) and Etaneracept for Rheumatoid arthritis (2). Half-life extension for biopharm drug candidates has been achieved in several ways; by expressing the drug as a genetic fusion with a protein which has long serum half-life, e.g., albumin (3, 4) or the Fc region of an antibody (5); by chemically attaching the drug to polyethylene glycol (PEG) which increases the hydrodynamic

Dirk Saerens and Serge Muyldermans (eds.), *Single Domain Antibodies: Methods and Protocols*,
Methods in Molecular Biology, vol. 911, DOI 10.1007/978-1-61779-968-6_28, © Springer Science+Business Media, LLC 2012

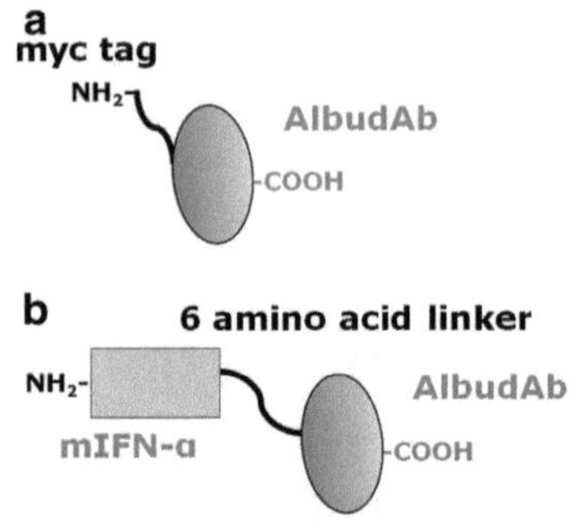

Fig. 1. A diagram of a Myc-tagged AlbudAb™ (**a**) and an AlbudAb™ fusion (mIFN-α AlbudAb™) (**b**) to illustrate the molecules used in the PK methods described.

size of the protein (6); and by selecting small binding domains that have affinity for serum albumin (e.g., AlbudAbs™) and fusing these albumin-binding domains to therapeutic drugs either by expression as a genetic fusion or by chemical means (7, 8) (as shown in Fig. 1). As albumin itself has a serum half-life in humans of 19 days (9) and is a well-validated carrier for many small molecule drugs, AlbudAbs™ fused to a drug allow these biopharm drugs to be carried around the body by albumin and to take on PK parameters similar to those of albumin itself.

Here we describe methods that could be used to detect AlbudAb™ levels in serum, for those AlbudAbs™ that are from Vk domain antibody (dAb™) phage libraries based on the DPk9 framework. These detection methods can be used to analyse serum from PK studies to determine whether candidate AlbudAbs™ (originally isolated from a phage display library(10)) have desirable preclinical *in vivo* PK characteristics. Such PK characteristics enable identification of AlbudAbs™ that could be selected for fusion to therapeutic moieties (e.g., interferon, IL-1ra). We describe the *in vivo* study designs that could be used for PK studies in rat and both an ELISA and an alternative Mesoscale Discovery (MSD) method based on electrochemiluminescent (ECL) detection of sulfo-tagged detection reagents (11, 12) that could be used to assay AlbudAb™ concentrations in serum. We have included the ELISA method as this requires equipment available in most molecular biology laboratories and also the alternative MSD method, as this tends to have higher sensitivity of detection (see Fig. 2 for a signal to background comparison), but does require the laboratory to have a specialist MSD sector 6000 instrument. For completeness, we have included protocols that could be used to generate bespoke reagents (both the immunization strategy that was used to generate a polyclonal anti-Vk reagent that binds all Vk AlbudAbs™ tested to date and the method that could be used to

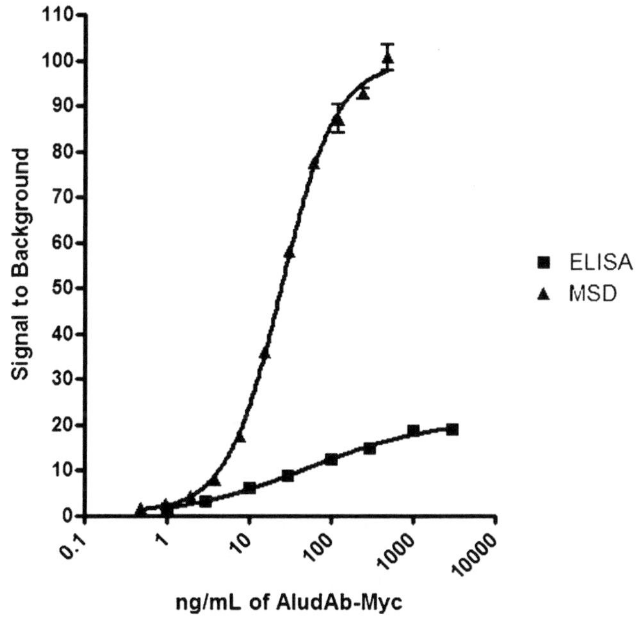

Fig. 2. A comparison plot of the signal to background values of a Myc-tagged AlbudAb™ reference standard when detected by either ELISA (see Subheading 3.3) or by the alternative MSD assay (see Subheading 3.5). The signal to background value was determined by dividing the signal obtained at each AlbudAb™ concentration by the mean assay background result (when no AlbudAb™ is present).

sulfo-tag this detection reagent for use in MSD). Also included is an example method that could be used to detect a surrogate therapeutic-AlbudAb™ fusion (mIFN-alpha, AlbudAb™) in serum. This is a method that could also been customized for a variety of other AlbudAb™ fusions, by using appropriate commercially available capture antibodies to capture whichever therapeutic moiety is in the fusion. Lastly, we have described noncompartmental analysis methods (13) which can be used to fit PK parameters to the AlbudAb™ concentration data generated by ELISA or MSD (example data shown in Fig. 3). Overall, the methods described here could be used to enable AlbudAbs™ and Therapeuitic-AlbudAbs™ to be optimised.

2. Materials

Prepare all solutions using ultrapure water (prepared by purifying deionized water to attain a sensitivity of 18 MΩ cm at 25°C) and analytical grade reagents. Prepare and store all buffer reagents at room temperature (unless indicated otherwise). AlbudAb™ material

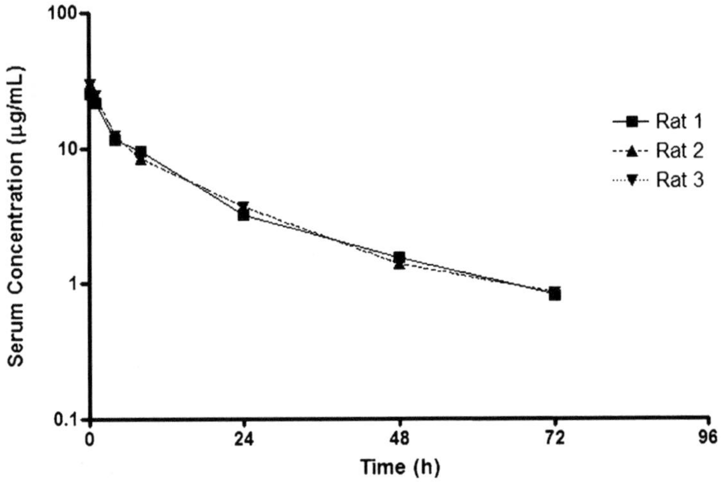

Fig. 3. An example PK profile of Myc-tagged AlbudAb™ DOM7h-11 when administered to rat as an intravenous bolus injection at a target dose of 2.5 mg/kg, as determined using the Myc capture ELISA (see Subheading 3.3).

should be kept at 4°C until use. Antibodies for assay can be stored short-term at 4°C or long-term at −20°C, unless stated otherwise by the manufacturer. Diligently follow all waste disposal regulations when disposing waste materials

2.1. Rat PK Studies: In Vivo Phase

1. Sterile Dulbecco's PBS: Sodium chloride 8.0 g/L, Potassium chloride 0.2 g/L, Di-sodium hydrogen phosphate 1.15 g/L, Potassium di-hydrogen phosphate 0.2 g/L, pH 7.3 ± 0.2 at 25°C.
2. Dosed AlbudAb™ material, produced to meet specifications (see Note 1).
3. Sprague–Dawley Rats (Charles River International, MA, USA).
4. Pellet diet, RMI (E) SQC, Special Diet Services, Witham, Essex, UK.
5. Plain tubes suitable for blood collection and preparation of serum, for example, Microcontainer serum tubes #365951 (BD, NJ, USA).

2.2. Developing Rabbit Anti-dAb™ Polyclonal Antibodies

1. White New Zealand Rabbits (Charles River International, MA, USA).
2. Dosed dAb™ material, produced to meet specifications (see Note 1).
3. Complete Freund's Adjuvant #F5881 (Sigma-Aldrich Company Ltd, Dorset, UK).

4. Incomplete Freund's Adjuvant #F5506 (Sigma-Aldrich Company Ltd, Dorset, UK).
5. Streamline rProtein A resin #17-1281-02 (GE Healthcare, Buckinghamshire, UK).

2.3. Myc Capture ELISA

1. Nunc Maxisorp ELISA Plates #439454 (Nalge Nunc International, NY, USA).
2. Goat anti-Myc polyclonal antibody #ab9132 (AbCam, Cambridge, UK).
3. 0.2 M Sodium carbonate-bicarbonate coating buffer pH 9.4 #28382 (Pierce/Thermo Scientific, IL, USA).
4. Dulbecco's PBS: Sodium chloride 8.0 g/L, Potassium chloride 0.2 g/L, Di-sodium hydrogen phosphate 1.15 g/L, Potassium di-hydrogen phosphate 0.2 g/L, pH 7.3 ± 0.2 at 25° C.
5. Tween-20 #BPR337 (Fisher Scientific UK, Loughborough, UK).
6. BSA #A7030 (Sigma-Aldrich Company Ltd, Dorset, UK).
7. Polyclonal rabbit anti-dAb™ reagent (see Subheading 3.2 for production).
8. AlbudAb™-Myc reference standard, usually produced to meet specifications (see Note 1).
9. Mouse anti-rabbit IgG HRP #A2074 (Sigma-Aldrich Company Ltd, Dorset, UK).
10. SureBlue TMB #52-00-00 (KPL Inc, Maryland, USA).
11. 1 M HCl #J/4320/21 (Fisher Scientific UK, Loughborough, UK).

2.4. Custom Labeling Rabbit Anti-dAb™ Polyclonal Antibodies with MSD Sulfo-Tag

1. Ruthenium MSD sulfo-tag NHS ester # R91AN-1 (MSD, Maryland, USA).
2. Zeba desalt columns #89890 (Pierce/Thermo Scientific, IL, USA).
3. BCA assay kit #23225 (Pierce/Thermo Scientific, IL, USA).
4. BGG standard #23212 (Pierce/Thermo Scientific, IL, USA).

2.5. Myc Capture Electrochemiluminescent Assay Using MSD

1. Standard bind 96-well uncoated MSD plates #L15XA-7 (MSD, Maryland, USA).
2. Goat anti-Myc polyclonal antibody #ab9132 (AbCam, Cambridge, UK).
3. Dulbecco's PBS: Sodium chloride 8.0 g/L, Potassium chloride 0.2 g/L, Di-sodium hydrogen phosphate 1.15 g/L, Potassium di-hydrogen phosphate 0.2 g/L, pH 7.3 ± 0.2 at 25°C.

4. Tween-20 #BPR337 (Fisher Scientific UK, Loughborough, UK).
5. BSA #A7030 (Sigma-Aldrich Company Ltd, Dorset, UK).
6. AlbudAb™-Myc reference standard, usually produced to meet specifications (see Note 1).
7. MSD sulfo-tagged polyclonal rabbit anti-dAb™ reagent (see Subheadings 3.2 and 3.4 for production).
8. MSD read buffer T with surfactant #R92TC-1 (MSD, Maryland, USA).

2.6. Example Assay to Detect Therapeutic-AlbudAb™ Molecules

1. Standard bind 96-well uncoated MSD plates #L15XA-7 (MSD, Maryland, USA).
2. Monoclonal rat anti-mouse IFNα #22100-1 (PBL InterferonSource, NJ, USA).
3. Dulbecco's PBS: Sodium chloride 8.0 g/L, Potassium chloride 0.2 g/L, Di-sodium hydrogen phosphate 1.15 g/L, Potassium di-hydrogen phosphate 0.2 g/L, pH 7.3 ± 0.2 at 25°C.
4. Tween-20 #BPR337 (Fisher Scientific UK, Loughborough, UK).
5. BSA #A7030 (Sigma-Aldrich Company Ltd, Dorset, UK).
6. AlbudAb™ reference standard, usually produced to meet specifications (see Note 1).
7. MSD sulfo-tagged polyclonal rabbit anti-dAb™ reagent (see Subheadings 3.2 and 3.4 for production).
8. MSD read buffer T with surfactant #R92TC-1 (MSD, Maryland, USA).

2.7. Noncompartmental Analysis

1. WinNonLin v5.2 (Pharsight, Missouri, USA).

3. Methods

3.1. Rat PK Studies: In Vivo Phase

1. Prepare AlbudAbs™ at a concentration suitable for dosing, formulated in sterile Dulbecco's PBS. If the aim of the study is to determine the PK parameters of AlbudAb™ alone, then Myc-tagged AlbudAb™ should be provided, if it is to test the PK parameters of a therapeutic-AlbudAb™ fusion then therapeutic-AlbudAb™ fusion should be provided (see Notes 2 and 3). Sufficient protein should be provided to dose all animals, assuming at least a 30% excess for syringe dead volume. Aim for an endotoxin level that is ≤40 EU/kg of animal. AlbudAbs™ should be kept chilled at 4°C from preparation until dosing (see Note 1).

2. Order sufficient male or female Sprague–Dawley rats to cover study requirements, plus spare animals in case of animal illness. Animals should arrive in the animal house weighing 200–350 g (see Notes 4 and 5).
3. Give each rat a unique identification number, marked onto the tail using permanent ink.
4. Examine rats for external signs of illness and exclude any unhealthy animals from the study.
5. House animals in groups of 4 in polypropylene cages in a thermostatically monitored room (21 ± 2°C) and exposed to 12 h of fluorescent light and 12 h of dark per day. Record temperature and relative humidity (55 ± 10%) continuously throughout the experiment.
6. Allow rats to settle into these conditions for a minimum of 3 days prior to dosing, with the health status of all animals monitored throughout and the suitability of the animal for use confirmed immediately before dosing.
7. A pellet diet and water from the domestic water supply should be available *ad libitum*.
8. Administer each AlbudAb™ under analysis into three rats at $t = 0$ h with a target dose for AlbudAb™ molecules of 2.5 mg/kg. Administer the dose by volume, based on the weight of the rat, as a single bolus injection into the tail vein.
9. At a range of time points, take serial blood samples from each individual rat. The time points typically used in rat studies of AlbudAbs™ are 10 min, 1, 4, 8, 24, 48, 72, 120, and 168 h postdose.
10. Collect serial blood samples into plain tubes and allow to clot at 4°C. Clotted samples should then be centrifuged at approximately 3,000 × *g* for 10 min. Serum is then pipetted into neutral tubes and immediately frozen and stored at −20°C until analysis.

3.2. Developing Rabbit Anti-dAb™ Polyclonal Antibodies

1. Generate anti-dAb™ antisera in white New Zealand rabbits (see Note 4). For each anti-dAb™ isotype reagent, use two groups of three rabbits. One group will receive a combination immunization strategy; the other will receive an alternating immunization strategy.
2. At $t = 0$, collect a predose blood sample from all animals for serum preparation. This sample will act as a baseline to monitor the immune response.
3. For each dAb™ isotype, provide two different dAbs™ for immunization. One should be dummy or germline dAb™ with no known activity, the other should be a therapeutic dAb™.

4. For the combination strategy group, mix both dAbs™ together at equal concentrations and immunized as follows:
   - Day 0 = Collect predose, followed by a 200 μg immunization of the dAb™ mixture (100 μg of each) in complete Freunds adjuvant (CFA)
   - Day 14 + 28 + 42 = booster immunization with 100 μg of the dAb™ mixture (50 μg of each) in incomplete Freunds adjuvant (IFA)
   - Day 49 = test bleed 1
   - Day 56 = booster immunization with 100 μg of the dAb™ mixture (50 μg of each) in IFA
   - Day 63 = test bleed 2
   - Day 70 = booster immunization with 100 μg of the dAb™ mixture (50 μg of each) in IFA
   - Day 77 = test bleed 3 + final bleed
5. For the alternating strategy group, keep both dAbs™ separate and dose as alternating boosters as follows:
   - Day 0 = Collect predose, followed by a 200 μg immunization of the therapeutic dAb™ in CFA
   - Day 14 = booster immunization, but with 100 μg of the dummy/germline dAb™ in IFA
   - Day 28 = booster immunization, but with 100 μg of the therapeutic dAb™ in IFA
   - Day 42 = booster immunization, but with 100 μg of the dummy/germline dAb™ in IFA
   - Day 49 = test bleed 1
   - Day 56 = booster immunization, but with 100 μg of the therapeutic dAb™ in IFA
   - Day 63 = test bleed 2
   - Day 70 = booster immunization, but with 100 μg of the dummy/germline dAb™ in IFA
   - Day 77 = test bleed 3 + final bleed
6. Monitor test bleeds for responses against a mixture of the immunized dAbs™ throughout the protocol using ELISA. Ensure the response is specific to the dAb™ isotype of choice by including a negative control screen against dAbs™ of an irrelevant isotype.
7. Assuming all animals are positive for a specific response, pool the final bleed serum from all rabbits of both immunization strategies. Purify to extract serum IgG using protein A and standard biochemical techniques.

3.3. Myc Capture ELISA

This ELISA is used to measure the concentration of Myc-tagged AlbudAbs™ in serum samples.

1. Ensure that this assay is sufficiently sensitive for detecting the AlbudAb™ of choice when in serum (see Note 6).
2. Administer AlbudAbs™ that have been expressed with an N-terminal Myc-tag (see Notes 1 and 2) to animals based on the study designs described in Subheading 3.1. Maintain serum samples from the animal studies at −20°C until required.
3. Coat 96-well Nunc Maxisorp ELISA plates overnight in the fridge with 100 μL per well of a polyclonal goat anti-Myc antibody at 1:500 in 0.2 M sodium carbonate-bicarbonate coating buffer pH 9.4 (see Note 7).
4. The next day, wash plates three times with Dulbecco's PBS + 0.1% Tween-20, 300 μL per well, followed by three washes with Dulbecco's PBS, 300 μL per well.
5. Block wells with 200 μL of assay buffer, consisting of 5% BSA in Dulbecco's PBS + 1% Tween-20 for 1 h at room temperature on an orbital rocker.
6. Wash plates as before.
7. Add serum samples at a range of dilutions in duplicate, diluted in assay buffer, 100 μL per well. A Myc-tagged AlbudAb™ reference standard is added to each plate in duplicate at a range of known concentrations, 100 μL per well (see Note 8). Samples and reference standards are incubated for 1 h at room temperature on an orbital rocker.
8. Wash plates as before.
9. Detect captured Myc-tagged AlbudAb™ by adding 100 μL per well of unconjugated polyclonal rabbit anti-dAb™ reagent at 1:1,000 in assay buffer (Immunization schedule used to raise this antibody described in Subheading 3.2). Incubate plates for 1 h at room temperature on an orbital rocker.
10. Wash plates as before.
11. Detect bound anti-dAb™ by adding 100 μL per well of mouse anti-rabbit IgG HRP at 1:10,000 in assay buffer. Incubate plates for 1 h at room temperature on an orbital rocker.
12. Wash plates as before.
13. Add 100 μL of SureBlue TMB and incubate the plates at room temperature for approximately 10 m until a sufficient blue color has developed.
14. Stop the colorimetric reaction by the addition of 100 μL of 1 M HCl.
15. Measure the absorbance of all wells at 450 nm using a suitable microplate absorbance reader.

16. Prepare a standard curve by plotting the average absorbance value of the reference standard against the known concentration at each point. Fit a standard curve through the data using a 4PL nonlinear regression model.
17. Interpolate the absorbance values of samples against the standard curve to determine the concentration of Myc-tagged AlbudAbs™ in the sample, taking into account any sample dilution factors.

3.4. Custom Labeling Rabbit Anti-dAb™ Polyclonal antibodies with MSD Sulfo-Tag

1. Ensure that the unlabeled antibody meets the following specifications before labeling with the MSD sulfo-tag: The concentration should be ≥0.2 mg/mL, the volume should be ≥200 μL, and the antibody must be in preservative-free PBS. Also, the antibody should not contain any carrier proteins such as BSA (see Notes 9–11).
2. Calculate the amount of MSD sulfo-tag required based on Eqs. 1 and 2 below:

$$\text{Tag required (nmoles)} = 1{,}000 \times \frac{\text{Antibody conc (mg/mL)}}{\text{Antibody weight (Da)}} \times \text{Challenge ratio} \times \text{volume } (\mu\text{L}) \quad (1)$$

$$\mu\text{L of MSD Sulfo-tag stock required} = \frac{\text{nmoles of tag required}}{\text{Concentration of MSD Sulfo-tag stock}} \quad (2)$$

3. For rabbit anti-dAb™ antibodies, use a challenge ratio of 1:12. A challenge ratio is the molar ratio of sulfo-tag NHS-Ester to unlabeled protein.
4. Immediately prior to use, add 50 μL of ice-cold distilled water to a vial of MSD sulfo-tag. Swirl the vial gently to ensure all the lyophilized material is dissolved. Place the vial on wet ice until use (see Note 12).
5. Add the calculated volume of the reconstituted MSD sulfo-tag stock to the antibody solution and vortex immediately. Discard any remaining sulfo-tag stock.
6. Place the antibody and sulfo-tag mixture into a dark drawer at room temperature and incubate for 2 h.
7. Approximately 20 min before the end of the conjugation incubation, equilibrate Zeba desalt columns with Dulbecco's PBS according to the manufacturer's instructions.
8. Once the conjugation reaction is complete and the columns have been prepared, add the antibody and sulfo-tag mix dropwise to the center of the compacted resin in the desalt column. To ensure maximal antibody recovery, add a stacker to the resin once the antibody and sulfo-tag mix has been added and absorbed into the resin. For a 2 mL Zeba desalt column, this is only required if the volume of antibody added is ≤350 μL, where a stacker of 40 μL of Dulbecco's PBS should be added. For volumes >350 μL, no stacker is required.

9. Place the column in a 15 mL Falcon tube into a centrifuge and spin at 1,000 × *g* for 2 min.
10. The purified labeled antibody will now be at the bottom of the Falcon tube and should have a slight orange color to it. Remove and discard the desalt column but retain the Falcon tube. Briefly mix the Falcon on a vortex and retain for use.
11. Measure the concentration of the purified antibody using a BCA colorimetric protein quantification assay with a BGG (bovine gamma globulin) standard. Test samples at a suitable dilution depending on expected concentration. Prepare a standard curve by plotting the average absorbance value of the BGG standard against the known concentration at each point. Fit the curve with a 4PL nonlinear regression model. Interpolate the absorbance values of test samples against the standard curve to determine the concentration of antibody in the sample, taking into account any sample dilution factors.
12. Measure the absorbance of the purified labeled antibody at 455 nm at a 1 cm pathlength, using Dulbecco's PBS as a blank reference. Calculate the MSD sulfo-tag concentration, in moles per liter, according to Eq. 3 below:

$$\text{Concentration of MSD sulfo-tag (M)} = \frac{\text{OD @ 455 nm (1 cm)}}{15{,}400\ \text{M/cm}} \quad (3)$$

13. Calculate the incorporation ratio of the MSD sulfo-tag to antibody according to Eq. 4. This value will give an indication of the success of the labeling (see Note 13).

$$\text{Incorporation ratio (Sulfo-tag:protein)} = \frac{\text{Concentration of MSD sulfo-tag (M)}}{\text{Concentration of protein (M)}} \quad (4)$$

14. For long-term storage, it is generally wise to aliquot the labeled antibody into working vials and freeze at −20 or −80°C.

3.5. Myc Capture Electro-chemiluminescent Assay Using MSD

1. Ensure that this assay is sufficiently sensitive for detecting the AlbudAb™ of choice when in serum (see Note 6).
2. Administer AlbudAbs™ that have been expressed with an N-terminal Myc-tag (see Notes 1 and 2) to rats based on the study designs described in Subheading 3.1. Maintain serum samples at −20°C until required.
3. Coat 96-well standard bind bare MSD plates overnight in the fridge with 50 μL per well of a polyclonal goat anti-Myc antibody at 1:250 in Dulbecco's PBS (see Note 7).
4. The next day, wash plates three times with Dulbecco's PBS + 0.1% Tween-20, 300 μL per well, followed by three washes with Dulbecco's PBS, 300 μL per well.
5. Block wells with 150 μL of assay buffer, consisting of 5% BSA in Dulbecco's PBS + 1% Tween-20 for 1 h at room temperature on an orbital rocker.

6. Wash plates as before.
7. Add serum samples at a range of dilutions in duplicate, diluted in assay buffer, 25 μL per well. Also add a Myc-tagged AlbudAb™ reference standard to each plate in triplicate at a range of known concentrations, 25 μL per well. Incubate samples and reference standards for 1 h at room temperature on an orbital rocker (see Note 8).
8. Wash plates as before.
9. Detect captured Myc-tagged AlbudAb™ by adding 50 μL per well of labeled polyclonal rabbit anti-dAb™ reagent at 1:1,000 in assay buffer (Immunization schedule used to raise this antibody described in Subheading 3.2). These antibodies should be labeled with the MSD sulfo-tag as described in Subheading 3.4. Incubate plates for 1 h at room temperature on an orbital rocker.
10. Wash plates as before.
11. Dilute the MSD Read buffer T with surfactant 1:4 with distilled water and add 150 μL of this to each well, ensuring no bubbles are in the well.
12. Immediately read the plates on a SECTOR 600 MSD imager.
13. Prepare a standard curve by plotting the average count value of the reference standard against the known concentration at each point, after applying a double log transformation of $X = \log X$ and $Y = \log Y$ to the data. Fit a standard curve through the transformed data using a 4PL nonlinear regression model.
14. Interpolate the transformed count values of samples against the standard curve to determine the concentration of Myc-tagged AlbudAbs™ in the sample, taking into account reverse transformation and any sample dilution factors.

3.6. Example Assay to Detect Therapeutic-AlbudAb™ Molecules

1. Ensure that this assay is sufficiently sensitive for detecting the AlbudAb™ of choice when in serum (see Note 6).
2. Administer mouse IFNα-AlbudAbs™ to animals based on the study designs described in Subheading 3.1, reducing dose where required due to mouse IFNα activity. Maintain serum samples at −20°C until required.
3. Coat 96-well standard bind uncoated MSD plates overnight in the fridge with 50 μL per well of a monoclonal rat anti-mouse IFNα antibody at 1 μg/mL in Dulbecco's PBS (see Note 14).
4. Wash plates the next day three times with Dulbecco's PBS + 0.1% Tween-20, 300 μL per well.
5. Block all wells with 150 μL of assay buffer, consisting of 5% BSA in Dulbecco's PBS + 1% Tween-20 for 1 h at room temperature on an orbital rocker.
6. Wash plates as before.

7. Add serum samples at a range of dilutions in duplicate, diluted in assay buffer, 25 μL per well. Include an IFNα-AlbudAb™ reference standard on each plate in triplicate at a range of known concentrations, 25 μL per well. Incubate samples and standard curves for 1 h at room temperature on an orbital rocker (see Note 8).
8. Wash plates as before.
9. Detect captured IFNα-AlbudAb™ by adding 50 μL per well of labeled polyclonal rabbit anti-dAb™ reagent at 1:1,000 in assay buffer (Immunization schedule used to raise this antibody described in Subheading 3.2). These antibodies should be labeled with the MSD sulfo-tag as described in Subheading 3.4. Incubate plates for 1 h at room temperature on an orbital rocker.
10. Wash plates as before.
11. Dilute MSD Read buffer T with surfactant 1:4 with distilled water and add 150 μL of this to all wells, ensuring no bubbles are in the well.
12. Immediately read plates on a SECTOR 6000 MSD imager.
13. Prepare a standard curve by plotting the average count value of the reference standard against the known concentration at each point, after applying a double log transformation of $X = \log X$ and $Y = \log Y$ to the data. Fit a curve through the transformed data using a 4PL nonlinear regression model.
14. Interpolate the transformed count values of samples against the standard curve to determine the concentration of Myc-tagged AlbudAbs™ in the sample, taking into account reverse transformation and any sample dilution factors.

3.7. Non-compartmental Analysis

1. Obtain a copy of WinNonLin version 5.2 and an associated license.
2. Enter final concentration and time data (from Subheadings 3.3, 3.5 or 3.6) into a new worksheet and enter other variables such as animal ID, dose, and study reference number, etc., to allow for correct data sorting prior to the fit.
3. Load noncompartmental model 201, for intravenously dosed studies (see Notes 15 and 16)
4. Enter data variables, identifying data for the X axis, Y axis, and any sort variables.
5. Enter dose information.
6. Select the lambda z ranges for each PK profile displayed. Typically select the appropriate time points of the terminal phase of the profile by eye, rather than allowing WinNonLin to decide this for itself.
7. Enter any partial areas or therapeutic range information.

8. Start modeling the data to obtain data outputs.
9. Diagnostics for NCA can be used to assess the quality of your fit and the study design. For example, aim for at least three data points to determine lambda z and an extrapolated $AUC_{0-\infty}$ of ≤10%. Also aim for the half-life to be fitted over a period of sampled time that is ≥2.5 times that of the determined half-life.
10. If the extrapolated $AUC_{0-\infty}$ is over 10% or the ratio of half-life to fit period is under 2.5, it suggests that the assay was not sufficiently sensitive for the dose given and/or the study design was not appropriate and would have benefitted from a longer sampling schedule.
11. Data can also be modeled using compartmental models (see Note 17).

4. Notes

1. Acceptable QC prior to injection of AlbudAbs™ includes endotoxin testing, SDS-PAGE gel, mass spec size determination of protein, and an activity assay to confirm that the AlbudAb™ binds to serum albumin. If a therapeutic-AlbudAb™ fusion is being tested, then a second activity assay to confirm the activity of the therapeutic partner is also desirable.
2. It is usual to clone AlbudAbs™ with a Myc-tag at the N terminus. The sequence for this tag is N-EQKLISEEDL-C. Alternative tag peptides that could be used are FLAG-tag (N-DYKDDDDK-C) or His-tag (N-HHHHHH-C).
3. As an alternative to using Myc or flag-tagged AlbudAbs™ for PK analysis, untagged AlbudAbs™ labeled via a lysine residue and NHS chemistry with *N*-Succinimidyl(2,3-^{3}H) propionate(NSP) could be used. Serum samples from the study are then analyzed by liquid scintillation counting, rather than by ELISA or MSD as described here.
4. *In vivo* phases may be outsourced to an appropriate Contract Research Organisation.
5. PK studies in mice may be used as an alternative to the rat study described in Subheading 3.1. The study design and dose would be very similar to that already described for rat, although modification of the sampling times will be required, for example: predose, 10 min, 1, 8, 24, 48, 72, and 96 h postdose. Rather than serially sampling mice, it may be necessary to use terminal sampling, where up to three animals are sacrificed and sampled at each time point. Whilst it is possible to take more than one

time point sample from a single mouse, the feasibility of this depends on the sensitivity of the detection assay. It is vital to have sufficient serum sample to run the assay more than once to allow for any repeat assays that are needed. Using three mice per time point should provide sufficient n numbers to give confidence in your results whilst complying with good ethical principles. Typically the sampling schedule up to 96 h is long enough post-dosing to provide an accurate fit of the data and reliable pharmacokinetic information.

6. After a 2.5 mg/kg intravenous dose, we would expect a maximum AlbudAb™ concentration of 40–65 μg/mL in serum at the first time point of 0.17 h. The assay must therefore have sufficient range to detect this concentration after dilution and must be also sensitive enough to detect lower concentrations at later time points. Typically a sensitivity of at least 20–50 ng/mL in whole serum is advisable for the best probability of obtaining an interpretable result (with good pharmacokinetic fit).
7. By their very nature, AlbudAbs™ in plasma or serum samples will be in complex with serum albumin. For this reason, it has been found that capturing the AlbudAb™ with serum albumin using standard immunoassay techniques (i.e., ELISA) for quantification is problematic and variable. Therefore tags or the drug fusion partner can be used to capture AlbudAb™ for quantification.
8. Each sample can be tested at three or more dilutions. As not all the dilutions used will give a result within the quantifiable range of the reference standard, the dilution used will vary depending on the time point being tested, with later time points requiring less dilution. However, the amount of serum in all diluted samples and in the reference standard should be fixed to a predetermined amount by the addition, where necessary, of control serum.
9. Custom labeling of detection antibodies with the ECL ruthenium MSD sulfo-tag allows users to develop a wide variety of assays using commercially available reagents or those generated internally, such as our own rabbit polyclonal reagents. Directly labeling detection antibodies has the benefit of reducing the assay duration, with the removal of a requirement for a species-specific secondary detection reagent.
10. If the antibody to be labeled with the sulfo-tag is in a storage buffer containing preservative such as sodium azide or EDTA or if they contain tris or glycine, it must be buffer exchanged into PBS before labeling.
11. If the antibody to be labeled contains a carrier protein (such as BSA), then the carrier protein will be labeled by the sulfo-tag

in addition to the antibody. Such proteins cannot be removed from antibody solutions by buffer exchange, so it is best to request carrier-free when ordering your antibody or when creating your own as described in Subheading 3.6.

12. The 150 nmole vial of MSD-tag is sufficient for most small-scale labeling procedures. The use of 500 nmole vials is more suitable for large-scale labeling.
13. We would typically expect an incorporation ratio of 1–5.
14. When AlbudAbs™ are conjugated to therapeutic peptides or proteins, the therapeutic partner can be used to confer the specificity required for capture from serum samples using standard immunoassay techniques, rather than a small peptide-tag as discussed in Subheadings 3.3 and 3.5.
15. Noncompartmental models may be used in WinNonLin v5.2 for fitting basic pharmacokinetic parameters and may be of particular use when comparing several potential lead molecules early in the life of a project.
16. Use model 200 for extravascular administration (such as subcutaneous). Mouse data, with terminal sampling, can be fitted using sparse sampling.
17. Compartmental models (14) may also be used in WinNonLin v5.2 to determine the PK characteristics of AlbudAbs™, with the benefit that more pharmacokinetic information can be obtained which may be of particular use, for example, for dose prediction in humans. However, this modeling approach is more complicated and may not be necessary for early stage drug discovery work. Typically attempt using models 1 and 7 for intravenous PK data or models 3 and 11 for subcutaneous PK data. Enter data as previously described but include any initial estimates for the model parameters, or else allow WinNonLin to choose these for itself. To decide on a final suitable model, fit the data with both suggested models, using an appropriate weighting strategy, and make a note of the determined AIC values. Select the most appropriate model by choosing the model that results in the lowest AIC result overall. %CV values for the determined parameters and plots of residuals (for example) can be used as a diagnostic of the final fit.

Acknowledgements

The authors were employees of Domantis Limited, and then subsequently of GlaxoSmithKline, at the time that this work was carried out.

References

1. St Onge EL, Miller SA (2010) Albiglutide; a new GLP-1 analogue for the treatment of type 2 diabetes. Expert Opin Biol Ther 10:801–806
2. Lee H (2003) Population pharmacokinetic and pharmacodynalic modelling of etanercept using logistic regression analysis. Clin Pharmacol Ther 73:348–365
3. Syed S et al (1997) Potent antithrombin activity and delayed clearance from the circulation characterise recombinant hirudin genetically fused to albumin. Blood 89:3243–3252
4. Osborn BL et al (2002) Pharmacokinetic and pharmacodynamic studies of a human serum albumin-interferon-alpha fusion protein in cynomolgus monkeys. J Pharmacol Exp Ther 303:540–548
5. Mohler KM et al (1993) Soluble tumor necrosis factor (TNF) receptors are effective therapeutic agents in lethal endotoxemia and function simultaneously as both TNF carriers and TNF antagonists. J Immunol 151: 1548–1561
6. Pasut G, Veronese FM (2009) PEGylation for improving the effectiveness of therapeutic biomolecules. Drugs Today 45:687–695
7. Holt LJ et al (2008) Anti-serum albumin domain antibodies for extending the half- lives of short lived drugs. Protein Eng Des Sel 21:283–288
8. Walker A et al (2010) Anti-serum albumin domain antibodies in the development of highly potent, efficacious and long-acting interferon. Protein Eng Des Sel 23:271–278
9. Peters T Jr (1985) Serum albumin. Adv Protein Chem 37:161–245
10. Ward ES et al (1989) Binding activities of a repertoire of single immunoglobulin variable domains secreted from *Eschericia Coli*. Nature 341:544–546
11. RhynePWetal(2009)Electrochemiluminescence in bioanalysis. Bioanalysis 1:919–935
12. Miao W (2008) Electrogenerated chemiluminescence and its biorelated applications. Chem Rev 108:2506–2553
13. DiStefano III (1982) Non-compartmental vs compartmental analysis: some bases for choice. Am J Physiol 243:R1–R6
14. Jacquez JA, Simon SP (1993) Qualitative theory of compartmental analysis. SIAM Rev 35:43–79

Chapter 29

Fluorescent Protein Specific Nanotraps to Study Protein–Protein Interactions and Histone-Tail Peptide Binding

Garwin Pichler, Heinrich Leonhardt and Ulrich Rothbauer

Abstract

Fluorescent proteins are widely used to study protein localization and protein dynamics in living cells. Additional information on peptide binding, DNA binding, enzymatic activity, and complex formation can be obtained with various methods including chromatin immunoprecipitation (ChIP) and affinity purification. Here we describe two specific GFP- and RFP binding proteins based on antibody fragments derived from llama single domain antibodies. The binding proteins can be produced in bacteria and coupled to monovalent matrixes generating so-called Nanotraps. Both Nanotraps allow a fast and efficient (one-step) isolation of fluorescent fusion proteins and their interacting factors for biochemical analyses including mass spectroscopy and enzyme activity measurements. Here we provide protocols for precipitation of fluorescent fusion proteins from crude cell extracts to identify and map protein–protein interactions as well as specific histone tail peptide binding in an easy and reliable manner.

Key words: Green fluorescent protein, Red fluorescent protein, Immunoprecipitation, Mass spectrometry, Peptide binding, Protein interactions

1. Introduction

Fluorescent proteins (FP) are widely used to study protein localization and dynamics in living cells (1, 2). The validation and interpretation of these data, however, require additional information on biochemical properties of the investigated fluorescent fusion proteins, e.g., enzymatic activity, DNA binding, and interaction with other cellular components. For these biochemical analyses proteins are mostly fused with a small epitope tag (e.g., Histidine-tag, c-Myc, FLAG, or hemaglutinin, HA-tag). Monomeric derivates of the green fluorescent protein (GFP) and the red fluorescent protein (RFP) are the most widely used labeling tags in cell biology

Dirk Saerens and Serge Muyldermans (eds.), *Single Domain Antibodies: Methods and Protocols*,
Methods in Molecular Biology, vol. 911, DOI 10.1007/978-1-61779-968-6_29, © Springer Science+Business Media, LLC 2012

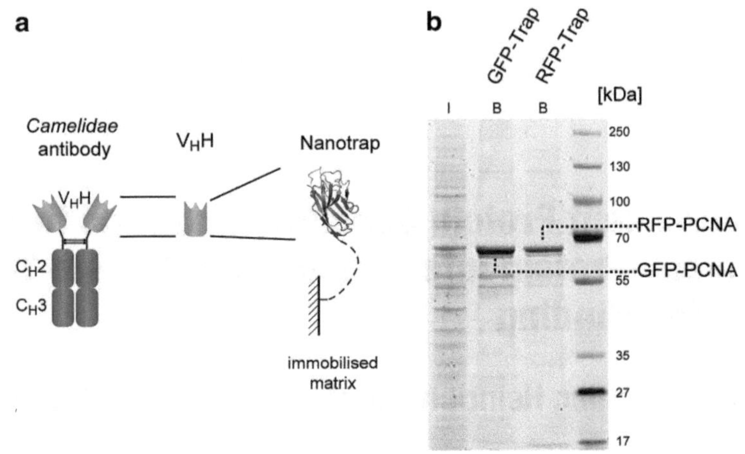

Fig. 1. Immunoprecipitation of fluorescent fusion proteins (FP). (**a**) Schematic drawing of a Nanotrap derived from camelid heavy-chain antibody. (**b**) Immunoprecipitation of GFP- or RFP-PCNA with the GFP- or RFP-Trap, respectively. 1% of input and 20% of bound fractions were subjected to a SDS PAGE and detected by Coomassie staining. The molecular size of the proteins (kDa) is indicated.

but are rarely used for biochemical analyses although various mono- and polyclonal antibodies are available (3, 4) (Abcam, Cambridge, UK; Sigma, St. Louis, USA; Roche, Mannheim, Germany, ChromoTek, Martinsried, Germany).

We recently generated specific GFP- and RFP binding proteins (GFP-Trap, RFP-Trap) based on single domain antibodies derived from *Llama alpaca* (5). Those binding proteins are characterized by a small barrel-shaped structure (approximately 13 kDa, 2.5 nm×4.5 nm) and very high stability (stable up to 70°C, functional in 2 M NaCl or 0.5% SDS). From detailed *in vitro* binding analysis we determined that one molecule of the GFP- or RFP-Trap binds one molecule GFP or RFP in stable stoichiometric complexes, respectively (see Fig. 1). The equilibrium dissociation constants (K_D) of both binding molecules are in the subnanomolar range comparable to conventional antibodies. Our binding analysis showed that the GFP-Trap exclusively binds to wtGFP, eGFP, and GFP^{S65T} as well as to YFP and eYFP, while no binding to RFPs derived from DsRed was detectable. Those RFP derivates including mRFP, mCherry or mOrange are recognized exclusively by the RFP-Trap without any cross-reaction to GFP derivates.

Here we demonstrate the application of both FP-Traps to investigate interacting factors as well as histone-tail peptide binding of fluorescent fusion proteins. For immunoprecipitations of fluorescent fusion proteins we coupled the GFP- or RFP-binding proteins covalently to monovalent matrices (e.g., agarose beads or magnetic particles). A direct comparison of the FP-Trap with conventional antibodies for immunoprecipitation of FP from crude cell lysates reveal that the FP-Traps allow a very fast (approximately 5–30 min) depletion of fluorescent fusion proteins from tested samples, which cannot be achieved with conventional antibodies even after 12 h of incubation. Moreover, after precipitation with the FP-Traps only the antigen (FP-fusion) was detectable on a Coomassie gel, whereas the typical antibody fragments (light chain, 25 kDa; heavy chain, 50 kDa) could be detected in the bound fraction after precipitation with conventional mono- and polyclonal antibodies (5).

The lack of unspecific binding or contaminating antibody fragments is one major advantage of the FP-Traps, because unspecific protein fragments in the bound fraction often interfere with subsequent mass spectrometry analysis of interacting complex partners. For the FP-Traps we demonstrated that they are versatile tools to purify FP-fusions and their interacting factors for biochemical studies including mass spectrometry and enzyme activity assays (6–9). Moreover, the FP-Traps are also suitable for chromatin immunoprecipitations (ChIPs) (5, 10, 11) in cells expressing fluorescent DNA binding proteins. In conclusion the protocol below can be used to perform immunoprecipitation of fluorescent fusion proteins from crude cell extracts to identify and map protein–protein interactions as well as specific peptide binding in an easy and reliable manner.

2. Materials

Prepare all solutions using ultrapure water (prepared by purifying deionized water to attain a resistance of 18 MΩ cm at 25°C) and analytical grade reagents. Prepare and store all reagents at room temperature (unless indicated otherwise). Ready-to-use buffers once prepared should be stored at 4°C. Diligently follow all applicable waste disposal regulations when disposing of waste materials.

2.1. Immuno-precipitation of FP

1. Phosphate buffer saline (PBS): 137 mM NaCl, 2.7 mM KCl, 10 mM Na_2HPO_4, 2 mM KH_2PO_4, pH 7.4.
2. Cell lysis buffer: 10 mM Tris–HCl, pH 7.5, 150 mM NaCl, 0.5 mM EDTA, 0.5% Non-Ident 40 (NP 40), 1 mM PMSF, Protease Inhibitor cocktail (e.g., provided by Roche, Mannheim, Germany).
3. Optional for nuclear proteins/chromatin proteins: DNaseI (f.c) 1 mg/mL, 2.5 mM $MgCl_2$.
4. RIPA buffer: 10 mM Tris–HCl, pH 7.5, 150 mM NaCl, 5 mM EDTA, 0.1% SDS, 1% Triton X-100, 1% Deoxycholate, 1 mM PMSF, Protease Inhibitor cocktail (e.g., provided by Roche, Mannheim, Germany).

5. Dilution buffer: 10 mM Tris–HCl, pH 7.5, 150 mM NaCl, 0.5 mM EDTA, 1 mM PMSF, Protease Inhibitor cocktail (e.g., provided by Roche, Mannheim, Germany).
6. Wash buffer 1: 10 mM Tris–HCl, pH 7.5, 150 mM NaCl, 0.5 mM EDTA, 1 mM PMSF, Protease Inhibitor cocktail (e.g., provided by Roche, Mannheim, Germany).
7. Wash buffer 2: 10 mM Tris–HCl, pH 7.5, 0.5 M NaCl, 0.5 mM EDTA, 1 mM PMSF, Protease Inhibitor cocktail (e.g., provided by Roche, Mannheim, Germany).
8. Elution buffer: 0.2 M glycine-HCl, pH 2.5.
9. Neutralization buffer: 1 M Tris-base, pH 10.4.
10. SDS-PAGE sample buffer (3×): 150 mM Tris–HCl pH 6.8, 300 mM DTT, 6% SDS, 0.3% Bromphenol blue, 30% glycerol.
11. Coomassie solution: 50% methanol, 40% H_2O, 10% acetic acid, 0.25% Coomassie Blue R-250.
12. FP-Trap gta-20 (agarose coupled), gtm-20 (magnetic particles) (ChromoTek, Martinsried, Germany)
13. FP-Trap rta-20 (agarose coupled), rtm-20 (magnetic particles) (ChromoTek, Martinsried, Germany).

Nanotraps based on specific binding proteins as provided by ChromoTek are most consistently effective; however, Nanotraps can be generated and used from other sources.

2.2. Histone-Tail Peptide Binding Assay

1. Dilution buffer: 10 mM Tris–HCl, pH 7.5, 150 mM NaCl, 0.5 mM EDTA, 1 mM PMSF, Protease Inhibitor cocktail (e.g., provided by Roche, Mannheim, Germany).
2. Wash buffer 3: 10 mM Tris–HCl, pH 7.5, 300 mM NaCl, 0.5 mM EDTA, 1 mM PMSF, Protease Inhibitor cocktail (e.g., provided by Roche, Mannheim, Germany).
3. Histone-tail peptides.
4. All histone-tail peptides are C-terminal labeled with fluorescent carboxytetramethylrhodamine succinimidyl ester (TAMRA) or Biotin. Absorptions- and emission wavelengths of TAMRA are 544 and 570 nm, respectively.
5. H3(1-20)K9me3-TAMRA, H3(1-20)K9me3-Biotin, H3 (1-20)K9ac-Biotin were purchased from Peptide Specialty Laboratories (PSL, Heidelberg, Germany).
6. Microplate 96-well (e.g., Greiner Bio-One GmbH, Frickenhausen, Germany)

2.3. Evaluation of Binding Ratios

1. Microplate reader (e.g., Tecan Infinite M1000) (TECAN, Männedorf, Switzerland).

3. Methods

Carry out all procedures at 4°C unless otherwise specified.

3.1. Immunoprecipitation of FP

The following step-by-step immunoprecipitation protocol is based on about 1×10^7 cells (HEK293T or HeLa) transiently transfected with expression vectors coding for fluorescent fusion proteins of interest. The transfection efficiency should be in the range of 60–90% determined by fluorescence microscopy.

1. Wash the cells two times with 5 mL of PBS on ice. Scrape the cells off. Transfer the cells to a tube and centrifuge at $800 \times g$ and 4°C for 3 min.
2. Wash the cells with 1 mL of PBS and centrifuge again (see Subheading 3.1, step 1).
3. Resuspend cell pellet in 200 μL of cell lysis buffer (see Note 1).
4. For lysis incubate cells on ice for 30 min Resuspend the cells every 10 min by gently pipetting.
5. Clear lysate by centrifugation at $20{,}000 \times g$ and 4°C for 10 min (see Note 2).
6. Adjust volume to 500 μL with dilution buffer (see Note 3).
7. Take an aliquot which corresponds to 5–10% of your diluted sample (referred to as input fraction (IP)) and add SDS-PAGE sample buffer.
8. Add 20–40 μL of GFP-Trap or RFP-Trap (gta-20, gtm-20 or rta-20, rtm-20) and incubate for 10 min to 2 h at 4°C with constant mixing. Binding reaction can also be performed on a microcolumn (see Notes 4 and 5).
9. Harvest immunocomplexes bound to the monovalent matrix by centrifugation for 2 min at $5{,}000 \times g$ and 4°C or magnetic separation using a specially designed rack (e.g., from Chemicell, Berlin, Germany).
10. Collect an aliquot of the supernatant or flow through (referred to as nonbound fraction (NB)) and add SDS-PAGE sample buffer.
11. Wash beads with 1 mL of wash buffer 1.
12. Repeat washing step with 1 mL of wash buffer 2 (see Note 6).
13. Resuspend the beads in 50–100 μL of SDS-PAGE sample buffer (referred to as bound (B)).
14. Elute proteins by boiling at 95°C for 10 min (see Note 7).
15. For immunoblot analysis subject 1% of input and, e.g., 20% of bound fractions to SDS-PAGE. Transfer to a nitrocellulose or PVDF membrane.

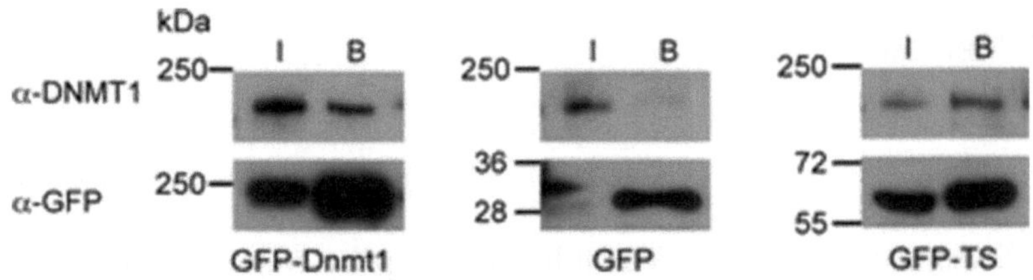

Fig. 2. Immunoblots after coimmunoprecipitations illustrate the interaction between GFP-Dnmt1 and endogenous DNMT1, whereas precipitation of GFP alone was used as negative control. 1% of input and 30% of bound fractions were subjected to immunoblot analysis. The molecular size of the proteins (kDa) and the antibodies used are indicated. Mapping the Dnmt1 dimerization region to the TS domain of Dnmt1: Immunoblot after coimmunoprecipitation showing that the N-terminal TS domain of Dnmt1 can coprecipitate endogenous DNMT1 (data taken from Fellinger et al. Dimerization of DNA methyltransferase 1 is mediated by its regulatory domain. J Cell Biochem 106(4):521–528, Copyright 2009© Wiley-Blackwell).

16. Detect precipitated GFP- or RFP-fusion proteins with an anti-GFP or anti-RFP antibody (e.g., from Roche, Mannheim, Germany, ChromoTek, Martinsried, Germany) and interacting proteins with the respective antibodies (see Fig. 2).

3.2. Histone-Tail Peptide Binding Assay

The following step-by-step histone-tail peptide binding protocol for FP-fusions continues after the washing step of the immunoprecipitation with the FP-Traps (see Subheading 3.1, step 11).

1. Equilibrate the beads with 1 mL of dilution buffer.
2. Add TAMRA-labeled histone-tail peptide to a final concentration of 0.15 μM (see Note 8).
3. Incubate for 15 min at room temperature with constant mixing (see Note 9).
4. Harvest the beads by centrifugation for 2 min at 5,000 × *g* and 4°C.
5. Wash the beads two times with 1 mL of wash buffer 3 (see Note 9).
6. Resuspend the beads in 100 μL of dilution buffer.
7. Transfer the beads to a 96-well plate.

3.3. Evaluation of Binding Ratios

For quantification, fluorescence intensity measurements are adjusted using standard curves from labeled probes with known concentrations. Fluorescence intensities (FI) were measured with a microplate reader Tecan Infinite M1000 (TECAN, Männedorf, Switzerland) (12). Following settings were used:

1. GFP: 490 ± 10 and 511 ± 10 nm
2. TAMRA: 560 ± 5 and 586 ± 5 nm
   - Measure fluorescence intensities (see Note 10).

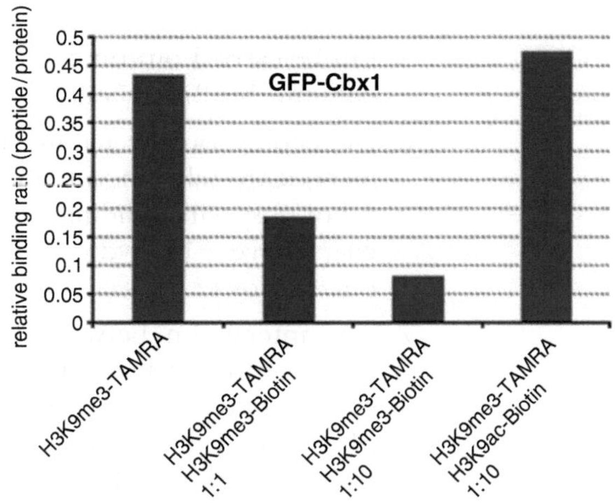

Fig. 3. Histone-tail binding properties of mouse Cbx1 (*Drosophila* HP1 beta). GFP-Cbx1 was purified with the GFP-Trap and incubated with TAMRA-labeled H3(1-20)K9me3 histone-tail peptide in competition with either biotinylated H3K9me3 or H3K9ac in different molar ratios.

- Calculate GFP- and TAMRA concentration using standard curves (see Note 10).
- Calculate relative binding ratio histone-tail peptide/protein (see Fig. 3).

4. Notes

1. The given example of buffer recipes can be modified according to the experimental needs. One can use different buffer recipes (e.g., phosphate buffered saline or HEPES) comprising higher salt concentrations or containing DNase I (AppliChem, Darmstadt, Germany) or MNase S7 (Roche, Mannheim, Germany) to release chromatin proteins or RIPA buffer to release chromatin or membrane bound fluorescent fusion proteins.
2. The centrifugation step to clarify the lysate can be shortened up the 2–5 min for highly soluble proteins. Such proteins will be transferred to the supernatant after 2–5 min of centrifugation.
3. If necessary the protein sample can be diluted in larger volumes. Accordingly, one should elongate the incubation time with the FP-Traps up to 12 h over night incubation at 4°C. Alternatively, one can increase the amount of GFP- or RFP-Trap in the pulldown reaction.
4. In some cases it was observed that N-terminal GFP-tagged proteins were better recognized as C-terminal tagged ones. If that is the case you can achieve a comparable efficiency with a prolonged incubation time.

5. As an alternative to batch purification the pulldown reaction can be carried out on columns like microcolumns (e.g., 1 mL column, MoBiTec GmbH, Göttingen, Germany).
6. Depending on the nature of the protein complexes one can increase the salt concentration (e.g., up to 500 mM NaCl to get rid of unspecific binding). Alternatively if transient interactions characterized by hydrophilic interactions have to be analyzed one can lower the salt concentration in the wash buffer 2.
7. The interaction between the FP-Traps and the fluorescent epitope can be released by acidic elution. It is recommended to elute bound proteins by adding 100 μL of 0.2 M glycine-HCL, pH 2.5 for 1 min. Acidic eluate should be immediately neutralized by adding 5–10 μL of 1 M Tris-base (pH 10.4).
8. As an alternative to TAMRA conjugates one can use every fluorescent label whose specific fluorescence characteristics do not interfere with GFP or RFP.
9. Depending on the nature of the protein and the histone-tail peptide one can vary the incubation time, temperature and salt concentrations for washing. In this case best results were observed at room temperature for 15 min and washing with 300 mM NaCl.
10. Calibration curves for the fluorescent DNA substrates and proteins were determined by measuring the fluorescence signal of known concentrations of the TAMRA-coupled histone-tail peptides and purified GFP and calculated by linear regression.

Acknowledgements

This work was supported by the GO-Bio Program of the BMBF (Federal Ministry of Science, Germany) and the Deutsche Forschungsgemeinschaft (SFB 646).

References

1. Baird GS, Zacharias DA, Tsien RY (2000) Biochemistry, mutagenesis, and oligomerization of DsRed, a red fluorescent protein from coral. Proc Natl Acad Sci U S A 97:11984–11989
2. Campbell RE, Tour O, Palmer AE, Steinbach PA, Baird GS, Zacharias DA, Tsien RY (2002) A monomeric red fluorescent protein. Proc Natl Acad Sci U S A 99:7877–7882
3. Cristea IM, Williams R, Chait BT, Rout MP (2005) Fluorescent proteins as proteomic probes. Mol Cell Proteomics 4:1933–1941
4. Rottach A, Kremmer E, Nowak D, Leonhardt H, Cardoso MC (2008) Generation and characterization of a rat monoclonal antibody specific for multiple red fluorescent proteins. Hybridoma (Larchmt) 27:337–343
5. Rothbauer U, Zolghadr K, Muyldermans S, Schepers A, Cardoso MC, Leonhardt H (2008) A versatile nanotrap for biochemical and functional studies with fluorescent fusion proteins. Mol Cell Proteomics 7:282–289
6. Trinkle-Mulcahy L, Boulon S, Lam YW, Urcia R, Boisvert FM, Vandermoere F, Morrice NA, Swift S, Rothbauer U, Leonhardt H, Lamond A (2008) Identifying specific protein interaction partners using quantitative mass spectrometry and bead proteomes. J Cell Biol 183: 223–239

7. Agarwal N, Hardt T, Brero A, Nowak D, Rothbauer U, Becker A, Leonhardt H, Cardoso MC (2007) MeCP2 interacts with HP1 and modulates its heterochromatin association during myogenic differentiation. Nucleic Acids Res 35:5402–5408
8. Schermelleh L, Haemmer A, Spada F, Rosing N, Meilinger D, Rothbauer U, Cristina Cardoso M, Leonhardt H (2007) Dynamics of Dnmt1 interaction with the replication machinery and its role in postreplicative maintenance of DNA methylation. Nucleic Acids Res 35: 4301–4312
9. Frauer C, Leonhardt H (2009) A versatile non-radioactive assay for DNA methyltransferase activity and DNA binding. Nucleic Acids Res 37:e22
10. Bergbauer M, Kalla M, Schmeinck A, Gobel C, Rothbauer U, Eck S, Benet-Pages A, Strom TM, Hammerschmidt W (2010) CpG-methylation regulates a class of Epstein-Barr virus promoters. PLoS Pathog 6:e1001114
11. Munoz IM, Hain K, Declais AC, Gardiner M, Toh GW, Sanchez-Pulido L, Heuckmann JM, Toth R, Macartney T, Eppink B, Kanaar R, Ponting CP, Lilley DM, Rouse J (2009) Coordination of structure-specific nucleases by human SLX4/BTBD12 is required for DNA repair. Mol Cell 35:116–127
12. Rottach A, Frauer C, Pichler G, Bonapace IM, Spada F, Leonhardt H (2010) The multi-domain protein Np95 connects DNA methylation and histone modification. Nucleic Acids Res 38:1796–1804

Chapter 30

Site-Specific Labeling of His-Tagged Nanobodies with ^{99m}Tc: A Practical Guide

Catarina Xavier, Nick Devoogdt, Sophie Hernot, Ilse Vaneycken, Matthias D'Huyvetter, Jens De VOS, Sam Massa, Tony Lahoutte, and Vicky Caveliers

Abstract

^{99m}Tc-tricarbonyl chemistry provides an elegant technology to site-specifically radiolabel histidine-tagged biomolecules. Considering their unique biochemical properties, this straightforward technology is particularly suited for Nanobodies. This chapter gives a detailed guide to generate highly specific Nanobody-derived radiotracers for both in vitro binding studies and in vivo molecular imaging.

Key words: Radiochemistry, ^{99m}Tc, Site-specific labeling

1. Introduction

The growth of nuclear medicine has been due mainly to the availability of Technetium-99m (^{99m}Tc) organometallic radiopharmaceuticals. This single isotope, the 43rd element in the periodic table, is used in over 80% of all diagnostic procedures. The availability of short-lived ^{99m}Tc (half-life 6.01 h) from widespread $^{99}Mo/^{99m}Tc$ generators, as the daughter product of long lived ^{99}Mo (half-life 67 h), is a major factor behind the universal use of this radioisotope. ^{99m}Tc emits γ-rays with 140 keV of energy that are detectable by clinical and particularly high-resolution small-animal single photon emission computed tomography (SPECT) cameras.

^{99m}Tc-radiopharmaceuticals are used in several diagnostic procedures, from the use of simple $^{99m}TcO_4^-$ (pertechnetate, the eluate of the $^{99}Mo/^{99m}Tc$ generator) to evaluate thyroid uptake (1), ^{99m}Tc-MIBI (Sestamibi) for cardiac imaging (2), to more complex molecules such as ^{99m}Tc-labeled antibodies for imaging infection and

Dirk Saerens and Serge Muyldermans (eds.), *Single Domain Antibodies: Methods and Protocols*, Methods in Molecular Biology, vol. 911, DOI 10.1007/978-1-61779-968-6_30, © Springer Science+Business Media, LLC 2012

inflammation (e.g., antigranulocyte antibody, Scintimun®, IBA Molecular) (3). Owing to its multiple oxidation states, ^{99m}Tc has a versatile chemistry, making it possible to produce a variety of complexes with specific desired characteristics, which is a major advantage of ^{99m}Tc for radiopharmaceutical development (4). Such complexes can be easily formulated from kits with long shelf lives, containing freeze-dried products that are prepared in authorized manufacturing facilities. The IsoLink™ kit (Covidien, St Louis, USA) for instance contains all components to reduce and carbonylate $^{99m}TcO_4^-$ into $(^{99m}Tc(CO)_3(H_2O)_3)^+$ (^{99m}Tc-tricarbonyl) after boiling, thereby avoiding the necessity to work in a CO atmosphere (5). ^{99m}Tc-tricarbonyl was soon discovered to serve as a precursor for simple labeling procedures of biomolecules. Indeed, imidazoles and histidines have proven to coordinate efficiently to the tricarbonyl core (6), which forms the basis for site-specific labeling of histidine-tagged recombinant proteins (7). This method is particularly elegant because the His-tag is genetically expressed for ease of purification of the protein on a nickel affinity column and has been successfully applied to site-specifically label peptides (8), antibody-derivatives (9), and artificial targeting proteins such as DARPins (10) and Affibodies (11). Nanobodies, the small antigen-binding fragments that are derived from camelid heavy-chain-only antibodies (12), are particularly suited for ^{99m}Tc-labeling via tricarbonyl-chemistry. Crystallography studies have shown for instance that its carboxyterminal His-tag is located on the opposite side of the paratope (13), hence minimizing interference with antigen-binding activity. High thermal and chemical stabilities have been shown to be essential for efficient complexation of ^{99m}Tc-tricarbonyl to His-tagged antibody-fragments (9). High stability properties are a typical feature of Nanobodies (14).

^{99m}Tc-Nanobodies have been shown to be highly stable in both PBS and serum (15). The short half-life of ^{99m}Tc also fits with the fast blood clearance of Nanobodies via the renal route (15, 16), whereby fast imaging, as early as 1 h post injection is possible, thereby generating good contrast-images (17). Finally, ^{99m}Tc-Nanobodies retain their high affinity and specificity, both in vitro in binding studies and in vivo upon targeting biomarkers on cancer or immune cells while uptake in nontargeted tissue is low (16–20). A more detailed description of our preclinical findings with ^{99m}Tc-labeled Nanobodies is available by Devoogdt et al. (see Chapter 35).

The current chapter gives a step-by-step description of a generic method to efficiently radiolabel Nanobodies via ^{99m}Tc-tricarbonyl chemistry. It starts with the generation and purity assessment of the ^{99m}Tc-tricarbonyl precursor. This is then followed by a straightforward protocol to complex the precursor with the His-tag of Nanobodies, and different ways to evaluate the radiochemical purity of the hence obtained Nanobody-derived radiotracer.

2. Materials

2.1. Preparation of ^{99m}Tc-Tricarbonyl Precursor

1. Lyophilized kit (IsoLink™, Covidien, St Louis, USA) containing 4.5 mg of sodium boranocarbonate, 2.85 mg of sodium tetraborate·$10H_2O$, 8.5 mg of sodium tartrate·$2H_2O$, and 7.15 mg of sodium carbonate, pH 10.5.
2. Hydrochloric acid (HCl): 1 M solution in water.
3. ^{99}Mo/^{99m}Tc generator (Drytec; GE Healthcare).
4. Well-ventilated hoods and lead shielding.
5. Water bath or dry heating block.

2.2. Assessment of Radiochemical Purity of ^{99m}Tc-Tricarbonyl Precursor

1. HPLC-system equipped with a radiometric γ-detector.
2. HPLC column: PLRP-S 300 Å, 5 μm, 250×4.6 mm (Agilent Technologies, Diegem, Belgium).
3. HPLC solvents: 0.1% trifluoracetic acid (TFA) in H_2O (solvent A) and acetonitrile (solvent B).

2.3. Labeling of His-Tagged Nanobodies with ^{99m}Tc-Tricarbonyl

1. Nanobody: 1 mg/mL in phosphate buffered saline pH 7.4 (see Note 1).
2. *fac*-$[^{99m}Tc(CO)_3(H_2O_{)3})^+$: 0.74–3.7 GBq/mL (see Subheading 3.1)
3. Eppendorf tubes.
4. Water bath (50°C).
5. Disposable NAP-5 columns (GE Healthcare, Diegem, Belgium), equilibrated with 10 mL phosphate buffered saline pH 7.4.
6. 0.22 μm membrane filter (4 mm, Millipore, Brussels, Belgium).

2.4. Assessment of Radiochemical Purity of ^{99m}Tc-Tricarbonyl Nanobody by HPLC Analysis

1. HPLC-system equipped with a UV and a radiometric γ-detector connected in series.
2. HPLC column: PLRP-S 300 Å, 5 μm, 250×4.6 mm (Agilent Technologies, Diegem, Belgium).
3. HPLC solvents: 0.1% TFA in H_2O (solvent A) and acetonitrile (solvent B).

2.5. Assessment of Radiochemical Purity of ^{99m}Tc-Tricarbonyl Nanobody by ITLC Analysis

1. Instant thin layer chromatography (ITLC) using silica gel impregnated glass fiber sheets (Pall Corporation, Life Sciences).
2. ITLC eluent: acetone.
3. Dose calibrator or gamma counter.

3. Methods

3.1. Preparation of ^{99m}Tc-Tricarbonyl Precursor

1. Add 1 mL of the $^{99m}TcO_4^-$ solution (^{99}Mo/^{99m}Tc generator eluate; 0.74–3.7 GBq) to the IsoLink™ kit.
2. Incubate the mixture at 100°C for 20 min.
3. Cool the reaction mixture in water.
4. Add 1 M HCl until pH 7.4.

3.2. Assessment of Radiochemical Purity of ^{99m}Tc-Tricarbonyl Precursor

1. For HPLC analysis, inject 2–5 μL of the ^{99m}Tc-Tricarbonyl (3–5 μCi) into the injection loop. Run the following HPLC gradient, at 1 mL/min:
   - 0–5 min: 75% solvent A/25% solvent B.
   - 5–7 min: linear gradient of 75% solvent A/25% solvent B to 66% solvent A/34% solvent B.
   - 7–10 min: linear gradient of 66% solvent A/34% solvent B to 100% solvent B.
   - 10–25 min: 100% solvent B.
2. The ^{99m}Tc-tricarbonyl precursor shows a retention time of 5–6 min, whereas unreacted $^{99m}TcO_4^-$ shows a retention time of 4 min. Typical purity of $[^{99m}Tc(CO)_3(H_2O)_3]^+$ (^{99m}Tc-tricarbonyl) is >95%.

3.3. Labeling of His-Tagged Nanobodies with ^{99m}Tc-Tricarbonyl

1. Mix 50 μL (50 μg; 1 mg/mL) of purified Nanobody with 500 μL of *fac*-$[^{99m}Tc(CO)_3(H_2O)_3]^+$ at pH 7.4.
2. Incubate at 50°C for 60–90 min (see Note 2).
3. Separate the labeled Nanobody from free ^{99m}Tc-Tricarbonyl and $^{99m}TcO_4^-$ by gel filtration methods such as the NAP-5 column using phosphate buffered saline (see Note 3).
4. Pass the purified solution through a 0.22 μm membrane filter to eliminate possible aggregates.
5. Evaluate radiochemical purity by RP-HPLC (see Subheading 3.4) and/or by ITLC (see Subheading 3.5 and Note 4).

3.4. Assessment of Radiochemical Purity of ^{99m}Tc-Tricarbonyl Nanobody by HPLC Analysis

1. Inject 2–5 μL of the ^{99m}Tc-Tricarbonyl Nanobody (3–5 μCi) into the injection loop. Run the following HPLC gradient, at 1 mL/min:
   - 0–5 min: 75% solvent A/25% solvent B.
   - 5–7 min: linear gradient of 75% solvent A/25% solvent B to 66% solvent A/34% solvent B.
   - 7–10 min: linear gradient of 66% solvent A/34% solvent B to 100% solvent B.
   - 10–25 min: 100% solvent B.

2. The ^{99m}Tc-Tricarbonyl Nanobody shows a retention time of 13 min. The ^{99m}Tc-tricarbonyl precursor shows a retention time of 5–6 min, and $^{99m}TcO_4^-$ has a retention time of 4 min.

3.5. Assessment of Radiochemical Purity of ^{99m}Tc-Tricarbonyl Nanobody by ITLC Analysis

1. Spot 2 μL of ^{99m}Tc-Tricarbonyl Nanobody solution on a 15 mm × 200 mm silica gel impregnated glass fiber sheet.
2. Develop the chromatogram in acetone.
3. Analyze the distribution of radioactivity by scanning with a γ-radiation TLC scanner or counting the strip cut in three parts (application point, middle, solvent front) in a dose calibrator or gamma counter. The ^{99m}Tc-Tricarbonyl precursor and the $^{99m}TcO_4^-$ reveal a Rf (retention factor) of 1 and ^{99m}Tc-Tricarbonyl-Nanobody a Rf of 0.

4. Notes

1. The Nanobody solution should be free of imidazole as this substance will interfere with the labeling procedure.
2. Temperature of incubation depends on the thermostability of the Nanobody, if possible always determine the melting temperature (Tm) of Nanobody to be labeled.
3. If the labeled Nanobody is more lipophilic, there might be some ^{99m}Tc-Tricarbonyl-Nanobody activity sticking on the NAP-5 column.
4. Radiochemical purity before gel filtration, as determined by either method, usually ranges from 90 to 98%, and depends on protein concentration. At 0.1 mg/mL final concentration, labeling will be complete after 60 min. After gel filtration and microfiltration, radiochemical purity should be >98% before in vivo assessment.

References

1. Andros G, Harper PV, Lathrop KA (1965) Pertechnetate-99m localization in man with applications to thyroid scanning and the study of thyroid physiology. J Clin Endocrinol Metab 25:1067–1076
2. Mandalapu BP, Amato M, Stratmann HG (1999) Technetium Tc 99m sestamibi myocardial perfusion imaging: current role for evaluation of prognosis. Chest 115:1684–1694
3. Richter WS et al (2011) ^{99m}Tc-besilesomab (Scintimun) in peripheral osteomyelitis: comparison with 99mTc-labelled white blood cells. Eur J Nucl Med Mol Imaging 38:899–910
4. Schibli R, Schubiger PA (2002) Current use and future potential of organometallic radiopharmaceuticals. Eur J Nucl Med Mol Imaging 29:1529–1542
5. Alberto R et al (2001) Synthesis and properties of boranocarbonate: a convenient in situ CO source for the aqueous preparation of [(99m) $Tc(OH_2)_3(CO)_3]^+$. J Am Chem Soc 123: 3135–3136
6. Egli A et al (1999) Organometallic ^{99m}Tc-aquaion labels peptide to an unprecedented high specific activity. J Nucl Med 40: 1913–1917

7. Waibel R et al (1999) Stable one-step technetium-99m labeling of His-tagged recombinant proteins with a novel Tc(I)-carbonyl complex. Nat Biotechnol 17:897–901
8. Du J et al (2001) Technetium-99m labelling of glycosylated somatostatin-14. Appl Radiat Isot 55:181–187
9. Willuda J et al (1999) High thermal stability is essential for tumor targeting of antibody fragments: engineering of a humanized anti-epithelial glycoprotein-2 (epithelial cell adhesion molecule) single-chain Fv fragment. Cancer Res 59:5758–5767
10. Zahnd C et al (2010) Efficient tumor targeting with high-affinity designed ankyrin repeat proteins: effects of affinity and molecular size. Cancer Res 70:1595–1605
11. Orlova A et al (2006) Comparative in vivo evaluation of technetium and iodine labels on an anti-HER2 affibody for single-photon imaging of HER2 expression in tumors. J Nucl Med 47:512–519
12. Hamers-Casterman C et al (1993) Naturally occurring antibodies devoid of light chains. Nature 363:446–448
13. Vincke C et al (2009) General strategy to humanize a camelid single-domain antibody and identification of a universal humanized nanobody scaffold. J Biol Chem 284:3273–3284
14. Dumoulin M et al (2002) Single-domain antibody fragments with high conformational stability. Protein Sci 11:500–515
15. Tchouate Gainkam LO et al (2011) Localization, mechanism and reduction of renal retention of technetium-99m labeled epidermal growth factor receptor-specific nanobody in mice. Contrast Media Mol Imaging 6:85–92
16. Vaneycken I et al (2011) Preclinical screening of anti-HER2 nanobodies for molecular imaging of breast cancer. FASEB J 25: 2433–2446
17. Vaneycken I et al (2011) Immuno-imaging using nanobodies. Curr Opin Biotechnol 22:877–881
18. Tchouate Gainkam LO et al (2011) Correlation between epidermal growth factor receptor-specific nanobody uptake and tumor burden: a tool for noninvasive monitoring of tumor response to therapy. Mol Imaging Biol 13: 940–948
19. Vaneycken I et al (2010) In vitro analysis and in vivo tumor targeting of a humanized, grafted nanobody in mice using pinhole SPECT/ micro-CT. J Nucl Med 51:1099–1106
20. De Groeve K et al (2010) Nanobodies as tools for in vivo imaging of specific immune cell types. J Nucl Med 51:782–789

Chapter 31

Nanobody-Based Chromatin Immunoprecipitation

Trong Nguyen Duc, Gholamreza Hassanzadeh-Ghassabeh, Dirk Saerens, Eveline Peeters, Daniel Charlier, and Serge Muyldermans

Abstract

Chromatin immunoprecipitation (ChIP), followed by microarray hybridization (ChIP-chip) or high-throughput sequencing (ChIP-seq), is becoming a widely used powerful method for the analysis of the in vivo DNA–protein interactions at genomic scale.

The success of ChIP largely depends on the quality of antibodies. Although polyclonal antibodies have been successfully used for ChIP, their production requires regular immunization and they exhibit high aspecificity and batch to batch variability. These problems can be circumvented by generating monoclonal antibodies (mAbs) via hybridoma technology. However, such mAbs do not often capture DNA–protein complexes and are not amenable to engineering.

Nanobodies are recombinant single domain antibody fragments derived from camelid Heavy-Chain antibodies. Nanobodies exhibit high affinity and specificity towards their cognate antigens and often capture their target antigens in solution. Moreover, the Nanobody genes can be easily tailored to streamline ChIP.

Here, we describe a Nanobody-based ChIP protocol which we have successfully used for genome-wide identification of the binding sites of the low-abundant transcription factor Ss-LrpB from the hyperthermoacidophilic archaeon *Sulfolobus solfataricus*.

Key words: Chromatin immunoprecipitation, DNA–protein interaction, Nanobody, Single domain antibody, *Sulfolobus solfataricus*

1. Introduction

Chromatin immunoprecipitation (ChIP) is a powerful technique to identify regions of the genome associated with regulatory proteins such as transcription factors, cofactors, etc. under in vivo conditions. The ChIP assay typically comprises five steps: (1) in situ protein–DNA cross-linking, (2) DNA fragmentation by sonication, (3) immunoprecipitation or immunocapturing of the protein target (cross-linked to its cognate protein or DNA partners), (4) post-ChIP DNA elution, purification, and amplification, and (5) identification of the ChIP enriched DNA.

Dirk Saerens and Serge Muyldermans (eds.), *Single Domain Antibodies: Methods and Protocols*, Methods in Molecular Biology, vol. 911, DOI 10.1007/978-1-61779-968-6_31, © Springer Science+Business Media, LLC 2012

1.1. Culture of Sulfolobus solfataricus P2

S. solfataricus is a hyperthermoacidophilic archaeon growing optimally at 80°C and pH of approximately 3.0 (1). The sequence of the *S. solfataricus* 3 Mbp genome has been published (2).

1.2. In Vivo Cross-Linking

In order to stabilize DNA–protein interactions, a formaldehyde-induced cross-linking step is performed. Formaldehyde is a reversible and high resolution (2 Å) cross-linker that can tether protein to DNA, RNA, or protein (3). The efficiency of formaldehyde DNA–protein cross-linking varies among different cell types (4).

1.3. Sonication

Before performing ChIP, cross-linked DNA molecules need to be sheared into small fragments of about 0.5–1 kb by sonication. These sonication conditions must be determined empirically for each cell or tissue type, and sonicator model (5). Large DNA fragments can carry both target and nontarget sequences and therefore insufficient sonication can result in aspecificity of ChIP.

1.4. Immuno-precipitation

Antibodies are very important factors for a successful ChIP experiment. Polyclonal antibodies are easy and fast to obtain and usually recognize several epitopes of the cognate antigen, thereby increasing signal levels of low-abundant targets. However, polyclonal antibodies might exhibit cross-reactivity towards nontarget molecules and there is always batch to batch variability so that conditions have to be optimized for each batch (6). In contrast to polyclonal antibodies, monoclonal antibodies have high specificity. For example, if the protein under investigation contains a highly conserved domain that is also present in other proteins, polyclonal antibodies raised against full length protein can fail in specifically capturing the target protein. In this case, a specific monoclonal antibody which does not bind to the common epitope is required to overcome the problem. Monoclonal antibodies can be obtained by hybridoma technology or recombinant DNA approaches. Monoclonal antibodies obtained by recombinant DNA technology, as compared with those obtained by hybridoma approach, are more amenable to extensive engineering, and therefore allow improving sensitivity and/or target specificity.

Nonspecific co-precipitated DNA fragments are a major source of aspecificity in ChIP experiments, especially when studying the whole genome which has large size and high complexity (7). Improving washing conditions may help to decrease aspecificity due to co-precipitated DNAs (7).

1.5. Post-ChIP DNA Elution, Purification, and Amplification

To use the ChIP-enriched DNA pool for further analysis by microarray, sequencing, etc., the DNA should not be associated with proteins and formaldehyde. Moreover, the amount of material obtained by ChIP is usually insufficient for further analysis. DNA elution, purification, and amplification steps provide sufficient DNA of high quality for downstream analysis.

1.6. ChIP Downstream Analysis

ChIP downstream analysis methods include small-scale and genome-wide approaches. For small-scale approaches, there are tools to assess the enrichment of both DNA and protein. Examples of methods for DNA analysis on a small scale are Southern blotting and quantitative real-time PCR (q-PCR) (8, 9). The q-PCR method is used more often and is considered as a standard method for the validation of ChIP. However, these approaches are limited because of the requirement for prior knowledge of genomic regions that are targeted by the protein under investigation. Methods for protein analysis are Western blotting and mass spectrometry (10).

Sequence tag analysis of genomic enrichment (ChIP-STAGE), serial analysis of chromatin occupancy (ChIP-SACO), ChIP-paired end tag (ChIP-PET), whole genome tilling arrays (ChIP-chip), and ChIP combined with depth-sequencing (ChIP-seq) allow genome-wide identification of DNA target sequences (11–13). In parallel with the advances in high-throughput technologies and bioinformatics tools, the ChIP-chip and ChIP-seq methods have gained popularity.

2. Materials

Prepare all solutions using pure water and analytical grade reagents. Prepare and store all reagents at room temperature (unless indicated otherwise). Diligently follow all waste disposal regulations when disposing waste materials.

2.1. Culture of S. solfataricus P2

1. *S. solfataricus* P2 (DSMZ 1617)
2. Brock I (for 200 mL): 14 g $CaCl_2{\cdot}2H_2O$, H_2O up to 200 mL, autoclave.
3. Brock II (for 1 L): 130 g $(NH_4)_2SO_4$, 25 g $MgSO_4{\cdot}7H_2O$, 1.5 mL of 50% H_2SO_4, H_2O up to 1 L, autoclave.
4. 2 mM $MnCl_2$ solution: 25 mg $MnCl_2$, H_2O up to 100 mL, autoclave.
5. 1 mM $CuCl_2{\cdot}2H_2O$ solution: 17 mg $CuCl_2{\cdot}2H_2O$, H_2O up to 100 mL, autoclave.
6. 2 mM $Na_2MoO_4{\cdot}2H_2O$ solution: 48 mg $Na_2MoO_4{\cdot}2H_2O$, H_2O up to 100 mL, autoclave.
7. 2 mM $VOSO_4{\cdot}2H_2O$ solution: 33 mg $VOSO_4{\cdot}2H_2O$, H_2O up to 100 mL, autoclave.
8. 0.6 mM $CoSO_4{\cdot}7H_2O$ solution: 16.9 mg $CoSO_4{\cdot}7H_2O$, H_2O up to 100 mL, autoclave.
9. 18 mM $NiSO_4$ solution: 47 mg$NiSO_4$, H_2O up to 100 mL, autoclave.

10. Brock III (for 500 mL): 27.2 g KH_2PO_4, 0.5 mL of 2 mM $MnCl_2$ solution, 4.6 mg $Na_2B_4O_7 \cdot 10H_2O$, 18.4 mg $ZnSO_4 \cdot 7H_2O$, 50 μL of 1 mM $CuCl_2 \cdot 2H_2O$ solution, 5 μL of 2 mM $Na_2MoO_4 \cdot 2H_2O$ solution, 5 μL of 2 mM $VOSO_4 \cdot 2H_2O$ solution, 5 μL of 0.6 mM $CoSO_4 \cdot 7H_2O$ solution, 5 μL of 18 mM $NiSO_4$ solution, 750 μL 50% H_2SO_4, H_2O up to 500 mL, autoclave.
11. 20 g/L Fe-solution (for 40 mL): 0.8 g $FeCl_3 \cdot 6H_2O$, H_2O up to 40 mL, filter-sterilize.
12. Brock medium (1 L): 900 mL of sterile H_2O, 1 mL of Brock I, 10 mL of Brock II, 5 mL of Brock III, 1 mL of 20 g/L Fe-solution, 90 μL of 95% H_2SO_4, pH 3–3.5, sterile H_2O up to 1 L.
13. 20% Tryptone: 20 g Tryptone (Duchefa Biochemie, Brussels, Belgium), H_2O up to 100 mL, autoclave.
14. 100-mL sterile glass flask
15. 500-mL sterile glass flask

2.2. In Vivo Cross-Linking

1. 36.5% (v/v) Formaldehyde (Sigma-Aldrich, St. Louis, MO)
2. Phosphate buffered saline (PBS) (for 1 L): 8.0 g NaCl, 0.2 g KCl, 1.8 g $Na_2HPO_4 \cdot 2H_2O$, 0.24 g KH_2PO_4, H_2O up to 1 L, autoclave.
3. 2 M glycine (100 mL): 18.8 g glycine, H_2O up to 100 mL, filter-sterilize.

2.3. Sonication

1. 5 M NaCl (500 mL): 146.1 g NaCl, H_2O up to 500 mL, autoclave.
2. 1 M Tris–HCl (for 1 L): 121.1 g Tris (Sigma-Aldrich), 900 mL H_2O, adjust pH to 8.0 with HCl (±10 mL of 37% HCl solution), add H_2O up to 1 L.
3. 10% Deoxycholate (100 mL): 10 g Deoxycholate (Sigma-Aldrich), H_2O up to 100 mL, filter-sterilize.
4. IP buffer (50 mL): 1.5 mL of 5 M NaCl solution, 2.5 mL of 1 M Tris–HCl solution, 0.5 mL of Triton x-100 (Sigma-Aldrich), 0.25 mL of NP-40 (Sigma-Aldrich), 5 mL of 10% Deoxycholate solution.
5. Reference DNA (10 ng/μL): PCR product of *Escherichia coli* gDNA amplified using primer pair DC821 and DC822 (the sequence of primers is given in Subheading 2.6, item 2).
6. 15-mL polystyrene conical tube (BD Falcon, Erembodegem, Belgium).

2.4. Immunoprecipitation

1. His-Select Nickel Affinity Gel (Sigma-Aldrich).
2. Purified antigen-specific Nanobody solution (1 mL): 1 mg/mL Nanobody in PBS buffer.

3. IP buffer (see Subheading 2.3, item 4).
4. PBS (see Subheading 2.2, item 2).
5. BSA blocking solution: 0.5 g BSA, 100 mL of IP buffer (see Subheading 2.3, item 4), filter-sterilize (see Note 1).
6. 10% SDS (100 mL): 10 g SDS, ddH_2O up to 100 mL, filter-sterilize.

2.5. Post-ChIP DNA Elution, Purification, and Amplification

1. DNase-free ddH_2O (50 mL): ddH_2O passed through a 0.2 μm filter, then autoclaved. Aliquot into 1 mL in 1.5 mL sterile tubes.
2. Elution buffer (100 mL): 10 mL of 10% SDS solution, 3 mL of 5 M NaCl solution, 3.4 g Imidazole (Sigma Aldrich), IP buffer up to 100 mL, filter-sterilize.
3. PCR grade Proteinase K solution: 20 mg Proteinase K (Roche Applied Science, Basel, Switzerland), 1 mL of ddH_2O.
4. 1 M Tris–HCl, pH 8.0.
5. 0.5 M EDTA (50 mL): 9.3 g EDTA (Duchefa Biochemie), ddH_2O up to 50 mL, autoclave.
6. 10× TE buffer (for 100 mL): 10 mL of 1 M Tris–HCl pH 8.0, 2 mL of 0.5 M EDTA, 88 mL ddH_2O, filter-sterilize or autoclave.
7. 1× TE buffer (for 10 mL): 1 mL of 10× TE buffer, 9 mL of ddH_2O.
8. Protein lysis solution (3 mL): 2.8 mL of 1× TE, 140 μL of Proteinase K solution, 60 μL of 10 mg/mL glycogen (Roche Applied Science), prepare freshly before use.
9. Extraction buffer 1: phenol, equilibrated with TE, pH 8.0 (Sigma-Aldrich)
10. Extraction buffer 2: chloroform–isoamyl alcohol (24:1) (Sigma-Aldrich)
11. 3 M sodium acetate (for 100 mL): 80 mL of ddH_2O, 40.8 g $NaOAc{\cdot}3H_2O$, adjust pH to 5.2 with glacial acetic acid, add ddH_2O to final volume of 100 mL, filter-sterilize.
12. 100% ethanol: absolute ethanol (Sigma-Aldrich), store at 4°C.
13. 70% ethanol (100 mL): 70 mL of 100% ethanol, 30 mL of ddH_2O, store at 4°C, prepare freshly before use.
14. RNase solution (1 mL): 16.5 μL of 20 mg/mL RNase (Invitrogen, San Diego, CA), ddH_2O up to 1 mL, prepare freshly before use.
15. GenomePlex Complete Whole Genome Amplification (WGA) Kit (Sigma-Aldrich WGA2-50RXN)
16. QIAquick PCR purification kit (Qiagen, The Netherlands)

2.6. ChIP Downstream Analysis

1. iCycler instrument equipped with the real-time detector MyIQ™ (Bio-Rad, Nazareth Eke, Belgium)
2. Primers to amplify reference DNA (*E. coli* K12 genomic position: 28223-28387): DC821 (5′-CGGGATCCAGTCATTCATCGACTCATGCC-3′), DC822 (5′-CGGGATCCATGCATAGCTATTCTCTTTTGTTAATTTGC-3′).
3. Primers to amplify negative control DNA (*S. solfataricus* P2 genomic position:612829-613008): DC701-f (5′-TGGGAAAAATCCCTTACAAGC-3′), DC702-r (5′-GCCTCTTCCGCCCTAATATC-3′)
4. Primers to amplify positive control DNA, the known binding site of Ss-LrpB (14) (*S. solfataricus* P2 genomic position : 1958904-1959007): SS2131-f (5′-CATTATCAAACATAAAAGGATTATTG-3′), SS2131-r (5′-GGGTTGCAAAATTATCAAACAAAG-3′).
5. SYBR green master mix (Invitrogen)
6. MilliQ water

3. Methods

3.1. Culture of S. solfataricus P2

1. Work under sterile conditions.
2. Prepare 20 mL of Brock medium in a 50-mL sterile glass flask.
3. Add 100 μL of 20% tryptone (final concentration 0.1%)
4. Add 200 μL of a glycerol stock of *S. solfataricus P2*.
5. Measure the optical density at 600 nm ($OD_{600\ nm}$) by a spectrophotometer.
6. Grow culture at 80°C while shaking at 200 rpm.
7. Regularly measure $OD_{600\ nm}$, and stop the growth of the culture when $\Delta OD = OD_{600\ nm}$ (obtained in Subheading 3.1, step 7)—$OD_{600\ nm}$ (obtained in Subheading 3.1, step 5) is about 0.2 (see Notes 2 and 3).
8. When the starter culture has reached ΔOD of about 0.2, prepare 200 mL of Brock medium in a 500-mL sterile glass flask.
9. Add 1 mL of 20% tryptone (final concentration 0.1%).
10. Add 10 mL of the *S. solfataricus P2* starter culture.
11. Measure $OD_{600\ nm}$ by a spectrophotometer.
12. Grow culture at 80°C at 200 rpm.
13. Regularly measure $OD_{600\ nm}$, and stop the growth of the culture when $\Delta OD = OD_{600}$ (obtained in Subheading 3.1, step 13)—OD_{600} (obtained in Subheading 3.1, step 11) is about 0.6 (see Notes 2 and 3).

3.2. In Vivo Cross-Linking

1. Work in the fume hood; wear gloves (see Note 4).
2. When the culture has obtained the desired density (see Subheading 3.1, step 13), cool it down on a shaker at 50 rpm until the culture temperature reaches 37°C.
3. Add 5.4 mL of 36.5% formaldehyde (1% of final volume) slowly to the culture while still shaking at 50 rpm for 1 min (see Note 5).
4. Add 12.5 mL of 2 M glycine solution to quench the cross-linking reaction. Continue the incubation with shaking for 5 min (see Note 6).
5. Transfer the cross-linked mixture to 50-mL polypropylene conical tubes, centrifuge at 3,300 × *g* for 10 min.
6. Discard the supernatant and resuspend the cell pellet in 30 mL of cold PBS. Centrifuge at 3,300 × *g* for 10 min. Repeat this step twice. Finally, recover the pellet for next step.
7. The pellet can be stored at −80°C or can be processed immediately as described below.

3.3. Sonication

1. Resuspend each pellet in 3 mL of fresh IP buffer.
2. Transfer the cell suspension to a 15-mL polystyrene conical tube.
3. Keep the sample at 4°C.
4. Add 2 μL of reference DNA to each sample.
5. Wash the microtip of the sonicator extensively with 70% ethanol followed by ddH_2O.
6. Position the microtip of the sonicator inside the tube, approximately 0.5–1.0 cm above the bottom of the tube. Make sure that the microtip is centered and does not touch any part of the tube.
7. Wear hearing protection during sonication.
8. Set the parameters of the Bioblock Scientific-Vibracell sonicator at operation time of 12 min and 20% amplitude. The sonication process is done in pulses: 3 s/pulse with 9 s time in between (see Notes 7 and 8).
9. Transfer the sonicated mixture to a 2-mL conical tube, centrifuge at 21,000 × *g* at 4°C for 15 min to separate debris and other insoluble materials.
10. Carefully transfer the supernatant into a sterile 5-mL polystyrene round-bottom tube (BD falcon) using a micropipette. Do not touch the pellet. The clear supernatant, which is ChIP input sample, is used for immunoprecipitation (see Note 9 and Subheading 3.4, step 9).

11. Keep 2 × 50 μL aliquots (at −80°C) from the supernatant, named QC and IP-R (input reverse cross-linking), which will be used as quality control (QC tube) and ChIP input (IP-R tube) later in the procedure (see Note 10).

3.4. Immuno-precipitation

1. Wear gloves and take all precautions to avoid sample contamination.
2. Resuspend the His-Select™ Nickel Affinity Gel carefully, and then transfer the appropriate amount (1 mL per sample) of His-Select Nickel Affinity Gel suspension to a 50-mL conical tube (BD Falcon) and centrifuge at 1,500 × *g* for 3 min.
3. Carefully remove and discard the supernatant.
4. Add 10 mL of PBS buffer per 1 mL of gel suspension, resuspend, and centrifuge at 1,500 × *g* for 5 min. Carefully remove and discard the supernatant.
5. Repeat previous step twice. Remove and discard the supernatant.
6. Add 20–40 mL of BSA Blocking Solution, close the tube carefully and seal with parafilm.
7. Place the tube horizontally on a shaker and shake at 150 rpm and 4°C overnight (see Note 11).
8. Add 0.5 mL of the purified antigen-specific Nanobody solution (1 mg/mL) to a 5-mL polystyrene round-bottom tube containing 3 mL of ChIP input sample (see Subheading 3.3, step 10).
9. Close the tubes carefully and seal with parafilm. Label tubes carefully, if handling more than one sample at the same time.
10. Place the tubes horizontally on a shaker and shake at 150 rpm at 4°C overnight to allow the formation of nanobody–antigen complexes (see Note 11).
11. Centrifuge the tube containing the affinity gel prepared previously in Subheading 3.4, step 7 at 1,500 × *g* for 5 min.
12. Remove and discard supernatant.
13. Add 30 mL of IP buffer to the affinity gel pellet obtained above. Resuspend and centrifuge again at 1,500 × *g* for 5 min.
14. Remove and discard the supernatant. Add IP buffer at ratio of 1:1 of the original gel volume (see Note 12) to resuspend the affinity gel.
15. Transfer 1 mL of the affinity gel suspension to a 5-mL polystyrene round-bottom tube containing 3.5 mL of Nanobody–ChIP sample mixture (see Subheading 3.4, step 8).
16. Close the tubes carefully and seal with parafilm. If handling more than one sample at the same time, label the tubes carefully.

17. Place the tube horizontally on a shaker at 150 rpm, at room temperature for 2–3 h to allow the binding of Nanobody–antigen complexes to the affinity gel.
18. Centrifuge the tube containing Nanobody–antigen complexes captured by affinity gel (see Subheading 3.4, step 15) at 800 × *g* for 2 min.
19. Remove and discard supernatant carefully. Add 4 mL of IP buffer to the affinity gel pellet and close the tubes very well.
20. Incubate the tubes horizontally on a shaker and shake at 150 rpm at room temperature for 5 min to perform a washing step.
21. Repeat Subheading 3.4, steps 18–20 two more times. Centrifuge the tubes at 800 × *g* for 2 min to obtain a clear affinity gel pellet. This gel pellet will be processed immediately as follows.

3.5. Post-ChIP DNA Elution, Purification, and Amplification

1. Wear gloves and work carefully to avoid contamination.
2. Add 400 μL of elution buffer to the affinity gel pellet previously obtained in Subheading 3.4, step 21. Close the tube very well, seal with parafilm. Incubate the tube horizontally on a shaker and shake at 150 rpm at room temperature for 1 h to elute Nanobody-DNA–protein complexes from the affinity gel.
3. Centrifuge at 1,800 × *g* for 10 min.
4. Carefully transfer the clear supernatant(s) to a 1.5-mL sterile Eppendorf tube. Incubate at 55°C overnight (16 h) to obtain the soluble de-cross-linked ChIP-enriched DNA.
5. In parallel, thaw the IP-R tube from Subheading 3.3, step 11. Add 300 μL elution buffer and incubate at 55°C overnight (16 h) to obtain soluble de-cross-linked ChIP-input DNA.
6. Add 400 μL of protein lysis solution to each tube from Subheading 3.5, steps 4 and 5. Mix gently by vortexing.
7. Incubate at 37°C for 2 h, without shaking.
8. At this stage, each tube contains approximately 800 μL solution. Divide the solution from each tube into two new 1.5-mL Eppendorf tubes in order to proceed with DNA extraction. Each tube now contains 400 μL of solution.
9. Add 400 μL of extraction buffer 1 and vortex well.
10. In parallel, thaw the QC tube from Subheading 3.3, step 11. Add 400 μL of extraction buffer 1 and vortex well.
11. Centrifuge the tube from Subheading 3.5, steps 9 and 10 for 10 min at 21,000 × *g*.
12. Carefully transfer the upper aqueous phase to a new 1.5-mL tube. It is important to avoid contamination from the lower

phenol phase. Therefore, retrieve only 300–350 μL of upper aqueous phase from the original 400 μL sample.

13. Repeat the process in Subheading 3.5, from steps 9 to 12, but replace the extraction buffer 1 by the extraction buffer 2. Finally, about 300 μL of extracted solution from each sample tube will be obtained.
14. Add 30 μL of 3 M sodium acetate, pH 5.2 to each sample.
15. Add 700 μL of 100% ethanol and mix well.
16. Incubate for 30 min at –80°C or overnight at –20°C.
17. Centrifuge for 20 min at 21,000 × *g*, and at 4°C.
18. Discard supernatant and add 500 μL of 70% ethanol, centrifuge for 5 min at 21,000 × *g*, and at 4°C.
19. Decant the supernatant; remove all excess liquid with a micropipette. Keep the cap of the Eppendorf tubes open to let the pellets dry under the laminar flow for about 5 min. Do not let the DNA dry too long since extensively dried DNA is difficult to dissolve.
20. Resuspend each sample in 50 μL of RNase solution.
21. Incubate for 2 h at 37°C.
22. Purify the DNA using QIAquick PCR purification kit; elute the DNA in 30 μL of DNase-free ddH_2O.
23. Determine the concentration of the purified DNA using a spectrophotometer (e.g., NanoDrop, Isogen Life Sciences). Store all samples at –20°C or continue as below.
24. The DNA in the ChIP-input (IP-R tube), the -quality control (QC tube), and the ChIP-enriched DNA in Subheading 3.5, step 23 are subject to amplification (see Note 13).
25. Clean the working surface of the laminar flow with 70% ethanol, turn on the UV light for at least 10 min to destroy contaminating DNA.
26. Wear gloves and work carefully in laminar flow to avoid contamination.
27. For each DNA sample, prepare at least 30 μL of a 3 ng/μL sample in DNase-free ddH_2O. If the concentration of the ChIP-enriched DNA sample is lower than 3 ng/μL, use the maximum concentration that is available (see Note 14).
28. For each DNA sample, use 10 μL of a 3 ng/μL sample for one amplification reaction. Follow the procedure as described by the supplier of the GenomePlex Complete Whole Genome Amplification (WGA2) Kit (Sigma Aldrich) starting from the library preparation step (see Subheading 2 Library Preparation from Kit manual GenomePlex Complete Whole Genome Amplification (WGA2) Kit (Sigma Aldrich), item 5).

29. Purify the amplified DNA using a QIAquick PCR purification kit (Qiagen); elute the DNA in 50 μL of DNase-free ddH_2O.
30. Determine the concentration of purified DNA using a spectrophotometer (e.g., NanoDrop, Isogen Life Sciences).
31. For each amplified DNA sample, prepare 200 μL of a 1 ng/μL sample using DNase-free ddH_2O. These samples will be used for quantitative real-time PCR analysis.
32. Store all samples at −20°C until further analysis.

3.6. ChIP Downstream Analysis

1. Clean the working-surface of the laminar flow with 70% ethanol, and turn on the UV light for at least 10 min to destroy contaminating DNA.
2. Wear gloves and work carefully in laminar flow to avoid contamination.
3. Put all PCR reaction components in a cooling box.
4. For each PCR reaction, combine 6.5 μL of MiliQ water, 12.5 μL of SYBR green master mix (Invitrogen), 0.5 μL of forward primer (20 μM), 0.5 μL of reverse-primer (20 μM), and 5.0 μL of DNA template (1 ng/μL) (see Note 15).
5. Spin down the PCR tubes or microtiter-plate. Place the tubes or plate in the Bio-Rad iCycler thermo-cycler. Set up a standard two-step program for 40 cycles including a melting curve analysis step after the PCR reaction. The fluorescent signal is detected by Bio-Rad My-iQ™ Single Color Real-time PCR detection system.
6. We use the 2-[Δ][Δ]CT method (15) to assess the quality of the ChIP-input sample and the ChIP enrichment from the ChIP-enriched sample, as compared to the ChIP-input sample. The method requires PCR data from both ChIP-input and ChIP-enriched samples. For each sample, two Ct values are determined: (1) Ct_{ref} = Ct value obtained from the reaction using the reference primer pair (DC821 and DC822); (2) Ct_{test} = Ct value obtained from the reaction using the primers specific for the region to test enrichment which, in this case, is the positive control (amplified using primers SS2131-f and SS2131-r) and negative control (amplified using primers DC701-f and DC702-r).
7. When the PCR reaction is finished, export the data obtained from MyIQ software to Excel spreadsheets. Turn off the thermo-cycler and the fluorescence detector.
8. Work on the Excel spreadsheets software to calculate the delta Ct values for the ChIP-input samples (ΔCt_{input}); the QC samples (ΔCt_{QC}); the ChIP-enriched ($\Delta Ct_{enriched}$). Also calculate [delta][delta]Ct values (ΔΔCt).
   - $\Delta Ct_{input} = Ct_{ref} - Ct_{test}$ (Ct_{ref} and Ct_{test} come from the reactions of the input DNA samples)

- $\Delta Ct_{enriched} = Ct_{ref} - Ct_{test}$ (Ct_{ref} and Ct_{test} come from the reactions of the ChIP-enriched DNA samples)
- $\Delta Ct_{QC} = Ct_{ref} - Ct_{test}$ (Ct_{ref} and Ct_{test} come from the reactions of the QC DNA samples)
- $\Delta\Delta Ct = \Delta Ct_{input} - \Delta\Delta Ct_{enriched}$ (see Note 16).
- $\Delta\Delta Ct_{QC} = \Delta\Delta Ct_{input} - \Delta\Delta Ct_{QC}$

9. For enrichment analysis, the $-[\Delta\Delta Ct]$ value is the $\log_2$[ratio of the ChIP-enriched DNA to the ChIP-input DNA] or the $\log_2$[fold-enrichment] of a certain genomic region. Make a graph with a horizontal axis deciphering genomic regions which are tested for ChiP-enrichment or for other experimental factors and a vertical axis deciphering $\log_2$[fold-enrichment] ($-[\Delta\Delta Ct]$) (see Note 17).
10. For input quality control analysis, the $-[\Delta\Delta Ct_{QC}]$ is the $\log_2$[ratio of free DNA to total DNA]. For a good quality ChIP-input sample, the $-[\Delta\Delta Ct_{qc}]$ is negative, indicating that the level of free DNA is very minor, as compared to the total DNA (free DNA + cross-linked DNA) (see Note 18)

4. Notes

1. Excessive vortexing of the solution can lead to irreversible denaturation of BSA. Prevent excessive foaming when mixing the BSA solution. Prepare this solution prior to use.
2. It may take 12–36 h for the starter culture to reach a $\Delta OD_{600\ nm}$ of about 0.2, and for the culture to reach a $\Delta OD_{600\ nm}$ of about 0.6.
3. The physiological state of the cells strongly affects the protein–DNA interaction. Therefore, in order to have reproducible results, the growth conditions among biological replicates need to be controlled as tightly as possible.
4. Formaldehyde is a known carcinogen and irritant, particularly at air concentrations above 20 ppm. Perform all work with formaldehyde in a chemical fume hood. The odor threshold for formaldehyde is 1 ppm.
5. The optimal conditions for cross-linking are different from protein to protein. For cross-linking using formaldehyde, the time and temperature are critical parameters. Excessive cross-linking can lead to the reduction of the availability of epitopes for antibody binding and to changes in epitopes.
6. Glycine is acting as a primary amine donor to absorb the excess cross-linking capacity of the formaldehyde present in the reaction and to "quench" the cross-linking reaction. Working

stocks can be stored at room temperature for several weeks, if prepared under sterile conditions. The solution can be filter-sterilized using 0.2 μm filter or autoclaved.

7. Sonication rapidly increases the temperature of the cell suspension which can damage the chemical linking between DNA and protein. A resting time between sections is necessary to cool down the cell suspension.
8. Extensive sonication of the ChIP-input sample could increase the enrichment of target in output sample because the IP of specific protein-bound regions is unaffected by fragment size, whereas the IP of background genomic regions decreases progressively with a reduced fragment size due to fewer nonspecific binding sites (16). However, overextensive sonication can lead to the dissociation of DNA–protein complexes.
9. The supernatant could be stored at −80°C but with this protocol, fresh extract is preferred for immunoprecipitation.
10. It is critical to save the two tubes of 50 μL extract samples; these tubes will be used to check the quality of the sample after cross-linking and sonication, and will be used as ChIP input control on the microarray.
11. The preparation of affinity gel and Nanobody–IP mixture should be performed on the same day because both procedures require an overnight incubation step. The shaking speed should be adjusted to prevent extensive foaming.
12. The volume of IP buffer added should be equal to the original volume of the affinity gel suspension taken from the storage bottle.
13. The amount of ChIP-enriched DNA is usually not sufficient for subsequent labeling and array hybridization. Therefore, in order to perform the microarray analysis, the ChIP-enriched DNA sample should be amplified. The DNA samples in the ChIP-input (IP-R tube) and the quality control (QC tube) are also treated the same way as ChIP-enriched DNA to be able to perform enrichment analysis in Subheading 3.6.
14. The formaldehyde treatment and sonication result in a significant amount of damaged DNA in the ChIP-input and ChIP-enriched DNA samples. Therefore, in order to have a good quality and an acceptable yield (4 μg amplified DNA in this case), sufficient amount of starting DNA sample is required. We usually obtain good amplification results when 90 ng or higher amounts of starting DNA are used. We recommend performing the amplification process in replicates in order to have access to quality control of the DNA sample.
15. Depending on the number of PCR reactions, one can prepare a master mix which contains all the components except the

DNA template. The master mix is aliquoted into PCR tubes or a microtiter-plate. Finally, the DNA templates are added to the corresponding wells/tubes. For each DNA sample, at least three replicates are needed in order to have reliable results.

16. If more than one reference and test regions are used, the ΔΔCt value has to be calculated from the value obtained from the same reference and test regions from ChIP-input and ChIP-enriched samples.
17. In qPCR analysis, genomic regions with a fourfold enrichment or higher are considered as ChIP-enriched regions. The samples that show good enrichment by relative quantitative-PCR analysis are good for genome-wide analysis using microarray or high throughput sequencing.
18. The quality control analysis can be performed immediately after the sonication step. If one would do so, IP and IP-R tubes are subject to DNA elution, purification, and amplification (see Subheading 3.5). The amplification step is optional for these two samples, if the quality control is the only purpose. Moreover, to be more confident about the quality of the ChIP-input sample, one could perform a 1% agarose-gel electrophoresis analysis to visualize the distribution range of sonicated DNA fragments. A ChIP input sample of good quality should have a length-range of about 400–800 bp.

References

1. Grogan DW (2000) The question of DNA repair in hyperthermophilic archaea. Trends Microbiol 8:180–185
2. She Q et al (2001) The complete genome of the crenarchaeon *Sulfolobus solfataricus* P2. Proc Natl Acad Sci USA 98:7835–7840
3. Orlando V (2000) Mapping chromosomal proteins in vivo by formaldehyde-crosslinked chromatin immunoprecipitation. Trends Biochem Sci 25:99–104
4. Orlando V, Strutt H, Paro R (1997) Analysis of chromatin structure by in vivo formaldehyde cross-linking. Methods 11:205–214
5. Nelson JD, Denisenko O, Bomsztyk K (2006) Protocol for the fast chromatin immunoprecipitation (ChIP) method. Nat Protoc 1:179–185
6. Haring M et al (2007) Chromatin immunoprecipitation: optimization, quantitative analysis and data normalization. Plant Methods 3:11
7. Weinmann AS, Farnham PJ (2002) Identification of unknown target genes of human transcription factors using chromatin immunoprecipitation. Methods 26:37–47
8. Dahl JA, Collas P (2007) Q2ChIP, a quick and quantitative chromatin immunoprecipitation assay, unravels epigenetic dynamics of developmentally regulated genes in human carcinoma cells. Stem Cells 25:1037–1046
9. Mukhopadhyay A et al (2008) Chromatin immunoprecipitation (ChIP) coupled to detection by quantitative real-time PCR to study transcription factor binding to DNA in *Caenorhabditis elegans*. Nat Protoc 3:698–709
10. Wells J, Farnham PJ (2002) Characterizing transcription factor binding sites using formaldehyde crosslinking and immunoprecipitation. Methods 26:48–56
11. Carroll JS et al (2006) Genome-wide analysis of estrogen receptor binding sites. Nat Genet 38:1289–1297
12. Impey S et al (2004) Defining the CREB regulon: a genome-wide analysis of transcription factor regulatory regions. Cell 119:1041–1054
13. Robertson G et al (2007) Genome-wide profiles of STAT1 DNA association using chromatin immunoprecipitation and massively parallel sequencing. Nat Methods 4:651–657

14. Peeters E et al (2004) Ss-LrpB, a novel Lrp-like regulator of *Sulfolobus solfataricus* P2, binds cooperatively to three conserved targets in its own control region. Mol Microbiol 54: 321–336
15. Livak KJ, Schmittgen TD (2001) Analysis of relative gene expression data using real-time quantitative PCR and the 2-[Delta][Delta]CT method. Methods 25:402–408
16. Fan X et al (2008) Extensive chromatin fragmentation improves enrichment of protein binding sites in chromatin immunoprecipitation experiments. Nucl Acids Res 36:e125

Chapter 32

User-Friendly Expression Plasmids Enable the Fusion of VHHs to Application-Specific Tags

Ario de Marco

Abstract

One of the advantages of using recombinant instead of conventional antibodies is that these can be easily manipulated by means of standard molecular biology techniques. Therefore this opportunity can be exploited to prepare fusion constructs composed of VHHs and suitable tags. According to the applications in which the antibodies will be applied, molecules such as fluorescent probes, biotin, and PEG can be either covalently or non-covalently linked to the antibodies. Within this chapter, practical tips for the choice and expression of the most appropriate among the available plasmids are listed, keeping in mind the experimental conditions in which usually the fusion antibodies will be applied.

Key words: Affinity purification, Detection tags, Expression systems, Multiple labeling, Recombinant antibodies, VHH

1. Introduction

Recombinant antibody technology offers exclusive advantages over the conventional monoclonal antibody technology. These include the possibility of performing subtractive panning, selecting binders for toxic or non-immunogenic molecules and, in the case of VHHs, even identifying competitive enzyme inhibitors (1, 2). Furthermore, standard molecular biology techniques enable easy manipulation of recombinant antibodies. Consequently, VHHs can be cloned in frame with any kind of tag for producing reagents with optimal features for specific applications (see Table 1). According to the experimental design and application purpose, the same VHH can be subcloned and expressed fused to different tags or tag combinations with the aim of simplifying the downstream protocols (3). This strategy for generating user-friendly

Dirk Saerens and Serge Muyldermans (eds.), *Single Domain Antibodies: Methods and Protocols*, Methods in Molecular Biology, vol. 911, DOI 10.1007/978-1-61779-968-6_32, © Springer Science+Business Media, LLC 2012

Table 1
Overview of the described VHH vectors and corresponding applications. The presence of the conserved *NcoI-NotI* recognition sequences allows the cut-and-paste subcloning of the same VHH from the original pHEN4 phagemid. The antibody is in frame with different tags designed for facilitating the down-stream applications

Purpose	Vectors	Reagents	Applications	References
Cytoplasmic expression	pSNAPcv	pETM90-Eco pSS26b	1:1 covalent labeling	(12, 17)
Periplasmic expression	pSNAPpv	pET22b+ pSS26b	1:1 covalent labeling	(12)
Cytoplasmic expression	pAOD-GFP	pETM82	Intrabody identification	(13)
Secretion at the cell surface	pVUB-prescVHH	pVUB4	Antibody microarray	(20)
Bivalent/bispecific antibodies	pFuseVHH (h/r/m)	pFuse-xFc2-scFv	Light and electron microscopy	(17)
Multifunctionality	pHEN8	pHEN2	IMAC and immunotechniques	This paper
SRP secretion pathway	pHEN7	pHEN6	Improved yields	(26)
Cellulose binding	pCBD	pET22b+, pET3 Zephyrin	Microarray, immunopurification	This paper

reagents is particularly useful for some applications, such as multiple labeling necessary for correlative microscopy or simultaneous labeling with a chromophore and PEG of antibodies used for preparing liposomes. Tags can be also used for inducing multimerization of VHH molecules and subsequently increasing the avidity of such antibodies.

Another advantage is that the presence of tags allows site-specific labeling. In contrast to what is frequently observed when using conventional IgGs, i.e., lower functionality after chemical labeling, VHH-tag fusion constructs can be labeled exclusively at the tag moiety (4). This strategy avoids the modification of amino residues involved in the active site of the antibody and consequent reduction of the antibody binding capacity. Therefore, the combination of VHHs and tags can widen the range of antibody applications by allowing manipulations not easily performable with conventional antibodies.

2. Materials

2.1. Preparation of the Universal Cytoplasmic Expression System Derived from the pETM90-Eco Vector—the Example of the pSNAPcv

1. pETM90-Eco vector (see Table 1) (5).
2. Template DNA (SNAP tag, GFP, biotin recognition site, etc,). For SNAP tag, use the plasmid pSS26b (Covalys Biosciences, Witterswil, Switzerland).
3. Primers (SNAP tag):

   Fw: 5′AATTTTGTTTAACTTTAAGAAGGA**GATATC**ATGG ACAAAGATTGCGAAATGAAACG TACC3′

   Rev1:5′GAATGATGATGATGATGGTGCATA**TGGCCA***CC* AGGTCCCAGACCCGGTTTACC CAGA3′

   Rev2: 5′TAGCAGCCGGATCTCAGTGGTGGTGGTGGTG GTG**CTCGAG***TCATCA***GCGGCCGC**GGTACCTTA TTCAGAGGC3′
4. Thermocycler for PCR reaction.
5. *Taq* DNA polymerase.
6. Polymerase buffer (Fermentas, St. Leon-Roth, Germany).
7. Restriction enzymes: *Dpn*I, *Eco*RV, *Xho*I.
8. DNA maxi-prep purification kit (Machery-Nagel, Düren, Germany).
9. Wizard SV Gel and Clean-Up System (Promega, Mannheim, Germany).
10. T4 DNA polymerase.
11. T4 DNA ligase buffer.
12. 10 mM dCTP.
13. T7 terminator and T7 promoter primers (Novagen).
14. Competent DH5α cells.

2.2. pSNAPpv Vector Preparation

1. pET22b+ vector (see Table 1).
2. Template DNA for SNAP tag: pSS26b vector (Covalys Biosciences, Witterswil, Switzerland).
3. Primers:

   Fw: 5′CCC**AAGCTTGCGGCCGC**GGTAGTGGTCCTGG TCTGGAAGTTCTGTTCCAGGGG CCC*GGC*ATGGA CAAAGATTGCGAAATGAAACGTA3′

   Rev: 5′CCG**CTCGAG**ACCAGAAGAGCCCTGAAAATAAA GATTCTCAGGTCCCAGACCCGGTTTACCCAGACG ATGACCTTCATGGCCAGCAGCCA3′
4. Thermocycler for PCR reaction.
5. *Taq* DNA polymerase.
6. Polymerase buffer (Fermentas, St. Leon-Roth, Germany).

7. DNA maxi-prep purification kit (Machery-Nagel, Düren, Germany).
8. Restriction enzymes: *Hind*III, *Xho*I.
9. Competent DH5α cells.

2.3. pVUBprescVHH Vector for Antibody Microarray Preparation

1. pVUB4 vector (see Table 1).
2. pETM14 (6).
3. Primers:

   Fw: 5′GGAAGATCTCACTGGAAGTTCTG3′

   Rev: 5′GCTCTAGATCAGTGGTGGTGGTGGTGGTGGTGTACT3′
4. Restriction enzymes: *Bgl*II, *Xba*I, *Nco*I, *Not*I.
5. BL21 bacterial cells.
6. Epoxy- or TiO_2-coated slides.
7. Microarray spotter (AD1500, BioDot, Irvine, CA).
8. Microarray scanner (GenePix 4000B, Molecular Device, Sunnyvale, CA).
9. Fluorochrome labeling kit.
10. Phosphate Buffered Saline (PBS), pH 7.2.

2.4. pFuseVHH (R/M/H) Vectors

1. pFUSE-xFc2-adapt-scFv vectors (see Table 1).
2. Primers:

   Fw: 5′ATCGGCCATGGCTGAGGTGCAGCTG3′

   Rev: 5′GGAGG**AGATCTGCGGCCGC**TGGAGA3′
3. Thermocycler for PCR reaction.
4. *Taq* DNA polymerase.
5. Polymerase buffer (Fermentas, St. Leon-Roth, Germany).
6. Competent DH5α cells.
7. Restriction enzymes: *Nco*I, *Not*I, *Bgl*II.
8. GST template.

2.5. pHEN8 Vector

1. pHEN2 vector (see Table 1).
2. Primers:

   Fw: 5′ATAAGAAT**GCGGCCGC***GG*AC ATCATCAT3′

   Rev: 5′CGC**GGATCC**TCATTAAAGCCAGAATGGA3′
3. Restriction enzymes: *Not*I, *BamH*I, *Nco*I.
4. Thermocycler for PCR reaction.
5. *Taq* DNA polymerase.
6. Polymerase buffer (Fermentas, St. Leon-Roth, Germany).
7. Competent DH5α cells.

2.6. pHEN7 Vector

1. pHEN6 vector (see Table 1).
2. DsbA template.
3. Oligonucleotides:

   Fw: 5′**agctt**gcatgcaaattctatttcaaggagacagtcataatgaaaaagatctggc tggcgctggctggtttagcg tttagcgcatcggc3′

   Rev: 5′**catgg**ccgatgcgctaaacgctaaaactaaaccagccagcgccagccagat ctttttcattatgactgtctcc ttgaaatagaatttgcatgca3′
4. Annealing buffer: 10 mM Tris–HCl, pH 7.5, 50 mM NaCl, 1 mM EDTA in MilliQH_2O.
5. Restriction enzymes: *Hind*III, *Nco*I.
6. Thermocycler for annealing reaction.
7. Competent DH5α cells.

2.7. pCBD Vector

1. pET22b+ vector (Novagen, Darmstadt, Germany).
2. Carbohydrate binding domain (CBD) template such as the pET3 Zephyrin (4).
3. Primers:

   Fw: 5′CGGATCCGAATTCGAGCTCCGTCGACAAGCTT **GCGGCCGC***TCCGCGGG TCTGGAA*ATGGCAAATA CACCGGTATCAGG3′

   Rev: 5′TAGCAGCCGGATCTCAGTGGTGGTGGTGGTGG TG**CTCGAG**TACTACACTG CCACCGGGTTCTT3′.
4. Restriction enzymes: *Not*I, *Xho*I.
5. Thermocycler for PCR reaction.
6. *Taq* DNA polymerase.
7. Polymerase buffer (Fermentas, St. Leon-Roth, Germany).
8. Competent DH5α cells.

3. Methods

3.1. Preparation of the Universal Cytoplasmic Expression System Derived from the pETM90-Eco Vector—The Example of the SNAPcv

The pETM90-Eco vector (5) is an optimal backbone to develop different VHH cytoplasmic expression vectors (see Note 1) that can be created by exchanging suitable cassettes between the *Eco*RV-*Msc*I sites. We advice using SLIC technology for optimizing the results (see Note 2).

1. Prepare a SLIC-compatible PCR fragment (7) corresponding to the tag sequence (SNAP, GFP, biotin recognition sequence, etc.) plus the recognition sites *Eco*RV (5′) end *Msc*I (3′) and clone it in a correspondingly digested pETM-Eco vector to obtain the pETM-Int vector (see Note 3). In the case of SNAP tag, perform SLIC using the Fw and Rev1 primers (see Subheading 2.3 and Note 4).

2. Prepare a PCR product suitable for SLIC using the pETM-Int vector as a template (8). For the cloning of the SNAP tag and if SLIC has already been used for the first PCR reaction, use the same forward primer in combination with the primer Rev2 (see Note 4).
3. Digest the PCR product by adding 20 U of *Dpn*I in 100 μL of reaction mix and incubate 60 min at 37°C.
4. Run the digested PCR product in 1% agarose gel and purify it using the Wizard SV Gel and Clean-Up System.
5. Digest 1 μg of the pETM-Int vector *EcoR*V-*Xho*I (*Ava*I).
6. Incubate separately 1 μg of the PCR product (insert) and 1 μg of the digested vector with 0.5 U of T4 DNA polymerase in a total volume of 20 μL of T4 ligase buffer for 45 min at 22°C to chew back one strand and reveal ssDNA overhangs (see Note 5).
7. Stop the reaction in both tubes by adding 2 μL of 10 mM dCTP to each of them. Incubate the tubes on ice.
8. Prepare the annealing reactions using 150 ng of the vector and the sufficient amount insert for reaching the molar ratios (1:1), (1:3), (1:6) in a total volume of 10 μL of ligation buffer. Incubate 30 min at 37°C.
9. Transform competent DH5α cells.
10. Confirm the presence of the construct by colony PCR using the T7 terminator and T7 promoter primers.
11. Recover the plasmid using a DNA maxi-prep purification kit.
12. The resulting pSNAPcv vector can be used for the cytoplasmic expression of VHH antibodies (intrabodies) (see Notes 1 and 6) and provides SNAP tag, 6× His tag, TEV recognition site, *Nco*I and *Not*I recognition sequences, and an in-frame stop codon (see Fig. 1a).
13. A staffer sequence corresponding to GST can be cloned between the *Nco*I-*Not*I sites for simplifying the evaluation of vector digestion efficiency and relegation (see Note 7).

The same plasmid construction strategy can be used to engineer a biotin recognition site and obtain in vivo biotinylated VHHs (see Note 8).

3.2. pSNAPpv Vector Preparation

The pET22b+ vector links a *pelB* secretion sequence to the proteins cloned downstream. Therefore, it enables the periplasmic accumulation of the mature product. However, some modifications must be introduced to obtain a vector compatible for direct VHH subcloning from pHEN4 and expression of SNAP-fused antibodies.

1. Perform a PCR reaction using the recommended primers (see Subheading 2.2, item 3) and the vector pSS26b as a template. The fw primer incorporates the *Hind*III and *Not*I recognition sites (bold), the recognition sequence for the 3C protease (9),

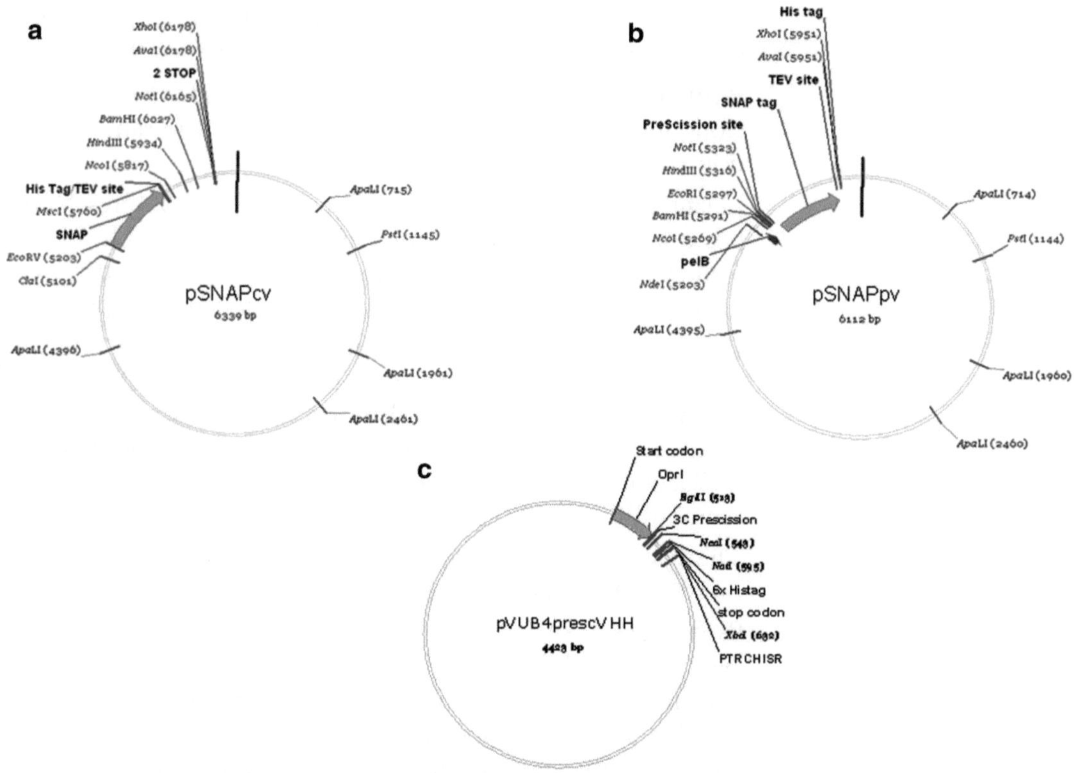

Fig. 1. Representation of the relevant features of the plasmids pSNAPcv, pSNAPpv, and pVUB4prescVHH.

a GGC codon for avoiding the creation of a *Nco*I site (italic), and the starting sequence of the SNAP tag (underlined). The rev primer corresponds to a recognition sequence for *Xho*I (bold), a TEV protease recognition site and the C-term of the SNAP tag.

2. Digest the PCR fragment *Hind*III-*Xho*I and clone it in a pET22b+ digested with the same enzymes (8).
3. Ligate and transform (8).

The resulting plasmid (see Fig. 1b) is suitable for the periplasmic expression of VHH-SNAP fusion constructs (see Notes 6 and 9).

3.3. pVUBprescVHH Vector for Antibody Microarray Preparation

The pVUBprescVHH vector (see Fig. 1c) has been designed for direct subcloning of VHH sequences from pHEN4 vectors and their expression as cleavable domains anchored to the external side of the bacteria outer membrane (see Note 10). This material is suitable for flow cytometry and antibody microarray preparation (see Note 11).

1. Amplify the cassette containing the sequences corresponding to the 3C recognition site, the *Nco*I/*Not*I restriction sites, and the 6× His tag by PCR using the pETM14 vector (6) as a template

and the primer pair that introduce the *Bgl*II and *Xba*I restriction sites at the 5′ and 3′ sides of the cassette sequence (8).

2. Purify the PCR product, digest with *Bgl*II and *Xba*I, and subclone into the pVUB4 vector digested with the same restriction enzymes.
3. Ligate and plate (8). The resulting vector, pVUB4prescVHH, possesses the *Nco*I/*Not*I restriction enzyme pair suitable for subcloning the VHH sequences from the pHEN4 vector and expressing them as fusions with the transmembrane protein OprI.
4. Once cloned the chosen VHH in the pVUB4prescVHH vector, transform BL21 competent cells. Inoculate LB medium (8) with a single colony and induce recombinant expression when the $OD_{600\ nm}$ is roughly 0.5. Let cells grow overnight at 28°C, collect the bacteria by centrifugation and resuspend them in PBS (8).
5. The bacteria can be directly spotted on epoxy or nanostructured TiO_2 surfaces. The VHHs expressed by the pVUB-prescVHH vector are exposed at the cell surface, active and suitable for binding their antigen (see Note 11).
6. Specific antibody–antigen binding can be detected directly (labeled antigen) or indirectly by using a labeled binder that recognizes an epitope different from the one recognized by the VHH on the antigen surface.

3.4. pFuseVHH R/M/H Vectors

The pFuseVHH vectors (see Fig. 2a) enable to obtain constructs formed by one Fc domain plus the VHH domain. Therefore, the resulting constructs allow the dimerization of VHH antibodies (bivalent VHHs with higher avidity and increased signal: see Fig. 2b, c), a further tag when multiple detections are necessary, and the possibility to select the optimal Fc domain (rabbit, mouse, or human) for reducing unspecific signals according to the used biological sample (see Note 12). Furthermore, bispecific combinations are possible (see Note 13).

1. Digest the pFUSE-xFc2-adapt-scFv vectors (10) with *Nco*I and *Bgl*II (8).
2. Prepare a PCR product using the indicated primers and the sequence of a VHH (2C1) as a template.
3. Ligate and transform (8).
4. Remove the original VHH sequence using the restriction sites *Nco*I- *Not*I and insert a staffer (GST-sequence) of mass differing significantly from VHHs (see Note 7).

3.5. pHEN8 Vector

The VHHs selected during panning using the HA-tagged phagemid pHEN4 are usually subcloned into pHEN6 for obtaining 6× His-tagged recombinant antibodies that can be easily purified by metal

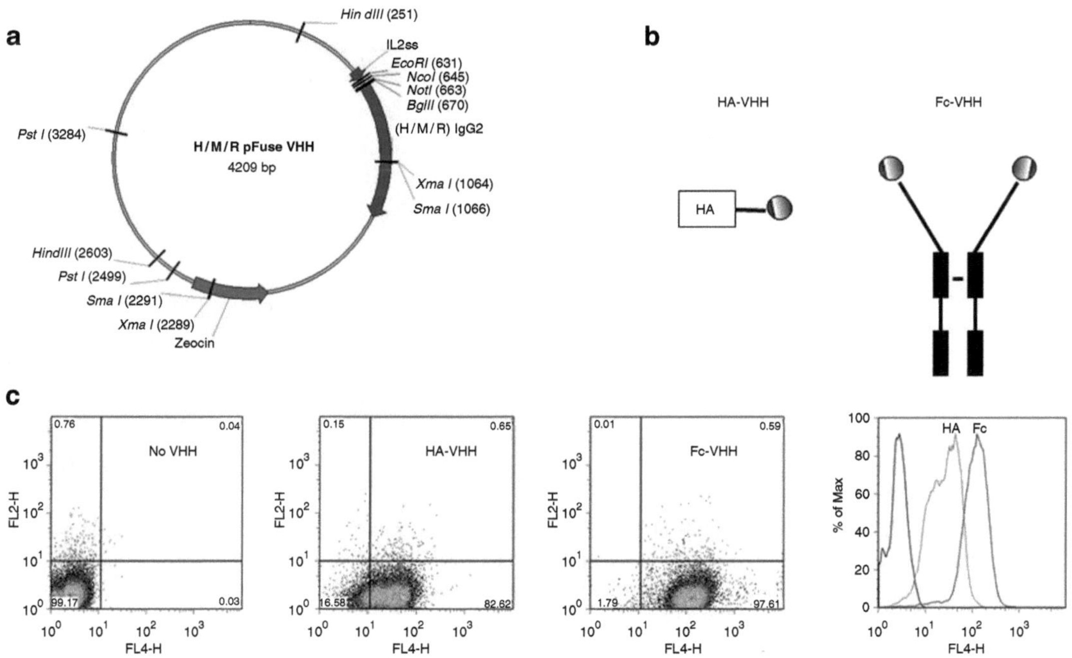

Fig. 2. Characteristic and application example of the pFuseVHH plasmids. (**a**) Schematic representation of the pFuseVHH plasmids. The three versions differ in providing Fc domains from human (H), mouse (M), and rabbit (R). (**b**) The fusion to an Fc domain induces the dimerization of the antibody molecule during the maturation step. Therefore, VHHs become bivalent when fused to Fc, whilst remain monovalent when fused to tags like HA. (**c**) Bivalent VHHs show higher avidity than monovalent VHHs and consequently give stronger signal when used in flow cytometry. The signal increase allows the complete separation of the labeled cell population with respect to the control.

affinity chromatography. However, 6× His is a poor tag for immunofluorescence and, therefore, accurate antibody characterization would be more conveniently performed whether VHHs would have both the 6× His and another tag suitable for immunofluorescence and immunoprecipitation. pHEN8 (see Fig. 3a) allows the expression of VHHs fused to a double tag 6× His-myc (see Note 14).

1. Prepare a PCR product using the indicated primers and the pHEN2 vector as a template (see Note 14). The recognition sites *Not*I and *BamH*I are in bold and the two extra GG introduced for obtaining the frameshift compatible with VHH cut-and-paste from pHEN4 are in italic.
2. Digest both the PCR product and the pHEN2 plasmid *Nco*I-*BamH*I (8).
3. Ligate and transform.
4. Remove the original VHH sequence using the restriction sites *Nco*I-*Not*I and insert a staffer (GST-sequence) of mass differing significantly from VHHs (see Note 7).

The yields of VHHs expressed in pHEN6 and pHEN8 are comparable and the antibody functionality is preserved (see Fig. 3b).

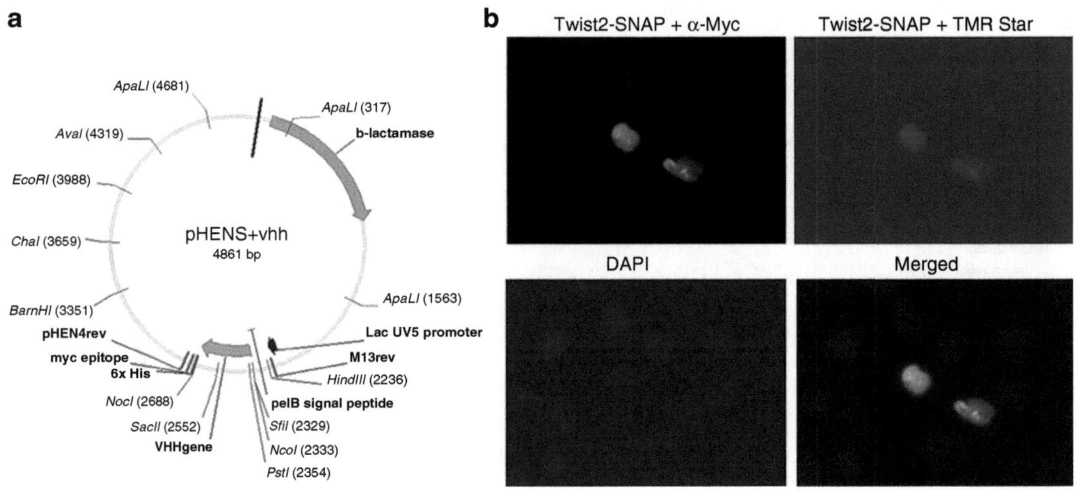

Fig. 3. Characteristic and application example of the pHEN8 plasmid. (**a**) Schematic representation of the pHEN8 plasmid. (**b**) Immunofluorescence experiment. The target fusion protein Twist2-SNAP was detected with perfectly overlapping signal patterns using both an anti-myc secondary antibody targeting the myc-VHH primary antibody and the cell-permeable fluorescent probe that covalently binds the SNAP tag.

3.6. pHEN7 Vector

The pHEN vector family shares a common Sec leader peptide for protein export in the periplasm. Although this strategy of using the posttranslational secretion pathway can be convenient for some constructs, it could prevent the export of constructs with particularly favorable thermodynamic (see Note 15). In this case, the SRP-mediated co-translational protein secretion route should be more suitable since it avoids the cytoplasmic accumulation of partially folded and export-incompetent polypeptides. The pHEN7 vector has the same features of pHEN6, but an SRP instead of a Sec leader peptide (*dsbA* and *pelB*, respectively). The preliminary experiments performed in our lab indicate that pHEN7 can improve the yields of some VHHs (see Note 16).

1. Digest the pHEN6 vector *Hind*III-*Nco*I (8).
2. Resuspend each of the two complementary and phosphorylated oligonucleotides designed for reproducing "digested-like" ends in annealing buffer to reach the same molar concentration. The sticky ends for *Hind*III and *Nco*I are indicated in bold.
3. Mix equal volumes of the oligonucleotides in a PCR tube.
4. Heat the oligo solution at 90°C in a thermocycler for 3 min and then let cool down to room temperature.
5. Ligate and transform (8).

3.7. pCBD Vector

This vector (see Fig. 4) enables the preparation of constructs in which the VHHs are fused to a CBD that allows the directional immobilization of the antibodies on a cellulose solid support (see ote 17). The pCBD vector has been created using the pET22b+ as a backbone.

1. Digest the pET22b+ vector *Not*I-*Xho*I (8).
2. Prepare a PCR product using the pZephyrin vector (4) as a template and the indicated primer pair. The primers possess long SLIC-compatible homology regions for the plasmid, the recognition sites for *Not*I and *Xho*I (bold), the homology regions for the tag and a linker region (italic).
3. Perform SLIC, ligate, and transform (7, 8).

The resulting vector is compatible with direct subclone of VHH sequences from the phagemid pHEN4 using the *Nco*I-*Not*I sites and expresses VHH-CBD fusions in which the two domains are connected by a flexible linker. No recognition sequences for protease have been added since the constructs have been envisaged for direct purification on immobilized supports where they can be used for immune-binding of the corresponding antigens.

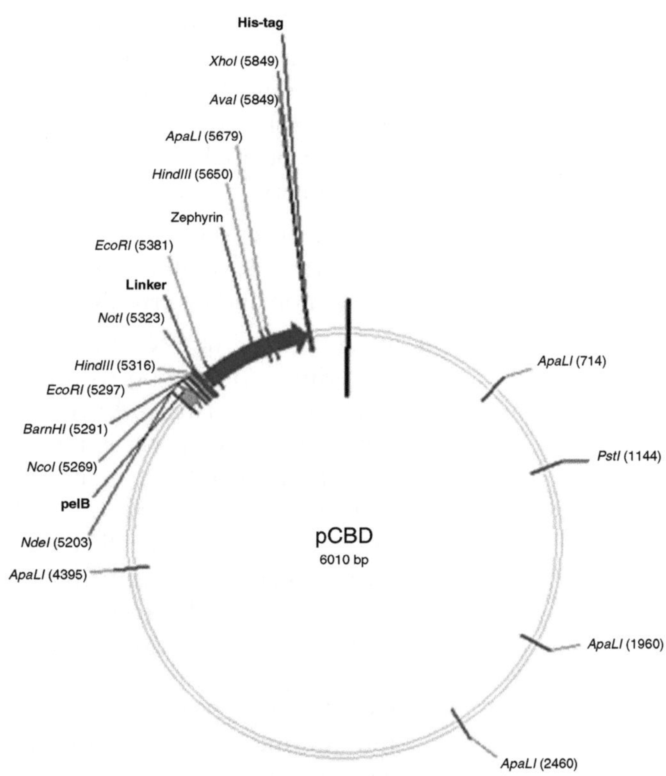

Fig. 4. Representation of the relevant features of the plasmid pCBD.

4. Notes

1. In our experience, roughly 50% of the llama VHH isolated from naïve libraries are soluble when expressed as intrabodies (11–13). The VHH native folding in the cytoplasm can be further increased by co-expressing the disulfide isomerase DsbC and by using strains that promotes disulfide bond formation in their cytoplasm (13–15). It can be expected that the excellent cytoplasmic yields of disulfide-bond-dependent proteins obtained co-expressing the yeast sulphydryl oxidase Erv1p (15) will strongly support the future production of VHHs using cytoplasmic vectors.

   The subcloning of VHH sequences into a cytoplasmic vector expressing a GFP reporter fused at the antibody C-term has been used for direct optical discrimination between VHHs that are functional as intrabodies and the others that are aggregation-prone (13).

2. The protocol describes a plasmid modification strategy suitable for preparing vectors enabling direct subcloning and expression of VHHs originally cloned *Nco*I-*Not*I into a pHEN4 phagemid library. SLIC (7) is a cloning procedure that allows the assembly of a single or multiple DNA fragments by exploiting in vitro homologous recombination and single-strand annealing. Single-strand DNA with overlapping sequences (30-bp) must be provided for efficient recombination. SLIC is suitable for introducing any modification into a given sequence and can be applied to any sequence by opportunely adapting the primers.

3. Both restriction enzymes cut blunt. SLIC is a convenient alternative to conventional cloning since it avoids plasmid re-ligation and inverse PCR fragment insertion.

4. In the case of the SNAP-tag vector, the first 30-bp of the SLIC Fw primer correspond to the vector backbone, whilst the tag starts with its natural ATG. The *Eco*RV recognition site is in bold. The same primer is suitable for both PCR reactions.

   The primer Rev1 is intended for the first PCR reaction, namely for the preparation of the tag insert to clone by SLIC into pETM-Eco. The first 30-bp corresponds to the vector backbone, whilst the remaining anneal to the terminal sequence of the tag. The *Msc*I recognition site is in bold. Two extra bases (italic) have been introduced to restore the frame.

   The primer Rev2 is designed for the second PCR reaction, namely for preparing the insert that enables the conversion of the intermediate vector into an expression vector compatible with direct subcloning of VHH sequences from pHEN4.

   It comprises the backbone homology region, the *Xho*I recognition site (bold), two stop codons (italic), and the recognition site for *Nco*I (bold). The sequence homology with *Ava*I has been used to insert the *Xho*I recognition site.

5. The Taq DNA polymerase was selected after comparison with other exonucleases since it provided the best reproducibility (7).
6. Applications for VHHs expressed using pSNAPcv and pSNAPpv vectors (see Table 1).
   (a) Covalent binding of *O*(6)-benzylguanine (BG) groups (16). The SNAP tag allows the efficient and rapid 1:1 covalent labeling with any molecule possessing a BG group. A large variety of reagents used in biology and biotechnology applications are already commercially available for conjugation, such as fluorochromes, biotin, PEG, building blocks (http://www.neb.com/nebecomm/products/category140.asp?#141). Any other chemical can be customized for SNAP conjugation. More recently it has been proposed the CLIP tag that has the same features of the SNAP tag, but binds *O*(6)-benzylcysteine groups and, consequently, a set of orthogonal substrates. CLIP tag can be simply exchanged with SNAP in the pSNAP vectors using the *Eco*RV-*Msc*I sites. The reliability of SNAP-tag technology in combination with VHHs has been recently demonstrated (12, 17).
   (b) Light microscopy. Each VHH-SNAP constructs can be labeled with a wide array of fluorochromes and the combination of different constructs labeled in vitro allows multiple staining.
   (c) Electron microscopy. VHH-SNAP covalent labeling with biotin enables recognition using gold-streptavidin and consequent detection by electron microscopy.
   (d) Correlative microscopy. The unique derivatization site of SNAP can be used for biotinylation and gold-streptavidin binding, whereas anti-SNAP antibodies are labeled with a fluorochrome. Both commercial polyclonal anti-SNAP antibodies and recombinant anti-SNAP VHHs (17) are available.
   (e) PEGylation. The modification of a molecule by the addition of a PEG chain can be used to decrease its clearance rate in vivo or to build up liposomes.
7. Cloning an irrelevant DNA sequence of 1,000-bp as a stuffer between the first and the second restriction sites of the multicloning site improves the vector digestion efficiency and simplifies the evaluation of the digestion after gel electrophoresis since the size of the exceeded stuffer will discriminate between uncut, single-cut, and double-cut vectors. Furthermore, the band corresponding to the stuffer will be easily identified in the agarose gel. Avoid using stuffer with a size close to the VHH

insert (500-bp) because it would complicate the possibility to discriminate between relegated and VHH-cloned vectors.

8. Biotin can be used as a tag in combination with streptavidin reagents such as enzyme and antibodies, gold particles, chromophores, and sepharose (magnetic) beads. Usually, protein sequences are fused to a short sequence (10–13 aa) recognized by BirA, the enzyme that catalyzes the biotinylation of the target lysine. The enzyme can be co-expressed with the target protein to obtain in vivo biotinylation of the target protein. VHH in vivo biotinylation can be obtained using both mammalian systems (pBigBirA plasmid, *18*) and bacterial platforms. The pUR5850 plasmid (18) has a biotinylation site and, in combination with the bivalent pUU-11 vector, has been used to obtain bispecific and multi-tagged VHH constructs (19).

9. The TEV recognition site has been used as a linker and because of the necessity to obtain primers of equal length. Its presence, however, can increase the application flexibility of the resulting construct since it allows the selective removal of the 6× His tag. Sometimes SNAP-fused proteins can be expressed poorly in the periplasm.

10. The expressed construct presents also a 3C recognition sequence that allows the protease-dependent cleavage of the exposed VHHs. Therefore, the system could be also considered for recovering highly pure antibodies from the medium. However, in our experience the yields remained relatively low in comparison to intracellular expression strategies.

11. The Purification Independent Microarray (PIM) platform has been described recently in detail (20).

12. The Fc domain is suitable for any kind of labeling based on secondary anti-Fc antibodies and protein A conjugates. The contemporary use of antibodies fused to different Fcs allows sample multilabeling.

    Furthermore, a second and independent labeling epitope can be created by cloning the entire VHH-Fc domain into the pBigBirA vector that enables the fusion of a biotinylated sequence to the main construct (21). However, a PCR reaction is necessary for transferring the VHH-Fc domain instead of simple cut-and-paste subcloning and, in our experience, the yields of the secreted constructs remain very low. However, since these constructs are expressed in mammalian cells, molecule glycosylation can further contribute to the immunological response in vivo.

13. Tandem vectors in which the same VHH (or two different VHHs) is cloned twice in sequence, using a myc or HA tag as a linker in between the two cassettes, can be also created. In this case, however, either *ad hoc* PCR products or successive

cloning steps are necessary to achieve the aim (18, 22). This makes the procedure cumbersome and, furthermore, the linker length can strongly influence the effectiveness of the probe.

14. Other similar vectors already exists, such as the pHEN2 (6× His+myc tag for scFvs), the pUR5850 (6× His+myc tag and biotinylation sequence for VHHs), or the pUR4676 (VHH phagemid with 6× His+myc tag) (18, 23). However, either the frame or the available restriction sites do not allow the direct cut-and-paste subcloning of VHH sequences from the pHEN4 phagemid.
15. The advantage of shifting to an SRP phage display vectors has been demonstrated in the case of DARPins (24). Concerning recombinant antibodies, a comparison between Sec and SRP vectors has been performed (25), but using one single scFv. Consequently, no general rule can be inferred.
16. Although we limited our analysis to the yields of already selected VHHs, it could be interesting to use an SRP phagemid (the corresponding version of the pHEN4) for investigating whether this phage display strategy could favor some fast-folding VHHs that could be potentially lost when expressed using the conventional pHEN4.
17. Both microarrays and immunopurification columns can be prepared using the CBD-VHH constructs. The immobilization support can be directly used for CBD-VHH purification from total lysates. The fusion constructs are expressed in bacteria periplasm with yields in the order of the mg/L culture.

Acknowledgements

The author thanks E. Morag for having provided the pET3 Zephyrin vector, P. Massa for the flow-cytometry data, and F. Perez who made available the modified pFuse vectors.

References

1. De Genst E et al (2006) Molecular basis for the preferential cleft recognition by dromedary heavy-chain antibodies. Proc Natl Acad Sci USA 103:4586–4591
2. Desmyter A et al (2002) Three camelid VHH domains in complex with porcine pancreatic alpha-amylase inhibition and versatility of binding topology. J Biol Chem 277:23645–50
3. Mertens N et al (2004) New strategies in polypeptide and antibody synthesis: an overview. Cancer Biother Radiopharm 19:99–109
4. Ofir K et al (2005) Versatile protein microarray based on carbohydrate-binding modules. Proteomics 5:1806–1814
5. de Marco A et al (2004) Recombinant proteins fused to thermostable partners can be purified by heat incubation. J Biotechnol 107: 125–1336
6. Dümmler A, Lawrence AM, de Marco A (2005) Simplified screening for the detection of soluble fusion constructs expressed in *E. coli* using a modular set of vectors. Microb Cell Fact 4:34

7. Li MZ, Elledge SJ (2007) Harnessing homologous recombination *in vitro* to generate recombinant DNA via SLIC. Nat Methods 4:251–256
8. Sambrook J, Russell PW (2001) Molecular Cloning: a laboratory manual. Cold Spring Harbor Laboratory Press, New York
9. Libby RT et al (1988) Human rhinovirus 3C protease: cloning and expression of an active form in *Escherichia coli*. Biochemistry 27:6262–62
10. Moutel S et al (2009) A multi-Fc-species system for recombinant antibody production. BMC Biotechnol 9:1410
11. Monegal A et al (2009) Immunological applications of single-domain llama recombinant antibodies isolated from a naive library. Protein Eng Des Sel 22:273–280
12. Bossi S et al (2010) Antibody-mediated purification of co-expressed antigen-antibody complexes. Protein Expr Purif 72:55–58
13. Olichon A, Surrey T (2007) Selection of genetically encoded fluorescent single domain antibodies engineered for efficient expression in *Escherichia coli*. J Biol Chem 282:36314–36320
14. de Marco A (2009) Strategies for successful recombinant expression of disulfide bond-dependent proteins in *Escherichia coli*. Microb Cell Fact 8:26
15. Nguyen VD et al (2010) Pre-expression of a sulphydryl oxidase significantly increases the yields of eukaryotic disulfide bond containing proteins expressed in the cytoplasm of *E. coli*. Microb Cell Fact 10:1
16. Keppler A et al (2003) A general method for the covalent labeling of fusion proteins with small molecules *in vivo*. Nat Biotechnol 21: 86–89
17. Aliprandi M et al (2010) The availability of a recombinant anti-SNAP antibody in VHH format amplifies the application flexibility of SNAP-tagged proteins. J Biomed Biotechnol 658954. doi:10.1155/2010/658954
18. de Haard HJ et al (2005) Llama antibodies against a lattococcal protein located at the tip of the phage tail prevent phage infection. J Bacteriol 187:4531–4541
19. Klooster R et al (2009) Selection and characterization of KDEL-specific VHH antibody fragments and their application in the study of ER resident protein expression. J Immunol Methods 342:1–12
20. De Marzi M et al (2012) Antibody Purification-Independent Microarrays (PIM) by direct bacteria spotting on TiO_2-treated slides. Methods 56(2):317–25
21. Predonzani A et al (2008) *In vivo* site-specific biotinylation of proteins within the secretory pathway using a single vector system. BMC Biotechnol 8:41
22. Conrath K et al (2001) Camel single-domain antibodies as modular building units in bispecific and bivalent antibody constructs. J Biol Chem 276:7346–50
23. Dolk E et al (2005) Isolation of llama antibody fragments for prevention of dandruff by phage display in shampoo. Appl Environ Microbiol 71:442–450
24. Steiner D, Forrer P, Plückthun A (2008) Efficient selection of DARPins with sub-nanomolar affinities using SRP phage display. J Mol Biol 382:1211–1227
25. Thie H et al (2008) SRP and Sec pathway leader peptides for antibody phage display and antibody fragment production in *E. coli*. Nat Biotechnol 25:49–54
26. Monegal A et al (2012) Single heavy chain antibodies with VH hallmarks are positively selected during panning of llama (Lama glama) naïve libraries. Develop Comp Immunol 36: 150–156

Chapter 33

Application of Single-Domain Antibodies in Tumor Histochemistry

Kien T. Maik and C. Roger MacKenzie

Abstract

High avidity, pentameric, single-domain antibodies, oligomerized through the B subunit of verotoxin, are excellent immunohistochemical reagents. The resulting molecules are termed pentabodies. Here, we describe the immunostaining of tissue sections with ES1, a pentabody recognizing CEACAM6 which is overexpressed in several cancers. The advantages of pentabodies, compared to conventional antibody reagents, in immunohistochemical studies are highlighted.

Key words: Single-domain antibodies, Pentabodies, CEACAM6, Lung carcinomas, Imunohistochemistry, Tissue arrays

1. Introduction

The analysis of the human proteome in normal and diseased states is largely dependent on the availability of affinity reagents yet currently available reagents cover only a small fraction of the proteome (1). In vitro generation strategies are widely seen providing a means of obtaining affinity reagents that bind to any member of the human proteome; a variety of antibody and non-antibody scaffolds have been identified for this purpose (2, 3). Fusion of non-aggregating single-domain antibodies (sdAbs) to a pentamerization domain, generating pentabodies, has been shown to be a very effective means of generating high avidity antibody reagents that show much improved binding to surface presented antigen when compared to their monomeric counterparts (3). Protocols for the generation and characterization of pentabodies are described elsewhere in this volume (see Chapter 27).

A pentabody, ES1, specific for CEACAM6 (4) has been shown to be an excellent reagent for the clinical evaluation of lung

Dirk Saerens and Serge Muyldermans (eds.), *Single Domain Antibodies: Methods and Protocols*, Methods in Molecular Biology, vol. 911, DOI 10.1007/978-1-61779-968-6_33, © Springer Science+Business Media, LLC 2012

adenocarcinomas (5). Compared to other antibodies used for this purpose, ES1 is less immunoreactive with normal tissues, more lung carcinoma specific, and more sensitive in terms of staining poorly differentiated adenocarcinomas, which are typically associated with distant metastases (5). CEACAM6 expression is elevated in many solid tumors and may be a good target for antibody-based therapy since it is thought to play a role in tumor invasiveness and the formation of distant metastases (6, 7). Here we describe an immunohistochemistry staining protocol for pentabodies using ES1 as an example.

2. Materials

Prepare all solutions using distilled and deionized water (ddH_2O) with a sensitivity of 18 MΩ cm at 25°C and analytical grade reagents. Prepare and store all reagents at room temperature (unless indicated otherwise). Diligently follow all waste disposal regulations for hazardous waste materials.

2.1. Tissue Embedding and Sectioning

1. Resection and resection/biopsy specimens containing tumors with or without surrounding "normal" tissue.
2. Autopsy organ tissue, not harboring tumor, from autopsy cases performed prior to 24 h after patient death and with minimal autolytic changes.
3. Formalin.
4. Standard histology laboratory embedding supplies.
5. Leica RM 2255 microtome or similar instrument.

2.2. Tissue Section Staining

1. Primary antibody: ES1 pentabody, 10 mg/mL used at a dilution of 1:100 in antibody dilution buffer (see Subheading 2.2, item 7, and Notes 1 and 2).
2. Primary antibody: MIB1 (Dako, Glostrup, Denmark), an anti-Ki67 nuclear protein mouse monoclonal antibody: Use at a dilution of 1:100 in antibody dilution buffer (see Notes 2 and 3).
3. Primary antibody: Anti-TTF-1 antibody (Dako): Use at a dilution of 1:50 in antibody dilution buffer (see Notes 2 and 4).
4. Secondary antibody: Rabbit anti-verotoxin antiserum; use at a dilution of 1:100 in antibody dilution buffer (see Note 2).
5. Tertiary antibody: Swine anti-rabbit antiserum (Dako) used at a dilution of 1:100 in antibody dilution buffer (see Note 2).

6. Phosphate buffered saline solution (PBS), pH 7.4: Dissolve 8 g NaCl, 0.2 g KCL, 1.44 g Na_2HPO_4, and 0.24 g KH_2PO_4 in 1 L of ddH_2O.
7. Antibody dilution buffer solution (Dako, Carpinteria, CA, USA).
8. Decloaking chamber (Biocare Medical, Concord, CA, USA) (see Note 5).
9. Antigen retrieval buffer: antigen decloaker, 1:10, (Biocare Medical).
10. Hydrogen peroxide: 3% in ddH_2O.
11. Chromogen and peroxidase substrate: 5-(4-Dimethylamino-benzylidene) rhodanine (D1801, Sigma-Aldrich Canada, Oakville, ON, Canada).
12. Hematoxylin–eosin stain.
13. MACH 4 Universal HRP Polymer Detection (Biocare Medical).
14. Blue buffer (SurgiPath, Richmond, IL, USA) diluted in ddH_2O in a 3:20 ratio.
15. Adhesive glass slides.

2.3. Morphological Evaluation

This requires a microscope that meets histology laboratory standards.

3. Methods

3.1. Tissue Embedding and Sectioning

1. Fix fresh surgical or autopsy specimens in 10% formalin in PBS for at least 12 h (see Note 6).
2. Remove 2–3 mm diameter portions from the specimens and process by dehydration and paraffin embedding using standard histology laboratory procedures.
3. Remove 2 mm diameter tissue cores from representative areas of the paraffin blocks (see Note 7).
4. Deparaffinize and re-embed, using standard histology laboratory procedures, the removed portions to make a tissue array containing up to 15 different tissue cores.
5. Cut 4 μm thick sections for hematoxylin–eosin staining and immunostaining.
6. Mount sections from warm ddH_2O onto slides and dry.
7. Deparafinize and rehydrate tissue sections using standard methods.

3.2. Tissue Section Staining

The staining process is the same whether performed manually or in an automatic stainer.

1. Treat sections with antigen retrieval system (Decloaker chamber) at 25 psi and 125°C for 5 min (see Note 8).
2. Wash slides well with ddH_2O.
3. Block endogenous peroxidase with 3% peroxidase for 20 min (see Note 9).
4. Wash slides well with ddH_2O and rinse in PBS.
5. Incubate with primary antibody for 30 min at room temperature (see Note 10).
6. Wash slides in PBS for 10 min.
7. Incubate with secondary antiserum for 10 min at room temperature.
8. Wash slides in PBS for 10 min.
9. Incubate with third antiserum for 20 min at room temperature.
10. Wash slides in PBS for 10 min.
11. Incubate slides in chromogenic substrate for 5 min.
12. Wash slides in ddH_2O.
13. Counterstain nuclei in hematoxylin for 45 s, wash slides with in ddH_2O and place in blue buffer for 15 s.
14. Wash in ddH_2O.
15. Dehydrate and mount slides using standard histology laboratory procedures.

3.3. Morphological Evaluation

1. Assess immunoreactivity of lung specimens with ES1 pentabody with reference to nuclear staining and immunoreactivity with MIB1 and anti-TTF-1 antibodies and with reference to the immunoreactivity of other tumor and normal specimens with ES1 (see Notes 11 and 12).
2. Score negative immunoreactivity in the absence of any antibody-mediated staining (see Fig. 1).
3. Score weak reactivity if there is discontinuous membranous or weak cytoplasmic staining.
4. Score 1 if there is continuous membranous and/or cytoplasmic staining of less than 10% of cells.
5. Score 2 if there is continuous membranous and/or cytoplasmic staining of more than 10% of cells but less than 50% of cells.
6. Score 3 if there is continuous membranous and/or cytoplasmic staining of more than 50% of cells (see Note 13).

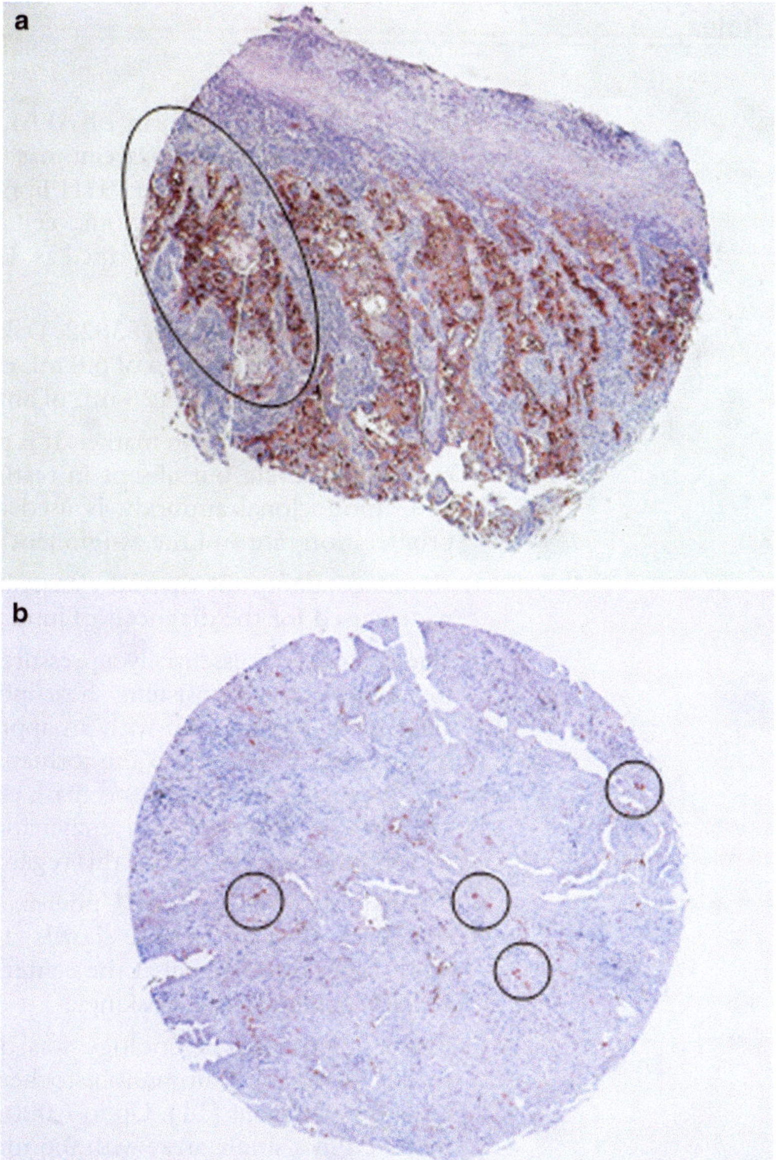

Fig. 1. (**a**) Lung adenocarcinoma, at low (×25) magnification, displaying strong (score of 3) reactivity for ES1. Regions showing immunopositivity, of which one of several is indicated, are stained an intense *reddish-brown color*. At higher magnification strong and diffuse membranous and cytoplasmic reactivity was evident (not shown). (**b**) Lung adenocarcinoma, at low magnification, displaying moderate (score of 2) reactivity for ES1. Regions showing immunopositivity, of which several of many are indicated, are stained an intense *reddish-brown color*. At higher magnification strong and focal membranous and cytoplasmic reactivity was evident (not shown). In both specimens the nuclei are stained *blue* but are not clearly defined at this low magnification.

4. Notes

1. ES1 is a pentameric form of AFAI, a VHH with excellent specificity for lung adenocarcinomas (4, 5). AFAI was isolated by panning a nonimmune VHH library (8) against the A549 non-small cell lung carcinoma cell line (4). ES1 was constructed, expressed, and purified as described elsewhere in this volume (see Chapter 27).
2. Antibody dilution buffer (S3022, Dako) is sold "ready-to-use" and does require addition of 6.0 mL of cold fish gelatin (Sigma G 7765–250 mL) into 125 mL of antibody dilution buffer.
3. Ki67 is cell proliferation marker. It is present in all stages of the cell growth cycle but absent in resting cells. MIB1, an anti-Ki67 monoclonal antibody, is used clinically to measure cell proliferation rate and the assignment of tumor grade (9).
4. Immunostaining for thyroid transcription factor-1 (TTF-1) is widely used for the diagnosis of lung adenocarcinomas (10).
5. The decloaker is essentially a pressure cooker and is employed for optimized, consistent heat-induced epitope retrieval (HIER) in conjunction with an appropriate buffer. Formalin fixation typically leads to the formation of methylene bridges which cross-link proteins and mask epitopes. Antigen retrieval can also be achieved with enzymatic protocols; trypsin is a commonly used enzyme in this regard.
6. The fixation time is critical. Under-fixation can result in uneven staining with more intense signals at the edge of a specimen and weaker or no signal at the center. Over-fixation can result in irreversible epitope masking.
7. Tissue microarray technology was developed as a means of readily performing immunohistochemistry on large numbers of tissue specimens (11). Up to 1,000 specimens can be accommodated in a single array with 0.6 mm diameter cores. Larger cores (2 mm) were employed here to achieve better representation of the original specimen.
8. Five minutes is a typical antigen retrieval time and can be adjusted as required. Suboptimal times will result in weak staining whereas antigen retrieval times that are too long result in nonspecific background binding.
9. With tissues that have endogenous peroxidase activity the use of HRP-conjugated antibodies will result in high, nonspecific, background binding. However, endogenous peroxidase can be irreversibly inactivated by incubation with saturating amounts of hydrogen peroxide.

10. Three antibodies (ES1, MIB1, and the anti-TTF-1 antibody) served as the primary antibody so that the immunoreactivity of lung adenocarinoma specimens with ES1 could be compared with immunoreactivity with the other two antibodies which are widely used in the clinical diagnosis and staging of lung adencarcinomas.
11. Positive immunoreactivity with ES1 was characterized by membranous staining. Some cells also showed cytoplasmic staining.
12. The interpretation of immunohistochemical staining results is inherently subjective. Results should therefore be evaluated by at least two independent observers. It is highly preferable that all observers are anatomical pathologists.
13. CEACAM6 is well recognized as a colorectal cancer marker (12) but less so as a lung cancer marker. However, ES1 shows somewhat higher immunoreactivity for lung adenocarcinoma than for colon carcinoma (5). A possible explanation for this observation is that ES1 recognizes an epitope, not readily accessible by conventional IgGs, which is more abundant on lung adenocarcinoma cells than on colon adenocarcinoma cells. It has been established that camelid sdAbs, also termed nanobodies, can recognize uncommon or hidden epitopes (13).

Acknowledgments

We thank Jianbing Zhang for providing the rabbit anti-verotoxin antiserum. The authors declare no financial conflict of interest.

References

1. Taussig MJ et al (2007) ProteomeBinders: planning a European resource of affinity reagents for analysis of the human proteome. Nat Methods 4:13–17
2. Dübel S et al (2010) Generating recombinant antibodies to the complete human proteome. Trends Biotechnol 28:333–339
3. Zhang J et al (2004) Pentamerization of single-domain antibodies from phage libraries: a novel strategy for generation of high-avidity antibody reagents. J Mol Biol 335:49–56
4. Zhang J et al (2004) A pentavalent single-domain antibody approach to tumor antigen discovery and the development of novel proteomics reagents. J Mol Biol 341:161–169
5. Mai KT et al (2006) ES1, a new lung carcinoma antibody – an immunohistochemical study. Histopathology 49:515–522
6. Blumenthal RD et al (2007) Expression patterns of CEACAM5 and CEACAM6 in primary and metastatic cancers. BMC Cancer 7:2
7. Duxbury MS et al (2004) CEACAM6 is a determinant of pancreatic adenocarcinoma cellular invasiveness. Br J Cancer 91:1384–1390
8. Tanha J et al (2002) Selection by phage display of llama conventional V_H fragments with heavy chain antibody V_HH properties. J Immunol Methods 263:97–109
9. Bryant RJ, Banks PM, O'Malley DP (2006) Ki67 staining pattern as a diagnostic tool in the

evaluation of lymphoproliferative disorders. Histopathology 48:505–515

10. Du MZ et al (2004) TTF-1 expression is specific for lung adenocarcinoma in typical and atypical carcinoids: TTF-1-positive carcinoids are predominantly in peripheral location. Hum Pathol 35:825–831
11. Kononen J et al (1998) Tissue microarrays for high-throughput molecular profiling of tumor specimens. Nat Med 4:844–847
12. Jantscheff P et al (2003) Expression of CEACAM6 in resectable colorectal cancer: a factor of independent prognostic significance. J Clin Oncol 21:3638–3646
13. Revets H, De Baetselier P, Muyldermans S (2004) Nanobodies as novel agents for cancer therapy. Expert Opin Biol Ther 5: 111–124

Part VI

Case Studies

Chapter 34

Nanobodies as Structural Probes of Protein Misfolding and Fibril Formation

Erwin De Genst and Christopher M. Dobson

Abstract

The deposition of peptides and proteins as amyloid fibrils is a common feature of nearly 50 medical disorders affecting the brain or a variety of other organs and tissues. These disorders, which include Alzheimer's disease, Parkinson's disease, the prion diseases, and type II diabetes, have an enormous impact on the public health and economy of the modern world. Extensive research is therefore taking place to determine the underlying molecular mechanisms and determinants of the pathological conversion of amyloidogenic proteins from their soluble forms into fibrillar structures. The use of molecular probes and biophysical techniques, such as X-ray crystallography and particularly NMR spectroscopy, are allowing detailed analysis of the mechanism of fibril formation and of the underlying structural and chemical features of the associated pathogenicity. Nanobodies, the antigen-binding domains derived from camelid heavy-chain antibodies, are excellent tools to probe protein aggregation as a result of their exquisite specificity and high affinity and stability, along with their ease of expression and small size; the latter in particular allows them to be used very efficiently in combination with NMR spectroscopy and X-ray crystallography. In this chapter we present an overview of how nanobodies are being used to obtain detailed information on the mechanisms of amyloid formation and on the nature and origin of their links with human diseases.

Key words: Nanobody, Amyloidosis, Parkinson's disease, Alzheimer's disease, Fibril

1. Introduction

The misfolding and aggregation of otherwise soluble proteins into fibrillar deposits is associated with the pathogenesis of a range of neurological and systemic disorders, including Alzheimer's disease (AD), Parkinson's disease (PD), Huntington's disease (HD), type II diabetes, and a variety of systemic amyloidoses (1). Neurodegenerative diseases such, as AD and PD, are increasingly recognized to be one of the greatest medical challenges of our time (http://www.dementia2010.org/). Although the impact of these diseases on the public health and economy of the modern world is broadly recognized (2–4), relatively little has been known until

Dirk Saerens and Serge Muyldermans (eds.), *Single Domain Antibodies: Methods and Protocols*, Methods in Molecular Biology, vol. 911, DOI 10.1007/978-1-61779-968-6_34, © Springer Science+Business Media, LLC 2012

recently of the determinants of these disorders at the molecular level. This knowledge is, however, crucial for understanding the links between the increasingly well-established principles of protein misfolding and aggregation and the underlying origins of pathogenesis, and for rational therapeutic strategies designed to combat the diseases associated with these aberrant processes.

The molecular mechanisms of amyloid formation and its associated toxicity have been extensively investigated in vitro and in vivo for a number of different proteins (5–12). From the information accumulating from such studies, it is generally believed that the events leading to the formation of the amyloid form of proteins have similar characteristics and involve several key steps. The first step involves the formation of species that have a high propensity for self-association, for example as the result of the exposure of hydrophobic residues. Such species can be partially unfolded intermediates populated on the folding or unfolding pathways of globular proteins, or partially folded aggregation-prone members of the ensemble of structures in intrinsically disordered proteins (12). In subsequent steps, such species self-assemble into a variety of oligomeric aggregates that then convert into highly organized mature fibrils, through a series of complex steps typically involving various types of nucleation conformational rearrangements, aggregate growth and fragmentation (13). The resulting fibrillar structures have remarkably similar or “generic” features, such as a characteristic “cross-beta” structure, which can be readily established through X-ray fiber diffraction studies, and the ability to bind dyes such as Congo red or thioflavin T. These generic features of amyloid fibrils can be explained by the fact that the atomic interactions resulting in these structures are primarily mediated through those features of polypeptide chains that are common to all proteins; by contrast, the native states of globular proteins are the result of the dominance of specific side-chain interactions characteristic of their unique individual sequences (14, 15). Indeed, the amyloid structure can be considered a generic fold, accessible in principle under appropriate conditions by all proteins regardless of their sequences, although the propensity to convert into this state can vary widely (15).

An extremely important, but only recently recognized, characteristic of the amyloid diseases is that the highly ordered fibrillar structures, which are one of their primary hallmarks, appear in many cases not be the most pathogenic forms of these misfolded proteins. Rather, it appears that relatively small, soluble oligomeric species with high surface-to-volume ratios and exposed hydrophobic residues are likely to be the underlying mediators of cytotoxicity (9, 16). It is therefore vital to obtain detailed information on the structures and stabilities of such oligomers to increase our understanding of both the mechanism of their formation and their role in pathogenesis, and hence to design strategies to block their formation, hasten their degradation or neutralize their toxicity. The structural characterization of such species is, however, extremely challenging because of the transient and highly heterogeneous nature of these assemblies. Moreover, the peptides or proteins associated with amyloid conditions are often intrinsically disordered, as is the case for the Aβ-peptides in AD and α-synuclein in PD. Such polypeptides typically adopt highly diverse and dynamically inter-converting sets of conformational states that make the use of conventional techniques, such as X-ray crystallography and NMR spectroscopy, for their structural characterization particularly demanding, as these techniques require highly concentrated and homogeneous samples of the protein of interest. Molecular tools that are highly specific and sensitive to structural motifs that are transiently populated would therefore be extremely useful for the purpose of investigating the structural aspects of such species, along with defining the variety of aggregated assemblies that are formed during the process of fibril formation (17).

In this context, antibodies in particular are characterized by high specificity and high affinity for their antigens, allowing them to be used as selective and extremely sensitive probes (18–20). Antibodies can, in addition, stabilize or solubilize certain forms of aggregates, and thereby potentially allow them to be studied by well-established structural techniques. Thus, for example, nanobodies have been used very successfully to solubilize and crystallize membrane proteins as well as dynamic protein complexes. The latter are inherently difficult to crystallize and often have large regions of ill-defined electron density. The value of nanobody-aided crystallization of such types of complexes has been very clearly demonstrated by the structure determination of the β_2 adrenoceptor in its active conformation and in complex with the G-protein (21). Alternatively, nanobodies can also help to crystallize the monomeric units of large linear or two-dimensional multimeric complexes, by preventing self-polymerization and promoting three-dimensional crystallization. This phenomenon has been demonstrated in the recent report on the structure of the full-length S-protein from *Geobacillus stearothermophilus* (22).

Nanobodies constitute the smallest antigen recognition unit of a heavy-chain antibody molecule (23). Their small single domain format, exceptional stability, specificity and affinity, and high expression levels and solubilities, make nanobodies excellent tools to probe and stabilize selected protein molecules along with their aggregates. In addition to their potential for characterizing structural features of the process of protein misfolding, these nanobodies have, like conventional forms of antibodies, applications as diagnostic markers (24, 25) and nanobodies that are capable of influencing the aggregation pathway of a disease-related protein, either by inhibiting the formation of particular intermediates or by neutralizing their neurotoxic effects, could also serve as potential therapeutics. Nanobodies have additional properties that make them particularly attractive as therapeutic and diagnostic agents, including low immunogenicity due to high sequence similarities with human VH family III (26, 27) and, of particular relevance for their potential use in neurodegenerative disorders, they have been shown to be able in some cases at least to cross the blood–brain barrier efficiently (28).

In this chapter we present an overview of how nanobodies can be used in combination with NMR spectroscopy and other biophysical techniques to study protein misfolding and aggregation and potentially to act as medical agents in the pathology of protein misfolding.

2. Nanobodies as Diagnostic Probes for the Investigation of the Process of Amyloid Formation

Nanobodies have been used to study the mechanism of amyloid formation for a variety of systems, including human lysozyme, the Aβ-peptides, α-synuclein and β_2-microglobulin (29–35). In most cases the nanobodies involved in these studies were raised against the native monomeric form of the amyloidogenic protein. In the case of human lysozyme and α-synuclein, for example, the wild-type soluble protein was either injected into camels or llamas to obtain maturated nanobodies, after panning of the immunized phage-display libraries (29, 31–33). In the case of $A\beta_{1\text{–}42}$, a mixture of the monomer and oligomers was injected into llamas (34, 36). By contrast, a nanobody was raised against $A\beta_{1\text{–}40}$ fibrils by panning a naïve/synthetic nanobody library (30) using streptavidin beads coated with biotinylated $A\beta_{1\text{–}40}$ fibrils and in an excess of $A\beta_{1\text{–}40}$ monomer. To investigate the effect of nanobodies on β2-microglobulin aggregation, a panel of nanobodies was raised against the wild-type protein as well as against the amyloidogenic proteolytic fragment, ΔN6β2m, which lacks the first six amino acids of the full-length protein and is found in 25–30 % of the β2-microglobulin amyloid deposits of dialysis-related amyloidosis (DRA) patients (35). Other single domain antibodies were obtained through protein engineering of scFv fragments, to obtain VL domains against huntingtin or Aβ-peptides (36–38).

We discuss below the way these nanobodies have been used to characterize the fibril formation process in their respective systems, and the nature of the information that could be obtained from these studies, and then discuss potential approaches to use nanobody technology in investigations of amyloid formation and its consequences.

2.1. Parkinson's Disease: Nanobody Binding to Monomer and Fibrillar Assemblies of α-Synuclein

Parkinson's disease is characterized neuropathologically by the deposition of fibrils of human α-synuclein, a pre-synaptic 140-residue protein, in intracellular inclusions called Lewy bodies (39, 40). There is very significant genetic evidence implicating α-synuclein in the pathogenesis of PD, with three point mutations (A30P, E46K, and A53T) and gene triplication (39, 40) of α-synuclein known to cause dominantly inherited early onset PD. Despite the clear presence of α-synuclein fibrils in the brain of PD patients, it is becoming increasingly evident, as in other amyloid systems, that these fibrils may not be the most toxic forms of the aggregated protein, and that instead smaller oligomers are likely to be the more damaging species (41–43).

There have been several reports describing the generation of scFv molecules against α-synuclein (44–48), but so far only a small number of studies has been carried out to explore the use of nanobodies in the investigation of α-synuclein fibril formation and toxicity. In De Genst et al. (29) a nanobody, NbSyn2, was raised against monomeric α-synuclein through dromedary immunization and through a phage-display selection strategy using monomeric α-synuclein. The interaction of α-synuclein with NbSyn2 was comprehensively characterized; the affinity and thermodynamics of the binding were measured using isothermal calorimetry, and secondary structure changes resulting from the interaction were evaluated by circular dichroism. These measurements reveal that NbSyn2 binds to α-synuclein with nanomolar affinity, with the interaction being primarily enthalpically driven and without any measurable secondary structure changes in either protein (29).

In order to define the epitope of NbSyn2, both protein crystallography and NMR spectroscopy were used (Figs. 1 and 2). NMR spectroscopy is an extremely powerful technique that is able to obtain both structural and dynamical information for proteins in solution and at the atomic level. In the two-dimensional (^{1}H and ^{15}N) Heteronuclear Single Quantum Correlation (HSQC) spectrum of ^{15}N labeled α-synuclein, each amide group is represented by a single cross-peak, with its position (its chemical shifts in both the ^{1}H and ^{15}N dimensions) and intensity depending respectively on the chemical environment and the dynamics of the residue with which it is associated (Fig. 1a, left panel). Addition of NbSyn2 selectively changes the chemical shifts and the signal intensities of certain peaks as the interacting residues experience changes in their conformational, environmental or dynamical properties (Fig. 1). Such perturbations can, however, also include secondary effects, such as those resulting from concerted movements of residues far from the binding site as a result of interactions with the nanobody.

The HSQC spectrum (as well as the analogous CON spectrum (Fig. 1a, right panel)), in which each cross-peak is associated with

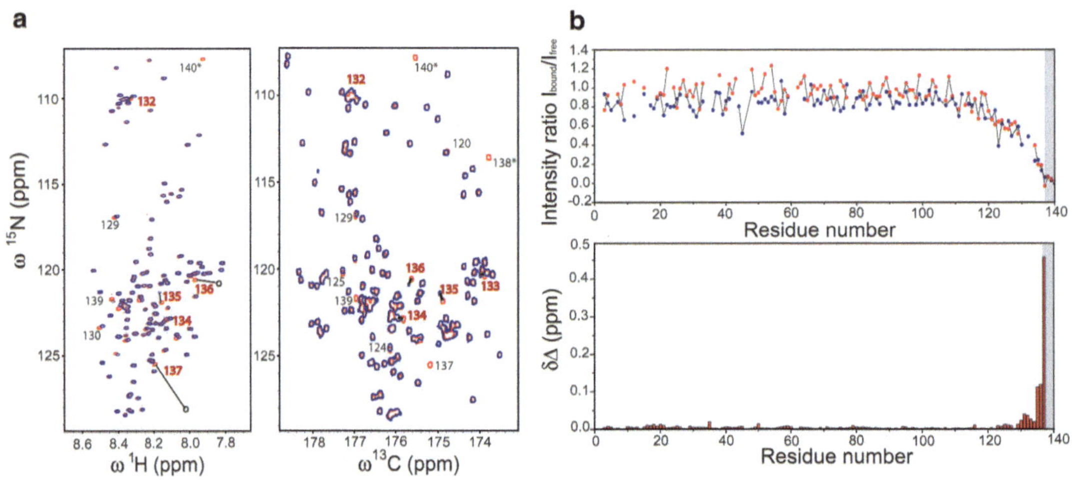

Fig. 1. NMR analysis of ^{14}N NbSyn2 binding to ^{15}N and ^{13}C α-synuclein. (**a**) ^{15}N-^{1}H HSQC (*left*) and ^{13}C-^{1}H CON spectra (*right*) of free α-synuclein (*red*) overlaid on the spectra of NbSyn2-bound α-synuclein (*blue*). The resonances of the residues that significantly shift on binding are indicated by *red labels*. (**b**) The ^{15}N resonance intensity ratios (*top*) for bound:free α-synuclein residues (*red*, HSQC; *blue*, CON), and, the chemical shift changes (*below*) of resonances of α-synuclein residues in the HSQC spectra resulting from binding to NbSyn2 (figure adapted from De Genst et al. (28)).

the carbonyl carbon and the amide nitrogen to which it is attached (49), in the presence or absence of NbSyn2 enabled the epitope to be defined as being located at the C-terminal region of the α-synuclein sequence, as the resonances of the last ten residues of the protein are significantly perturbed in the presence of NbSyn2 (Fig. 1). Indeed, the resonances of the four C-terminal residues are broadened beyond detection in the NMR spectrum, indicating that these residues have greatly perturbed dynamical behavior and therefore are likely to be key components of the epitope. This conclusion is confirmed by determination of the crystal structure of NbSyn2 in complex with a ten-residue peptide corresponding to residues 131–140 of α-synuclein. Clear electron density was evident for the five C-terminal residues of the peptide, indicating the existence of a well-defined conformation in the binding site for these otherwise disordered residues. Analysis of the structure reveals further that the four c-terminal residues (that are highly broadened in the NMR spectrum) make direct contact with the nanobody while the fifth residue is involved in crystal packing contacts (Fig. 2a).

The amide resonances of NbSyn2 that are perturbed as a result of binding to α-synuclein have in addition been mapped onto the X-ray structure of the complex of NbSyn2 with the peptide encompassing the last ten residues of α-synuclein (Fig. 2b); this analysis reveals that apart from the residues that are in direct contact with α-synuclein in the crystal structure, significant shifts are also observed for several residues of the nanobody that are located far away from the binding site; these shifts can be attributed to long

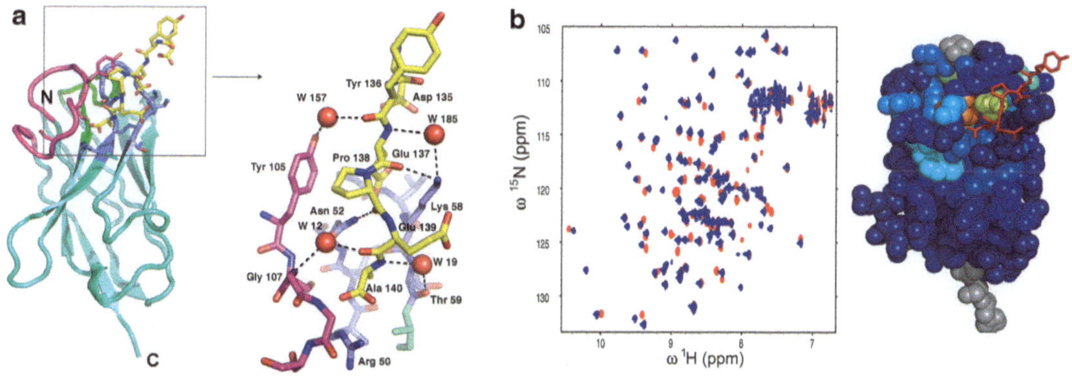

Fig. 2. (**a**) Crystal structure of NbSyn2 bound to a peptide fragment of α-synuclein. The structure of NbSyn2 is shown in *cyan*, with the antigen-binding loops, H1, H2, H3 colored in *green*, *blue* and *magenta*, respectively. The atoms of the peptide fragment are color coded as: C, *yellow*, N, *blue*, O, *red*. On the right of the structure a close up of the binding region is shown, displaying the details of the peptide-NbSyn2 interaction (*blue*). (**b**) *Left*: ^{15}N-^{1}H HSQC of NbSyn2, in its free state (*red*) and in complex (*blue*) with α-synuclein. *Right*: mapping the chemical shift perturbations due to binding of α-synuclein onto the crystal structure of NbSyn2 in complex with the peptide fragment. The peptide is shown in *red* and the residues of NbSyn2 is color coded from *dark blue* to *red* according to the extent of the difference in chemical shift (*dark blue*: no shift, *red*: large shift) (figure adapted from De Genst et al. (28)).

range conformational changes that are transmitted through the cooperative nature of the native structure of the protein. Such NMR measurements are particularly straightforward to carry out as the small, stable and soluble nanobodies are in general easily expressed in minimal media enriched with ^{15}N and ^{13}C isotopes, and their NMR spectra are typically of high quality and resolution. As a result well-resolved NOESY-HSQC spectra can readily be obtained, providing a means of defining in detail their structures and dynamics (50, 51).

NMR spectroscopy has also been used to characterize the binding of NbSyn2 to other states of α-synuclein, including those of the aggregated protein. Of particular interest are the results of experiments in which the well-defined fibrillar form of the protein was added to a sample of ^{15}N enriched nanobodies in solution and the HSQC spectrum recorded. The results reveal that the spectrum broadens beyond detection when the nanobody is present, an effect that can be attributed to the rapid transverse spin relaxation rates resulting from the slow tumbling of the high molecular weight fibrillar structure, indicating that NbSyn2 binds to the fibrils with an affinity that can be estimated by monitoring the progressive disappearance of the spectrum of the free nanobody (Fig. 3a). The results reveal that, on average, four molecules of α-synuclein in the fibril interact with just one molecule of nanobody, a finding consistent with the proposed structure for α-synuclein fibrils based on solid state NMR studies (52). In these latter studies it has been proposed that α-synuclein folds into five anti-parallel β-sheet structures, orthogonal to the fibril axis, with both termini

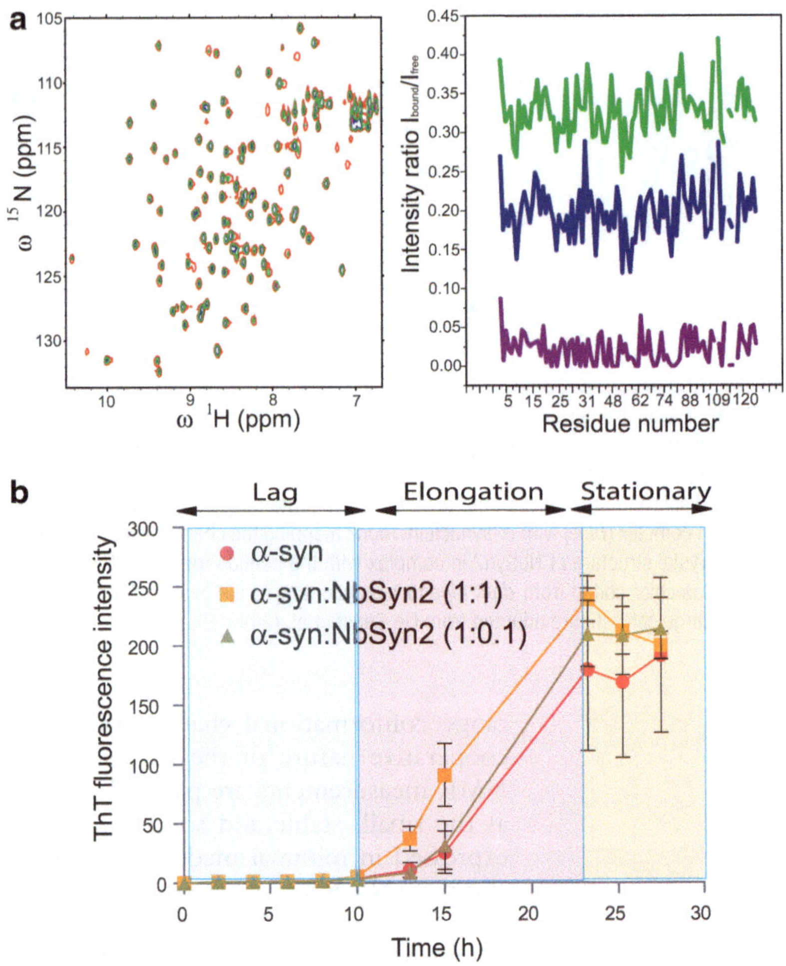

Fig. 3. NbSyn2 binding to α-synuclein fibrils and the effect of NbSyn2 on fibril formation by α-synuclein. (**a**) *Left*: ^{15}N-^{1}H HSQC spectra of NbSyn2, free (*red*), and following the addition of one (*green*), two (*blue*) and four (*purple*) molar equivalents of fibrillar α-synuclein. *Right*: The intensity of the respective ^{15}N-^{1}H HSQC spectra as a function of the sequence of NbSyn2. (**b**) The effect of NbSyn2 on the ThT fluorescence curves associated with α-synuclein aggregation and of NbSyn2 binding to α-synuclein fibrils. ThT fluorescence detection reflects the kinetics of α-synuclein fibril formation of the free protein (*red*); in the presence of 0.1 molar equivalent of NbSyn2 (*green*); and in the presence of 1 molar equivalent of NbSyn2 (*orange*) (figure adapted from De Genst et al. (28)).

lying on either side of the fibril cores. The stacking of these molecular units then forms a protofilament; the lateral packing of two protofilaments then forms each protofibril, and two protofibrils then intertwine to form the mature fibrillar structure. As this arrangement will result in just one in four termini being accessible to solvent, this model is in accord with the NMR experiments discussed above.

The presence of NbSyn2 does not generate any significant perturbation of the kinetics of the aggregation reaction of α-synuclein as shown by measuring the fluorescence intensity of thioflavin T (ThT) for samples taken at different time points during aggregation either in the presence or absence of NbSyn2 (Fig. 3b). These results reveal that the binding of NbSyn2 does not hinder fibril formation, a result consistent with the lack of direct involvement of this part of the C-terminal region of α-synuclein in the aggregation process. Taken together with the fact that NbSyn2 does not have any significant effect on the kinetics of the generation of α-synuclein fibrils or on their morphology and structure (Fig. 3b). This nanobody can therefore be used in principle as a "silent probe" for the further investigation of the nature of α-synuclein aggregation both in vitro and in vivo, as it should report on α-synuclein fibril formation with minimal perturbations to the kinetics of the process and to the structures of the species formed along the aggregation pathway.

2.2. Alzheimer's Disease: The Interaction of Nanobodies with Aβ-Peptides

Alzheimer's disease (AD) is characterized neuropathologically by the formation of amyloid plaques, made up of amyloid fibrils of the 40 or 42 residue Aβ-peptides ($A\beta_{1-40}$; $A\beta_{1-42}$), that are products of the proteolytic cleavage of the APP precursor protein by β- and γ-secretases, and are located predominantly in extra-cellular environments. The two peptides differ substantially in their rate of aggregation, with $A\beta_{1-42}$ being significantly more amyloidogenic than $A\beta_{1-40}$. It is therefore believed that $A\beta_{1-42}$ is the key mediator of AD pathogenesis although it has been shown that the two peptides are present in amyloid plaques (53) and that the ratio of the levels of the two peptides plays an important role in the development of AD (54). As is the case for α-synuclein in PD, in AD, hereditary variations are linked to early onset of the disease, notably, the E693G, A692G, A673V, V717I and the double mutation K670N/M671L of the APP gene, as these mutations result in increased levels of the $A\beta_{1-42}$ peptide (55, 56). In addition to the Aβ-peptides, the intracellular protein tau is strongly associated with AD (57). In AD, tau forms intracellular tangles, which are also fibrillar aggregates within neurons and may also cause cell death (58–64). It appears however that the misfolding and aggregation of tau is a downstream process initiated by the misfolding and aggregation of the Aβ-peptides (65, 66).

A nanobody, B10, has been raised against $A\beta_{1-40}$ fibrils and isolated through a naïve/synthetic nanobody library, i.e., a library of entirely man-made antigen combining sites, which interacts also with fibrils of $A\beta_{1-42}$ (30). By panning with streptavidin beads coated with biotinylated $A\beta_{1-40}$ fibrils, and in the presence of an excess of the $A\beta_{1-40}$ monomer, a specific selection of nanobodies that bind to aggregated species of $A\beta_{1-40}$ rather than to the monomer was obtained. Indeed B10 has been shown to bind to $A\beta_{1-40}$ fibrils without detectably interacting with the monomer, and with only weak binding to $A\beta_{1-40}$ oligomers. These oligomers are

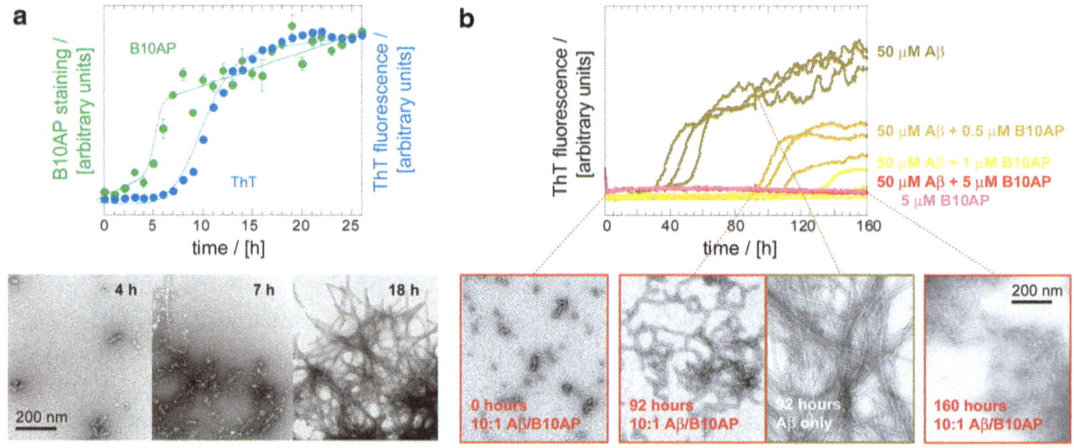

Fig. 4. A B10 alkaline phosphatase conjugate (B10AP) prevents fibril formation by $A\beta_{1-40}$ through stabilization of protofibrillar structures. (**a**) Kinetics of fibril formation monitored using ThT fluorescence at 490 nm (*blue*), B10AP immunoblots (*green*) and TEM images from aliquots taken at the time points indicated; the data are fitted to a sigmoidal model. Incubation conditions: 1 mg/mL $A\beta_{1-40}$ in 50 mM HEPES (pH 7.4), 50 mM NaCl at 37 °C. (**b**) $A\beta_{1-40}$ fibril formation in the presence and absence of B10AP monitored at 37 °C with ThT and TEM imaging (figure adapted from Habicht et al. (30)).

non-fibrillar aggregates of $A\beta_{1-40}$, with diameters of 10–60 nm and can be detected by another antibody, A10 (67). Measurements of such interactions have been carried out using surface plasmon resonance (SPR) and dot blot assays, the latter using B10 as an alkaline phosphatase conjugate. B10 also recognized fibrils formed from a variety of peptides and proteins with unrelated sequences, including serum amyloid A protein and immunoglobulin light chains, demonstrating that the epitope of B10 must be a structural not sequential motif common to all such fibrils.

The B10 nanobody has also been shown to inhibit very effectively the formation of mature $A\beta_{1-40}$ fibrils that are able to bind ThT. TEM data indicate that this inhibition occurs as a consequence of the stabilization of $A\beta_{1-40}$ protofilaments that results from their interaction with B10. These protofilaments are much less efficient in binding ThT than are the mature fibrils, but immunoblots, using B10 as an alkaline phosphatase conjugate, reveal that one can detect in the aggregation assay the presence of protofibrils, which precede the appearance of the mature fibrils that bind ThT strongly (Fig. 4). The use of this nanobody therefore makes it possible to increase the resolution of experiments designed to characterize the steps in the aggregation reaction and hence to enhance the quality of information that can be extracted concerning the mechanism of the reaction. In addition, by using SPR, the stoichiometry of the binding of B10 molecules to the fibrils has been estimated to be ca. 1:10 (B10: $A\beta_{1-40}$ peptide), a value that is consistent with the dimensions of a homology model of the B10 nanobody and the structure of the fibrils. In this model, the CDR loops

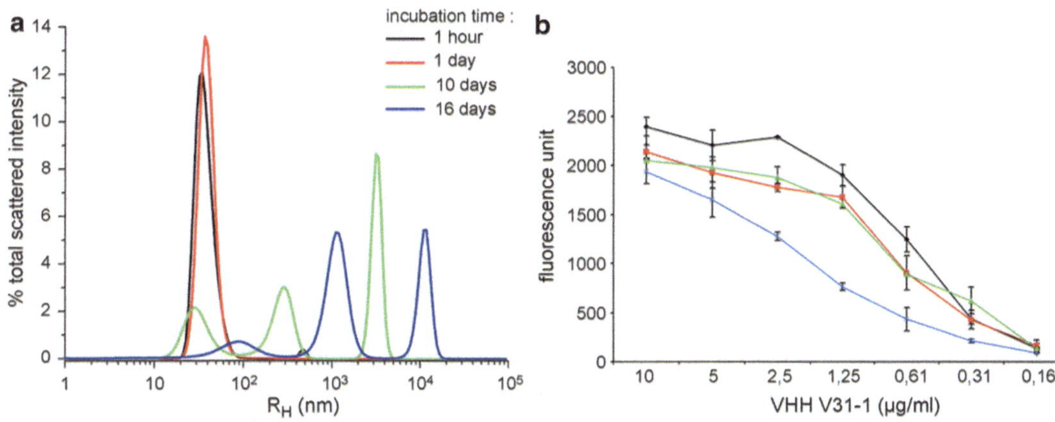

Fig. 5. Time-dependence of the binding of VHH V31-1 to $A\beta_{1-42}$. Aliquots of $A\beta_{1-42}$ were taken after incubation at 37 °C for 1 h, 1 day, 10 days, and 16 days. (**a**) The R_H distribution of $A\beta_{1-42}$ (0.2 μM) was determined by dynamic light scattering (DLS). The data are representative of at least three independent experiments. (**b**) The binding of V31-1 to the same fractions of $A\beta_{1-42}$ was analyzed using ELISA. The coating of $A\beta_{1-42}$ and incubation with VHH V31-1 (two wells per VHH dilution) was performed at 4 °C. The means and standard deviations are again representative of three independent experiments (figure adapted from Lafaye et al. (34)).

span a distance of 31 Å, and X-ray diffraction studies of $A\beta_{1-40}$ amyloid fibrils reveal a peptide repeat of 4.76 Å in the fibril structure (68). Therefore one B10 nanobody is estimated to cover approximately seven residues of $A\beta_{1-40}$, which is close to the 1:10 B10: $A\beta_{1-40}$ stoichiometry observed by SPR; the discrepancy can readily be rationalized by the presence of unoccupied sites on the fibril and imperfections in the B10 binding density (30).

Three other nanobodies against Aβ peptides have been isolated from llamas, following immunization and phage display (34). The immunogen was a sample of $A\beta_{1-42}$, which had been incubated overnight at 37 °C, and was therefore a mixture of monomeric and a variety of oligomeric and fibrillar states of $A\beta_{1-42}$. The binder with the highest affinity isolated from the immunization library, VHH V31-1, stains efficiently intra-neuronal deposits of $A\beta_{1-42}$ on tissue slices taken from the brains of diseased individuals, whereas it stains extracellular amyloid plaques only very faintly. In a separate experiment, $A\beta_{1-42}$ samples were incubated in vitro for different lengths of time and then analyzed by DLS and fluorescence methods to determine the size and distribution of the aggregates in these samples. For this purpose, dot blot, western blot and ELISA techniques were used to characterize the reactivity of the nanobody, which was found to bind preferentially to the molecular species that are in the samples that were incubated for only one h (Fig. 5). For samples incubated for longer times the nanobody progressively lost reactivity, suggesting that VHH V31-1 binds preferentially to low molecular weight oligomers, and not to fibrillar forms of $A\beta_{1-42}$. VHH V31-1, however, was also found to inhibit ThT binding to the aggregates, an observation consistent with the view that the nanobody blocks the formation of fibrils by binding preferentially to the species that are formed early during the aggregation of $A\beta_{1-42}$. This conclusion is supported by DLS measurements showing that in the presence of VHH V31-1, high molecular weight species could not be detected during the time of the aggregation experiment, in complete contrast to the situation in the absence of the nanobody. VHH V31-1 also showed a marked inhibition of the cellular toxicity of $A\beta_{1-42}$ samples incubated for one day, for which DLS measurements show that these samples contain a large quantity of oligomers of, on average, 40 nm in diameter. Unlike the B10 nanobody, VHH V31-1 is specific to $A\beta_{1-42}$, and does not recognize $A\beta_{1-40}$. Although the nanobody binds to monomeric $A\beta_{1-42}$ as determined by western blot, it appears to be more reactive towards low molecular weight $A\beta_{1-42}$ oligomers that are 30–40 nm in diameter. The nanobody does not react with $A\beta_{1-42}$ in fibrillar form nor does it, for example, recognize the PrP protein (34).

Following a previous study, where it was observed that naturally occurring antibodies of the IgM subtype and their isolated light-chain subunits hydrolyze $A\beta_{1-40}$ by a mechanism typically found for serine proteases, in accord with the presence of a serine protease-like catalytic triad in the IgM molecule and by the observed inhibition of IgM-induced proteolysis by electrophilic serine-protease inhibitors. This proteolytic activity of the IgM auto-antibodies impedes the aggregation of $A\beta_{1-40}$ and suppresses its induced neurotoxicity (69, 70). A large (10^7) library of variable domains of immunoglobulins (IgV) was constituted from mRNA isolated from patients suffering from the autoimmune disease lupus (36). This library consists of scFv (VH-linker-VL), $IgVL_2$ (VL-linker-VL) and IgVL (VL) constructs cloned in a phagemid vector, to allow the expression of the IgV on the tip of a phage. The library was then screened for the ability to hydrolyze $A\beta_{1-40}$, either randomly or by a covalent selection mechanism using electrophilic phosphonate sites incorporated into the $A\beta_{1-40}$ molecule in conjunction with phage-display methods. In the latter strategy, potential nucleophilic centra (proteolytic active sites) in the IgV constructs can react with the phosphonate groups efficiently if the IgV also binds specifically to the $A\beta_{1-40}$ molecule. Using phage-display and the covalent linkage strategy, IgV constructs were obtained with high $A\beta_{1-40}$ hydrolyzing activity. The IgV constructs that were selected from the library with the highest hydrolyzing activity were, surprisingly, VL domains suggesting that these domains might be used to aid clearance of $A\beta_{1-40}$ in AD, as in other passive immunization strategies (36). The mechanism and the therapeutic potential of these domains, however, remain to be evaluated.

2.3. Systemic Amyloid Disease: Nanobodies Binding to Human Lysozyme

Human lysozyme (HuL) is a 130 residue globular protein that hydrolyses the β1-4 glycosidic bonds between *N*-acetylmuramic acid and *N*-acetyl-D-glucosamine residues in peptidoglycans, and between *N*-acetyl-D-glucosamine residues in chitodextrins (71).

Several natural mutational variants of lysozyme have been found to be linked with hereditary systemic amylodosis, a disease in which misfolded lysozyme aggregates are deposited in a variety of organs, including the liver, spleen and kidney (72, 73), and indeed lysozyme was the first protein whose misfolding and fibril formation was studied by using nanobodies as probes of the structural properties of the species present during the reaction. Two lysozyme specific nanobodies have so far been characterized (31–33), known as cAb-HuL6 and cAb-HuLB22, both of which have been shown to bind to disease-related amyloidogenic variants of lysozyme and to inhibit their aggregation, despite being raised by immunization with wild-type lysozyme rather than the amyloidogenic variants. Relative to the WT protein, the disease-related lysozyme variants have decreased stabilities and higher propensities to form partially structured intermediates, in which the β-domain and the adjacent C-helix of the protein are simultaneously unfolded (72).

This locally cooperative unfolding transition increases the aggregation propensity of lysozyme very significantly and is therefore thought to be the key event that triggers the formation of amyloid fibrils (72). Evidence for this conclusion comes from the finding that both nanobodies have been observed to be able to restore the global cooperativity of the lysozyme molecule. The most direct information comes from H-D exchange experiments using NMR and mass spectrometry (31–33, 72). These experiments rely on the fact that the well-folded and highly stable WT lysozyme molecules only very gradually exchange thier amide hydrogens for hydrogen atoms of solvent water molecules; under physiological conditions this exchange of the WT species occurs as the result of local conformational fluctuations. However, any partially unfolded intermediate populated to a significant level by the amyloidogenic variants will allow readier access of solvent to the unfolded region of the structure resulting in more rapid exchange of labile hydrogens. Such behavior can be monitored particularly readily by measuring the change in mass, resulting from the exchange of hydrogen and deuterium atoms in the protein structure by using mass spectrometry. Addition of the nanobodies to the amyloidogenic variant proteins was found to restore their behavior to that of the WT protein, indicating that binding results in the suppression of the formation of the intermediate and, in addition, directly inhibits the aggregation process (Fig. 6b).

A variety of biophysical methods, such as SPR and isothermal calorimetry, has also been used to characterize the kinetics and thermodynamics of the cAb-HuL22–HuL binding interaction

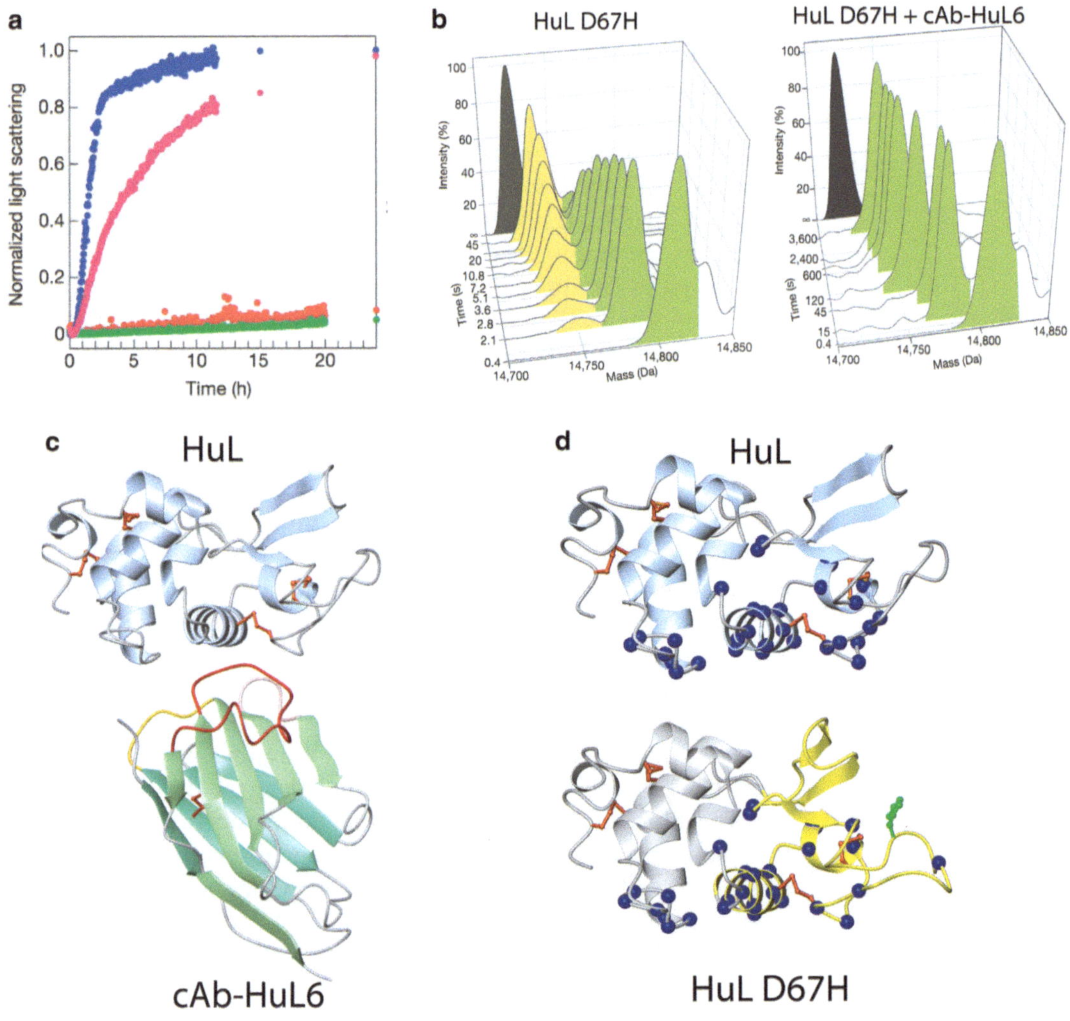

Fig. 6. Inhibition of the formation of human lysozyme fibrils by cAbHuL6. (**a**) Time course of the aggregation of D67H lysozyme (HuL D67H) in the absence (*blue*) and presence of cAbHuL6 (HuL D67H:cAbHuL6 1:1 (*green*), HuL D67H:cAbHuL6 1:0.5 (*pink*)) monitored by light scattering. Data are also shown for WT human lysozyme in the absence of cAb-HuL6 (*red*). (**b**) Electrospray mass spectra of HuL D67H in the absence (*left*) and presence (*right*) of an equimolar quantity of cAb-HuL6. The peaks observed in spectra of control samples, recorded after complete hydrogen–deuterium exchange, are shown in *black*. (**c**) Ribbon representation of the X-ray structure of HuL in complex with cAbHul6. The β-strands in cAb-HuL6 are colored *green*, the HuL molecule is shown in *gray* and the disulfide bridges are colored *orange*. (**d**) Chemical shift perturbations of the NMR resonances of HuL (*top*) and HuL D67H (*bottom*) due to binding to cAbHuL6. The Cα atoms of residues for which the resonances experience significant perturbations due to the formation of the cAbHuL6 lysozyme complex are shown in a *blue* space-filling representation on the ribbon diagram, *top panel*, of HuL; *bottom*, of HuL D67H. The regions of the Hul D67H that cooperatively unfold to form the amyloidogenic intermediate are colored *yellow*, and the side-chain residue (H) at position 67 is shown in a ball-and-stick representation (figure adapted from Dumoulin et al. (32)).

(31–33), and X-ray crystallography and NMR spectroscopy have been used to characterize in detail the specific binding sites of both nanobodies. In the case of cAb-HuL6, a crystal structure of the nanobody in complex with the wild-type protein has enabled the identification of the residues of both proteins that interact directly with each other in the complexes, and the existence of the same interactions in solution has been confirmed using NMR spectroscopy (Fig. 6c, d). This latter technique has also revealed that additional residues, including many that are located far from the binding site, including those in the vicinity of the amyloidogenic mutations, are affected by the binding, indicating that the latter restores the global cooperativity of the amyloidogenic variants rather than simply shielding the aggregation-prone residues.

The second nanobody investigated in detail so far in studies of lysozyme, cAb-HuLB22, has been found to bind in the active site of the enzyme. Evidence for this mode of binding comes from the demonstration of competition between the binding of the nanobody and that of the substrate inhibitor N-acetyl-chitotriose $(GlcNAc)_3$. In addition, HSQC NMR experiments with ^{15}N labeled human lysozyme show that the chemical shifts of many resonances of residues located in the active site of human lysozyme are perturbed on cAb-HuLB22 binding, including those of the catalytic residues. The crystal structure of a different nanobody cAbLys3, in complex with hen lysozyme reveals that this nanobody binds in the active site of the protein, with direct contacts that include the catalytic residues of hen lysozyme (74). The chemical shifts in the hen lysozyme spectrum that are significantly perturbed by binding of cAb-Lys3 are comparable to those found by binding of cAb-HuLB22 to human lysozyme and show that the epitopes for both nanobodies consist of closely similar residues in the protein from both species (31). In both cases, chemical shift perturbations are also found for resonances of residues located far from the epitopes, including the β-domain and the residue positions corresponding to the amyloidogenic variants, again suggesting that the inhibition mechanism proceeds through the restoration of the global cooperativity of the human lysozyme molecule.

The analysis of nanobody binding to human lysozyme in these two cases has, therefore, provided crucial evidence that the population of the partially unfolded unfolded intermediate state is a key event triggering self-association and fibril formation by human lysozyme. Indeed both nanobodies efficiently block human lysozyme fibril formation by restoring the wild-type behavior of the amyloidogenic mutants of lysozyme by inhibiting the formation of the aggregation-prone partially unfolded intermediate.

2.4. Dialysis Related Amyloidosis: Nanobody Binding to β2-Microglobulin

DRA occurs in patients who undergo regular haemodialysis as a consequence of renal failure (75). During dialysis treatment, a specific protein β2-microglobulin (β2m), a component of the Major Histocompatibility Complex I (MHC I), which is a cell-surface protein assembly that occurs on all nucleated cells and that presents the epitopes to cytotoxic T cells. Upon prolonged dialysis treatment, the β2m protein increases in concentration as a result of inefficient permeability of the dialysis membrane, and forms amyloid deposits in skeletal tissue (76). The protein has a seven-stranded immunoglobulin fold and 25–30 % of the amyloid material extracted from patients suffering from DRA, consists of ΔN6β2m, a truncated form of β2m, which lacks the first six residues of the A strand of the β2m β-barrel and which, unlike the wild-type protein, spontaneously forms fibrils at physiological pH (77).

A panel of nanobodies has been raised against wt β2m and ΔN6β2m and several of these nanobodies have been shown to inhibit very potently the spontaneous fibril formation by ΔN6β2m. SDS page analysis has revealed that inhibition of fibril formation results from the solubilization of ΔN6β2m as a result of its interactions with the nanobodies (35). Crystallization and structural analysis of one of the nanobodies, Nb24, in complex with ΔN6β2m reveals the existence of a hetero-tetramer, involving a domain-swapped dimer of ΔN6β2m molecules in the crystal (Fig. 7). The crystal structure reveals that the dimer of the ΔN6β2m molecules is formed by exchanging the residues 91–94, which normally make up the G-strand of the linear β2m molecule, for the corresponding residues of the other ΔN6β2m molecule, hence resulting in a G-strand swapped dimer of ΔN6β2m. Due to this C-terminal G-strand swap, residues 83–89 (with sequence NHVTLSQ) of both monomer adopt an extended conformation, and interact with each other to form a two-stranded anti-parallel β-sheet. In the native monomeric structure of β2m, this region forms a loop connecting the F- and G-strands of the protein. In the ΔN6β2m swapped dimer structure, the backbone NH and CO groups of H84, T86 and S88 of one monomer are hydrogen-bonded to the CO and NH groups of residues S88, T86 and H84 of the other monomer (Fig. 7). In addition, the backbone NH and CO groups of residues V85 and L87 are solvent exposed and accessible for interacting with a second swapped dimer through hydrogen bonding. This dimer structure is then a possible nucleus for self-templated addition of further molecules of a ΔN6β2m to generate protofilaments. Growing oligomers may start to pack together and interdigitate as the newly formed β-sheet interactions by the two hinge regions, resulting in the exposure of a hydrophobic patch formed by the side-chain atoms of V85 and L87 (Fig. 7) (35).

This structure offers important insights into the process of β2m fibril formation, and the structural details are consistent with previously published and more recent work on the possible determinants of β2m fibril formation (78–84). This work further demonstrates the power of nanobodies as crystallization aids for transiently populated species along the fibril formation pathway (21, 85, 86).

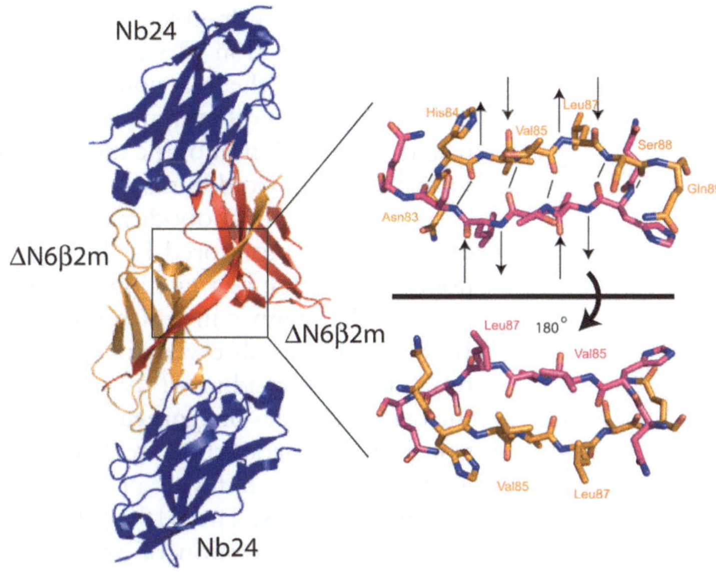

Fig. 7. The crystal structure of the domain-swapped dimer of ΔN6β2m in complex with Nb24. *Left*: Ribbon representation of the hetero-tetramer of ΔN6β2m in complex with Nb24. The Nb24 molecules are colored *blue* and the ΔN6β2m molecules *orange* and *pink*. The hinge region in the ΔN6β2m swapped dimer is shown within a *square*. *Right*: Structure of the open interface of the ΔN6β2m dimer, showing the positions of residues 83–89 in both molecules. *Top*: The main chain NH and CO groups of H84, T86, and S88 are hydrogen-bonded to the carbonyl and the amide groups of S88, T86, and H84 on the adjacent strand, respectively. The backbone donor and acceptor sites of V85 and L87 are exposed to solvent (indicated by *arrows*). *Bottom*: 180° rotation of the top view, showing the hydrophobic patch at one face of the hinge region that is exposed upon forming the new β-sheet (figure adapted from Domanska et al. (35)).

3. Probing the Mechanism of Fibril Formation Using Nanobodies

Formation of amyloid fibrils involves a characteristic nucleation-dependent polymerization reaction, which can be conveniently followed on a macroscopic scale by monitoring the enhancement of fluorescence that results from binding of ThT to the amyloid structure (87–90); in addition, Congo red staining (91–93), electron microscopy, atomic force microscopy (94–99) and X-ray fiber diffraction (100) are techniques commonly used to follow fibril formation by proteins. We can distinguish three broad regions in the kinetic profiles, the lag phase, the elongation phase and the stationary or plateau phase (Fig. 3b).

The lag phase represents the initial stage of the aggregation reaction, and is characterized by the assembly of aggregation-prone monomeric species into small oligomers. These oligomers then grow by further self-association and rearrangement steps, to generate larger aggregates, generally termed pre-fibrillar species, and also proliferate by fragmentation and potentially other forms of secondary nucleation (13). All of the species populated during these phases of the reaction are extremely heterogeneous, and often only transiently populated, before the stationary phase that results from depletion of the monomeric species and ultimately the formation of amyloid fibrils.

The effects of nanobodies on the overall rate of fibril formation can readily be monitored by adding the species at different time points during the aggregation reaction probed by ThT, therefore probing the manner in which they influence the different phases. In this way it was observed, for example, that NbSyn2, which binds to the last four residues of α-synuclein, has no significant effect on the overall kinetics of aggregation, therefore leading to the conclusion that this part of the C-terminal sequence is not involved, or at least is not associated with a rate-limiting step, in the formation of α-synuclein fibrils. The B10 antibody, by contrast, has been found to block the conversion of protofilaments of $A\beta_{1-40}$ into mature fibrils (30). Therefore, the epitope bound by B10 must be formed only at the protofilament stage of the assembly reaction and be involved in the formation of the final mature fibrils. Indeed, as we have discussed above, the reactivity of the B10 nanobody coincides with the appearance of the protofilaments of $A\beta_{1-40}$ and blocks the formation of the multi-filamentary mature fibrils that are able to bind to ThT.

In the case of lysozyme, the nanobodies cAb-Hul6 and cAb-HulB22 were found to inhibit fibril formation strongly. This result can be attributed to the restoration of the global cooperativity of the native lysozyme structure as a result of binding (31–33), strongly supporting the idea that the formation of a partially folded aggregation-prone species is the key step in initiating the fibril formation reaction (101). And in the case of the Nb24 nanobodies raised against ΔN6β2m, it is evident that inhibition of fibril formation results from the stabilization of the initial ΔN6β2m dimer, which then blocks amyloid formation (35). By using the nanobody as a modulator of the fibril formation process, we can therefore alter the rate determining steps along the reaction pathway. Furthermore, if the detailed nature of the epitope of the nanobody is known, the significance of different regions of the sequences of aggregating proteins can be assessed, as well as the nature of any conformational changes involved in the various molecular species of the protein prior to the emergence of the fully formed fibrils.

Despite the value of the ThT assay for probing, the overall formation of fibrils, defining the detailed microscopic events within each phase of the reaction requires additional techniques to be defined at high resolution. Some information on the rates of the formation of such species can, however, be obtained by means of nanobody probes, as has been shown for the B10 species, which binds to Aβ protofilaments (30). Similarly the rates of formation and reaction of oligomeric species of Aβ peptides can be explored through the interaction with VHH VH31-1 (34).

One approach to obtaining more detailed microscopic data about the assembly reaction, however, is to monitor the appearance and disappearance of individual molecular species e.g. by fluorescence measurements (102–105). These experiments involve labeling with a specific fluorophore, and are proving of great value for following the events taking place within the crucial early stages of the assembly reaction (29, 106). This approach is particularly powerful for studying protein aggregation because it can be applied to probe single molecules, whilst most bulk biophysical techniques can only measure the average characteristics of all molecules in the sample, and it is able to distinguish different molecular species in a highly heterogeneous mixtures such as those present at the beginning of the fibril formation process. Such single molecule techniques detect individual particles as they diffuse into a very small volume, and allow the detection of particles that are present only transiently (43, 106, 107). One powerful approach for studying aggregation behavior is to label aliquots of a given sample of protein with two fluorescent dyes of different colors. A burst of fluorescence will be generated each time a labeled molecule diffuses through the flow-cell and is excited by a laser beam of the correct wavelength. The amplitude of each fluorescence flash is related to the number of labels that are excited and hence the sizes of the oligomeric aggregates that are present in a given solution at a given time. Moreover the different fluorophores can exchange energy when excited and if close to each other in space, a phenomenon known as Förster resonance energy transfer (FRET), enabling information to be obtained on the way that the molecules are assembled within specific oligomeric species (108–111). During the course of an aggregation experiment one therefore can in principle follow the process in real time of an ensemble of different species formed along the pathway as the aggregation proceeds, and also determine the size of the species and their relative populations, as well as the stability and structural compactness of the various species at any given time. Addition of fluorescently labeled conformationally specific antibodies can give additional information on the accessibility of the epitopes in the various aggregates as well as their number and orientation (112). Binding of the antibodies could also modify the rates of formation and structure of the different species of aggregates formed by an amyloidogenic protein. As any influence on the rate of oligomer formation can affect dramatically the toxicity of species formed during the aggregation process, and such an experiment can in principle permit the identification of antibodies that hold significant therapeutic potential.

4. Nanobodies as Probes for In Situ Aggregation and Cellular Toxicity

The high affinity, solubility and expression levels of nanobodies, complemented by their exquisite specificity, make them ideal probes for monitoring the process of misfolding and aggregation of amyloidogenic proteins in situ or in vivo. In living systems, nanobodies can readily be engineered to meet specific requirements for expression within specific cells or organisms such as *Caenorhabditis elegans*, and can be linked to fluorophores, such as the green fluorescent protein (GFP), for visualization of the targeted protein as it diffuses and detects aggregates in the cell (113–115). Such nanobody-GFP fusions could, for example be expressed throughout an organism in an appropriate vector, allowing visualization and location of the protein within the cell.

The nature of the epitope with which the nanobody interacts, and the effect of the latter on the aggregation reaction, will determine its role either as a structural marker or as modulator of the aggregation process. For example NbSyn2, which binds to the C-terminal region of α-synuclein, does not significantly affect the course of the aggregation of the protein even though it binds to a variety of different intermediate species as the protein converts into fibrils (29). Such a nanobody, therefore, should be an ideal probe for following aggregation in cells and organisms without significantly perturbing the process itself, hence acting as a "silent reporter" of the formation of α-synuclein fibrils. Other nanobodies, such as B10, stabilize prefibrillar forms of the material of Aβ peptides and therefore could moderate its toxicity under different conditions providing key information for the rational design of potential therapeutics (30).

The use of nanobodies as in-cell modulators of the cytotoxic effect of protein aggregation has indeed been investigated for a number of model systems for amyloid disorders, such as Huntington's and Parkinson's diseases (116–121), and nanobodies have been shown in several cases to reduce protein misfolding and protect against toxicity and cell death. In addition to the information that these model systems can provide on the mechanism of cytotoxicity, these nanobodies, therefore, potentially have a significant intrinsic therapeutic value, although a number of important issues will need to be addressed before they can be developed for clinical use. A major hurdle is likely to be associated with delivery to the central nervous system because of the existence of the blood–brain barrier through which the diffusion of large hydrophilic molecules is very much restricted. A number of reports have shown, however, that nanobodies can be designed to cross the blood-brain-barrier through active transport either by direct binding to a endothelial receptor or through fusion to proteins that bind to specific receptors designed for transport of molecules through the endothelial barrier (28, 122–124).

5. Conclusions

In this chapter we have given an overview of how nanobodies can be used in the investigation of the mechanism of protein misfolding and aggregation and its associated cellular toxicity. We have shown that nanobodies can constitute excellent probes through which to obtain structural information on the multiple types of aggregates formed during the misfolding process, and that nanobodies that modulate the aggregation kinetics can provide key information on the mechanism of such processes. The facile generation of nanobodies and their implementation in standard biophysical techniques such as NMR and X-ray crystallography has been demonstrated to be able to enhance significantly our understanding of the structural and mechanistic principles of the formation of transient and toxic complexes. In addition, we have discussed the fact that nanobodies are currently being explored for their potential value as therapeutics, also following an *in cell* expression (an "intra-cellular antibody" or "intrabody") approach. Although this approach is still in the developmental stage, it holds great promise in the search for the means to combat amyloid diseases in general and neurodegenerative diseases, in particular for Huntington's disease and Parkinson's disease, where the formation of toxic aggregates and their effects are clearly mediated within the cellular environment.

Acknowledgements

This work was supported by the Medical Research Council, the Wellcome Trust, the Leverhulme Trust, and Parkinson's UK.

References

1. Chiti F, Dobson CM (2006) Protein misfolding, functional amyloid, and human disease. Annu Rev Biochem 75:333–366
2. Souetre EJ, Qing W, Vigoureux I, Dartigues JF, Lozet H, Lacomblez L, Derouesne C (1995) Economic analysis of Alzheimer's disease in outpatients: impact of symptom severity. Int Psychogeriatr 7:115–122
3. Sloane PD, Zimmerman S, Suchindran C, Reed P, Wang L, Boustani M, Sudha S (2002) The public health impact of Alzheimer's disease, 2000–2050: potential implication of treatment advances. Annu Rev Public Health 23:213–231
4. Small GW, McDonnell DD, Brooks RL, Papadopoulos G (2002) The impact of symptom severity on the cost of Alzheimer's disease. J Am Geriatr Soc 50:321–327
5. Dobson CM (1999) Protein misfolding, evolution and disease. Trends Biochem Sci 24:329–332
6. Dobson CM (2003) Protein folding and misfolding. Nature 426:884–890
7. Luheshi LM, Crowther DC, Dobson CM (2008) Protein misfolding and disease: from the test tube to the organism. Curr Opin Chem Biol 12:25–31
8. Luheshi LM, Dobson CM (2009) Bridging the gap: from protein misfolding to protein misfolding diseases. FEBS Lett 583: 2581–2586

9. Stefani M, Dobson CM (2003) Protein aggregation and aggregate toxicity: new insights into protein folding, misfolding diseases and biological evolution. J Mol Med 81:678–699
10. Vendruscolo M, Zurdo J, MacPhee CE, Dobson CM (2003) Protein folding and misfolding: a paradigm of self-assembly and regulation in complex biological systems. Philos Transact A Math Phys Eng Sci 361: 1205–1222
11. Wright CF, Teichmann SA, Clarke J, Dobson CM (2005) The importance of sequence diversity in the aggregation and evolution of proteins. Nature 438:878–881
12. Ecroyd H, Carver JA (2008) Unraveling the mysteries of protein folding and misfolding. IUBMB Life 60:769–774
13. Knowles TP, Waudby CA, Devlin GL, Cohen SI, Aguzzi A, Vendruscolo M, Terentjev EM, Welland ME, Dobson CM (2009) An analytical solution to the kinetics of breakable filament assembly. Science 326:1533–1537
14. Dobson CM (2001) Protein folding and its links with human disease. Biochem Soc Symp 68:1–26
15. Fandrich M, Fletcher MA, Dobson CM (2001) Amyloid fibrils from muscle myoglobin. Nature 410:165–166
16. Bucciantini M, Calloni G, Chiti F, Formigli L, Nosi D, Dobson CM, Stefani M (2004) Prefibrillar amyloid protein aggregates share common features of cytotoxicity. J Biol Chem 279:31374–31382
17. Dumoulin M, Dobson CM (2004) Probing the origins, diagnosis and treatment of amyloid diseases using antibodies. Biochimie 86:589–600
18. Borrebaeck CA (2000) Antibodies in diagnostics—from immunoassays to protein chips. Immunol Today 21:379–382
19. Hudson PJ, Souriau C (2003) Engineered antibodies. Nat Med 9:129–134
20. Valle RP, Jendoubi M (2003) Antibody-based technologies for target discovery. Curr Opin Drug Discov Devel 6:197–203
21. Rasmussen SG, Choi HJ, Fung JJ, Pardon E, Casarosa P, Chae PS, Devree BT, Rosenbaum DM, Thian FS, Kobilka TS, Schnapp A, Konetzki I, Sunahara RK, Gellman SH, Pautsch A, Steyaert J, Weis WI, Kobilka BK (2011) Structure of a nanobody-stabilized active state of the beta(2) adrenoceptor. Nature 469:175–180
22. Baranova E, Fronzes R, Garcia-Pino A, Van Gerven N, Papapostolou D, Pehau-Arnaudet G, Pardon E, Steyaert J, Howorka S, Remaut H (2012) SbsB structure and lattice reconstruction unveil Ca(2+) triggered S-layer assembly. Nature 487(7405):119–122
23. Muyldermans S, Cambillau C, Wyns L (2001) Recognition of antigens by single-domain antibody fragments: the superfluous luxury of paired domains. Trends Biochem Sci 26:230–235
24. Huang L, Muyldermans S, Saerens D (2010) Nanobodies(R): proficient tools in diagnostics. Expert Rev Mol Diagn 10:777–785
25. Revets H, De Baetselier P, Muyldermans S (2005) Nanobodies as novel agents for cancer therapy. Expert Opin Biol Ther 5:111–124
26. Muyldermans S (2001) Single domain camel antibodies: current status. J Biotechnol 74:277–302
27. Muyldermans S, Atarhouch T, Saldanha J, Barbosa JA, Hamers R (1994) Sequence and structure of VH domain from naturally occurring camel heavy chain immunoglobulins lacking light chains. Protein Eng 7:1129–1135
28. Jones DR, Taylor WA, Bate C, David M, Tayebi M (2010) A camelid anti-PrP antibody abrogates PrP replication in prion-permissive neuroblastoma cell lines. PLoS One 5:e9804
29. De Genst EJ, Guilliams T, Wellens J, O'Day EM, Waudby CA, Meehan S, Dumoulin M, Hsu ST, Cremades N, Verschueren KH, Pardon E, Wyns L, Steyaert J, Christodoulou J, Dobson CM (2010) Structure and properties of a complex of alpha-synuclein and a single-domain camelid antibody. J Mol Biol 402:326–343
30. Habicht G, Haupt C, Friedrich RP, Hortschansky P, Sachse C, Meinhardt J, Wieligmann K, Gellermann GP, Brodhun M, Gotz J, Halbhuber KJ, Rocken C, Horn U, Fandrich M (2007) Directed selection of a conformational antibody domain that prevents mature amyloid fibril formation by stabilizing Abeta protofibrils. Proc Natl Acad Sci U S A 104:19232–19237
31. Chan PH, Pardon E, Menzer L, De Genst E, Kumita JR, Christodoulou J, Saerens D, Brans A, Bouillenne F, Archer DB, Robinson CV, Muyldermans S, Matagne A, Redfield C, Wyns L, Dobson CM, Dumoulin M (2008) Engineering a camelid antibody fragment that binds to the active site of human lysozyme and inhibits its conversion into amyloid fibrils. Biochemistry 47:11041–11054
32. Dumoulin M, Canet D, Last AM, Pardon E, Archer DB, Muyldermans S, Wyns L, Matagne A, Robinson CV, Redfield C, Dobson CM (2005) Reduced global cooperativity is a common feature underlying the amyloidogenicity of pathogenic lysozyme mutations. J Mol Biol 346:773–788

33. Dumoulin M, Last AM, Desmyter A, Decanniere K, Canet D, Larsson G, Spencer A, Archer DB, Sasse J, Muyldermans S, Wyns L, Redfield C, Matagne A, Robinson CV, Dobson CM (2003) A camelid antibody fragment inhibits the formation of amyloid fibrils by human lysozyme. Nature 424:783–788
34. Lafaye P, Achour I, England P, Duyckaerts C, Rougeon F (2009) Single-domain antibodies recognize selectively small oligomeric forms of amyloid beta, prevent Abeta-induced neurotoxicity and inhibit fibril formation. Mol Immunol 46:695–704
35. Domanska K, Vanderhaegen S, Srinivasan V, Pardon E, Dupeux F, Marquez JA, Giorgetti S, Stoppini M, Wyns L, Bellotti V, Steyaert J (2011) Atomic structure of a nanobody-trapped domain-swapped dimer of an amyloidogenic beta2-microglobulin variant. Proc Natl Acad Sci U S A 108:1314–1319
36. Taguchi H, Planque S, Sapparapu G, Boivin S, Hara M, Nishiyama Y, Paul S (2008) Exceptional amyloid beta peptide hydrolyzing activity of nonphysiological immunoglobulin variable domain scaffolds. J Biol Chem 283:36724–36733
37. Colby DW, Garg P, Holden T, Chao G, Webster JM, Messer A, Ingram VM, Wittrup KD (2004) Development of a human light chain variable domain (V(L)) intracellular antibody specific for the amino terminus of huntingtin via yeast surface display. J Mol Biol 342:901–912
38. Schiefner A, Chatwell L, Korner J, Neumaier I, Colby DW, Volkmer R, Wittrup KD, Skerra A (2011) A disulfide-free single-domain V(L) intrabody with blocking activity towards huntingtin reveals a novel mode of epitope recognition. J Mol Biol 414:337–355
39. Cookson MR, Xiromerisiou G, Singleton A (2005) How genetics research in Parkinson's disease is enhancing understanding of the common idiopathic forms of the disease. Curr Opin Neurol 18:706–711
40. Singleton AB, Farrer M, Johnson J, Singleton A, Hague S, Kachergus J, Hulihan M, Peuralinna T, Dutra A, Nussbaum R, Lincoln S, Crawley A, Hanson M, Maraganore D, Adler C, Cookson MR, Muenter M, Baptista M, Miller D, Blancato J, Hardy J, Gwinn-Hardy K (2003) Alpha-synuclein locus triplication causes Parkinson's disease. Science 302:841
41. Bucciantini M, Giannoni E, Chiti F, Baroni F, Formigli L, Zurdo J, Taddei N, Ramponi G, Dobson CM, Stefani M (2002) Inherent toxicity of aggregates implies a common mechanism for protein misfolding diseases. Nature 416:507–511
42. Olofsson A, Ostman J, Lundgren E (2002) Amyloid: morphology and toxicity. Clin Chem Lab Med 40:1266–1270
43. Cremades N, Cohen SI, Deas E, Abramov AY, Chen AY, Orte A, Sandal M, Clarke RW, Dunne P, Aprile FA, Bertoncini CW, Wood NW, Knowles TP, Dobson CM, Klenerman D (2012) Direct observation of the interconversion of normal and toxic forms of alpha-synuclein. Cell 149:1048–1059
44. Emadi S, Barkhordarian H, Wang MS, Schulz P, Sierks MR (2007) Isolation of a human single chain antibody fragment against oligomeric alpha-synuclein that inhibits aggregation and prevents alpha-synuclein-induced toxicity. J Mol Biol 368:1132–1144
45. Emadi S, Kasturirangan S, Wang MS, Schulz P, Sierks MR (2009) Detecting morphologically distinct oligomeric forms of alpha-synuclein. J Biol Chem 284:11048–11058
46. Emadi S, Liu R, Yuan B, Schulz P, McAllister C, Lyubchenko Y, Messer A, Sierks MR (2004) Inhibiting aggregation of alpha-synuclein with human single chain antibody fragments. Biochemistry 43:2871–2878
47. Lynch SM, Zhou C, Messer A (2008) An scFv intrabody against the nonamyloid component of alpha-synuclein reduces intracellular aggregation and toxicity. J Mol Biol 377:136–147
48. Zhou C, Emadi S, Sierks MR, Messer A (2004) A human single-chain Fv intrabody blocks aberrant cellular effects of overexpressed alpha-synuclein. Mol Ther 10:1023–1031
49. Bermel W, Bertini I, Felli IC, Lee YM, Luchinat C, Pierattelli R (2006) Protonless NMR experiments for sequence-specific assignment of backbone nuclei in unfolded proteins. J Am Chem Soc 128:3918–3919
50. Tanha J, Xu P, Chen Z, Ni F, Kaplan H, Narang SA, MacKenzie CR (2001) Optimal design features of camelized human single-domain antibody libraries. J Biol Chem 276:24774–24780
51. Vranken W, Tolkatchev D, Xu P, Tanha J, Chen Z, Narang S, Ni F (2002) Solution structure of a llama single-domain antibody with hydrophobic residues typical of the VH/VL interface. Biochemistry 41: 8570–8579
52. Vilar M, Chou HT, Luhrs T, Maji SK, Riek-Loher D, Verel R, Manning G, Stahlberg H, Riek R (2008) The fold of alpha-synuclein fibrils. Proc Natl Acad Sci U S A 105: 8637–8642
53. Selkoe DJ (2001) Alzheimer's disease: genes, proteins, and therapy. Physiol Rev 81: 741–766

54. Kuperstein I, Broersen K, Benilova I, Rozenski J, Jonckheere W, Debulpaep M, Vandersteen A, Segers-Nolten I, Van Der Werf K, Subramaniam V, Braeken D, Callewaert G, Bartic C, D'Hooge R, Martins IC, Rousseau F, Schymkowitz J, De Strooper B (2010) Neurotoxicity of Alzheimer's disease Abeta peptides is induced by small changes in the Abeta42 to Abeta40 ratio. EMBO J 29:3408–3420
55. Bertram L, Tanzi RE (2008) Thirty years of Alzheimer's disease genetics: the implications of systematic meta-analyses. Nat Rev Neurosci 9:768–778
56. Tanzi RE, Bertram L (2005) Twenty years of the Alzheimer's disease amyloid hypothesis: a genetic perspective. Cell 120:545–555
57. Ittner LM, Gotz J (2011) Amyloid-beta and tau—a toxic pas de deux in Alzheimer's disease. Nat Rev Neurosci 12:65–72
58. Diana FF, Silva Esteves AR, Oliveira CR, Cardoso SM (2011) Mitochondria: the common upstream driver of abeta and tau pathology in Alzheimer s disease. Curr Alzheimer Res 8(5):563–572
59. LaFerla FM (2010) Pathways linking Abeta and tau pathologies. Biochem Soc Trans 38:993–995
60. Reiniger L, Lukic A, Linehan J, Rudge P, Collinge J, Mead S, Brandner S (2011) Tau, prions and Abeta: the triad of neurodegeneration. Acta Neuropathol 121:5–20
61. Small SA, Duff K (2008) Linking Abeta and tau in late-onset Alzheimer's disease: a dual pathway hypothesis. Neuron 60:534–542
62. Blurton-Jones M, Laferla FM (2006) Pathways by which Abeta facilitates tau pathology. Curr Alzheimer Res 3:437–448
63. LaFerla FM, Oddo S (2005) Alzheimer's disease: Abeta, tau and synaptic dysfunction. Trends Mol Med 11:170–176
64. Hutton M, McGowan E (2004) Clearing tau pathology with Abeta immunotherapy—reversible and irreversible stages revealed. Neuron 43:293–294
65. Seino Y, Kawarabayashi T, Wakasaya Y, Watanabe M, Takamura A, Yamamoto-Watanabe Y, Kurata T, Abe K, Ikeda M, Westaway D, Murakami T, Hyslop PS, Matsubara E, Shoji M (2010) Amyloid beta accelerates phosphorylation of tau and neurofibrillary tangle formation in an amyloid precursor protein and tau double-transgenic mouse model. J Neurosci Res 88:3547–3554
66. St George-Hyslop PH, Petit A (2005) Molecular biology and genetics of Alzheimer's disease. C R Biol 328:119–130
67. Kayed R, Head E, Thompson JL, McIntire TM, Milton SC, Cotman CW, Glabe CG (2003) Common structure of soluble amyloid oligomers implies common mechanism of pathogenesis. Science 300:486–489
68. Sachse C, Xu C, Wieligmann K, Diekmann S, Grigorieff N, Fandrich M (2006) Quaternary structure of a mature amyloid fibril from Alzheimer's Abeta(1–40) peptide. J Mol Biol 362:347–354
69. Liu R, McAllister C, Lyubchenko Y, Sierks MR (2004) Proteolytic antibody light chains alter beta-amyloid aggregation and prevent cytotoxicity. Biochemistry 43: 9999–10007
70. Taguchi H, Planque S, Nishiyama Y, Symersky J, Boivin S, Szabo P, Friedland RP, Ramsland PA, Edmundson AB, Weksler ME, Paul S (2008) Autoantibody-catalyzed hydrolysis of amyloid beta peptide. J Biol Chem 283:4714–4722
71. Prager EM, Jolles P (1996) Animal lysozymes c and g: an overview. EXS 75:9–31
72. Booth DR, Sunde M, Bellotti V, Robinson CV, Hutchinson WL, Fraser PE, Hawkins PN, Dobson CM, Radford SE, Blake CC, Pepys MB (1997) Instability, unfolding and aggregation of human lysozyme variants underlying amyloid fibrillogenesis. Nature 385:787–793
73. Pepys MB, Hawkins PN, Booth DR, Vigushin DM, Tennent GA, Soutar AK, Totty N, Nguyen O, Blake CC, Terry CJ et al (1993) Human lysozyme gene mutations cause hereditary systemic amyloidosis. Nature 362:553–557
74. Desmyter A, Transue TR, Ghahroudi MA, Thi MH, Poortmans F, Hamers R, Muyldermans S, Wyns L (1996) Crystal structure of a camel single-domain VH antibody fragment in complex with lysozyme. Nat Struct Biol 3:803–811
75. Floege J, Ehlerding G (1996) Beta-2-microglobulin-associated amyloidosis. Nephron 72:9–26
76. Garrett TP, Saper MA, Bjorkman PJ, Strominger JL, Wiley DC (1989) Specificity pockets for the side chains of peptide antigens in HLA-Aw68. Nature 342:692–696
77. Jones S, Smith DP, Radford SE (2003) Role of the N and C-terminal strands of beta 2-microglobulin in amyloid formation at neutral pH. J Mol Biol 330:935–941
78. Jahn TR, Parker MJ, Homans SW, Radford SE (2006) Amyloid formation under physiological conditions proceeds via a native-like folding intermediate. Nat Struct Mol Biol 13:195–201

79. Radford SE, Gosal WS, Platt GW (2005) Towards an understanding of the structural molecular mechanism of beta(2)-microglobulin amyloid formation in vitro. Biochim Biophys Acta 1753:51–63
80. Ami D, Ricagno S, Bolognesi M, Bellotti V, Doglia SM, Natalello A (2012) Structure, stability, and aggregation of beta-2 microglobulin mutants: insights from a Fourier transform infrared study in solution and in the crystalline state. Biophys J 102:1676–1684
81. Colombo M, de Rosa M, Bellotti V, Ricagno S, Bolognesi M (2012) A recurrent D-strand association interface is observed in beta-2 microglobulin oligomers. FEBS J
82. Azinas S, Colombo M, Barbiroli A, Santambrogio C, Giorgetti S, Raimondi S, Bonomi F, Grandori R, Bellotti V, Ricagno S, Bolognesi M (2011) D-strand perturbation and amyloid propensity in beta-2 microglobulin. FEBS J 278:2349–2358
83. Colombo M, Ricagno S, Barbiroli A, Santambrogio C, Giorgetti S, Raimondi S, Bonomi F, Grandori R, Bellotti V, Bolognesi M (2011) The effects of an ideal beta-turn on beta-2 microglobulin fold stability. J Biochem 150:39–47
84. Fogolari F, Corazza A, Varini N, Rotter M, Gumral D, Codutti L, Rennella E, Viglino P, Bellotti V, Esposito G (2011) Molecular dynamics simulation of beta(2)-microglobulin in denaturing and stabilizing conditions. Proteins 79:986–1001
85. Koide S (2009) Engineering of recombinant crystallization chaperones. Curr Opin Struct Biol 19:449–457
86. Abskharon RN, Soror SH, Pardon E, El Hassan H, Legname G, Steyaert J, Wohlkonig A (2011) Combining in-situ proteolysis and microseed matrix screening to promote crystallization of PrPc-nanobody complexes. Protein Eng Des Sel 24(9):737–741
87. Biancalana M, Koide S (2010) Molecular mechanism of Thioflavin-T binding to amyloid fibrils. Biochim Biophys Acta 1804:1405–1412
88. Ban T, Hamada D, Hasegawa K, Naiki H, Goto Y (2003) Direct observation of amyloid fibril growth monitored by thioflavin T fluorescence. J Biol Chem 278:16462–16465
89. LeVine H III (1999) Quantification of beta-sheet amyloid fibril structures with thioflavin T. Methods Enzymol 309: 274–284
90. Rogers DR (1965) Screening for amyloid with the thioflavin-T fluorescent method. Am J Clin Pathol 44:59–61
91. Klunk WE, Jacob RF, Mason RP (1999) Quantifying amyloid by congo red spectral shift assay. Methods Enzymol 309:285–305
92. Turnell WG, Finch JT (1992) Binding of the dye congo red to the amyloid protein pig insulin reveals a novel homology amongst amyloid-forming peptide sequences. J Mol Biol 227:1205–1223
93. Benditt EP, Eriksen N, Berglund C (1970) Congo red dichroism with dispersed amyloid fibrils, an extrinsic cotton effect. Proc Natl Acad Sci U S A 66:1044–1051
94. Goldsbury C, Baxa U, Simon MN, Steven AC, Engel A, Wall JS, Aebi U, Muller SA (2011) Amyloid structure and assembly: insights from scanning transmission electron microscopy. J Struct Biol 173:1–13
95. Chen B, Thurber KR, Shewmaker F, Wickner RB, Tycko R (2009) Measurement of amyloid fibril mass-per-length by tilted-beam transmission electron microscopy. Proc Natl Acad Sci U S A 106:14339–14344
96. Legleiter J, Kowalewski T (2004) Atomic force microscopy of beta-amyloid: static and dynamic studies of nanostructure and its formation. Methods Mol Biol 242:349–364
97. Ding TT, Harper JD (1999) Analysis of amyloid-beta assemblies using tapping mode atomic force microscopy under ambient conditions. Methods Enzymol 309:510–525
98. Kowalewski T, Holtzman DM (1999) In situ atomic force microscopy study of Alzheimer's beta-amyloid peptide on different substrates: new insights into mechanism of beta-sheet formation. Proc Natl Acad Sci U S A 96: 3688–3693
99. Goldsbury C, Kistler J, Aebi U, Arvinte T, Cooper GJ (1999) Watching amyloid fibrils grow by time-lapse atomic force microscopy. J Mol Biol 285:33–39
100. Serpell LC, Fraser PE, Sunde M (1999) X-ray fiber diffraction of amyloid fibrils. Methods Enzymol 309:526–536
101. Chiti F, Dobson CM (2009) Amyloid formation by globular proteins under native conditions. Nat Chem Biol 5:15–22
102. Hohlbein J, Gryte K, Heilemann M, Kapanidis AN (2010) Surfing on a new wave of single-molecule fluorescence methods. Phys Biol 7:031001
103. Rigler R (2010) Fluorescence and single molecule analysis in cell biology. Biochem Biophys Res Commun 396:170–175
104. Joo C, Balci H, Ishitsuka Y, Buranachai C, Ha T (2008) Advances in single-molecule fluorescence methods for molecular biology. Annu Rev Biochem 77:51–76

105. Michalet X, Weiss S, Jager M (2006) Single-molecule fluorescence studies of protein folding and conformational dynamics. Chem Rev 106:1785–1813
106. Orte A, Birkett NR, Clarke RW, Devlin GL, Dobson CM, Klenerman D (2008) Direct characterization of amyloidogenic oligomers by single-molecule fluorescence. Proc Natl Acad Sci U S A 105:14424–14429
107. Narayan P, Orte A, Clarke RW, Bolognesi B, Hook S, Ganzinger KA, Meehan S, Wilson MR, Dobson CM, Klenerman D (2012) The extracellular chaperone clusterin sequesters oligomeric forms of the amyloid-beta(1–40) peptide. Nat Struct Mol Biol 19:79–83
108. Yengo CM, Berger CL (2010) Fluorescence anisotropy and resonance energy transfer: powerful tools for measuring real time protein dynamics in a physiological environment. Curr Opin Pharmacol 10:731–737
109. Kenworthy AK (2001) Imaging protein-protein interactions using fluorescence resonance energy transfer microscopy. Methods 24:289–296
110. Matyus L (1992) Fluorescence resonance energy transfer measurements on cell surfaces. A spectroscopic tool for determining protein interactions. J Photochem Photobiol B 12:323–337
111. Selvin PR (2000) The renaissance of fluorescence resonance energy transfer. Nat Struct Biol 7:730–734
112. Bieschke J, Giese A, Schulz-Schaeffer W, Zerr I, Poser S, Eigen M, Kretzschmar H (2000) Ultrasensitive detection of pathological prion protein aggregates by dual-color scanning for intensely fluorescent targets. Proc Natl Acad Sci 97:5468–5473
113. Cao M, Cao P, Yan H, Ren F, Lu W, Hu Y, Zhang S (2008) Construction and characterization of an enhanced GFP-tagged anti-BAFF scFv antibody. Appl Microbiol Biotechnol 79:423–431
114. Didier P, Weiss E, Sibler AP, Philibert P, Martineau P, Bigot JY, Guidoni L (2008) Femtosecond spectroscopy probes the folding quality of antibody fragments expressed as GFP fusions in the cytoplasm. Biochem Biophys Res Commun 366:878–884
115. Schots A, van der Wolf JM (2002) Green fluorescent protein fluobody immunosensors. Immunofluorescence with GFP-antibody fusion proteins. Methods Mol Biol 183: 265–273
116. Colby DW, Chu Y, Cassady JP, Duennwald M, Zazulak H, Webster JM, Messer A, Lindquist S, Ingram VM, Wittrup KD (2004) Potent inhibition of huntingtin aggregation and cytotoxicity by a disulfide bond-free single-domain intracellular antibody. Proc Natl Acad Sci U S A 101:17616–17621
117. Messer A, McLear J (2006) The therapeutic potential of intrabodies in neurologic disorders: focus on Huntington and Parkinson diseases. BioDrugs 20:327–333
118. Miller TW, Messer A (2005) Intrabody applications in neurological disorders: progress and future prospects. Mol Ther 12: 394–401
119. Cardinale A, Biocca S (2008) Combating protein misfolding and aggregation by intracellular antibodies. Curr Mol Med 8:2–11
120. Butler DC, Messer A (2011) Bifunctional anti-huntingtin proteasome-directed intrabodies mediate efficient degradation of mutant huntingtin exon 1 protein fragments. PLoS One 6:e29199
121. Butler DC, McLear JA, Messer A (2012) Engineered antibody therapies to counteract mutant huntingtin and related toxic intracellular proteins. Prog Neurobiol 97:190–204
122. Abulrob A, Sprong H, Van Bergen en Henegouwen P, Stanimirovic D (2005) The blood–brain barrier transmigrating single domain antibody: mechanisms of transport and antigenic epitopes in human brain endothelial cells. J Neurochem 95: 1201–1214
123. Boado RJ (2008) A new generation of neurobiological drugs engineered to overcome the challenges of brain drug delivery. Drug News Perspect 21:489–503
124. Muruganandam A, Tanha J, Narang S, Stanimirovic D (2002) Selection of phage-displayed llama single-domain antibodies that transmigrate across human blood–brain barrier endothelium. FASEB J 16: 240–242

Chapter 35

Molecular Imaging Using Nanobodies: A Case Study

Nick Devoogdt, Catarina Xavier, Sophie Hernot, Ilse Vaneycken, Matthias D'Huyvetter, Jens De Vos, Sam Massa, Patrick De Baetselier, Vicky Caveliers, and Tony Lahoutte

Abstract

Molecular imaging is a noninvasive method to measure specific biological processes in animal models and patients using imaging. In recent years there has been a tremendous evolution in hardware and software for imaging purposes. This progress has created an urgent need for new labeled targeted molecular probes. The unique physicochemical and pharmacokinetic properties of Nanobodies match the requirements of the ideal molecular imaging tracer. Preclinical studies show strong and specific targeting in vivo with rapid clearance of unbound probe resulting in high contrasted images at early time points after intravenous administration. These data suggest that the Nanobody platform might become a generic method for the development of next generation molecular imaging probes.

Key words: Molecular imaging, Biodistribution, SPECT, PET, Radiochemistry, Radionuclide, Fluorescence

1. Introduction

Molecular imaging is aimed at the noninvasive investigation of cellular and molecular events in living subjects. The key advantage of this imaging methodology is that a biological process can be investigated in its native environment in the intact living individual (animal or human) (1). The most sensitive methods are currently based on radionuclide and optical imaging. The cameras that are used for radionuclide molecular imaging include Single Photon Emission Computed Tomography (SPECT) and Positron Emission Tomography (PET) systems often in combination with an anatomical imaging device such as an X-ray based Computed Tomography (CT) scanner or Magnetic Resonance Imaging system (see Fig. 1). Optical imaging is performed using a sensitive cooled charge coupled device (CCD).

Dirk Saerens and Serge Muyldermans (eds.), *Single Domain Antibodies: Methods and Protocols*,
Methods in Molecular Biology, vol. 911, DOI 10.1007/978-1-61779-968-6_35, © Springer Science+Business Media, LLC 2012

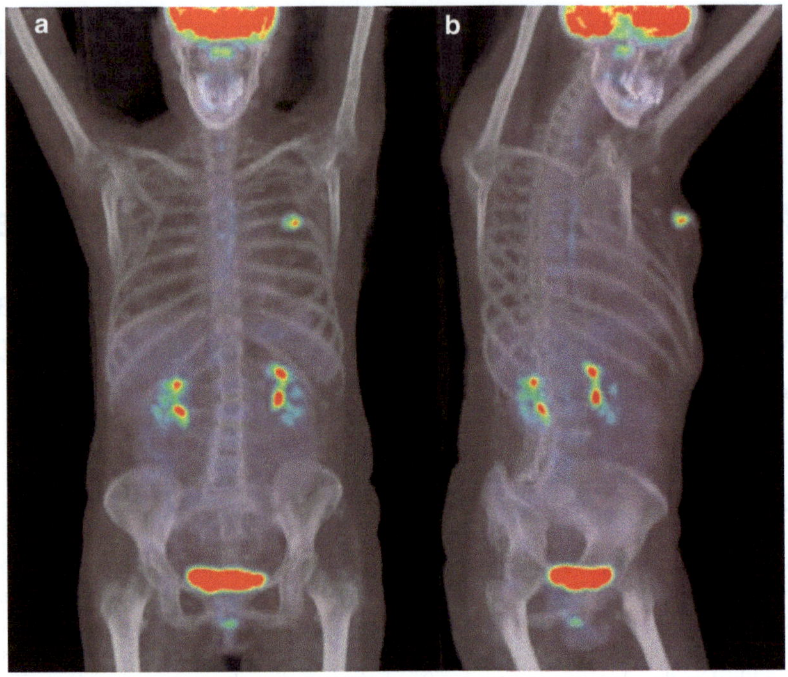

Fig. 1. PET/CT scan of a patient with breast cancer. A trace amount of radiolabeled glucose (^{18}F-Fluorodeoxyglucose) was injected intravenously 1 h prior to the scan. The CT scan enables the visualization of the anatomical structures such as the bone in grayscale. The color-coded image represents the distribution of the molecular tracer in the body. The radiolabeled glucose shows normal uptake in brain and elimination via kidneys into the bladder. At the level of the left breast there is an intense signal signifying the presence of hypermetabolic cells in the breast cancer. On the left (**a**) is the anterior view and on the right (**b**) is the right oblique view of a 3D reconstructed image.

The imaging procedure mostly involves the intravenous administration of a tracer molecule that will specifically target a certain molecular event or cell type. Once the biological event is identified, the tracer molecule needs to be retained in relation with the intensity of the molecular process or the number of cells. The target can only be imaged when there is sufficient contrast between the target and the surrounding tissues. This imposes a number of pharmacokinetic requirements for an ideal tracer: avid and specific targeting combined with fast clearance of unbound tracer from the blood and the nontargeted tissues. These characteristics are hallmarks of Nanobodies. The small size and the physicochemical properties of Nanobodies results in an extremely fast distribution of the molecules throughout the different body compartments, except for the brain (2, 3). High affinity Nanobodies find and bind their target within minutes after intravenous administration and unbound molecules are rapidly eliminated via the kidneys. This makes Nanobodies not only excellent probes for molecular imaging but also superior candidates for drug applications that require

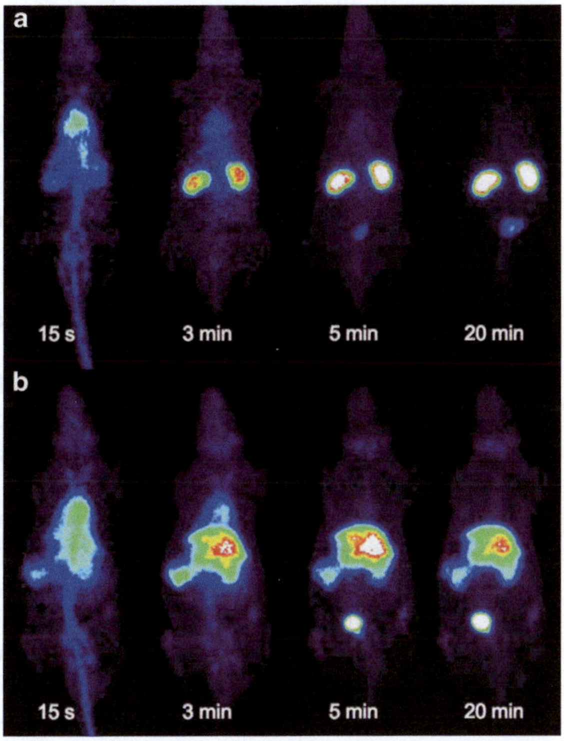

Fig. 2. Image sequence showing the rapid binding and elimination of ^{99m}Tc-labeled Nanobodies in rats. (**a**) Distribution of a Nanobody that has no target for binding in the rat. It shows an extremely fast distribution and subsequent elimination via the kidneys and filling of the bladder. (**b**) Images after intravenous injection of a Nanobody targeted at macrophages. Already at 3 min after injection a clear uptake can be seen in the liver, spleen, and bone marrow where the cell expressing the target are localized.

rapid and highly specific molecular interaction with a limited duration in time such as anti-coagulation or toxin neutralization (4–6). The speed of distribution and targeting of Nanobodies is illustrated in Fig. 2.

2. Generation and Selection of Nanobodies for Molecular Imaging

When generating "imaging Nanobodies" it is of interest to generate binders that are cross-reactive for both the human and rodent analogs of the targeted antigen. This is to allow for comprehensive preclinical testing before the new tracer is translated into the clinic. This might require immunization with both the human and mouse protein if the homology is limited. The generated phage library can then be screened for binding on both variants of the antigen. The double immunization can be avoided in case there is a knock-in model available or generated for the human protein to allow preclinical testing. Within the pool of generated Nanobodies that bind to the target, groups with similar composition of the antigen-binding loops can be found. Some groups will be more abundantly represented, whereas other groups might have only a few members or might even be found only once. Large groups usually exist of variants with only a few amino acid substitutions. Such small alterations should not affect the interaction with the targeted epitope significantly, but may have an important effect on the in vivo biodistribution pattern and labeling efficiency. Moreover, it can also influence the production yield. The fact that one can choose from an array of sequences is an important advantage for the development of an imaging probe compared to scFv or Fab fragments because it enables preselection of amino acid sequences that are more suitable for the application (3). In practice it is best to select for binders with a low nanomolar affinity (<10 nM) and sequences that contain one or more reactive lysine residues in the framework region because radionuclide or fluorescent labels are easily coupled to lysine residues using amine chemistry. Nanobodies with lysines in the antigen-binding loops are best excluded since couplings at the binding site would negatively affect the affinity of the interaction between the Nanobody and its target. Alternatively, it is also possible to introduce extra amino acids in the framework regions to allow for site-specific labeling. Histidine residues at the amino terminal side allows for site-specific labeling with ^{99m}Tc using tricarbonyl chemistry (2) or a well positioned cysteine residue enables the use of maleimide chemistry (7). However, these alterations might also influence the biodistribution significantly resulting in unwanted background activity such as increased renal uptake when a histidine tail is added.

Nanobodies with an agonistic effect are also best excluded as an imaging probe because the goal of imaging is to detect the presence of the antigen and not to induce a pharmacological effect (8). Agonistic effects would also raise toxicity concerns and might hamper the translation of the new tracer into a clinical application. Another consideration is that the Nanobody tracer should preferably not compete with any natural ligand or any known drug that also binds to the target. This is to avoid in vivo competition that would result in a lower specific binding of the imaging Nanobody and thus less contrasted images (3). In function of the application it might also be of interest to produce bivalent or bispecific Nanobodies (9, 10). This generally increases the avidity for the target and could have a positive effect on internalization. However, when reformatting one needs again to pay attention to the effects on pharmacokinetics and biodistribution. Large multimeric constructs or lifetime extended variants are generally not of interest for imaging since it increases the residence time of the probe in the blood (11) and thus results in poor specific contrast at the target, especially at early time points.

3. Labeling of Nanobodies

The most convenient isotope for radiolabeling Nanobodies is technetium-99 m (^{99m}Tc, $t_{1/2:}$ 6.01 h) for imaging with microSPECT in preclinical research. The hexahistidine tag (His$_6$-tag) inserted genetically for immobilized metal affinity chromatography purification is highly suited for site-specific labeling via ^{99m}Tc-tricarbonyl chemistry (2). This ($^{99m}Tc(CO)_3(H_2O)_3)^+$ intermediate, obtained after reduction of $^{99m}TcO_4^-$ forms stable complexes with histidines and imidazoles (12). A practical guide for ^{99m}Tc labeling of Nanobodies is given in a separate chapter in this book, authored by Xavier et al. (*see* Chapter 30). In vitro stability and binding studies demonstrated that the complexes are stable at least up to 24 h in PBS and serum and that the ^{99m}Tc-labeled Nanobodies retain their functionality (2, 3, 13, 14). The His$_6$-tag is located at the carboxy-terminal end of the Nanobody structure, opposite to the antigen-binding site (15) and thus the radiolabel will not interfere with the binding capacities of the Nanobody. Labeling procedures for other radioisotopes such as indium-111 (^{111}In, $t_{1/2}$: 2.6 days), gallium-68 (^{68}Ga, $t_{1/2}$: 67.7 min), copper-64 (^{64}Cu, $t_{1/2}$: 12.7 h), or ^{18}F (^{18}F, $t_{1/2}$: 110 min) are currently under investigated. The advantage of ^{111}In is that it allows imaging at later time points using microSPECT. This can be of interest for imaging targets in areas of inflammation where there can be a substantial extravasation of the radiolabeled Nanobody requiring more time for elimination of nonspecific accumulation. The other mentioned isotopes are positron emitters and are more ideal for clinical imaging using a PET camera.

For in vivo optical imaging with Nanobodies a coupling to a near infrared fluorophore (650–900 nm) is preferred. This is because tissue absorption of light is at its lowest in the "near infrared window" allowing deep tissue imaging (several cm depths) in mice (16). Fluorophores in the visible spectrum are limited to superficial applications (1 mm depth). In vivo optical imaging is possible in nude or shaved mice using dedicated NIRF-camera systems (see Fig. 3). Clinical applications of NIRF imaging are envisaged for intra-operative surgical guidance where the NIRF-labeled Nanobodies make cancer cells visible for the surgeon using a dedicated camera system during surgery, enabling more accurate tumor removal.

4. In Vivo Imaging Using Nanobodies

After intravenous injection radiolabeled Nanobodies distribute extremely fast throughout the body and are rapidly cleared from the blood via the kidneys. At 90 min postinjection, less than 1% IA/g remains present in the blood (3, 13). The preferential renal

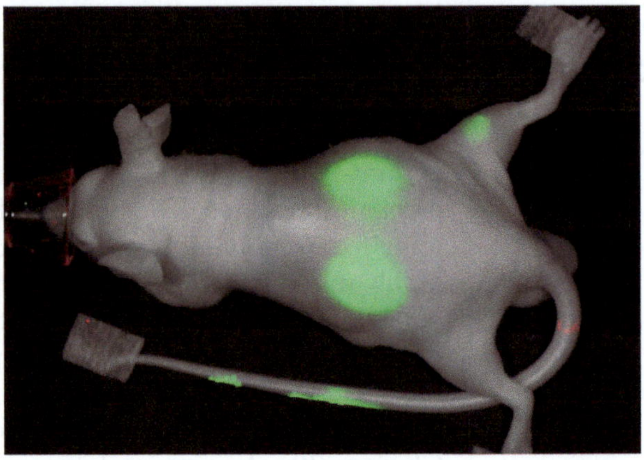

Fig. 3. In vivo fluorescence image of a mouse xenograft bearing a HER2 expressing tumor in the right hind limb. The animal was injected with an anti-HER2 Nanobody labeled with a near infrared emitting fluorophore. The image was acquired at 24 h postinjection and shows intense uptake in both kidneys and in the tumor. The fluorescence at the tail is situated at the site of intravenous injection.

elimination is explained by the relative hydrophilic nature of Nanobodies and because their size is below the renal threshold for glomerular filtration (50–60 kDa). After filtration, most of the Nanobody protein is taken up by the proximal tubuli cells. This is for a large part mediated by the megalin receptor and the internalized Nanobodies are then metabolized (17). The total kidney retention of the radiolabel signal can vary between 7% per gram to above 300% per gram kidney tissue. Factors that play a major role in this are the amino acid sequence of the Nanobody, the type of radiolabel and the choice of the linker or chelator that connects the Nanobody to the radiolabel. In other nontargeted tissues or organs we find only low levels of Nanobody retention. Targeted uptake depends on the level of expression at the target site, the affinity of the Nanobody, the internalization rate, and on the specific activity of the injected nanobody.

Nanobodies against the tumors markers CEA, EGFR, and HER2/neu have been already developed and evaluated for in vivo imaging (see Fig. 4) (2, 3, 13, 14, 18). In xenograft mice accumulation up to 9% IA/g in tumors was observed as soon as 1 h postinjection (2). Using the EGFR-targeted ^{99m}Tc Nanobodies, it was not only possible to detect the presence of the cancer but it also enabled to monitor the expression of the marker (19). It was also shown that the in vivo biodistribution of ^{99m}Tc-Nanobodies directed to markers of dendritic cells reflected the location of these immune cells in the body and could thus be used for in vivo cell tracking (20). Imaging in patients has not been reported at present. However, a lead selection for clinical translation was recently reported by Vaneycken and Devoogdt et al. (3). This lead compound—the 2Rs15d HER2-specific Nanobody—is currently produced under cGMP conditions and the first clinical trial is expected in the

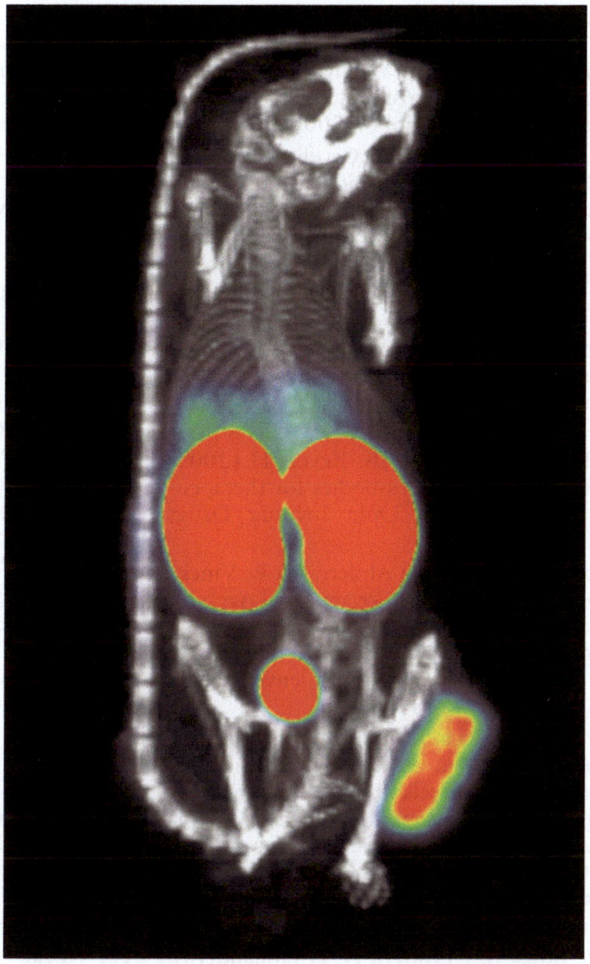

Fig. 4. MicroSPECT/CT image of a mouse xenograft bearing a subcutaneous CEA positive colon carcinoma at the left hind limb. Images were acquired at 1 h post intravenous injection of a ^{99m}Tc labeled anti-CEA Nanobody. The image shows intense uptake of the nanobody at the tumor site and clearance via the kidneys. A low level of liver accumulation is also visible.

near future. In this application an immunoPET scan using ^{68}Ga-2Rs15d will be performed in patients with breast cancer in order to detect HER2 expression in the cancer lesions. It is expected that the diagnostic PET scan can be done between 1 and 3 h post intravenous injection of the labeled Nanobody. This is in contrast with immunoPET using the zirconium-89 (^{89}Zr, $t_{1/2}$: 12.7 h) labeled trastuzumab, a monoclonal antibody targeting HER2, where imaging is only performed at 4 days postinjection (21). This tremendous shortening of the delay between tracer injection and diagnostic imaging is of utmost importance for the patient comfort, the speed of diagnosis and is expected to be a major clinical advantage of using nanobody-based tracers compared to conventional immunoPET techniques.

References

1. Pysz MA, Gambhir SS, Willmann JK (2010) Molecular imaging: current status and emerging strategies. Clin Radiol 65:500–516
2. Gainkam LO, Huang L, Caveliers V et al (2008) Comparison of the biodistribution and tumor targeting of two 99mTc-labeled anti-EGFR nanobodies in mice, using pinhole SPECT/micro-CT. J Nucl Med 49:788–795
3. Vaneycken I, Devoogdt N, Van Gamer N, Vincke C, Xavier C, Nennery U, Muyldermans S, Lahoutte T, Caveliers V (2011) Pre-clinical screening of anti-HER2 Nanobodies for molecular imaging of breast cancer. FASEB J 25: 2433–2446
4. Van Bockstaele F, Holz JB, Revets H (2009) The development of nanobodies for therapeutic applications. Curr Opin Investig Drugs 10:1212–1224
5. Hmila I, Saerens D, Ben Abderrazek R, Vincke C, Abidi N, Benlasfar Z, Govaert J, El Ayeb M, Bouhaouala-Zahar B, Muyldermans S (2010) A bispecific nanobody to provide full protection against lethal scorpion envenoming. FASEB J 24:3479–3489
6. Ulrichts H, Silence K, Schoolmeester A, de Jaegere P, Rossenu S, Roodt J, Priem S, Lauwereys M, Casteels P, Van Bockstaele F, Verschueren K, Stanssens P, Baumeister J, Holz JB (2011) Antithrombotic drug candidate ALX-0081 shows superior preclinical efficacy and safety compared to currently marketed antiplatelet drugs. Blood 118:757–765
7. Van de Broek B, Devoogdt N, D'Hollander A, Gijs HL, Jans K, Lagae L, Muyldermans S, Maes G, Borghs G (2011) Specific cell targeting with nanobody conjugated branched gold nanoparticles for photothermal therapy. ACS Nano 5:4319–4328
8. Roovers RC, Laeremans T, Huang L, De Taeye S, Verkleij AJ, Revets H, de Haard HJ, Van Bergen en Henegouwen PM (2007) Efficient inhibition of EGFR signaling and of tumour growth by antagonistic anti-EFGR Nanobodies. Cancer Immunol Immunother 56:303–317
9. Conrath K, Lauwereys M, Wyns L, Muyldermans S (2001) Camel single-domain antibodies as modular building units in bispecific and bivalent antibody constructs. J Biol Chem 276:7346–7350
10. Hmila I, Abdallah RB, Saerens D, Benlasfar Z, Conrath K, Ayeb ME, Muyldermans S, Bouhaouala-Zahar B (2008) VHH, bivalent domains and chimeric Heavy chain-only antibodies with high neutralizing efficacy for scorpion toxin AahI'. Mol Immunol 45:3847–3856
11. Tijink BM, Laeremans T, Budde M, Stigter-van Walsum M, Dreier T, de Haard HJ, Leemans CR, van Dongen GA (2008) Improved tumor targeting of anti-epidermal growth factor receptor Nanobodies through albumin binding: taking advantage of modular Nanobody technology. Mol Cancer Ther 7:2288–2297
12. Waibel R, Alberto R, Willuda J, Finnern R, Schibli R, Stichelberger A, Egli A, Abram U, Mach JP, Pluckthun A, Schubiger PA (1999) Stable one-step technetium-99 m labeling of His-tagged recombinant proteins with a novel Tc(I)-carbonyl complex. Nat Biotechnol 17:897–901
13. Vaneycken I, Govaert J, Vincke C, Caveliers V, Lahoutte T, De Baetselier P, Raes G, Bossuyt A, Muyldermans S, Devoogdt N (2010) In vitro analysis and in vivo tumor targeting of a humanized, grafted nanobody in mice using pinhole SPECT/micro-CT. J Nucl Med 51:1099–1106
14. Huang L, Gainkam LO, Caveliers V, Vanhove C, Keyaerts M, De Baetselier P, Bossuyt A, Revets H, Lahoutte T (2008) SPECT imaging with 99mTc-labeled EGFR-specific nanobody for in vivo monitoring of EGFR expression. Mol Imaging Biol 10:167–175
15. Vincke C, Loris R, Saerens D, Martinez-Rodriguez S, Muyldermans S, Conrath K (2009) General strategy to humanize a camelid single-domain antibody and identification of a universal humanized nanobody scaffold. J Biol Chem 284:3273–3284
16. Weissleder R, Ntziachristos V (2003) Shedding light onto live molecular targets. Nat Med 9:123–128
17. Gainkam LO, Caveliers V, Devoogdt N, Vanhove C, Xavier C, Boerman O, Muyldermans S, Bossuyt A, Lahoutte T (2011) Localization, mechanism and reduction of renal retention of technetium-99 m labeled epidermal growth factor receptor-specific nanobody in mice. Contrast Media Mol Imaging 6:85–92
18. Cortez-Retamozo V, Lahoutte T, Caveliers V, Tchouate-Gainkam O, Hernot S, Packeu A, De Vos F, Vanhove C, Muyldermans S, De

Baetselier P, Revets H (2008) 99mTc-labeled nanobodies: a new type of targeted probes for imaging antigen expression. Curr Radiopharm 1:37–41

19. Tchouate LO, Gainkam M, Keyaerts V, Caveliers N, Devoogdt C, Vanhove LV, Grunsven SM, Lahoutte T (2011) Correlation between epidermal growth factor receptor-specific nanobody uptake and tumor burden: a tool for noninvasive monitoring of tumor response to therapy. Mol Imaging Biol 13(5):940–948

20. De Groeve K, Deschacht N, De Koninck C, Caveliers V, Lahoutte T, Devoogdt N, Muyldermans S, De Baetselier P, Raes G (2010) Nanobodies as tools for in vivo imaging of specific immune cell types. J Nucl Med 51:782–789

21. Dijkers EC, Kosterink JG, Rademaker AP, Perk LR, van Dongen GA, Bart J, de Jong JR, de Vries EG, Lub-de Hooge MN (2009) Development and characterization of clinical-grade 89Zr-trastuzumab for HER2/neu immunoPET imaging. J Nucl Med 50:974–981

Chapter 36

Case Study on Live Cell Apoptosis-Assay Using Lamin-Chromobody Cell-Lines for High-Content Analysis

Kourosh Zolghadr, Jacqueline Gregor, Heinrich Leonhardt, and Ulrich Rothbauer

Abstract

The understanding of cellular processes and their physiopathological alterations requires comprehensive data on the abundance, distribution, modification and interaction of cellular components. On the one hand, artificially introduced fluorescent fusion proteins provide information about their distribution and dynamics in living cells but not on endogenous factors. On the other hand, antibodies can detect endogenous proteins, posttranslational modifications and other cellular components but mostly in fixed and permeabilized cells. Here we highlight a new technology based on the antigen-binding domain of heavy-chain antibodies (VHH) from *Camelidae*. We have demonstrated that these VHH domains can be fused with fluorescent proteins and expressed in living cells. Those fluorescent antigen-binding proteins-called chromobodies-can be used to detect and trace proteins and other cellular components *in vivo*. In principle chromobodies can detect any antigenic structure including posttranslational modifications or nonprotein components and thereby dramatically expand the quality and quantity of information that can be gathered in high-content analyses. Here we demonstrate the suitability of this technology to follow apoptosis in living cells in real time.

Key words: Antibodies, Chromobodies, High-content analysis, GFP, Fluorescent proteins, Live cell microscopy, Apoptosis, HCA assay

1. Introduction

In the early stage of pharmaceutical drug development, high-content analysis (HCA) is an important technology, aiming at maximal readout of cellular parameters in both, quality and quantity. This way, compound libraries are screened and analyzed for desired effects and/or possible side effects at cellular level. Based on high-throughput microscopy with automated image acquisition and computational pattern recognition in multi-well formats, HCA facilitates the simultaneous investigation of multiple cellular

Dirk Saerens and Serge Muyldermans (eds.), *Single Domain Antibodies: Methods and Protocols*,
Methods in Molecular Biology, vol. 911, DOI 10.1007/978-1-61779-968-6_36, © Springer Science+Business Media, LLC 2012

biomarkers in a statistically secured manner. However, HCA is still limited by the availability of reliable biomarkers.

One main application of HCA is the analysis of apoptosis induced by biological agents or chemical compounds. Apoptosis, the programmed cell death, is a multistep process involving cell shrinkage and rounding, chromatin condensation and nuclear envelope breakdown (1). These characteristic features, mainly the degradation of the nuclear lamina, are early events of apoptosis (2, 3).

Until now, apoptosis assays for HCA are static endpoint assays on fixed and permeabilized cells where laborious antibody stainings have to be performed. In principle these are powerful assays, however they do not provide information about dynamic processes in the cell. For a detailed understanding of the mode of operation of compounds this information is crucial. To obtain such information assays have to be performed in living cells.

So far, only in a few cases intracellular antibody derivatives have been successfully used for protein analysis *in vivo* (4–6). Those antibody derivates including monovalent antibody fragments (Fab, 50 kDa) or single-chain variable fragments (scFv, 25 kDa) are based on conventional antibodies (IgG, 150 kDa). However, as these antibody derivatives are composed of heavy and light chain domains, their application in living cells is still hampered by inefficient folding and disulfide bond formation in the reducing environment of the cytoplasm of the cell.

One alternative to conventional antibodies are the so-called heavy-chain antibodies (HCAbs) (7). They recognize and bind their antigen via a single variable domain, the VHH (variable heavy chain of a heavy chain antibody). VHHs provide a series of advantages in comparison to other antibody fragments such as Fab or scFv. First, only one single domain has to be cloned and expressed to generate an intact antigen-binding fragment. As such, VHHs can be isolated as *in vivo* affinity matured entities that do not need *in vitro* affinity maturation steps. Most often affinity maturation is required for binders isolated from naive or synthetic libraries. Second, due to their structure (8), VHHs are extremely stable, soluble and efficiently produced in heterologous expression systems (9, 10). Third, the antigen-binding affinities of VHHs are in the nanomolar range and comparable to those of conventional antibodies (11, 12). Last not least, due to their robustness and structural simplicity VHHs can be selected for functional analysis in living cells.

Based on these interesting characteristics, we established a new class of cellular biomarkers by genetically fusing VHHs with fluorescent proteins for visualization of antigens in living mammalian cells. Due to their chimeric structure these recombinant derivatives were termed "chromobodies" (see Fig. 1a). In a proof-of-concept study, chromobodies were introduced as novel tools in cell biology research (13). We demonstrated that chromobodies are able to detect antigens in chromatin and replication complexes as well as

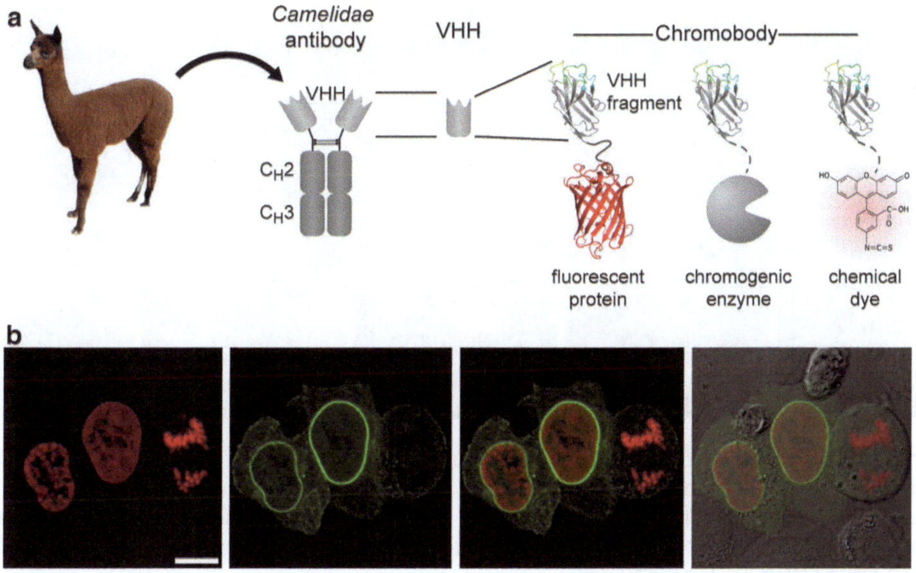

Fig. 1. The chromobody technology. (**a**) Schematic illustration of chromobodies, (**b**) detection of the nuclear lamina with lamin-chromobody in living cells. Confocal images of HeLa cells co-expressing lamin-chromobody (*green*) and red fluorescent histone H2B as mitosis marker. Shown are cells in prophase, G2-phase, and anaphase (from *left to right*), the latter displaying breakdown of the nuclear lamina, concomitant with chromosome separation (*right*). Scale bar: 10 μm.

the cytoskeleton and allowed the visualization of dynamic changes during the cell cycle in real time.

We generated a green fluorescent chromobody against the nuclear lamina (lamin-chromobody) (13) and demonstrated that this lamin-chromobody can be used to detect the nuclear envelope in live cells (see Fig. 1b).

In this case study we highlight that chromobodies can complement and extend existing HCA approaches by monitoring apoptosis in real time. For the cellular assay we generated a HeLa cell line stably expressing the green fluorescent lamin-chromobody detecting the integrity of the nuclear lamina as the cellular parameter of interest. Upon addition of apoptosis inducing agents the characteristic fragmentation of the nuclear envelope can be monitored in real time. Using automated image acquisition and computational pattern recognition a concentration dependent increase of apoptotic cells was detectable in real time.

2. Results

2.1. Detection of Apoptosis in Real Time with a Lamin-Chromobody

Recently we described the application of a specific lamin-chromobody to target and trace the dynamic changes of the nuclear envelope. In a more detailed analysis we demonstrated by fluorescence recovery after photobleaching (FRAP) that the lamin-chromobody binds to

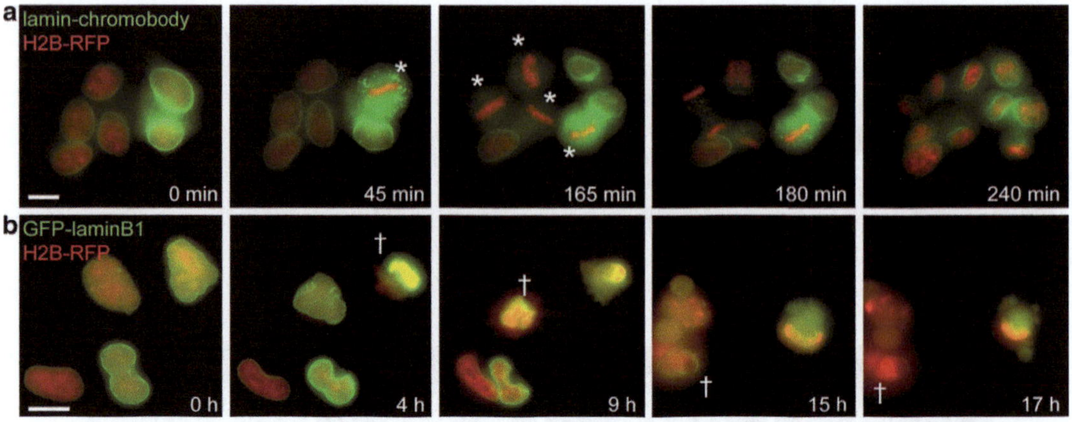

Fig. 2. Comparison of HeLa cells expressing lamin-chromobody and GFP-laminB1. (**a**) Time-lapse imaging of HeLa cells co-expressing red fluorescent histone H2B (*red*) as nuclear marker and lamin-chromobody (*green*). The cells progress through cell cycle and proliferate normally indicated by a *star*. (**b**) HeLa cells co-expressing GFP-laminB1 and histone H2B-RFP show abnormal morphology. Long-term observation shows cells going into apoptosis upon expression of the GFP-laminB1 fusion protein. Scale bars: 10 μm.

the nuclear lamina in a very transient manner (13). However, this binding is sufficient to visualize the nuclear envelope. Furthermore, expression of the lamin-chromobody does not influence the cellular morphology and does not hamper progression through the cell cycle. Moreover, the transient binding mode of the lamin-chromobody seems to minimize functional interference and allow cells to pass through mitosis (see Fig. 2a). This unique feature to detect the endogenous lamina without cytotoxic effects cannot be obtained with a fluorescent fusion protein as it is usually used for live cell imaging. In a comparative study we tested cells expressing the laminB1 fused to GFP (GFP-laminB1). Expression of GFP-laminB1 construct leads to dramatic changes in cellular morphology with strong blebbing of the nuclei and a reduced viability (see Fig. 2b).

Long-term observation of cells expressing the lamin-chromobody revealed a very characteristic distribution pattern of the protein throughout the cell cycle. By binding to the lamina the chromobody is enriched at this particular structure and clearly visualizes it. The fluorescent signal of unbound fraction is dispersedly distributed in the nucleus and the cytoplasm providing additional information on the cellular size and morphology.

During two cellular events the distribution of the lamin-chromobody changes significantly. First, during mitosis when chromatin condenses the lamin-chromobody visualizes the reversible process of depolymerization of the nuclear envelope. Second, during apoptosis the chromobody detects the characteristic process of disassembly of the nuclear envelope.

The process of apoptosis is controlled either by extrinsic or intrinsic cellular signals leading to the activation of specific signaling pathways including the mitochondrial release of cytochrome *c* and the activation of proteolytic caspases. Activation of Caspase 3, for example, directly leads to the cleavage of nuclear proteins including the lamina and the formation of cytoplasmatic vesicles comprising the degraded nuclear lamina (14, 15).

Those characteristic morphological changes can now be visualized with the lamin-chromobody. The quantitative detection of bright fluorescent vesicles comprising the degraded nuclear lamina can be easily analyzed with the appropriate HCA software and algorithms. In terms of high-content data, labeling of the lamina in combination with the enrichment of the chromobody protein in the nucleus enables an automated intensity-, shape-, and size-based segmentation of the cell. The unbound fraction of the chromobody is evenly distributed in the cytoplasm, leading to a weak fluorescent staining of the cytoplasm. Setting a threshold, this signal can be used to identify cellular size and shape. Alternatively, a fixed radius around the nucleus can be defined as the cytoplasm. The bright fluorescent vesicles formed during apoptosis are automatically segmented and counted on bases of their size (between 1 and 2 μm), their cytoplasmic localization, and their signal intensity.

2.2. Real Time Apoptosis Assay Based on a Human Cell Line Stably Expressing Lamin-Chromobody

Our live cell apoptosis assay is based on a cell line stably expressing the lamin-chromobody. Therefore we selected a HeLa cell clone comprising stable and homogenous expression levels of the lamin-chromobody with a sufficient signal-to-noise ratio for automated image analysis and a proliferation rate comparable to the wild type cell line.

Next we tested the cellular system by adding increasing concentrations of the apoptosis inducing drug/antibiotic (16) staurosporine (STS). Cells stably expressing the lamin-chromobody are seeded at 50–70% confluence in 96-well plates with optical bottom. Cells were treated with corresponding concentrations (0, 0.1, 1, and 5 μM) of STS. For an optical read-out, the plate is transferred to a high-content fluorescent microscope suitable for long-term observation of live cells (here: INCell Analyzer 1000, GE Healthcare, equipped with an environmental control module). To analyze and evaluate a statistically significant amount of cells, images from multiple fields of view per well were acquired. For an adequate temporal resolution of cellular events time intervals of 15 min of image acquisition were chosen (see Fig. 3a).

Computational image segmentation implemented exemplarily in the multi-target analysis module of the INCell Analyzer Workstation software results in identification of nuclei and cytoplasm. Furthermore, a basal level of vesicles is detectable. However, after induction of apoptosis this number of vesicles increases in a concentration dependent way over time. Those morphological changes can be quantitatively evaluated and the result provides real time information about the actual state each individual cell is in (see Fig. 3b). This live cell detection of apoptosis is a unique feature of the cell line stably expressing the lamin-chromobody.

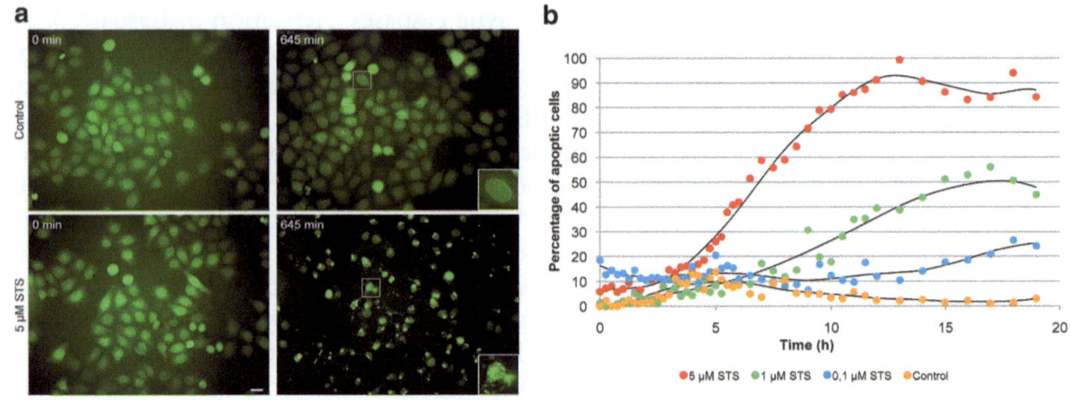

Fig. 3. Apoptosis assay with lamin-chromobody expressing cell line clone 4.1. (**a**) Time lapse imaging of untreated cells (*upper row*) and after addition of 5 μM staurosporine (STS). The nuclear lamina is visualized with a lamin-chromobody (*green*). Shown are selected images before and after (645 min) addition of STS. (**b**) Quantitative evaluation with automated image acquisition and computational pattern recognition. Morphological changes of the lamina (fragmentation and vesicle formation) were monitored in 15 min intervals. Shown is the percentage of apoptotic cells after treatment with increasing concentrations of STS (0–5 μM) over a time period of 20 h. Scale bar: 10 μm. (Data taken from Schmidthals et al. Novel antibody derivatives for proteome and high-content analysis. Anal Bioanal Chem J Cell Biochem 397(8):3203–3208, Copyright 2010© The Authors).

Additionally, parameters, such as shape, size, or morphology of either the whole cell or the nucleus, can be obtained from the same fluorescence channel.

3. Discussion

Here we demonstrated that the chromobody technology is applicable for real time HCA. The lamin-chromobody cell line is suitable for direct analysis of apoptosis in real time. In contrast to conventional apoptosis assays, there is no need for laborious fixation processes and antibody staining. However, multiplexed conventional antibodies can still be applied for additional analysis. The use of a stable cell line gives the assay the necessary robustness for HCA applications. Moreover, the chromobody technology allows live cell HCA assays providing an increased gain of spatial and temporal information.

Currently the chromobody technology does not yet allow the detection and visualization of every single cellular protein. Providing an optical readout of essential cellular processes such as apoptosis, cell cycle progression, or epigenetic regulation chromobodies are likely to become reliable biomarkers to detect and to follow such processes *in vivo*. Therefore we propose that the chromobody technology will become very interesting for live cell HCA assays. At present, the rate limiting factor is the limited availability of antigen specific chromobodies as the most suitable binders have to be generated in a time-consuming procedure from *in vivo* matured heavy-chain antibodies. Thus the development of better selection and *in vitro* maturation procedures for the isolation and engineering of highly specific binders is of utmost importance.

Acknowledgements

The authors declare competing financial interests. This work was supported by the GO-Bio Program of the BMBF (Federal Ministry of Science, Germany).

References

1. Elmore S (2007) Apoptosis: a review of programmed cell death. Toxicol Pathol 35: 495–516
2. Neamati N, Fernandez A, Wright S, Kiefer J, McConkey DJ (1995) Degradation of lamin B1 precedes oligonucleosomal DNA fragmentation in apoptotic thymocytes and isolated thymocyte nuclei. J Immunol 154:3788–3795
3. Oberhammer FA, Hochegger K, Froschl G, Tiefenbacher R, Pavelka M (1994) Chromatin condensation during apoptosis is accompanied by degradation of lamin A+B, without enhanced activation of cdc2 kinase. J Cell Biol 126:827–837
4. Biocca S, Pierandrei-Amaldi P, Cattaneo A (1993) Intracellular expression of anti-p21ras single chain Fv fragments inhibits meiotic maturation of *Xenopus* oocytes. Biochem Biophys Res Commun 197:422–427
5. Cardinale A, Lener M, Messina S, Cattaneo A, Biocca S (1998) The mode of action of Y13-259 scFv fragment intracellularly expressed in mammalian cells. FEBS Lett 439:197–202
6. Marasco WA, Chen S, Richardson JH, Ramstedt U, Jones SD (1998) Intracellular antibodies against HIV-1 envelope protein for AIDS gene therapy. Hum Gene Ther 9:1627–1642
7. Hamers-Casterman C, Atarhouch T, Muyldermans S, Robinson G, Hamers C, Songa EB, Bendahman N, Hamers R (1993) Naturally occurring antibodies devoid of light chains. Nature 363:446–448
8. Rothbauer U, Zolghadr K, Muyldermans S, Schepers A, Cardoso MC, Leonhardt H (2008) A versatile nanotrap for biochemical and functional studies with fluorescent fusion proteins. Mol Cell Proteomics 7:282–289
9. Muyldermans S, Baral TN, Retamozzo VC, De Baetselier P, De Genst E, Kinne J, Leonhardt H, Magez S, Nguyen VK, Revets H, Rothbauer U, Stijlemans B, Tillib S, Wernery U, Wyns L, Hassanzadeh-Ghassabeh G, Saerens D (2009) Camelid immunoglobulins and nanobody technology. Vet Immunol Immunopathol 128: 178–183
10. Olichon A, Schweizer D, Muyldermans S, de Marco A (2007) Heating as a rapid purification method for recovering correctly-folded thermotolerant VH and VHH domains. BMC Biotechnol 7:7
11. Sheriff S, Chang CY, Jeffrey PD, Bajorath J (1996) X-ray structure of the uncomplexed anti-tumor antibody BR96 and comparison with its antigen-bound form. J Mol Biol 259:938–946
12. van der Linden RH, Frenken LG, de Geus B, Harmsen MM, Ruuls RC, Stok W, de Ron L, Wilson S, Davis P, Verrips CT (1999) Comparison of physical chemical properties of llama VHH antibody fragments and mouse monoclonal antibodies. Biochim Biophys Acta 1431:37–46
13. Rothbauer U, Zolghadr K, Tillib S, Nowak D, Schermelleh L, Gahl A, Backmann N, Conrath K, Muyldermans S, Cardoso MC, Leonhardt H (2006) Targeting and tracing antigens in live cells with fluorescent nanobodies. Nat Methods 3:887–889
14. Susin SA, Daugas E, Ravagnan L, Samejima K, Zamzami N, Loeffler M, Costantini P, Ferri KF, Irinopoulou T, Prevost MC, Brothers G, Mak TW, Penninger J, Earnshaw WC, Kroemer G (2000) Two distinct pathways leading to nuclear apoptosis. J Exp Med 192:571–580
15. Kihlmark M, Imreh G, Hallberg E (2001) Sequential degradation of proteins from the nuclear envelope during apoptosis. J Cell Sci 114:3643–3653
16. Chae HJ, Kang JS, Byun JO, Han KS, Kim DU, Oh SM, Kim HM, Chae SW, Kim HR (2000) Molecular mechanism of staurosporine-induced apoptosis in osteoblasts. Pharmacol Res 42:373–381

Index

Dirk Saerens and Serge Muyldermans (eds.), *Single Domain Antibodies: Methods and Protocols*, Methods in Molecular Biology, vol. 911, DOI 10.1007/978-1-61779-968-6, © Springer Science+Business Media, LLC 2012

N

O

P

R

S

T

MIX
Papier aus verantwortungsvollen Quellen
Paper from responsible sources
FSC® C105338

If you have any concerns about our products,
you can contact us on
ProductSafety@springernature.com

In case Publisher is established outside the EU,
the EU authorized representative is:
Springer Nature Customer Service Center GmbH
Europaplatz 3, 69115 Heidelberg, Germany

Printed by Libri Plureos GmbH
in Hamburg, Germany